The Search for Mental Health

A History and Memoir of WFMH 1948–1997

The Search for Mental Health

A History and Memoir of WFMH 1948–1997

Eugene B. Brody

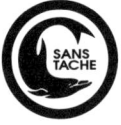

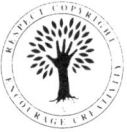

Brody, Eugene B.
    The search for mental health: a history and memoir of WFMH,
1948–1997 / Eugene B. Brody.
    p. cm.
    Includes bibliographical references.
    ISBN 0-683-18346-X
    1. World Federation for Mental Health—History.   I. Title.
RA790.A1B76   1998
362.2' 06' 01—DC21   98-23508
                                   CIP

Printed in the United States of America
(ISBN 0-683-18346-x)

98 99 00 01 02
1 2 3 4 5 6 7 8 9 10

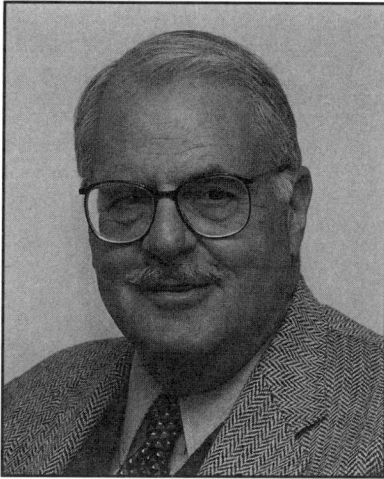

Eugene B. Brody was born on June 17, 1921 in the center of the United States. His father, a pioneer in the application of mathematics to biological processes, was a professor and research scientist at the University of Missouri in Columbia. Many factors, including close contact with a mentally ill family member, conspired to awaken his early interest in understanding human behavior, and, ultimately, his advocacy for the rights of patients and those at risk for illness. Columbia, burned by both sides in the Civil War, exposed him in the 1920s and 1930s to the culture of the racially segregated south. In contrast, the family values were politically liberal, his father maintained close connections with colleagues in other countries, and his graduate students came from all backgrounds and all parts of the world. Brody's view of the world through them was expanded when the award of a Guggenheim fellowship allowed his father to take the family to France for a year.

Despite his cosmopolitan experience, Brody regards himself primarily as a Midwesterner. He graduated from the University of Missouri "with distinction" in psychology, and in 1941 took an M.A. degree in Experimental Psychology. Fifty years later, in 1991, he returned to Missouri to be awarded an Honorary Doctor of Science degree.

In 1941 he abandoned the pursuit of a Ph.D. in psychology and shifted his interests to medicine. In pursuit of this goal he transferred to Harvard Medical School where he was awarded a prize for a paper entitled "Hormones and Behavior." Receiving his M.D. from Harvard in September 1944, he was married the following day. On the next day he began his psychiatric training at Yale while his wife, Marian, returned to Brown University in nearby Providence to complete her Master's Degree.

In 1946, the work at Yale was interrupted by military service in Germany where, in addition to other duties, he was the psychiatric consultant to the International Military Tribunal in Nuremberg. This intensified his interest in the sociocultural determinants of behavior and in human rights. Returning to Yale in January, 1948 he completed his assignment as Chief Resident in Psychiatry in July, 1949 and remained on the faculty . There he served from 1953–1957 as Associate Clinical Professor and the first Chief of the Neuropsychiatric Service at the Yale-affiliated West Haven VA Hospital. He also completed his studies at the New York Psychoanalytic Institute by commutation. He is now a Life Member of the American Psychoanalytic Association as well as a Life Fellow of the American Psychiatric Association. In 1997, he returned to New Haven to receive a Distinguished Alumnus award from the Yale Department of Psychiatry.

In 1957, Dr. Brody joined the University of Maryland Medical School, serving for the next 20 years as Professor and Psychiatrist-in-Chief of its affiliated hospitals, Chairman of its Department of Psychiatry, Director of its Institute of Psychiatry and Human Behavior, and Associate Dean of the School of Medicine for Social and Behavioral Studies. During this period, he initiated the development of a community mental health system for the Western Health District of Baltimore, the establishment of the Maryland Psychiatric Research Center and the psychiatric service of the Veteran's Administration Hospital, and was an active contributor to desegregating Maryland's state mental hospitals. After a year as a Fellow at Stanford's Center for Advanced Study in the Behavioral Sciences, he returned to Maryland as Professor of Psychiatry and Human Behavior, and in 1987, retired completely from the University with the title of Professor Emeritus.

In the 1950s and 1960s, Dr. Brody was on the boards of the Maryland and National Mental Health Associations. In 1981, he became President of the World Federation for Mental Health and since 1983 has served on a volunteer basis as the Secretary General of that organization. In 1987, he was appointed Senior Associate at the Johns Hopkins School of Hygiene and Public Health, and Senior Advisor to the Harvard Program in Refugee Trauma, and since 1997, has been a Visiting Professor at Harvard Medical School. He continues the post held since 1967 as Editor-in-Chief of the *Journal of Nervous and Mental Disease* which, appearing monthly since 1874, is the world's oldest independent journal of human behavior.

Dr. Brody's initial research interests were in thyroid and brain function in rats and monkeys. Clinical work in the preneuroleptic era directed his interest to psychotherapy with people diagnosed as schizophrenic and he was an early leader in this field. However, he soon became focused on the influence of social and cultural context on behavior (including that defined as mental illness), personal fertility regulation, and migration, with special reference to issues of inequality, including minority group status. In pursuit of these interests he was, in addition to his University duties, Director of the Interamerican Mental Health Studies Program (of the American and Pan American Psychiatric Associations) from 1966-1968. He has done field work resulting in book length monographs on Brazil and Jamaica, and has been a visiting professor in Australia, New Zealand, and Israel where he was a Fellow of the Institute for Advanced Study of Tel Aviv University. He has also been a visiting lecturer and consultant in many other countries, in Asia, Europe, the Middle and Far East, as well as consultant or advisor for the U.S. NIMH (schizophrenia, epidemiology, HIV prevention), the U.S. Veteran's Administration medical services, and the Hogg Foundation for Mental Health of the University of Texas. His United Nations consultancies and advisory roles have been in relation to PAHO, WHO, UNESCO, UNHCR, and the International Social Science Council, on which he served as a member of its executive committee. He has published some 250 scientific papers and reviews, and written or edited 10 books, some of which are listed in the bibliography of this volume.

Dr. and Mrs. Brody, who reside in Baltimore, have maintained a sailboat on nearby Chesapeake Bay for nearly 40 years. Their children and grandchildren live in Florida and Colorado.

Preface and Acknowledgments

CREATING A HISTORY

The search for mental health

What passes for normality in one group of people is not always accepted in another. As the Spanish philosopher, George Santayana, wrote, "we know that we are sane to the extent that our neighbors agree with us." Even within the Western cultures that formulate the human condition in terms of "mental health," it is not easy to achieve consensual definition. Most observers would agree that the abilities to adapt and cope are basic to optimal functioning. Most would also agree, however, that there is more to life and a feeling of fulfillment than adapting and coping. Some sense of this may have motivated the definition attributed to Brock Chisholm (see Chapter 2) and written into the WHO constitution in 1946: "Health is more than merely the absence of disease. It is a state of complete wellbeing, social, physical, and mental." The elusiveness of that much-desired state, especially when sought on an international and cross-cultural basis, and the difficulties in organizing to promote it, are reflected in this volume's title.

Telling the WFMH story presents another challenge. Our understanding of the present is always influenced by what has gone before. As Henri Bergson wrote in 1911: "We trail behind us, unawares, the whole of our past...." Our perception of today is determined by our interpretation of yesterday. Conversely, the apparent meaning of what has gone before is determined by what is happening today.

This account of the origins and life of the World Federation for Mental Health (WFMH) is written from the perspective of the late 1990s. It looks back to the Federation's prenatal development in the post-World War II period and ends as it enters its 50th year in the spring of 1997. The intervening years saw the evolution of a unique organization over a half-century marked by major changes in the scientific understanding of health and illness, and a proliferation of organizations laying claim to the field's varied constituencies.

The searchers

WFMH's increased worldwide prominence in the 1980s, and the global adoption of the American Psychiatric Association's diagnostic system, helped stimulate an increase in the number and variety of professional organizations with overlapping concerns. Until their appearance, WFMH was the only nongovernmental organization offering professionals as well as citizen volunteers an entry into the international world, including that of the United Nations. In the late 20th century, with readily available global communications and transport, international associations of psychiatrists, psychoanalysts, psychologists, social workers, nurses, and rehabilitation specialists all offer their members the kind of international contact previously found only through WFMH. So now do many of their national associations, particularly in the United States.

Associations of relatives have also drawn individuals and groups who, in an earlier era, might have affiliated with WFMH. They have become a powerful constituency, with aims not always congruent with those of the survivors of illness or users of mental health services themselves. The "users" and self-help organizations, some with sponsorship by WFMH beginning in the 1980s, have offered a home to people who, in an earlier era, might have become part of the Federation. The emergence of these new mental health constituencies has been facilitated by the Federation's global efforts to reduce the stigma of mental illness. In turn, they have exerted a powerful influence on the agenda of the contemporary WFMH.

Yet, despite the proliferation of new specialized organizations, the Federation remains the sole truly ecumenical international voluntary mental health association. Unlike the international unions of professionals, its constituency is not bound by economic or guild interests. It is not limited by the particular visions of mental health association volunteers, families of patients, or patients and ex-patients (users and survivors); nor must it be responsive to the concerns of any particular governmental or corporate entity. It is not obliged to increase the power and influence of a sponsoring nation or institution. Finally, unlike the agencies of the United Nations, it does not have to be cautious about the political sensitivities of those who control its budget or be concerned with interfering in the "internal affairs" of any sovereign state.

What has kept this geographically far-flung, ever-changing group of people, separated by national, cultural, social, and ethnic divisions, with no shared economic motivation, working together for the common ideal of positive mental health?

The human story

In the effort to answer this question, I have not limited this organizational biography to a simple chronicle of events, an account of achievements, or a description of an international mental health agenda. It is also a human story that recognizes the interpersonal conflicts as well as collaborations and the frustrations as well as the triumphs of the individuals who have comprised it. These people of undoubted good will and sincerity have sometimes embraced quite different perspectives about mental health related issues, mainly organizational, and defended them vigorously. Considerations of privacy preclude a totally frank account of the most emotional exchanges. Resolving conflicts is part of the persisting search for common ground that has bound us together.

It is evident that to achieve its goals the Federation's individual and organizational components must recognize the interdependence and the commonality of resources on which we all depend. Such recognition may be particularly important in the era after the 1983 establishment of the Baltimore-Washington Secretariat with our success in establishing decentralized sources of power and influence: topic-oriented committees, university-based collaborating centers, and regional councils. Our regional vice-presidents, in particular, are learning to serve simultaneously as agents of the global Federation and as leaders of the new constituencies embodied in their councils. I have written this history and memoir in the belief that their attachment to the Federation, and that of our other components, signifies commitment to a common goal and recognizes "a shared resonance of spirit in our common life which both transcends and permeates our own and the other's distinctiveness" (Daloz 1996, pp.76–77).

Sources and Acknowledgments

The President of the anonymous Foundation that subsidized this volume's publication and distribution deserves specific mention for a necessary investment of trust and money in WFMH. Without it this book would not have been created. I have agreed to say no more.

The book's title, *The Search for Mental Health*, was suggested by Marian Brody. It reflects the sympathetic intelligence with which she has experienced Federation life during the years beginning when I became president-elect in 1980. This experience has included not only patient and informed attention at major and minor meetings, but the occasional care and feeding of the Directors and Executive Committee. She has been a true participant-observer. She also deserves the acknowledgment because of her tolerance for the long hours in which I sequestered myself reading old WFMH documents and transferring them to the growing manuscript on my computer.

The written record

Time was a major consideration in the production of this story. It had to be a part-time task accomplished in bits and pieces of time snatched from other obligations and opportunities. Another constraint made it impossible to achieve a smooth flow of themes and events. That was the need to pack the account with as much archival material as possible. I leave it to some later student of our development to produce a more integrated history.

The basic written materials from which Federation-related events and impressions of the personal interactions involved have been reconstructed are the minutes of early Board meetings, Newsletters and Bulletins, and Annual Reports. Federation records before 1983, however, have not been systematically collected, and funds have not been available for the professional archiving essential for their long-term organization and preservation. Some events have simply not been recorded. Some records seem to be irretrievably missing. The data from the years between 1966 and 1975 are especially sparse, since records stored at UN Geneva were, reportedly, mistakenly discarded. Length requirements have made it impossible to utilize fully even the materials that are available. Most of the paper-filled crates in an Alexandria, Virginia storage facility—shipped there from Vancouver—have remained unopened. There is room, within the available materials, for a much longer and more detailed account of the origins and development of WFMH, and its efforts to define the mental health that it has tried to support. I have encouraged European leaders to produce a volume on the origins and development of the voluntary mental health movement on their continent.

Annual Reports were initially available from 1948–1949 to 1967. They were not available again until I began to write them myself in my capacity as Secretary General. Beginning in the mid-1980s I issued them at first in typewritten form for distribution only to the Board and a few others. In recent years the anonymous foundation previously mentioned has made it possible to publish the Reports in printed form for distribution to our total membership.

In the Rees years, Bulletins were initiated on a quarterly basis, but with lack of funding, and hence of personnel, they became irregular. Some of these are available in our archives. After a hiatus, they became available as Newsletters, again irregularly, beginning with an issue dated "1971/72," and continued until the establishment of the Baltimore-Washington Secretariat.. Our first Newsletters, initially five times yearly, then quarterly, were issued by my office beginning in March, 1984. Our effort was to include everything that might later become part of an Annual Report. At first I wrote most of them, but with time, Kathy McKnight, M.Ed. (currently Managing Editor of the *Journal of Nervous and Mental Disease),* and then, her successor in my office, Elena Berger, D. Phil., began to do more. In the 2 years before this publication, Dr. Berger has done the largest share of Newsletter writing.

The account of the Federation's prenatal period and founding in August, 1948 is based on several sources, all of which are referenced in the text itself. Among them is Rees' *Reflections,* published in 1966. Important information is contained in the 1948 proceedings of the Third International Congress, especially Volume IV, which is concerned with developments leading to the Congress, its Conference on Mental Health, the Federation, and its founding document, "Mental Health and World Citizenship."

The Margaret Mead files in the U.S. Library of Congress provided a wealth of relevant material, including minutes of the International Committee on Mental Hygiene as it debated concerns relevant to the 1948 Congress, and materials concerning the International Preparatory Commission which, meeting in Roffey Park for 2 weeks before the Congress, produced the founding document.

Interviews and memories: WFMH as history and as memoir

The history on the basis of written materials has, from 1972 forward, been increasingly supplemented by my own observations. These, inevitably, reflect lacunae or distortions in my memory. With this in mind, I decided to include the term "memoir" in the title, and to use the first person, as in this Preface, whenever it seemed to clarify possibly subjective elements in the narrative or make it a more human story. In this respect, some aspects of my account are, indeed, those of a personal memoir, just as that published in 1966 by my predecessor in the role of Federation Chief Executive, John R. ("Jack") Rees, M.D. Nonetheless, I believe that it provides an objective portrayal of a unique organization in the context of its times.

Several individuals have given generously of their time and effort to this enterprise. Special acknowledgment is due Dr. Calvin Saxton who spontaneously offered to send me his doctoral dissertation on education for worldmindedness. It contained rich material about the earliest impulses that led to the Congress and the Federation, discussed in Chapter 2. These were in the 1945 collaboration of the American psychiatrist Harry Stack Sullivan, M.D., and George Brock Chisholm, M.D., who, at his invitation, lectured in that year about peace and mental health. These impulses were also found in the early interests of UNESCO, and documented in 1946 and 1947, leading to the famous meeting on tensions affecting international understanding—of which Sullivan was a part. Saxton was also kind enough to read and comment on a semi-final draft of Chapter 2.

The Chapters on Regional activities have been reviewed by key figures in their development. The section in Chapter 9 on the Caribbean was reviewed by my friend and former colleague at the University of the West Indies (UWI, Jamaica), Professor Michael Beaubrun, M.D., now of Trinidad, who was WFMH President between 1972 and 1974. His letters and reprints supplemented by memories of my own experience as a Visiting Professor in his Department at UWI between 1972 and 1975 provided additional information useful in the development of Chapters 5 and 9.

Another helpful friend, whom I had not seen for at least 25 years, was Bertram Schaffner, M.D., a New York psychiatrist and psychoanalyst. Bert, a key figure in the Federation activities in New York and in the Caribbean during the Rees years, as well as the 1963–1967 period of the Geneva Secretariat, was most gracious and generous with his time, permitting a recorded interview at his home in the evening after he had been seeing patients all day. This took place on November 20, 1995. Documents from his work in that period are stored in the American Psychiatric Association's library in Washington, D.C. Bert Schaffner's interview also contributed to the section on the Caribbean in Chapter 9. The section on Latin America, also in Chapter 9, was reviewed by Federico Puente Silva, M.D., of Mexico, WFMH President, 1993–1995.

In Chapter 10, the section on Africa was reviewed by Lage Vitus, Director of the South African Federation for Mental Health, and Isaac Mwendapole, M.S.W., WFMH Regional Vice President for Africa; that on the Eastern Mediterranean by Gamal El Azayem, M.D., WFMH President, 1987-1989, and Ahmed El Azayem, M.D., Regional Vice President for the WFMH Eastern Mediterranean Region, both of Cairo; that on Oceania by Dr. Max Abbott of Auckland; those on Asia (Southeast Asia and Western Pacific) by Professor Tsung-yi Lin, M.D. and Mei-chen Lin, M.S.W. Sincere thanks are due to all.

Edith Morgan, O.B.E., active in WFMH since the 1960s and President in 1985–1987, was a most helpful contributor to Chapter 11 on the development of WFMH in Europe. She generously allowed me to read her materials, including minutes of the United Kingdom Committee for WFMH, when I visited her in London, October 6–8, 1996. She also reviewed in detail a late draft of Chapter 11 itself, before my arrival. We spent one long day, October 7th, at her kitchen table going over it sentence by sentence. As Founder President of the European Regional Council of WFMH she was eminently qualified to evaluate the contents of this Chapter, and I am most grateful for her willingness to do so and for the time she devoted to the task. She may wish, one day, to produce a more detailed and definitive history of the development of WFMH's European Region.

Rees' memoirs, containing accounts of the initial period of Federation life, from 1948 through his retirement at the end of 1961, were published by the United States Committee for the World Federation for Mental Health, Inc. William T. Beaty, II, Executive Director of that Committee and of the WFMH Regional Office in New York (covering North, Central and South America and the Caribbean) graciously allowed me to record an interview with him in New York on November 20, 1995. He also directed me to the WFMH papers he had contributed to the Diethelm Library at Cornell University Medical School, subsequently transferred to the New York Academy of Medicine. Unfortunately, time permitted only a single day's perusal of these materials. Beaty's interview material contributed to Chapters 3, 4, 5, and 6.

Chapter 4 also owes much to my old and valued friend, Dr. Henry David, who was, perhaps, the key contributor to the continued productivity of the Federation during its Geneva era. He generously permitted me to record an interview with him. His edited book of proceedings of a 1963 Federation conference also provided important information about aspects of its international mental health agenda. It was Henry who directed me to Dr. Pierre Visseur, WFMH

Director from 1965–1967, who kindly took the time to send me a long and interesting letter about the personalities with whom he came in contact during that period.

Vancouver lawyer-businessman, Gowan Guest, Esq., WFMH President from 1979–1981, wrote, in response to my request, a multipage letter including his own memories dating back to the first appearance in Vancouver of Professor Tsung-yi Lin, M.D., WFMH President from 1974–1979.

The contents of Chapter 8 on WFMH and the United Nations are largely derived from available historical materials. In addition, however, Dr. Kay C. Greene of New York supplied important information. More than anyone else, she was responsible for our contemporary organization at UN New York and generously wrote an account of her work from 1991–1995 during her period as our Senior Representative. Her successor, Nancy Wallace, C.S.W., reviewed the materials on UN New York after 1995. Thanks are also due to Dr. Maria Dorothea Simon, our representative to UN Vienna, for her notes on the WFMH role there.

Many others have contributed through notes, discussions, and their work in supporting the Federation. They begin with Eileen Potocki, my Secretary for many years at the University of Maryland; Kathy McKnight, M.Ed., in several roles, first as my University Secretary, then as my major Federation executive assistant, and finally, after 1992 as Managing Editor of the *Journal of Nervous and Mental Disease*, a role in which she has continued to be a major contributor to the Federation's work. As early as 1994, before I had finally decided to write this volume, Edward J. Pennington, General Director of the Canadian Mental Health Association was good enough to respond to my request for historical materials on mental health in Canada. Ms. McKnight's successor as my primary Federation assistant, Dr. Elena Berger, was an important aide in the volume's preparation. In Taiwan, in December 1996, informal conversations with Tsung-yi and Mei-chen Lin were rewarding.

Finally, my closest Federation associate, Richard C. ("Dick") Hunter, has been uniformly supportive—even reminding me that a "memoir" is not identical with a "history." He helped me locate old reports, and, on several occasions reviewed and recommended significant changes in Chapters 5 and 6. As I devoted less time to ongoing Federation work during 1995–1997 and more time to writing, Dick Hunter along with Elena Berger carried more and more of the everyday responsibility that kept us moving forward.

To all these and many more I express my gratitude in the hope and expectation that WFMH will continue its forward momentum and its search for mental health into the new millennium.

Eugene B. Brody
March, 1998

Contents

Part I

ORGANIZATIONAL DEVELOPMENT

Chapter 1

Precursors of Federation

The roots of the World Federation for Mental Health (WFMH) lie deep in the early efforts of men and women of good will to improve the lot of their fellows, recognized not as deliberate miscreants or possessed by demons, but as distressed persons, stigmatized by an illness that frightened or disgusted their families and communities. A detailed account of the precursors of the voluntary mental health movement is beyond the scope of this volume. It is apparent, however, that early efforts to improve the lot of mentally ill or distressed persons were nourished by at least two major streams of influence. These were, first, the writings and advocacy of a few exceptional leaders who had survived this affliction themselves and, second, a deep strain of morality impelling more fortunate citizens to try to better the lot of those less advantaged.

INDIVIDUAL SURVIVORS OF MENTAL ILLNESS: THE PASSION TO HELP

Among the earliest influences on constructive public concern with issues of mental health and illness was the advocacy of people who had suffered mental illness and, sometimes, hospital confinement. They were passionately impelled to improve the lot of those who had suffered similar difficulties. Discussions with contemporary survivors of episodes of mental illness, and with those whose parents, children, or siblings have been ill, reveal many possible motivations for their efforts. This is true for those who have become mental health professionals, as well as nonprofessional volunteers. For some it is a persisting effort to exorcise their own residual demons. For others it is part of a necessary effort to know and understand a persisting mystery. Some are tormented by frustration-induced aggression in their attempts to change society. Yet others, uniquely empathic because of their own experience, are simply compassionate and principled.

Two of the best-known individual survivors driven by their own experience of suffering to improve the lot of others were New Englanders, products of the morally assertive 19th century culture of the northeast coast of the United States. Their energy, education, and well-developed views of right and wrong, together with their personal experience of affliction, made them effective advocates for the mentally ill.

Dorothea Dix: The First Advocate

Dorothea Dix, of Boston, was the world's most prominent pioneer, a nonprofessional or "lay" advocate for the care of mentally ill persons. Her effort was to get them out of almshouses, prisons, and the hidden confinements of private homes and into specialized mental hospitals run by the State. In her heyday in the 1840s, having succeeded in her campaign to have state legislatures build such hospitals, she was known as the "Queen of the Asylums" and wielded great power over the appointment of their superintendents (Bell, 1849).

The intimate Dorothea Dix story is told, on the basis of previously unknown letters, in Gollaher's, *Voice for the Mad*(1995). With a background so disturbed that she could say that she "never knew childhood," she suffered from recurrent severe depressions. Never hospitalized, she dealt with them by temporarily retreating from the world. In the years 1836–1837, recuperating in England from what was termed a "nervous breakdown," she met, among other reformers, Samuel Tuke of the York Retreat for mentally ill Quakers. The Retreat was known for its noncoercive approach to psychotic persons, whom it tried to help by treating them in a way that increased their self-esteem and motivated them to manage their own behavior. Her visit there set the stage for her later explorations of American jails and other nontherapeutic places of confinement for chronically psychotic people.

Just two years later, in 1841, at the age of 39, she was prepared to become the "voice for the mad." In that year she began the epoch-making presentations to American state legislatures that led to the development of hospitals dedicated solely to the treatment of people called "insane." Her work was fueled by the conviction that the mentally ill were neither criminal nor morally bad, but capable, with adequate treatment, of leading normal lives. This intensely held conviction led her to address many state legislatures, exhorting them to appropriate funds for mental hospitals intended to replace the prevailing punitive, neglectful warehousing of patients with active treatment.

In 1843 her speech to the Massachusetts State Legislature foreshadowed the contemporary WFMH view of the mentally ill as a minority without a voice. In it she defined herself as "the advocate of helpless, forgotten, insane and idiotic men and women...." Her reports of these visits were "intended to establish the lunatic's humanity, and bridge the chasm, the strong sense of 'otherness,' that separated the mad from the rest of society.... Her empathy for the lunatic sprang from the deeper themes of abandonment, isolation, and broken family ties to which she had always been so exquisitely sensitive.... [She] was not merely concerned for the insane, she was fascinated by them as though she could see specters of herself in even the most hopeless cases. With a conviction wrung from personal experience, she constantly warned that reason could be dispossessed at any moment." She implored her readers to place themselves "in that dreary cage.... and imagine how they would want to be treated" (Gollaher, 1995, p. 153). The remedy, in her view, was "rightly organized Hospitals, adapted to the special care of the peculiar malady of the Insane" (Dix, 1843, 1847, cited in Grob, 1994). She was also concerned with the financing of these hospitals. In 1848 she became an advocate before the United States Congress for legislation to distribute five million acres of federal lands to the states, with proceeds to be used to care for the indigent insane (Grob, 1994, p. 97). Although this effort was unsuccessful, she was largely responsible for the development of a United States network of public state institutions for the care of the mentally ill. In time, her influence extended to Canada and Europe. This story, described in many places, is told in Albert Deutsch's *The Mentally Ill in America* (1937), and in a history of psychology written by J. C. Flugel (1948), a British psychologist who was one of the founders of the WFMH.

Dorothea Dix was one of those reformers driven by anger as well as empathy. Gollaher suggests that her success in the face of attacks by almshouse keepers and officials lay in "the angry personal narrative embedded in her text, a narrative that captured the meaning of insanity in human terms [implying] a mysterious affinity for these beings...represented as people....[S]he was the first in America to identify with their plight and to invest the insane with the dignity of individual identity" (Gollaher, 1995, pp. 5–6). Her special genius lay in the feeling and empathy stemming from her own private pain combined with the education, talent, and status enabling her to effectively promote her moral cause with the legislative and administrative leaders of her time. She "thrust what we have come to call mental disease and homelessness squarely into the center of public policy…[and] held that to provide a decent level of care for those so lost to reason that they could not care for themselves was an essential obligation of the modern state" (Gollaher, 1995, p. vii).

Clifford W. Beers: Grandfather of the WFMH

Another survivor of mental illness to become a major advocate was Clifford Whittington Beers, of Connecticut (1876–1943). His illness began, according to his own account (Beers, 1908) and that of Albert Deutsch (1937), with a longtime obsession with the idea that he was fated to suffer from epilepsy, as did an older brother. This developed into a delusional belief that he actually had the disease. In June of 1900, only three years after his graduation from Yale, having first intended to jump, he hung by his hands until he fell from a fourth story window, narrowly escaping death. The obsession with epilepsy disappeared, to be replaced by delusions of persecution and of grandeur. The next three years, except for a few months in the home of an attendant, were spent in Connecticut mental hospitals, both private and public.

Beers began writing his autobiographical account of his mental hospitalizations, *A Mind that Found Itself*, not long after being released from a hospital in September 1903. It was completed in 1906 when he was 30 years old and published two years later, in 1908. In it he gave a moving description of his illness, with episodes both of depression with feelings of being persecuted, and of manic overactivity with delusions of grandeur. He described the often abusive and punishing treatment, common at the time, to which he had been subjected as a hospital inmate. This included being beaten, spat upon, confined in isolation, and restrained in a straitjacket. At one point he scribbled on the wall of his room: "God bless our Home, which is Hell" (Beers, 1908; Deutsch, 1937, p. 303).

After the first two years of illness, burdened with the belief that he had committed some vague, unpardonable crime, he passed into a state of "extreme exaltation." It was, apparently, in this period that he conceived the idea of starting "a world-wide movement for the protection of the insane." However, he was sufficiently intact to be able to translate his idea into action. His advocacy efforts began before his hospital discharge with long letters to the Governor of Connecticut and other public officials. During this early phase of his recovery, presumably in order to thoroughly experience all aspects of asylum life so as to be able to expose them, he deliberately provoked attendants "to throw him into the worst of the 'violent' wards" (Deutsch, 1937, pp. 304–305).

Approximately one year after being finally discharged from hospital care he had a single mild period of elation that caused him to return voluntarily to the private hospital where he had been earlier in his illness. Otherwise, he remained free of major symptoms. However, he continued, even as he resumed the business career in which he had engaged before his hospitalizations, to be concerned with the possibility of starting a mental hospital reform movement. The idea of an autobiographical book as a means of changing public attitudes was reinforced by the example of *Uncle Tom's Cabin* as a stimulus to the anti-slavery movement. Later, he wrote, "Why cannot a book be written which will free the helpless slaves of all creeds and colors confined today in the asylums and sanitariums throughout the world…free them from unnecessary abuses to which they are now subjected."

By January 1907 he was devoting himself completely to writing his own book. He also outlined his plan for a "national society" to improve the care of the mentally ill. It would involve public education encouraging a more humane attitude toward sufferers, research into the causes of mental illness, and preventive services. Other exposés of asylum life had already been published in the United States, both by former patients and newspaper reporters searching for sensational stories. Only Beers, however, had had his manuscript reviewed by professionals and other leaders, so his veracity and motives were never in doubt. Looking for backers, he took the manuscript to Professor William James of Harvard, the leading psychological scholar of his day. James' enthusiastic letter of approval was, according to Beers, the turning point in his struggle. From that time on James was a major source of strength, writing letters, soliciting money, and enlisting academic colleagues and others in support of Beers' cause (Ridenour, 1961). Among the latter were America's first full-time Professor of Psychiatry, Adolph Meyer, M.D., and William H. Welch, M.D., Professor of Medicine, both at Johns Hopkins University in Baltimore, literary figures such as Booth Tarkington, and others. James wrote the introduction to the book's first edition, noting, "It reads like fiction but it is not fiction."

The personal magnetism that made Beers such an effective leader was rooted partly in his intelligence and grasp of public issues, partly in the expansive thinking of his "manic" episodes, but mainly—as in the case of Dorothea Dix—in the passionate conviction rooted in his period of personal trauma. He had learned from harsh, personal experience what it was like to be a patient in that era. Although he had spent three years in three Connecticut hospitals, and was deeply critical of their patient care (Beers, 1908; Dain, 1980; Deutsch, 1937; Mora, 1980), he did not question the validity of the concept of mental illness, the field of psychiatry, or the concept of mental hospitals. His aim was to make these places into truly healing institutions and psychiatry into a truly caring and scientifically enlightened profession. Yet, he could not rid himself of a lingering suspicion of psychiatrists and a wariness of their perceived need for power over him. This residual wariness and suspicion remained a source of difficulty in his later organizational efforts.

Nearly 90 years after his epoch-making book, 79 years after founding the International Committee on Mental Hygiene (see below), and 51 years after the Preparatory Commission for the WFMH began its work, the objectives put together in Connecticut in 1908 remain compatible with WFMH goals and those of mental health associations all over the world. They encompass such fundamental points as improving the delivery and quality of psychiatric care, promoting mental health, preventing mental disorders and ill health, and educating the public and influential leaders.

Truly, Clifford W. Beers was the effective grandparent of the WFMH. Sadly, in 1943, he was once more in the depths of a severe depression. He did not recover and, at the age of 67, died in a psychiatric institution, Butler Hospital, in Providence, Rhode Island. This time, though, the place was one of the world's leading private hospitals, and Beers was not listed as a patient, but as the guest of its distinguished Director, Dr. Arthur Ruggles—who in 1946, was part of the group to which George Brock Chisholm, M.D., suggested the formation of the WFMH (see Chapter 2).

ORIGINS OF THE CONTEMPORARY VOLUNTEER MOVEMENT

Human communities organize themselves to protect and improve the effectiveness and well-being of their members. The decisive step of civilization, as Sigmund Freud put it, is asserting the power of community (Freud, 1930). This is especially apparent with regard to the institutions and healers concerned with people perceived as afflicted, diseased, possessed, or under the spell of malignant nonhuman forces. In preindustrial communities, deviant persons were destroyed or subjected to rituals and deliberate punishments aimed at exorcising their demons and restoring them to accepted standards of behavior. Otherwise, they, especially the indigent, were allowed to wander at will and suffer whatever fate befell them.

In the industrializing world the initial emphasis in dealing with these deviant members was on isolating them for the protection of others in the community. Early places of isolation were in the cellars, attics, and barns of private dwellings, or in almshouses, poorhouses, pesthouses, or prisonlike asylums. Responsibility for these public places of sequestration was in the hands of local authorities, who were careful to ensure that the indigent insane from other areas did not remain with them and utilize their scarce resources.

In time, institutions of isolation acquired therapeutic goals. As progress was made in the scientific understanding of irrational behavior, "insanity" was recognized as a disease requiring treatment rather than banishment or exorcism. As the "insane" were converted into "patients," power was increasingly concentrated in the hands of medical practitioners, professors of psychiatry, hospital superintendents, and, in some urban centers, community health boards. Their health care philosophy was thoroughly paternalistic. Their initial emphasis, as before, was on isolating the most violent and agitated patients for the protection of others in the community. This was especially evident in their ability to commit persons to involuntary confinement on the grounds of mental illness.

Reform Movements in Europe and England

The seeds of early citizens' reform movements arising in the challenges to physician power and patient restraint came, mainly, from physicians. They were especially prominent during social crises with heightened emphasis on the values of individual freedom and self-determination (Brody, 1993a). It was in the climate of the French Revolution in 1792, for example, that Philippe Pinel tried to transform mentally ill men at Bicetre from chained "wild beasts" to patients with the dignity appropriate to human beings (Weiner, 1994). In Florence, Italy, at about the same time, a new law required a mental examination to be performed on people after their hospital commitment on grounds of insanity. The rules of the newest mental hospital, prepared under the direction of Vicenzo Chiarugi, stated: "It is a supreme moral duty and medical obligation to respect the insane individual as a person." In the same year, 1792, the Quakers in England were presented with a proposal by William Tuke, a grocer, for a refuge for treating the mentally ill that was based on moral principles. It depended on the absence of coercion and the psychotic patient's own desire for self-esteem. A basic aim was to provide its patients with the environment of a kindly and considerate family. Bloodletting, "the bane of centuries" (Deutsch, 1937, p. 94), was forbidden.

The new institution, in York, opened its doors in 1796. It was named The Retreat in order to avoid the stigma associated with such traditional designations as asylum and madhouse. Tuke and the York Retreat had a significant influence on the mental hospitals established in early America (Deutsch, 1937). This was most evident in the 1811 proposal for a Friends' Asylum, finally opened at Frankford, Pennsylvania, in 1817. It appears to have come from a Quaker minister, Thomas Scattergood, who had visited the Retreat near York in January of 1797. An abridged version of Samuel Tuke's *Description of the Retreat near York*, published in London in 1813, emphasizing the "moral treatment" it practiced, was widely circulated among prospective donors to the Asylum project.

These early efforts, in the same historical period when physicians were beginning to specialize and medical associations were gaining influence, created an atmosphere favorable to the eventual emergence of a nonofficial, nonmedical, citizen-based mental health movement led by nonsalaried, self-appointed individuals. Among the best-documented efforts at organized voluntary work were those in the United Kingdom.

Early voluntary bodies in the United Kingdom aimed at serving or protecting the mentally ill differed from those arising in the United States, as they still do in the 1990s, in their relationship with the government. While those in the United States are primarily advocacy and educational in nature and financially as well as administratively independent of the government, those in the United Kingdom receive funds from government agencies in return for actual services. Perhaps the earliest recorded example was the Society for Improving the Condition of the Insane, organized in London in 1842. Its first president was a famous social reformer, Lord

Shaftesbury, and its active leaders included Dr. D. Hack Tuke, of the Quaker family that had founded the York Retreat. The Society's aims included the diffusion of knowledge about the nature, causes, and treatment of "mental disorder," especially to medical practitioners; educating the attendants who had immediate contact with "insane patients"; and stimulating thought about the management of hospitals and asylums. This organization appears to have been merged with the Lunacy Law Reform Society of London (Deutsch, 1937, p. 311). However, it seems to have served as an inspiration while it lasted. Dr. Pliny Earle, an early American psychiatrist, was so impressed by the formation of voluntary associations in Britain that he wrote an account of the London Society in 1845 for the *American Journal of Insanity*. In it he challenged his compatriots: "When will a similar association be formed among the dignitaries of this land?" (Earle, 1845).

The Alleged Lunatics' Friend Society, founded in the same year, 1845, with a former patient as secretary, foreshadowed the trend toward an organized constituency of former and current mental health service users. However, having emerged in response to legal and press interest in the United Kingdom's Lunacy Law, it also anticipated the 20th century antipsychiatry movement. Neither the new Society nor the law was primarily concerned with improving the care and treatment of patients. Instead, they were concerned with civil liberties. The Society's focus on protecting citizens from wrongful mental hospital detention fitted a major press emphasis of the time. The press was engaged in "constant attack" upon Asylum doctors, implying not only that they were incompetent but that they drove previously normal persons crazy (Jones, 1993, p. 95). The Alleged Lunatics' Friend Society was termed the "first libertarian pressure group," as it aimed at "the protection of the British subject from unjust confinement on the grounds of mental derangement and for the redress of persons so confined" (Hansard, cited by Jones, 1993).

Similar concerns arose in France. The French mental health law of 1893 "took the greatest care to underline the fundamental difference existing between the restriction of freedom imposed on mentally ill patients and the restriction of freedom imposed on criminals by courts of justice" (Pichot, 1967). Yet, there too, criticism began almost immediately to focus on the risk of arbitrary confinement of presumably normal citizens, including commitment for ulterior reasons.

In 1879, in London, a Mental After-Care Association was formed by concerned citizens. This may have been the first to influence the emergence of similar movements in the young United States of America.

Although Britain seems to have been the home of the precursors of today's national voluntary mental associations, none of them persisted there. The first organization for the mentally ill, which has remained in continuous existence despite changes of name, was founded in Finland on 19 January 1897. It was primarily charitable, as indicated by its name, A Relief Organization for the Mad, and worked primarily to arrange accommodations, food, and employment for patients discharged from mental hospitals. However, it had a moral component in addition to its compassionate aims. In the absence of scientific knowledge, mental illness was seen as shameful, and families carefully isolated their sick relatives from the rest of society. The country already had psychiatrists among its medical practitioners, and they were prominent among the founders of the new organization. These professionals wished to use it to combat the stigma associated with mental illness. They were acutely aware of the general public ignorance about mental health and illness, and did what they could to remedy it. Prejudice against the mentally ill, indeed against all minorities, has continued as a major concern of the Association.

With time and experience, the Finnish association's activities and self-concept changed, and in 1919 it was renamed The Healthy Spirit Association. By the 1920s it had become sufficiently recognized for the state authorities to solicit its opinions regarding issues concerning mental illness. In 1939 it was again renamed, The Association for Fighting Nervous Diseases and Mental Illness. Its present name, The Finnish Association for Mental Health, dates from 1952 (Salonen et al., 1994).

Social and Mental Health Movements in North America

Pliny Earle's call for United States citizens to emulate the early English mental health movement was not answered for more than a generation. Albert Deutsch (1937) reviewed American developments during the decade beginning in 1872, nearly 30 years after Earle's letter. That period was exceptionally rich in the development of social movements and associations, many including both professionals and volunteers. These included the 1872 founding of the American Public Health Association which, though it was not remarkable for specific attention to mental health, was among the forces contributing to the growth of interest in preventive medicine and positive health, ultimately coming to include mental health.

The emergence of social work as a profession in the United States had a more positive and specific effect. One of its early emphases was on environmental factors contributing to social as well as psychological problems. The 1878 meeting of the National Conference of Social Work (established in 1874) included a paper on "The Prevention of Disease and Insanity." This influenced a public meeting in 1879 concerned with lunacy reform, where a more focused citizen's reform organization was conceived. This was The National Association for the Protection of the Insane and the Prevention of Insanity which, in retrospect, may be viewed as ecumenical in the WFMH sense, lacking only the consumer participation of the present era. Its founding membership in 1880 included social workers, neurologists, and psychiatrists, as well as nonprofessionals. The new reform group engaged vigorously in campaigns to alleviate abuses in institutional care, including legislative inquiries and supervisory offices. In so doing, however, it evoked the antagonism of the Association of Medical Superintendents of American Institutions for the Insane, forerunner of the American Psychiatric Association. This contributed to its failure to rally public support and it died in 1886 (Deutsch, 1937).

During these early stirrings of volunteers in continental Europe, England, and the United States, similar activities were taking place elsewhere in North America. Early volunteers in Canada included religious groups in the late 17th and early 18th centuries and a number of lay organizations established at least in part to help those disabled by disease as well as poverty (Griffin, 1989). Many prominent Canadians coupled their names with that of the crusading Dorothea Dix in petitioning their government to develop appropriate asylums for the insane. A voluntary after-care society modeled after that in England was proposed in 1898. Although it was never established, the proposal contributed to increased public interest in mentally retarded persons, especially those likely to have children.

The United States Voluntary Mental Hygiene Movement: Parent of the International Movement

The precursor of the international voluntary mental health movement was the formally organized National Committee for Mental Hygiene in the United States. As described above, this began with Clifford Beers more than a half-century after Dorothea Dix started her campaigns. It seems probable that the historically based atmosphere of free political discussion between citizens and government in the United States had been opened to social concerns by Dix's interventions with the state and federal legislatures.

Beers' book, *A Mind that Found Itself*, was unique in having immediately drawn the praise of the country's leading mental health scholars. It also made a profound impression on nonprofessional readers, particularly the residents of Beers' home state, Connecticut, where he had been hospitalized. Their receptivity made it easy for him, almost immediately after his discharge, to organize the Connecticut Society for Mental Hygiene. Nina Ridenour, later to become Executive Secretary of the International Committee for Mental Hygiene, described the first step toward Beers' new "national society": "It was the afternoon of May 6, 1908, that a little knot of people sat down together in a residence in New Haven, Connecticut upon the invitation of Clifford Whittingham Beers—a young man with a remarkable history—to organize the Connecticut Society for Mental Hygiene…the beginning of the organized mental health movement in America. According to his plan [this] was not only to be the first in a long line of societies to follow, but also to serve as a pilot effort to provide experience in organizing" (Ridenour, 1961, pp. 1–2). In the language of the day the Society's stated objectives were: "To work for the conservation of mental health; to help prevent nervous and mental disorders and mental defects; to help raise the standards of care…to secure and disseminate reliable information.…" These objectives included several of the cardinal aims of today's WFMH: public education, prevention of mental illness, improving standards of care, and promoting positive mental health.

Beers' book, coupled with his charismatic personality and his untiring efforts, allowed him to carry out the next stage of his plan on February 19, 1909, only nine months after founding the Connecticut Society. On that day he "invited a similar group of a dozen people to come together in New York City's Manhattan Hotel for the purpose of creating the National Committee for Mental Hygiene.…[H]is dreams for the future called for a growing network of state and local mental hygiene societies extending across the United States and eventually throughout the world…" (Ridenour, 1961, p. 2). The charter members included both William James and Adolph Meyer. Beers had originally intended to focus on asylum reform, but Meyer—foreshadowing the philosophy of the WFMH's founders—persuaded him that the prevention of mental illness and the promotion of "mental hygiene" were more important. The idea of prevention was inherent in the term mental hygiene, which had been used by William Sweetser, an American physician, as early as 1843, at the beginning of Dorothea Dix's advocacy (Rosen, 1968; Sweetser, 1843). Unfortunately, Beers' distrust of Meyer's perceived power led, in 1910, to a break in their relationship. However, due mainly, it seems, to Professor Meyer's equanimity and long-range view, it was not decisive. Meyer, though wary of Beers as a person, maintained a positive attitude toward his endeavor, and his (Meyer's) reputation remained a factor in the decision of many psychiatrists to become active in the new mental health organization (Rosen, 1968).

A favorable context for the new voluntary association was provided by the rapid pace of industrialization, the expansion of urban communities, and the U.S. National Child Labor Committee, which Beers proposed the new Committee should be modeled after (Beers, 1908; Rosen, 1968). The National Committee for Mental Hygiene acted rapidly to expose the negative conditions in most asylums and the problems of mentally ill persons in jails. It successfully exerted pressure for change on governmental bodies. It also played a role in the establishment of schools of social work and gave rise to the child guidance movement with a major focus on preventing mental illness. In the period between the two World Wars, prior to the establishment of the U.S. National Institute of Mental Health, the United States Association played a role in broadening the training of psychiatrists and their acceptance—and that of the relevance of psychopathology in daily life—by the general public (Dain, 1980).

Another possible factor favoring the establishment of a voluntary association in the United States was the rise of psychoanalysis. It had been greeted with skepticism and hostility by medical authorities in Freud's native Vienna (where the WFMH marked his home with a plaque in 1952) and, except for a limited group of intelligentsia, made little impression on the European public of the time. In the United States, however, the relatively rapid popular acceptance of Freudian thinking may have reflected the appeal of John Dewey's philosophy of self-improvement. After Freud's famous lectures at Clark University in Worcester, Massachusetts, his host, psychologist and educator G. Stanley Hall, wrote to him on 7 October 1909, asking for a publishable manuscript. In the letter he mentioned Adolph Meyer's positive response to the lectures and the likelihood that a "strong American school" could develop (Rosenzweig, 1992, p. 359). The popularization of Freud's volume *The Psychopathology of Everyday Life* (1905) contributed to public interest in individual psychology and the de-stigmatization of some types of psychiatric disorders. As deviant behavior became more understandable, the promise of relieving it seemed less remote.

During the years immediately following the establishment of the Connecticut society and the National Committee, mental health associations were formed in many of the United States, and in 1914 the first national meeting of state societies for mental hygiene was convened. It was attended and widely reported by E. H. Young, M.D., secretary of the Canadian Medical Association's Committee on Mental Hygiene, which was formed in the same year. In this way it came to the attention of Clarence Hincks, M.D., of Toronto (also present at the 1946 meeting with Chisholm) who was dissatisfied with his work in the outpatient clinic there and concerned with the poor quality of mental hospitals and the lack of interest in prevention in Canada. In 1917 he consulted leading medical, psychiatric, and neurological specialists in the United States. There, apparently by accident, he met Beers, who gave him a copy of his book and asked him to join in creating a worldwide mental hygiene movement. As reported by Griffin, "They both had a contagious enthusiasm which at times became excited exuberance.... Both were cyclothymic and subject to occasional periods of fatigue, anxiety, depression, and apathy. As long as they were not depressed at the same time they made an excellent team" (Griffin, 1989, p. 7).

Following his contacts with Beers, Hincks immediately began a campaign. The Canadian National Committee for Mental Hygiene, later to become the Canadian Mental Health Association, an early WFMH member, was established in 1918. Hincks became the Association's first Secretary and from 1926 to 1952 served as its General Director. He was succeeded in this post by Griffin, who served until 1971. Jack Griffin told me some of this story himself, as we came to know each other personally in the mid-1960s as members of the Interamerican Council of Psychiatric Associations. I became involved because of my work at the Federal University of Rio de Janeiro in that era. Daniel Blain, then Medical Director of the American Psychiatric Association, asked me to explore the possibility of forming an Interamerican Council with the Executive of the Associacion Psichiatrica de America Latina (APAL) meeting in Lima, Peru, in 1964. I spent two days talking with the APAL leadership, and gave a speech at their invitation in Lima's Alcade (the City Hall). Consequently, I became a founding member of the Council. Jack Griffin joined us later as a representative of Canada and we met together on several occasions in Latin America, where, among other matters, we compared the developing voluntarism in North and Latin America.

THE INTERNATIONAL CONNECTION, ICMH

Beers' seminal idea was the creation of a worldwide network of national mental hygiene committees, all with the same or similar constitutions. With this in mind, in 1919 he called together an organizing committee for a new International Committee for Mental Hygiene (Ridenour, 1961). The initial participants in the International Committee were the United States and Canadian national mental health organizations. Later, other educational and clinical leaders in the two countries—significantly, professors of psychiatry and well-known figures in psychology, health education, and the social sciences—were given key roles. These changed from time to time depending upon their relationship with the sometimes volatile and always expansive Beers. With this beginning it grew to include representatives of other countries. Its stationery in July 1924 shows William H. Welch, M.D., Professor of Medicine at Johns Hopkins, as Chairman. Other members at that time represented mental health associations in the United States, Canada, Great Britain, France, Belgium, China, Brazil, South Africa, and New South Wales and Tasmania, both of Australia.

Beers had hoped for an International Congress on Mental Hygiene in 1925. He was unsuccessful, however, in raising the needed $100,000. A philanthropic foundation to which he applied declined to help on "grounds of policy," not wishing "to establish the precedent of helping to finance international congresses," but he regarded this as only "a temporary setback." (Beers, 1924). He continued to dream of a gathering that would be "a clarion call for action on the treatment and prevention of mental disorders of all kinds, a call that could be heard around the world" (Griffin, 1989, p. 66). In the 1920s and 1930s he travelled extensively, carrying on a voluminous correspondence encouraging people in other countries to organize national mental hygiene societies. The 1917 version of the society in Finland, following its 1897 precursor group, was recognized as the second national organization, after the one in the United States, to focus directly on mental hygiene. Canada was the third, making the movement "officially international," as Beers said (Ridenour, 1961). The fourth society was that of the Union of South Africa in 1919.

It was not until 1930, 11 years after the International Committee was formed, that Beers' grand plan approached reality. By then, 21 more countries had formed mental health associations. Although Beers, the volunteer and former patient, had provided the inspiration and the energy, professional establishment figures, largely psychiatrists, assumed major responsibility for organizing the First International Congress on Mental Hygiene in that year. It was a historic landmark in the history of the voluntary mental health movement, attracting by various estimates from 3000 to more than 4100 people (this last and most expansive estimate from Rees, 1966) from 53 countries to Washington, DC, under the honorary patronage of President Herbert Hoover. This was the first time that anything approaching this number of people had come together to support the ideal of mental hygiene. The excitement it generated focused public attention on the subject and created the momentum leading to the formation of the WFMH, which has carried through to the end of the century.

Beers' vision and tireless enthusiasm were widely and specifically recognized and applauded during this Congress. This recognition came despite the organizational dominance of internationally known psychiatrists, all of whom did not share his, or the public's, enthusiasm for the meeting. As noted by Ridenour (1961), some of the professional leaders "were frank in expressing their doubts as to whether the solid gains for the mentally ill were commensurate with the fanfare." Thus, immediately following the Congress, in May 1930, Professor Welch wrote a letter to Dr. Simon Flexner that could have come from contemporary detractors of the international voluntary mental health movement. As Welch wrote: "That big mental hygiene congress which I attended recently in Washington was rather terrible and an example of arousing the public before the foundation of sound knowledge and doctrine has been laid. With good psychiatric and neurological institutes something might be done in mental hygiene, but it would have to be at first so elementary as to lack altogether the spectacular appeal now made for the subject" (Ridenour, 1961, p. 67).

At that Washington, DC, Congress a new International Committee for Mental Hygiene (ICMH) was founded on 6 May 1930. Now including representative groups and individuals from 29 countries, the first annual meeting of its governing board took place on 1 April 1932, when its bylaws were ratified. Its European members met as part of a "European Reunion on Mental Hygiene and Prevention" in Paris, 29-31 May 1932. The report of this meeting began by stating: "The world movement for mental hygiene, so successfully and actively begun at the First International Congress on Mental Hygiene at Washington in 1930, advanced a further step at the meeting held in Paris on 29 May at the Union Interalliée when Mr. Clifford Beers, founder and general secretary of the International Committee for Mental Hygiene, met over 40 European members representing more than a dozen different countries, namely: Austria, Belgium, Czecho-Slovakia, Finland, France, Germany, Great Britain, Italy, Netherlands, Norway, Spain, Switzerland, and the United States of America" (News and Notes, 1932, p. 22). The purposes of ICMH "as set forth in its bylaws" were detailed in the report: "They include the creation of an intelligent public opinion, to disseminate information, and to endeavor to secure local, state, federal, and foreign legislation regarding the care and treatment of cases of nervous or mental disorder or mental defect, and regarding mental problems involved in education, research, industry, unemployment, delinquency, crime, dependency, psychology, psychiatry, sociology, prostitution, drug addiction, and other subjects within the broad field of human behavior" (News and Notes, 1932, p. 24).

At that time, Beers summarized the financial status of ICMH in terms which, in retrospect, are reminiscent of similar summaries regarding the financial status of WFMH. It depended, except for one Canadian gift, entirely on gifts and grants from United States individuals and foundations, the volunteer, nonsalaried status of its officers, and the fact that it received rent-free quarters from the U.S. National Committee for Mental Hygiene. Beers, again in the optimistic tones of WFMH officers succeeding him, declared that "now that the International Committee has entered upon its active work, and has interested representatives in so many countries, it is hoped that persons in countries other than those mentioned will begin to help finance its work."

This new ICMH sponsored, along with French organizations, a Second International Congress on Mental Hygiene in France, planned for 1935, but not realized until 1937. By then, voluntary movements in many countries were trying to mobilize public support to improve the quality of care for the mentally ill, particularly those confined to hospitals. However, World War II intervened and progress toward international affiliation was halted.

Meanwhile, one of the areas in which major organizational activity had been stimulated was the United Kingdom (England, Wales, and Scotland). Organizations formed in the United Kingdom to deal with mental illness and retardation, as well as child guidance, had been merged in 1939 to form the National Association for Mental Health. This NAMH was the precursor of MIND, the national mental health association of England and Wales. The new association was not permanently established until 1946, after the end of the Second World War.

Similar organizations were forming and dissolving in the United States, where the war and its aftermath ended what might be called the heroic phase of the United States mental health movement. What has been described as a turning point in the United States national mental health movement (Sareyan, 1993) occurred in consequence of a national decision to permit "conscientious objectors" to military duty during World War II to serve as aides in public mental hospitals rather than bear arms. These objectors developed a strong sense of moral obligation to change the harsh and antitherapeutic conditions they encountered, and they found willing allies in a number of well-known professionals and public officials. Among the conscientious objectors was Richard C. Hunter, later to become a senior staff member of the U.S. National Mental Health Association and, after his retirement, the volunteer Deputy Secretary General of WFMH. He helped form the National Mental Health Foundation, which, in 1950, merged with the older National Committee for Mental Health and another developing body, the American Psychiatric Foundation, to form what became the present-day U.S. National Mental Health Association. In his work with the WFMH, Hunter embodied the initial moral roots of the mental health movement. This was most striking in his later and frequent references to what he termed our joint work for "the cause."

The 1940s and 1950s were characterized by a cluster of changes that had great significance for the evolving post-World War II culture of the United States. They included the socioeconomic dislocations attendant on national mobilization, the new self-awareness of many minorities drafted into military service or working for the first time in the war-related industrial boom, and the 1946 passage of the National Mental Health Act. These and other changes—all after Clifford Beers' final illness and death—contributed to a new, more broadly based model of voluntary organizational development. The new organizations were less dependent upon the recruiting efforts of individual, charismatic personalities and more upon the continuing, characteristically inadequate, support of dues-paying members of national associations and their local chapters, united in support of an idealistic cause.

The ICMH, which had been inactive during the war years, was reactivated to help plan what was at first called the "International Conference on Mental Health and World Citizenship," scheduled for 16–21 August, 1948, under ICMH auspices. This reactivation, the individuals involved, and the nature of the planning process are essential to an understanding of the early roots of the World Federation for Mental Health.

Chapter 2

The Founding of the WFMH

RENEWING THE INTERNATIONAL MENTAL HEALTH MOVEMENT

The international mental health movement, dormant since the outbreak of war in Europe, began to stir once more with the return of peace. Interested and committed volunteers and professionals—members of national mental health and professional associations and academic specialists—were eager to resume their prewar contacts. Their first goal was to convene the Third International Congress on Mental Hygiene. This would reestablish the momentum begun with the First Congress in Washington, DC in 1930, which, because of rising international tension in Europe, was already faltering by the time of the Second Congress in Paris in 1937.

A related and more fundamental goal was to revive the organization responsible for the two earlier congresses. This was the International Committee for Mental Hygiene (ICMH) formed with great effort by Clifford Beers in 1919. It had emerged from the mental hospital reform movement described in Chapter 1. But the post-World War II activists who founded the World Federation for Mental Health (WFMH) were not primarily interested in traditional mental hospital reform. Mainly psychiatrists who had emerged from military service, their ideas were generated within the World War II therapeutic philosophy of prevention, rapid treatment of casualties near the traumatic setting, and rapid return to one's unit. To this the Canadians, following a 1939 decision to emphasize personnel selection for their armed forces (Ferguson, 1993), added concern with the initial personalities and capacities of the people who became soldiers. Thus, the dominant perspective was one of creating alternatives to, rather than reform of, the traditional mental hospital, a perspective that had an early effect on North American psychiatry culminating in the U.S. Community Mental Health Act of 1963. It also reflected the postwar preoccupation with avoiding repetition of the kind of devastating global conflict that had just ended. This required a revitalized international mental health movement that would do much more than sponsor occasional world meetings, with a mission reaching beyond that of local mental health associations to encompass the preservation of world peace, considered an aspect of preventive mental health.

In the autumn of 1941 the Canadian army created a Directorate of Personnel Selection. Its leaders were to become influential in the postwar mental health movement. The first director was psychiatrist George Brock Chisholm, M.D., and second in command was psychologist

William Line, Ph.D. Line "was humanistic in his outlook and wanted to move the quality of military life in a more humane direction" (Ferguson, 1993, p. 9). In time, both became presidents of the new WFMH, but their ideas had impact preceding their achieving official status. Later they were joined by psychiatrist Jack Griffin, M.D., who after the war became General Director of the Canadian Mental Health Association. He, too, was on the WFMH executive board, although for a short time.

The natural leader of the Canadian personnel selection group was Chisholm, "...a man of great courage and inner strength...whose goals extended beyond the army and into society at large.... [H]e believed that problems of health, both physical and psychological, were to some extent social problems, that medicine was in part a social science" (Ferguson, 1993, pp. 8–9). He was a friend of John Rawlings "Jack" Rees, M.D., formerly Brigadier General and distinguished Senior Consultant in Psychiatry to the British Army during World War II who was suggested by Britain's NAMH to become the Congress President and its prime organizer.

Chisholm, according to Rees, was "the person primarily responsible" for suggesting the formation of a new organization, to be called the World Federation for Mental Health, in 1946 (WFMH Annual Report, 1957, p. 11). By then he had retired as the senior psychiatrist for the Canadian armed forces and was the Interim Secretary for the United Nations' (UN) embryonic World Health Organization (WHO), whose constitution had been approved in 1946 and put into force on 7 April 1948. He later became the first Director General of the WHO.

Rees' first act on behalf of the Third Congress was to travel to New York to recruit the North American psychiatric leadership, which he considered essential to its success. It was there that Chisholm's suggestion for the new body, WFMH (of which he became President, 1957–1958), came during a small gathering of old friends just after Rees had obtained the ICMH's agreement to sponsor the projected Congress (see below). They were at the headquarters of the U.S. National Committee for Mental Hygiene, in New York, in the small office of George Stevenson, M.D., the Committee's Medical Director, who was president-elect of the American Psychiatric Association (and became WFMH President, 1961–1962). Those present, besides Rees, Chisholm, and Stevenson, were two members of the generation who had worked with Clifford Beers in his original organizing attempts. They were Clarence Hincks, M.D., of Canada who, with Beers, had founded the original ICMH in 1919 (see Chapter 1), and Arthur Ruggles, M.D., Superintendent of Butler Hospital in Providence, Rhode Island who, along with Beers and Hincks, had also been active in helping with the historic 1930 Washington, DC International Congress (see Chapter 1). That pregnant moment, 1946, in which Chisholm's conception of the WFMH was accepted by his four colleagues, was dominated by the emerging intergovernmental organization, the UN, for which he was developing the new WHO. Rees immediately saw the potential of a new nongovernmental organization (NGO). By the following year, 1947, it was translated into formal Articles of Association. Its definition of purpose was crucial: "To promote among all peoples and nations the highest possible level of mental health...in its broadest biological, medical, educational and social aspects." All of the other specified goals, such as cooperation with UN agencies, were intended to support this central purpose.

The WFMH philosophy was further elaborated two years later, in the last week of July and the first week of August 1948, by the London Congress' International Preparatory Commission (IPC). The document it prepared for the Congress, *Mental Health and World Citizenship*, was one to which Chisholm and his close friend and confidant, psychiatrist Harry Stack Sullivan, M.D., were prominent contributors (see below). Its guiding principles of reciprocal international communication, cooperation, and support, loyalty to the entire human family rather than to only one of its subdivisions, and the nonviolent resolution of intergroup conflict provided an intellectual and spiritual context for resurgent nongovernmental transnational affiliations and processes. Within this context the ICMH was transformed into a WFMH dedicated less to the traditional mental illness concerns of national mental health associations than to positive mental health, including the international goal of world peace.

The new nongovernmental organization, WFMH, as described below, was officially founded on 19 August 1948 during the Congress, announced by Rees at a plenary session on 20 August, and ratified by the official delegates during another plenary session on the following day, 21 August 1948.

THE POST-WORLD WAR II CONTEXT

The Search for World Peace Through the UN

The resumption of international communication in mental health, and the formation of a new voluntary, international, interdisciplinary, and ecumenical mental health association, grew from that uniquely post-World War II phenomenon, the UN, dedicated to preventing or peacefully resolving conflict between nations. It represented the first attempt at a global deliberative body since the ill-fated League of Nations. The name United Nations had been suggested by President Franklin D. Roosevelt during a meeting on 1 January 1942, when representatives of 26 nations fighting the Axis powers (Germany, Italy, and Japan) proclaimed their support for the Atlantic Charter. The document they produced was called, following Roosevelt's idea, The Declaration by United Nations. The first detailed blueprint for the UN as an organization was prepared during discussions at Dumbarton Oaks in Washington, DC beginning 9 October 1944, before the end of hostilities. Roosevelt died on 12 April 1945, having just drafted a Jefferson Day address for delivery the next day. The last words he wrote were, "The only limit to our realization of tomorrow will be our doubts of today. Let us move forward with strong and active faith" (Bethell, 1996, p. 87).

Approximately a fortnight after Roosevelt's death, on 25 April 1945, with the Pacific war still in progress, the delegates of 50 countries met in San Francisco for the UN Conference on International Organization. The French delegation's preference was apparently for an organization built around a revived and reorganized International Institute of Intellectual Cooperation, an organization founded in Paris in 1925 as the executive body of the International Commission for Intellectual Cooperation of the League of Nations. That did not come to pass. The Charter of the United Nations was adopted on 25 June 1945 (Lacoste, 1994).

The founders of the WFMH were sensitive to the work of these peace-oriented political leaders, especially Roosevelt. The first number of the newly founded WFMH Bulletin, issued in January-February 1949 under the editorship of psychology professor Dr. J. C. Flugel, who had been Programme Director of the London Congress, quoted President Roosevelt who, like the Federation founders, expressed confidence in a developing "science of human relationships." "Today," declared Roosevelt, "we are faced with the pre-eminent fact that if civilization is to survive we must cultivate the science of human relationships; the ability of peoples of all kinds to live together and work together in the same world at peace." The hoped-for "science" did not achieve the power predicted for it, yet the UN lived to celebrate its 50th birthday in the autumn of 1995, as we in the WFMH began to discuss our own 50th anniversary to take place in 1998.

Flugel, in that initial number of the WFMH Bulletin, also quoted a pregnant statement from the Preamble to the Constitution of the United Nations Educational, Scientific, and Cultural Organization (UNESCO): "Since wars begin in the minds of men it is in the minds of men that the defenses of peace must be constructed." This was attributed to one of the United States delegates both to Dumbarton Oaks and San Francisco, Archibald MacLeish, the U.S. Librarian of Congress (Lacoste, 1994).

Among the UN's formal acts with a direct bearing on the new Federation's future agenda, perhaps most significant was its Declaration of Human Rights. The United Nations Universal Declaration of Human Rights was proclaimed on 10 December 1948, four months after the founding of the WFMH. It referred to the rights of "all members of the human family" as the foundation of freedom, justice, and world peace. The concept of a "human family" was an important link between the intergovernmental UN and the emerging nongovernmental organizations. For mental health associations it represented a thematic continuity from the motivation for social reform espoused by Dorothea Dix, herself inspired by the liberal religion of Boston's William Ellery Channing, the intellectual father of Unitarianism. Channing's concept of the brotherhood of man virtually mandated social action as an expression of religious philosophy.

UNESCO, WHO, Chisholm, and Sullivan in the Preorganizational Context of the WFMH

Chisholm's vision of a new nongovernmental mental health organization acting to reduce international tensions and preserve world peace had its roots within the two still-embryonic agencies first associated with the UN. They were the WHO, which Chisholm himself was shaping, and UNESCO. The idea contained in the preamble to UNESCO's constitution, that wars begin in the minds of men, and that is where the defenses of peace must be constructed, could have been the inspiration for *"Mental Health and World Citizenship"* written by members of the IPC for the 1948 London Congress. If the primary function of the UN was to promote peace and security throughout the world, then UNESCO's task was "to promote the same ends in the fields of education, science and culture" (Besterman, 1951, p. 6). More than that, and relevant to WFMH's later concerns with prejudice and discrimination, the preamble stated that it is "suspicion and mistrust between the peoples of the world through which their differences have all too often broken into war" and that a common cause of that suspicion and mistrust has been "ignorance of each other's ways and lives." It attributed World War II to the "denial of the democratic principles of the dignity, equality and mutual respect of men, and by the propagation in their place, through ignorance and prejudice, of the doctrine of the inequality of men and races." These points led Besterman (1951, p. 7) to emphasize the preamble's "remarkable" and insufficiently noticed conclusion that any secure international peace must be founded "upon the intellectual and moral solidarity of mankind."

The individual within the developing UN structure who was most vocal, articulate, and committed to mental health in relation to peace was not in UNESCO, however. He was Brock Chisholm, WHO's first leader, chairman of its interim committee, and later its first Director General. His thinking may well have been influenced by conversations with his close friend and intellectual confidant, Sullivan, leader of the William Alanson White Foundation and the Washington School of Psychiatry. Sullivan was already known as an outstanding therapist of young male schizophrenic patients, perhaps because of his ability to empathize and identify with them, arguably a consequence of his poverty-stricken rural background and his early isolation from supportive parental figures (Perry, 1982). In addition, he may have been unique among American psychiatrists in his intense interest in the development of harmonious relationships between socially defined groups, including nations. Again, a possible sense of being a discriminated-against outsider may have contributed to this. At any event, he and Chisholm shared many views, and close scrutiny of their joint activities suggests that he may have been a more significant influence on Chisholm's thinking than vice versa.

Chisholm, with the political influence stemming from his status as the leader of a major UN agency, was crucial to the inclusion of inspirational elements associated with the search for world peace in the founding articles and bylaws of the new WFMH and in its founding theme.

Perry (1982, pp. 405–407), in her definitive biography of Sullivan, also recognized Chisholm's global perspective and his developmental story. Born and reared in a small town in Ontario, he enlisted at age 18 as a private in the Canadian forces during World War I, serving as an infantryman, receiving several medals for gallantry, and ending his service with the rank of captain. He did not enter medical school until the age of 28. After a brief practice of general medicine he spent two years, 1931 to 1933, on the psychiatry staff at Yale, spending much time with colleagues in its Institute of Human Relations, the site of some of my own formative intellectual experiences a generation later. In 1938, aware of the threat of Nazism to world peace, he rejoined the Canadian army. By 1941 he was in charge of personnel selection as director of its personnel services and was a deputy adjutant general. Although he and Sullivan had met at earlier psychiatry meetings, that was the point at which they became friends. Sullivan was then a consultant to the U.S. Selective Service. He and Chisholm shared a common interest in the problems of selecting a civilian army—which required knowledge and sensitivity regarding the psychology of young males—maintaining national morale, and especially "in the conviction that war did not have to be inevitable for each generation" and that "the general public would need new and better resources for mental health after the war" (Perry, 1982, p. 405). They were already in the process of generalizing their conclusions from the study of interpersonal conflicts to social pathology in general, and international tensions in particular.

Immediately after the United States' atomic bombing of Hiroshima in 1945 (a year before the decisions were made to begin organizational work on the Third International Congress, and a year before the idea of WFMH emerged) Sullivan, in his directorial capacity with the William Alanson White Foundation, invited Chisholm, then a major general, the Director of Medical Services for the Canadian army, and Deputy Minister of National Health of Canada's Federal Department of National Health and Welfare, to give two lectures, followed by distinguished commentators. One was delivered in Washington on 23 October 1945 and the other in New York City on 29 October 1945, just two months after the end of the war. They were published under the title *The Psychiatry of Enduring Peace and Social Progress*. In them Chisholm expressed his idealistic postwar concept of global mental health and the role of psychiatry in achieving it. His words were consonant with those of the UNESCO preamble, and anticipated some of the themes of the new WFMH to be formed three years later: "We are all now, perforce, citizens of the world.... Can we identify the reasons why we fight wars or even enough of them to perceive a pattern? Many of them are easy to list—prejudice, isolationism, the ability emotionally and uncritically to believe unreasonable things, excessive desire for material or power, excessive fear of others, belief in a destiny to control others, vengeance, ability to avoid seeing and facing unpleasant facts and taking appropriate action. These...are all well known and recognized neurotic symptoms...."

Chisholm felt that the world might live in peace if its inhabitants, especially psychiatrists and psychologists with the ability to influence others, could achieve "maturity." This would involve a balance of "dissatisfaction with the status quo, which calls forth aggressive, constructive effort; and...social concern and devotion." He concluded with a challenge to his fellow psychiatrists: "With the other human sciences psychiatry must now decide what is to be the immediate future of the human race. No one else can. And this is the prime responsibility of psychiatry" (Chisholm, 1946).

This was the period when the draft constitution of WHO (approved in 1946, put into force 7 April 1948) was being created. While Chisholm's philosophy inevitably imbued it, his exact contribution to its entire wording cannot be stated with certainty. However, its definition of health, which has remained unchanged for more than a half century, was perfectly congruent with the sentiments expressed repeatedly in his public utterances. It has been attributed to him by Ridenour (1961, p. 70). "Health," according to the WHO constitution, "is a state of complete physical, mental and social wellbeing and not merely the absence of disease or infirmity." It goes on to state that "informed opinion and active cooperation on the part of the public are of utmost importance in the improvement of the health of the people."

Chisholm's 1945 lectures and his 1946 statement, together with the WHO definition, constitute a call for worldwide positive mental health, conceived as well-being in the absence of the "neurotic" behavior that had made it impossible for humankind in all its diversity to survive in peace. He offered his own profession, that of psychiatry, as the group most logically equipped to approach that goal. This message, which elicited strong responses in those immediate post-war months, presaged his later views on the importance of mental health as a tool for reducing international tensions. He believed that it was possible to gain and use knowledge for the humane raising of children everywhere, and that peace and social progress would depend upon raising children to value and achieve these goals. He and Sullivan were already thinking in terms of "a psychiatry of peoples" (Sullivan, 1948; Perry, 1982).

What about the specific contribution of UNESCO? The exact origins of the idea attributed to it by Rees "that a body representing voluntary services in the mental health field was needed to cooperate with UN agencies" and that it should be "thoroughly interprofessional and completely international" (Rees, 1966, p. 76) are unclear. There is no record of a committed individual advocate in its ranks comparable to Chisholm at WHO. (Chisholm, in fact, as noted below, expressed a similar idea in 1947, referring to the new NGO as providing a much needed bridge between the nongovernmental and the intergovernmental worlds). UNESCO's first official recorded message to the 1948 London Congress came at its end after the founding of the new WFMH. It was delivered by its first Director General, Julian Huxley, Ph.D., a world famous biologist, and although his intellectual approval of the idea was important to its later elaboration, there is no evidence that he, personally, was deeply involved in its genesis and development.

Calvin I. Saxton (letter to the author, 18 November 1996) suggests that crediting UNESCO may have been Rees' retrospective way of giving this UN agency, which had been very supportive of the WFMH, some credit for the origins of the Federation. His statement, after all, was not written until 1965, in his fourth year after resigning as WFMH director. Aside from specific attribution, though, it seems probable that the impetus for *Mental Health and World Citizenship* was facilitated by UNESCO's constitution and its project on Tensions Affecting International Understanding (see Sullivan, 1950; Perry, 1982). As reviewed by Saxton (1995) the First General Conference of UNESCO, convened in November 1946 (after Rees' meeting with Chisholm, Stevenson, Hincks, and Ruggles), included among its roles that of promoting international, interdisciplinary intellectual exchange. It directed its secretariat to initiate an investigation of social tensions. Shortly thereafter it circulated a memorandum outlining the project aimed at reducing intergroup, especially international hostility and increasing goodwill through mutual understanding. The first project director was sociologist Hadley Cantril, Ph.D., an outstanding scholar in the field of prejudice, stereotyped thinking, and nonviolent conflict resolution. There is no record, however, of his having been active in the founding of the WFMH. The next director, Otto Klineberg (WFMH president 1966–1967), was an influential figure in the preparatory work for the London Congress and later in the Federation, where he was Chairman of the Executive Board, 1960–1961. The project's preliminary organizational phase was in 1947, after the 1946 organization of national preparatory commissions for the London Congress (see below); an unpublished UNESCO memorandum of 12 May 1947 is entitled *Preliminary Outline of Project on Tensions Affecting International Understanding*. The project's major meeting, on "Tensions That Cause Wars," took place in Paris in 1948 shortly before the Roffey Park meeting of the IPC for the London International Congress on Mental Hygiene.

According to Klineberg (in Stanton et al., 1951) it was Cantril who invited the eight social scientists "brought together by UNESCO to consider the causes of nationalistic aggression and the conditions necessary for international understanding" (Common Statement, UNESCO Conference, in Saxton, 1995). The other participants were Sullivan, Dr. Gordon Allport, Professor of Social Relations at Harvard, a world authority on problems of prejudice; Dr. Gilberto Freyre, Professor of Sociology at the University of Bahia in Brazil; Dr. Georges Gurevitch, Professor of Sociology at the Sorbonne in Paris; Dr. Max Horkeimer, Director of the Institute for Social Research in New York City; Dr. Arne Naess, Professor of Philosophy at the University of Oslo in Norway; John Rickman, M.D., Editor of the *British Journal of Medical Psychology* and a psychoanalyst who, like Sullivan, was notably world-minded; and Dr.

Alexander Szalai, Professor of Sociology at the University of Budapest and President of the Hungarian Institute of Foreign Affairs. Sullivan was listed as M.D., with his official positions as Chairman, Council of Fellows of the Washington School of Psychiatry, and Editor of *Psychiatry, Journal for the Operational Statement of Interpersonal Relations*. His editorship was especially important to him as it provided him a vehicle, especially in his unsigned editorials, for the expression of views more difficult to place in more conventional psychiatric journals.

Many of the ideas contained in the conclusions of this group were repeated or reflected in the WFMH founding document. Among them was the view, written by Sullivan himself (Saxton, 1995), that education must oppose national self-righteousness, and that attitudes and loyalties acquired during development are no longer adequate to serve as effective guides to action in a changing world. The group did not recommend creation of a mental health NGO, but it did recommend the cooperation of social scientists on broad regional, intercultural (although they did not use that term), and international levels, the creation of an international university, and a series of world institutes of the social sciences under international auspices. Sullivan also attended a second UNESCO conference, "Educating Children for World Mindedness," held later in the summer in Podelbrady, Czechoslovakia, then behind the "iron curtain."

By 1947, as the work of the varied preparatory commissions for the Congress was well under way, Chisholm's international influence was further enhanced as he became Executive Secretary of the Interim Commission of the WHO, en route to becoming its Director General. He moved from inspiration to organization, promoting the idea of a new international, nongovernmental body to cooperate with UN agencies on matters related to mental (broadly interpretable as social) health. More concisely, he articulated the view that the new organization was needed as a bridge between the United Nations and the "grass roots." This new bridging entity would be launched at the Third International Congress of Mental Hygiene in 1948. Elaborating on this theme at the 1947 annual meeting of the American Psychiatric Association he stated that the London Congress could well be critical in the affairs of the world. Not surprisingly, a number of colleagues in psychiatry criticized him for his involvement in matters far beyond the domain of conventional clinical psychiatry. With limited responses from both WHO and the American Psychiatric Association, Sullivan, who still nourished dreams of an international network of psychiatrists and social scientists to advise the WHO in confronting the problems of an increasingly dangerous world, devoted increasing energy to promoting the London Congress (Sullivan, 1947). But, there was little enthusiasm for social science or mental health among physicians and health planners, and few representatives of these disciplines at the new WHO's first World Health Assembly attended by Sullivan, who shared Chisholm's disappointment (Sullivan, 1948).

In the following year, on 26 April 1948, shortly before the London Congress, Chisholm introduced another seminal concept to the ICMH governing board (now designated "Interim") at the Hotel Beekman in New York (MinBd). There he spoke directly of "world loyalty." (Although this was a theme articulated by Sullivan at the UNESCO Tensions Conference, there was no reference to that possible source or overlap.) Chisholm made this concrete for the interdisciplinary IPC process, which was approaching its last phase. In his words, these "...groups which never before came together are getting to know each other and learning to compromise in their definitions and use of language. Inevitably they will become more tolerant and more capable of living together in peace. If this Congress succeeds it will be one of the great historical occasions of the world. Its work will go on forever. It *must* work because many large groups of informed people are determined to make it work.... Until recently we did not think it mattered if millions of people throughout the world did not get beyond a provincial loyalty. Now it is imperative that no loyalty stop short of world loyalty.... [A]n amazing spirit has permeated this Congress organization from the outset. Almost nothing else could have commanded such a self-sacrificing attitude." Thus, the seeds of Federation and of its founding document were sown.

It has not been widely appreciated that Sullivan's suggestion led to the formation of the IPC, which produced *Mental Health and World Citizenship* (MM/LC; Perry, 1982; Saxton, 1995). Fresh from the first 1948 UNESCO conference, he was a prime mover in developing the ideas embodied in that founding document of the WFMH.

In 1949, Chisholm, now Director General of the WHO, wrote of the new Federation's social responsibility (Chisholm, 1949): "Only in the last few years has it become clear to the people in all countries who are capable of thinking independently of the hysteria of the media of mass communication that this old method of [military and commercial] competitive survival has become synonymous with racial suicide" (p. 27). He cited ICMH as having been a "most encouraging sign of this awakening concern...about the immediacy and importance of world problems of human relations and interhuman communication...There is now only one basic importance in the world, the one importance upon which the very existence of the race depends—the emotional relationship between the people of the world" (p. 30).

ORGANIZING THE INTERNATIONAL CONGRESS AND WFMH

Toward a Third International Congress on Mental Hygiene

With the United Nations blueprint for international political collaboration in place, professional and voluntary mental health organizations, university professors of psychiatry, and others accelerated their efforts toward building international scientific and professional bridges and developing world standards of care for the mentally ill. The concerns with the origins, prevention, and treatment of mental illness or emotional distress, given form at the 1930 Washington DC Congress, re-emerged in new guises. The anticipation and construction of a new, international, voluntary and all-embracing mental health association—including the new opportunities for international leadership it offered—have been described in retrospect with various emphases by different participants. In the immediate postwar autumn of 1945 many voices were being heard. After much meeting and discussion a number of mainly European-based international organizations, some brought together in the European League for Mental Health (ELMH), took the initiative. They asked NAMH, the National Association for Mental Health of England and Wales, later called MIND, to organize an international mental health congress. ELMH formally asked John Rees to do so, obtaining his consent to become the Congress' prime organizer and its president.

Volunteer leader Lady Priscilla Norman, who later became an honorary president of WFMH, perceived a particular opportunity: "Those of us who...had worked for the amalgamation of the voluntary mental health associations before the war, became aware after the war of the growing mental health problems of the world" (Norman, 1982, p. 151). Her close friend Robina Addis, one of the world's first psychiatric social workers, after attending the 1945 meeting of the Society for the Study of Child Victims of the War convinced her that the newly formed NAMH "should set its sights on the international field as well as the national." Addis persisted in her interests and was one of the half-dozen representatives from the United Kingdom who participated in the foundation meetings of WFMH on 18 and 19 August 1948 during the International Congress of Mental Hygiene. Norman adopted her perspective. "Here was a real chance for us [she wrote] to influence governments in war-weary Europe," as well as elsewhere, "in a great drive to make known to the governments of the world the unhappy state of the mentally sick and the mentally handicapped, as well as the needs of displaced persons, evacuees, refugees and returning P.O.W.s" (Norman, 1982, pp. 151–152).

More than that, postwar health and welfare workers, along with politicians, became imbued with the sense of participating in a moral cause insofar as their work required undoing the wrongs committed by the Nazi aggressors, recompensing their victims, and reconciling disparate peoples and viewpoints. I can remember such feelings in myself when, from the autumn of 1946 and throughout 1947, I was the only military psychiatrist working with German prisoners at the International Military Tribunal in Nuremberg. My tasks were narrowly psychiatry-oriented, dealing, for example, with those who claimed memory loss, or who appeared too depressed to testify. But the destruction of human lives in which they had participated, and the intuitive sense that what had happened in Germany could take place elsewhere, inevitably stimulated reflection on the nature of justice, and of right and wrong in terms of allegiance to a state versus to humanity. Even then, it was not clear that justice as defined by the victors in war provided the most rational and effective way of dealing with the losers, who had been the aggressors.

At the same time the theme of world peace continued as a major concern for the theoreticians, clinicians, and academicians who were interested in the forthcoming Congress, but did not have mental health association backgrounds. The initial Congress announcement, produced in June 1947 by Rees' developing staff, bracketed "human relations" with "mental health" as solutions to the vast postwar social problems: "In the present postwar period all of us are conscious of the aftermath of those very disturbed years [1939–1945]. Events seem at times to present a menace rather than a promise of peace.… [R]esocialization and reconstruction are urgent, and this is largely a problem in which human relations and considerations of mental health are predominant." Sullivan, influenced by his membership in the ICMH governing body, wrote in the August 1947 number of *Psychiatry*, which he edited, that psychiatry can aid the effort to ensure "enduring peace and social progress."

John Rawlings "Jack" Rees, Organizer for Mental Health

Rees, like many of the founders of the WFMH, had served as a medical officer in the military forces of his country, part of the victorious coalition that defeated the Axis powers. They conceived of improving "mental health" in terms of values much more encompassing than meeting conventional standards of psychiatric care. For them psychiatry was not viewed merely as a branch of medicine, a form of clinical practice, but as a "human science" with the potential of solving the problems leading to armed international conflict.

"J.R." or "Jack" Rees, as he was widely known, was a child of the turn of the century, born in 1889. He completed his medical training in 1920 as World War I was drawing to a close, and at the end of World War II became the primary figure in establishing the Federation and shepherding it through its first years. The affairs of the Federation occupied him through its preorganizational formative period from 1946 to its actual founding in 1948, and during his presidency and directorship from 1948 through 1961. After that he remained active, especially in the Caribbean (see Chapter 9) until illness forced his retirement from active work prior to his death on 11 April 1969. Perhaps his last official communication was a note in the Summer 1968 number of the *WFMH Bulletin* regarding the organization's 20th anniversary. In it he wrote that, since 1948: "The Federation has grown from 21 to 165 member associations in 63 countries…at present we are vividly reminded by the upsets and tensions of the world of the need for better mental health. We probably know it in ourselves also."

Key elements of Rees' professional career were outlined in an obituary in the *British Medical Journal* by H. V. Dicks, M.D., who had been one of the founders of the WFMH. After demobilization from military service in World War I in 1919, and working briefly on a private psychiatric service, he helped found, in 1920, what was then known as the Tavistock Square Clinic for Functional Nervous Disorders. It was intended as a new model for treating neuroses and behavior disorders in adults and children. As its deputy medical director he spent much time dealing with its precarious financing, fostering the new idea of a doctor-psychologist-social worker team, and in general building it into a British institution. In 1933 he became its medical director as its name was shortened to, simply, Tavistock Clinic. By 1939 he was planning to develop it into an Institute of Medical Psychology, but another war was consuming Europe and military service again interrupted his civilian life. A number of sources confirm that during World War

II, with a relatively small number of psychiatrists, he instituted successful plans incorporating group methods for dealing with heavy casualties in the armed forces. One of his most valued assistants was Ronald Hargreaves, M.D., later to become the first mental health advisor for WHO. After the war he was faced with the return of vast numbers of prisoners of war and the rehabilitation of former service people. Lawrence Kubie, M.D., a senior figure in American psychoanalysis (Brody, 1978) who had played a key role in bringing European psychoanalyst refugees fleeing Hitler to the United States, supplied an obituary for the Summer 1969 number of the *WFMH Bulletin* (thereafter discontinued to re-emerge as the *Newsletter*). There, he credited Rees with having achieved "remarkable results," due in part to his "exceptional personal qualities." These stemmed, in Kubie's opinion, from his family's religious tradition which allowed him to accept, without conflict, a self-image as a missionary. He also described him as having played a decisive role in developing psychiatric and psychoanalytic interest in both prolonged individual psychotherapy and in social and cultural issues. At Tavistock he was a leader in group work, with special reference to what he and others called "human relations." In Kubie's words, "his entire life was consecrated to research in peace…it was no accident that his missionary zeal in ordinary civil life informed his medical and psychiatric work, or that in the postwar years he struggled for the world peace without which humanity could not survive." His wife, Mary Heminway Rees, M.D., had a particular interest in spiritual factors in relation to mental health, which reinforced Rees' own investment. Her interests persist in a Mary Heminway Rees Memorial Lecture on spiritual factors in mental health, which is presented at each World Congress for Mental Health.

After the war Rees was instrumental in creating the new Tavistock Institute of Human Relations. However, he resigned in 1947 in order to devote his energies to the forthcoming 1948 International Congress on Mental Hygiene. His particular background made it natural for him not only to accept the task of organizing a Congress on mental hygiene, but also to accept the leadership of a new international voluntary association with idealistic goals. His appointment was determined in part by his reputation for having an international perspective and a grasp of individual and cultural differences. He also had a proven record as an organizer, teacher, and clinician. Perhaps most important was the fact that, as Chisholm put it in the 1966 volume *Reflections*, issued on the occasion of Rees' retirement, he was perceived "as a rebel, an innovator, a heretic," highly disturbing to those who believed that psychiatry should "concern itself only with the treatment of insane patients by the orthodox methods of the mental hospitals" (Chisholm, 1966).

Rees was, in a general sense, sympathetic to the perspectives expressed earlier by Sullivan and Chisholm although, despite Chisholm's description, he was a more conventional figure and known at least as well as an organizer as an inspirational thinker. Perhaps these contributed to his being given the Mary Lasker and Adolph Meyer Awards, and the most honorific, that of Commander of the British Empire, but his special character was his ability to combine organizational and leadership skills, with those of a visionary. The concept of human relations as a general discipline encompassing not only psychology and the social sciences, but clinical psychiatry, gained international credence significantly because of the Tavistock influence, in which he was a major figure. This influence reached across the ocean to New Haven, Connecticut (not far from the place where Clifford Beers had been hospitalized) to touch me when I was learning psychiatry in the early post-World War II era. The wards and clinics as well as the offices of the Yale University Department of Psychiatry where, after leaving Harvard Medical School, I became a house officer in 1944 were housed, along with psychology, child development, and several social science groups, in the Institute of Human Relations where Chisholm had spent two years. When I returned from Germany to become Chief Resident in Psychiatry in January 1948, Kubie, who commuted from his office in Manhattan, was my first supervisor in psychotherapy. In 1961, when he retired to become Psychiatrist-in-Chief at the Sheppard Pratt Hospital in Baltimore, it was my privilege to appoint him as a clinical professor in the Institute of Psychiatry and Human Behavior, which I then headed at the University of Maryland. It was at his home, just a few years later, that I met Jack Rees again. He was suffering from memory loss, with his pockets stuffed with reminder notes, but was cheerful and seemingly indomitable. This proved to be his last visit to the United States, and one of his last trips away from England before his death.

REACTIVATING ICMH

Rees Goes to New York

Although the official Congress instigator was the ELMH, and its local sponsor was the NAMH of England and Wales, Rees' first move upon accepting the organizing assignment in 1946 was to consult with the ICMH, headquartered in New York. The ICMH had been the parent body for the 1930 and 1937 World Congresses, and although it had been relatively inactive since then, was alive and sensitive to the new postwar possibilities. Initially, its ability to assume responsibility for a Third International Congress was in doubt because of an earlier commitment to a congress in Rio de Janeiro. However, that activity was subsequently canceled. Led by Frank Fremont-Smith, M.D., then president of the Josiah Macy, Jr. Foundation, which was dedicated to health promotion (Dr. Fremont-Smith later became WFMH president, 1954–1955) the ICMH was now able to promise Rees its full support, and it agreed to become the official sponsoring body of the Congress.

After gaining ICMH approval Rees moved to recruit leaders in psychiatry in the United States to work with him. As noted above, he met with a small group of interested colleagues in the New York office of Dr. George Stevenson. It was there that Brock Chisholm initially suggested the formation of a new organization to succeed the ICMH. Chisholm, by now, was executive secretary of the newly formed Interim Commission for the WHO, and well-launched on the work that caused him to be described by some as quite literally the "creator" of the WHO (Ridenour, 1961, p. 70).

The ICMH Reorganized

The Committee, which had never dissolved, but lay dormant during the years after the Paris World Congress of 1937, gradually awakened after Rees' 1946 visit. By 12 May 1947 a new governing board was in place, sufficiently confident to pass a resolution to change its name to the WFMH. Rees, looking to its future as the WFMH, had been persuaded to become ICMH president, replacing Fremont-Smith, who became its United States vice-president. The honorary president was Professor of Psychiatry Adolph Meyer of Johns Hopkins University, who had resigned after the 1930 World Congress, which he had characterized as "terrible," promising much too much in the name of mental health with insufficient evidence. The other vice-presidents were Jean L'Ermitte, M.D., of France, August Ley, M.D., of Belgium, Eugenio Medea, M.D., of Italy, Jonathan C. Meakins, M.D., of Canada, and Henrique Roxo, M.D., of Brazil. These were all academic or institutional psychiatrists. Of the 33 additional members of the governing board, all were physicians except for four with Ph.D. degrees, one with a doctorate in education, and one with a law degree. H. Edmond Bullis, its secretary general, was a former military colonel with a civilian background as a U.S. state mental health association executive.

A 12 May 1947 letter from Bullis to United States anthropologist Margaret Mead, one of the four with Ph.D. degrees who had been elected to the governing board (sometimes called the Interim Governing Board) (MM/LC) notes: "The reason for the great predominance of United States members on the Governing Board is that they have been elected to serve until the International Conference on Mental Hygiene…at which time delegates from various mental health societies and leagues from all over the world will elect a new Governing Board truly representative of the world…Federal departments of various governments will be invited to designate official observers to attend all meetings."

Bullis also described the reactivated ICMH's task. This was to help with the planning of the Third Conference of the forthcoming Congress now definitely scheduled for 16-21 August 1948 in London. It was now called the International Conference on Mental Health and World Citizenship and was to be held "under the auspices of ICMH." As he put it, the ICMH aim was "to outline proposed action on mental health problems for consideration at the 1948 Conference. The resultant recommendations on mental health matters will be then formally presented to the World Health Organization. It is expected that the ICMH will be the only mental health organization accredited to the World Health Organization. No national group or individual can present recommendations directly to WHO…[which] gives such prominence to mental health and to the psychological tasks involved in *preparing the way for individuals to become citizens of the world* [italics mine].… [I]t is important that activities be started at once so as to propose practical methods of action to the World Health Organization."

The new ICMH held its initial planning meeting at the Hotel Beekman in New York on 19 May 1947 (MinBd). It was attended by invited representatives of 52 agencies and institutions, all wanting to have their opinions known. They came from U.S. Government agencies, private groups, universities, and associations—most from the United States, but some from Europe—representing anthropology, medicine, psychiatry, social work, and psychoanalysis, as well as the WHO. The confused and lengthy discussions made it clear that a smaller, possibly more homogeneous group with more time was necessary to progress with planning. After this most meetings were confined to the governing board. Nonetheless, emerging differences of viewpoint, often engendered by the human rights violations of the war just past, sometimes led to emotionally charged discussions. In a 25 June 1947 letter to Fremont-Smith, Mead (MM/LC) referred to a 28 May 1947 meeting of the group as "bumpy" due to "the ghost of old Nuremberg quarrels" which were "putting the edge into people's voices."

The Justification for the Congress and the WFMH

Despite the careful preparations and general enthusiasm, minutes of ICMH governing board meetings suggest occasional uncertainties about the justification for and intentions of the forthcoming international conference. The minutes of a 17 September 1947 meeting at the Hotel Beekman in New York record that George Stevenson questioned "the springs" of the Congress, wondering if "the people of Europe" felt a "real need for it." Later, he expressed the view that "the London Congress is merely a warming-up for the more important job to be done later." This apparently followed Rees' perspective on the Congress and its hoped-for sequelae in the work of the WFMH, the now-agreed-upon successor of the ICMH. Acknowledging that the first and second international congresses, of 1930 and 1937, had produced international exchange and stimulation, Rees believed that, in order to go beyond this level, a permanent organization capable of constructive action was needed. This should be "a continuously functioning agency to promote world mental health whenever and by whatever means, including congresses, that conditions dictated…an agency that could sense problems, sense the timing of efforts at solutions, sense the persons or other agencies that should be activated as partners or as primary functionaries, and that could turn these sensings into programming and the carrying out of action" (Stevenson, 1966).

The ICMH Board agreed that this vision represented a new type of organization, bringing the world's mental health associations together into an effective force. As resolved at its 12 May 1947 meeting, it was to be transformed into the World Federation for Mental Health, WFMH (MinBd). At the 19 May 1947 Board meeting, only a week later, it was expected that rapid moves would be made to incorporate the new organization. However, Rees reported, after meeting with representatives of several mental hygiene groups in Europe, that they felt that the Board "was moving too fast and that they should have been consulted even though the incorporation of the Federation was only an enabling act with final organization on a democratic basis to be effected later." In consequence the Board rescinded the 12 May 1947 resolution to change the ICMH name to WFMH. An indication of the sensitivity of the Europeans was Fremont-Smith's feeling that he should apologize for prematurely announcing the incorporation of WFMH in the July issue of *Mental Hygiene*, the journal of the U.S. National Committee for Mental Hygiene. In deference to these apparent sensitivities a letter went to "all known mental hygiene societies to see how they feel about the plan for a Federation" (MinBd). But this did not end the matter, which Fremont-Smith saw as complicated by the inclusion in the proposed International Congress of special conferences on child psychiatry and on "medical psychotherapy" to be added to that already planned on mental hygiene, still expected to be the core of the Congress. Evidently this was done by the British without adequate consultation with other participants. As Fremont-Smith put it (MinBd): "One of the chief problems has been the difficulty of being sure on this side of the Atlantic just what the London group wanted and of keeping [them] accurately informed of what is being done here." The anticipated activities in London struck him as "a sort of three ring circus." Although travel by ship was a time-consuming affair he was sufficiently concerned to go to London from 8–25 October 1947 hoping "to resolve all misunderstanding and confusion" (MinBd).

At the October 1947 Board meeting a formal proposal to change the ICMH name was once more put forward. As reported in Bulletin Number 1 of the International Congress on Mental Hygiene in December 1947: A "World Federation for Mental Health" to be incorporated "within the next few months" was proposed as the replacement for the ICMH. It was expected that a permanent constitution and bylaws would be adopted by the new WFMH during the Congress, and that a board would be organized "consisting of democratically elected delegates from many countries. The new WFMH will then apply to UNESCO and the WHO of the UN for recognition as *the* [italics mine] official, international, voluntary organization in the field of mental health."

Announcing the Congress and its Tripartite Composition

As noted above, the proposed Third International Congress of Mental Hygiene, scheduled for London in 1948, was to include three conferences. These were announced in a 10 February 1948 press release to professional journals. The first, as described in the press release, was to be on child psychiatry, with a theme of "personality development in its individual and social aspects with special reference to aggression." The second was on medical psychotherapy with the central theme of "guilt." These two were planned to run concurrently from 11 to 14 August. The third and major meeting was on mental hygiene with the theme of "Mental Health and World Citizenship." This last, to run from 16-21 August, was described as "by far the largest and most important of the three" (Flugel et al., 1948d, p. iii).

The announcement suggested that the Congress, encompassing all three Conferences, would have a restricted audience with preference given to social scientists and scientifically trained clinicians. That is, it would be "open to trained workers in mental health and related subjects and to members of recognized organizations connected with such work." It also stated that "one, if not the chief, aim of the Congress is to facilitate the interchange of scientific knowledge and experience acquired in the social field during the war years."

It was planned that mornings would be devoted to plenary sessions and afternoons to small discussion groups. This led to further concern, expressed in the 10 February 1948 announcement, about the discussion process: the aim of exchanging scientific knowledge and experience "cannot be even remotely achieved in a crowded conference if a hundred interests are allowed to compete for the time and attention of 2000 members. This has led to the setting up of preparatory discussion groups…with the purpose of thinking beforehand about a number of topics chosen by agreement…. The Congress presents a great opportunity for the attainment of a larger collective wisdom through the pooling of information and escape from the limitations of a too-narrow national or professional point of view."

Despite these announcements, the projected gathering was perceived, both in its anticipation and in its realization, as more generally inclusive. "The Congress as a whole" (encompassing all three conferences) was seen by volunteer leaders as being "for all the organizations, associations and individuals who were willing to discuss the ways and means of improving the services for the mental health of the world" (Norman, 1982, p. 153).

THE PREPARATORY COMMISSIONS OR NATIONAL DISCUSSION GROUPS

Initial Ideas

Once ICMH and United States backing were assured, the actual work of organizing the Congress began. The preparations are described, with little reference to the intense interaction characterizing them, in Rees (1966); volume I of the proceedings dealing with the history and preparations for the Congress (Flugel et al., 1948b); and volume IV, concerned specifically with the ICMH (Flugel et al., 1948d). Flugel, a former Assistant Professor of Psychology at University College, London, and, as noted above, Chairman of the Programme Committee, was an active Congress participant, and personally familiar with its internal processes. Aware of existing doubts about the feasibility of the enterprise among potential participants, he addressed them in the third number of the "Preparatory Commissions' Bulletin" in October 1947: "Some individuals...are rather alarmed at the magnitude of the task...subjects such as World Citizenship and The Individual and Society seem to them pretentious.... [O]n the whole, however, the direction of the Congress towards social rather than purely individual issues has aroused great interest.... [W]orld Citizenship is, in fact, an immediate practical issue." The central place of the new UN in the thinking of the Congress planners was revealed in Flugel's hope that the Congress would "become a means by which WHO will inform itself about the authoritative facts and opinions relevant to mental health."

The crucial innovation that suffused and influenced all preparations stemmed from Rees' background in group work and the Tavistock human relations philosophy. Presaging the original concept of how WFMH might operate, he had what Margaret Mead described as "the imaginative idea of getting people from all over the world to identify problems" (Flugel, 1948b, p. 300). In practical terms this meant at least three people from different professions coming together to talk and prepare a report about what they thought were the world's leading mental health problems. They were designated, somewhat grandiloquently, as "national discussion groups" or "preparatory commissions." Rees' call resulted in 351 groups in 21 different countries. The ICMH, as reported by its executive officer, psychologist Nina Ridenour, Ph.D., was involved in the "mobilization of the several thousand" participants whose findings were later reported to the Congress (Ridenour, 1961, p. 68). Approximately 4100 men and women from 28 disciplines came together in small groups "of members of the different professions concerned with the study of human behavior [who] were to give careful thought to the themes of the Congress, to try and thrash out the points of agreement and disagreement, and to indicate the areas needing immediate research" (Flugel et al., 1948b). Flugel hoped that through their pooled knowledge and experience the groups would achieve "some understanding of the problems of sick societies." In his opening remarks to the Mental Health Conference he described the work of the Preparatory Commissions as "of import to everyone who is concerned with the better ordering of human life in every corner of the world" and of the "vast brotherhood of fellow workers" they brought together (Flugel et al., 1948d, p. 49). Their reports were to be presented to a summarizing group (later developed as the IPC) which would assimilate them for presentation in five keynote speeches to the Congress proper.

How to Organize a Commission and ICMH Debates about Their Topics

In the October 1947 number of the Preparatory Commissions' Bulletin, Flugel gave directions about how to form a Commission or study group. It should "consist of small numbers of individuals belonging to different professions or scientific disciplines which have bearing upon mental health. It has been agreed that this Congress shall be a forum of *combined* knowledge and wisdom." Groups were advised to begin by discussing the definition of a healthy or "good" society, starting with the family environment. However, it was not easy to persuade people to form groups. A 22 December 1947 minute, for example, records the difficulties in recruiting members of the American Society of Applied Anthropology to form some commissions.

The flavor of United States discussions regarding proposed preparatory commission themes is reflected in the minutes of various ICMH governing board meetings (MinBd). The informality and directness of the discussions were facilitated by the fact that many of the American psychiatrists on the board were also members of the newly formed Group for Advancement of Psychiatry (GAP), organized by former Brigadier General William Menninger, who had been the senior U.S. military officer concerned with psychiatric casualties and their prevention. These men, all professionals, had many opportunities to discuss Congress-related mental health issues outside of formal meetings. Their concerns switched back and forth between the desirability of emphasizing individual mental health issues on one hand and group and cultural processes on the other. The ICMH, affected by the war, was more concerned with social processes and peace than with psychiatric patients or hospital care. At the 17 September 1947 meeting Mead made a number of thematic suggestions for the work of the preparatory commissions. These included analyses of mental health problems according to age periods in the life cycle; socioeconomic and political situations, including housing, unemployment, and institutional practices; the "problems of alcoholism, delinquency, prostitution, homosexuality, addiction, illegitimacy and adoption"; and "the lunatic fringe in its manifestations in political and religious cults" (MM/LC).

As the year wore on other issues surfaced and were debated. In Preparatory Commission Bulletin No. 2 on 1 August 1947 editor Flugel was concerned with "values." This was in response to a letter from Professor Henry Murray, M.D., of Harvard to Jack Rees—which Rees then passed on to him. Murray believed that the Congress needed "an orienting principle on the top level...a positive conception of health in terms of energy, development and happiness...not merely freedom from symptoms" to be discussed in terms of its determinants for society and for the individual. He called for "one great session" to be devoted to "an overall ideology." This worried Flugel, who asserted that he too was concerned with "the general relation of mental health to values...in the sense of aims worth achieving, activities worth pursuing, problems worth solving, or beliefs worth holding." However, unlike Murray, he felt that "there must be imposed some limitation of our attitude with regard to the more ultimate moral values. The sphere of mental health...is yet not co-terminous with that of religion, moral philosophy, or economics." And he concluded that "it is here that Dr. Murray's demand for *positive* values raises an issue where it behooves us to tread warily...[because], given health and freedom, human beings will soon discover ends that seem to them worthwhile."

Ridenour was prominent among those suggesting that the Congress include a "practical focus" on children displaced by war. Mead, who agreed with her, told of reporting some data on war-damaged children to the executive committee of UNESCO, which responded hostilely, especially since some of the children were described in "mildly psychoanalytic terms." They were interested, she said, only in discussing "nationalism and internationalism."

Fremont-Smith declared that "psychiatry is not going to save the world." Instead, "what we need most desperately today is understanding and regulation of group relations. This is the function of the social sciences [but] they do not know how to do it. They do not know much about individual motivation...." Then he reverted to dependence upon his parent disciplines of medicine and psychiatry: "Dynamic psychiatry is the enzymatic agent by which we can coordinate the thinking of social sciences as a whole to make the basis of the science of human relations…. Out of [the preparatory commissions] can come studies of group motivation that will lead to management of group action." At the same time he spoke of the danger that its governing body "believes that ICMH and the Congress will change the world…. [E]veryone here is aware of the near impossibility of doing anything significant in time to prevent world disaster. However, this kind of effort seems to be the only hope there is."

Menninger felt that the proposals, insofar as they depended on the wisdom of psychiatrists, were "thin soup." It is premature, he suggested, to think that 10 psychiatrists could agree on five principles, for example, to instruct mothers of disturbed children. He was more optimistic about other disciplines. A possible solution would be to include laymen, economists, writers, and so forth in the international conference's discussion groups: "They may have more to contribute than psychiatrists" (MinBd).

The Central Preparatory Commissions

Five central preparatory commissions, all convened by British scholars, were also organized in London in order to provide leadership for the national commissions in every part of the world. Their themes, to be carried forward by the Congress, also set forth the philosophy expected to guide the new World Federation for Mental Health.

The first theme, anticipating the Federation's future founding document, was "World Citizenship and Good Group Relations," convened by psychoanalyst Edward Glover, M.D., Director of the Institute for the Scientific Treatment of Delinquency in London. Glover, uniquely open-minded among the United Kingdom psychoanalysts of his time, had been the analyst in 1928 for Lawrence S. Kubie, M.D. (Glover, 1969). He was one of the speakers at the mental hygiene conference.

Second, reflecting a concern shared by clinicians and psychosocial scientists, was "The Individual and Society," convened by social psychologist John Cohen, Ph.D., then a lecturer in psychology at the University of Leeds; he later served as technical secretary for the synthesizing International Preparatory Commission meeting at Roffey Park.

Third, reflecting the founders' interest both in development and in the context of behavior, was "Family Problems and Psychological Disturbances," convened by psychiatric social worker S. Clement Brown, M.A., a former tutor in mental health at the London School of Economics and Political Science who was Programme Secretary for the International Congress.

The importance the organizers granted to context, and especially to the workplace, was embodied in the fourth commission, "Mental Health in Industry and Industrial Relations," convened by J. D. Sutherland, M.D., of the Royal Edinburgh Hospital and a member of Morris Carstairs' faculty of psychiatry.

John Bowlby, M.D., then director of Tavistock's child guidance clinic, later to become the leading world authority on attachment behavior during development, convened the fifth commission on "Planning for Mental Health: Organization, Training, Propaganda."

Two central commissions were also set up in New York to coordinate the work of the American commissions. The first, again emphasizing the major concerns of the organizers in this postwar period, was on "Mental Health and World Citizenship," chaired by Lyman Bryson with Lawrence K. Frank as executive secretary. Frank, who had no graduate degree, but was an ardent and widely respected advocate for children and mental health, was director of the Caroline Zachry Institute of Human Development in New York City. He was described by Margaret Mead, supporting his nomination for the 1947 Lasker Award "for outstanding service in mental hygiene," as having had "the imagination and foresight 24 years ago to give an essential impetus to the whole field of child development and parent and family education" (MM/LC). This award had been given to William Menninger in 1944 for contributions to the mental health of people in the U.S. armed services, in 1945 to John Rees, and in 1946 to Brock

Chisholm. Frank was to chair the 14 day meeting of the IPC in Roffey Park in July and August 1948, with just a week intervening before the International Congress.

The other New York commission was on "The Effect of War on Children in the United States." It was chaired by psychoanalyst and research scientist David Levy, M.D., of Columbia University, who had done developmental research with particular reference to the impact of deprivation on sucking and other oral behaviors in both animals and humans. Its executive secretary was psychologist and social worker Helen Speyer, M.A.

In addition to Great Britain and the United States, preparatory commissions were formed in Belgium, Canada, Czechoslovakia, Finland, France, Greece, Holland, Ireland, Italy, Palestine (this was immediately before the birth of Israel), Portugal, Puerto Rico, South Africa, South America (countries not specified), Sweden, Switzerland, Turkey, and the West Indies (countries not specified). The North American and northern European contributions were clearly predominant. All commissions were asked to send their reports to the Congress office and many were published in a bulletin issued approximately monthly during 1947 and early 1948. The final reports were called for 31 March 1948. They were summarized and edited by a large team of volunteer specialists, and made available to the IPC (see below).

THE INTERNATIONAL PREPARATORY COMMISSION

Formation and Mission

The central group of planners, designated as the International Preparatory Commission (IPC) in residence, met for 14 days prior to the Congress from 24 July to 8 August 1948 to consider and amalgamate the reports of the national preparatory commissions. This Commission was the incubator from which the core themes of the Congress submitted by the planners and the commissions were to be extracted, and in which the anticipated new Federation's founding statement was to be generated. The formation of IPC, with its crucial tasks, is generally acknowledged to be the consequence of a suggestion by Sullivan (MM/LC). Brock Chisholm confirmed this, specifically crediting "the whole idea of the International Preparatory Commission to Sullivan" (Chisholm, 1948, p. 543).

The assignment to the IPC by the Congress program committee headed by Flugel was to produce a document intended to guide not only the discussions of the mental health conference (the Congress' third meeting), but the work of the projected World Federation for Mental Health as well. The site selected for this group by the program committee was a rural rehabilitation center in Roffey Park near Horsham, Sussex, outside of London. A 22 June 1948 letter from Flugel to the participants (MM/LC) described the setting. The main building was a rehabilitation center for "mild psychiatric cases from industry," but the group would be living and working in a building used for postgraduate training. It was "a pleasant, comfortable house with modern furniture...lakes for swimming...and tennis courts." He also noted that "we hope to provide a little light relief in the shape of excursions. If any members play the violin or piano we hope they will come prepared to give us the pleasure of hearing from them." Travel and accommodations were paid for "with the exception of alcoholic drinks."

IPC participants were selected from mental health association delegates to the Congress and outstanding mental health figures of the day by an informal process of networking and consensus. There was no significant representation of the biologically deterministic viewpoint, nor were there any representatives from the East, Far East, or Africa, only one from South America, and none, despite Rees' efforts, from the Soviet Union. Asian delegates were said to have been unable to afford travel expenses (Saxton, 1995, p. 27). Although lack of transportation in Japan was attributed to postwar shipping shortages there were Asians at the Podelbrady conference in Czechoslovakia not long thereafter (Saxton, letter to the author, 18 November 1996). The IPC, in any event, represented mainly the European and North American mental health elite of the era: prominent, educated, politically liberal clinicians, investigators, and administrators who shared a particular vision of positive mental health rather than of freedom from mental disease. This was an era before the development of clinical psychology and the professionalization of psychology, which was still a scholarly and research discipline. Psychiatry, as it had been in the late 19th and early 20th centuries was, effectively, the only mental health profession. Although most participants were physicians trained as psychiatrists, they shared a belief that the proper study of psychiatry was not disease as such, but human behavior, and that social scientists should be their natural collaborators.

It was a mixture, therefore, of socially inclined psychiatrists and psychosocial scholars that formulated both the new Federation's founding document, which the Roffey Park participants called their Manifesto, and their more clinically defined mission statement: "to promote the mental health of all of the world's peoples from the social, educational, medical and biological aspects." This last reflected their recognition of the social and cultural significance of the new Federation and their hope that ultimately it would "embrace all the social sciences as well as medicine" (Griffin, 1989, p. 147).

The Members and Their Philosophies

The IPC was comprised of 19 people including psychologists Flugel and Cohen and psychiatrist Sullivan, plus four Congress staff members and three advisors and consultants, one of whom was Rees. Their identities and backgrounds were certainly among the factors influencing the nature of the new Federation's founding document. Editor Flugel underscored the fact that most had "a wider background of training and experience than may be suggested by their present occupation" (Flugel et al., 1948b, p. 24). Thus they included people experienced in industrial, educational, and social psychology; sociology; philosophy; theology; cultural anthropology; political science; and general and medical administration; as well as psychiatry and psychoanalysis.

Oswaldo Camargo-Abib, M.D., Superintendent of Mental Health Services of the Brazilian state of Bahia, was perhaps the first of his country's psychiatrists to break away from traditional categorizing and hospital work to study the possibilities of mental health care in the community. I remember him during the year he spent at Yale studying social psychiatry while I was on the faculty there in the early 1950s. He impressed us as a very serious man, imbued with a pioneer spirit and enthusiastic about the possibilities of community-based psychiatric services in Bahia. He was also open-minded enough to see the potential usefulness of collaboration between conventionally trained psychiatrists and the traditional healers of the region. This open-mindedness was not displayed by some leading faculty members of the Bahia medical school during my visits in the decade of the 1960s when, based in Rio de Janeiro, I was engaged in research on social forces in relation to mental illness (Brody, 1973).

H.V. Dicks, M.D., a former professor of psychiatry at the University of Leeds, was Senior Psychiatrist at the Tavistock Clinic and imbued, as was Rees, with optimism about human relations as the proper field of study for mental health professionals. It was Dicks who, 21 years later in 1969, wrote Rees' obituary for the *British Medical Journal*.

Oscar L. Forel, M.D., was a lecturer in psychiatry at the University of Geneva.

Lawrence K. Frank, noted above, was a psychoanalytically inclined philanthropic foundation leader from the United States, interested in social welfare and child development. He was noted for his open-mindedness and creativity.

The IPC chairman, Frank Fremont-Smith, M.D., in addition to being Medical Director of the Josiah Macy, Jr. Foundation in New York, was vice-president of the ICMH and chairman of its executive board. His intimate involvement with the founding of the WFMH proved essential to its later support through contributions from the Macy Foundation.

Otto Klineberg, M.D., Ph.D., although a medical graduate in his native Montreal, was not further trained as a clinician or psychiatrist. With a Ph.D. from Columbia University in New York he functioned as a social psychologist investigator with a special interest in the relationships between nations and the reduction of violence. At the time of Roffey Park he was based in Paris as director of UNESCO's continuing project "Tensions Affecting International Understanding," which followed the conferences noted above. He also served as professor of psychology at Columbia University.

J. Koekebakker, Ph.D., was head of the Mental Health Division, Institute for Preventive Medicine, Leiden.

William Line, Ph.D., Professor of Psychology at the University of Toronto and Director of Research for Canada's National Committee for Mental Hygiene, became the Federation's third president in 1950.

Margaret Mead, Ph.D., perhaps the world's best-known cultural anthropologist, was Associate Curator of Ethnology at the American Museum of Natural History in New York City. Deeply concerned with human communication across all kinds of boundaries and human development in many cultural contexts, she had accepted membership in the U.S. National Committee for Mental Hygiene in 1945. In a 30 April 1945 letter of acceptance to its medical director, George Stevenson, she wrote: "I take [this] as an omen of closer cooperation between anthropology and the Mental Hygiene Movement in the years to come" (MM/LC). She became the WFMH President in 1956.

Professor D. Mitrany, D.Sc., was a social scientist and member of the Institute for Advanced Study at Princeton, New Jersey with a particular interest in peace research. His affiliation at the time was as an advisor on international affairs to a business, Lever Brothers and Unilever Ltd. of London.

The Reverend Eamonn F. O'Doherty, with B.D., M.A., and Ph.D. degrees, a Jesuit priest, was Professor of Psychology at University College in Dublin. A 10 September 1948 letter from him to Margaret Mead (MM/LC) indicates the exceptional nature of the IPC experience and the depth of feeling it engendered in some participants: "My sudden departure from London…meant that I failed to say *au revoir* to my dearest friends on the IPC. The IPC was a revelation of how lovable human beings can be. Never before in my life did I find so many completely lovable people in one place. I hope that my own occasional jaggedness and explosiveness will not be remembered too vividly." He referred to the "depth of emotion in old Harry Stack Sullivan [who] I believe, loved me as a son but always fought off any attempt to show it…John Cohen if he were a Catholic should be a saint, and so on down the list."

O'Doherty and I had a chance to discuss the WFMH founding period when he was a visiting lecturer in my Department of Psychiatry at the University of Maryland in the early 1960s. In Baltimore as a guest of the leading Catholic psychiatrist, Leo Bartemeier, M.D., who at one time was a substitute member of the WFMH Executive Board, he was always concerned with the role of religion in mental health. He was especially fond of making two points: first, religion is not a neurosis, but it can be used neurotically; second, the problem with many psychiatrists is that "they do not differentiate real guilt from neurotic guilt."

A. Querido, M.D., a community psychiatry specialist, was Director, Department of Mental Hygiene of the Public Health Services of Amsterdam.

Professor Carlo de Sanctis, M.D., was Assistant Director of the Psychiatric Hospital in Rome.

T.S. Simey, M.A., was Professor of Social Science, University of Liverpool.

Torgny Segerstedt, Ph.D., was Professor of Sociology at the University of Uppsala.

Jean Stoetzel, D. es L., was Professor of Social Science at the University of Bordeaux.

Members of the Congress staff who participated in the Roffey Park deliberations included Dr. Nina Ridenour, Ms. S. Clement Brown, and Helen Speyer, already mentioned above. A fourth was psychiatric social worker E. N. Goldberg, Assistant Programme Secretary for the Congress. The advisors and consultants included, in addition to Rees, Daniel Blain, M.D., Medical Director of the American Psychiatric Association, and George S. Stevenson, M.D. Two world-famous social scientists were listed as consultants in Flugel's June 1948 letter, but there is no record of their participation. They were sociologist Professor Hadley Cantril, Ph.D., the first director of UNESCO's project "Tensions Affecting International Understanding," and Professor Gordon W. Allport who, as noted above, participated with Sullivan and Cantril in the UNESCO "tensions project" shortly before the opening of the London Congress.

Among the Federation founders gathered at Roffey Park, only Sullivan was known for his clinical creativeness with individual patients rather than groups. He was already famous as the creator of the concepts of "interpersonal relations" and "participant observation." He was also the one most experienced and concerned, in that pre-neuroleptic era, with available and accessible treatment for the world's greatest psychiatric public health problem, schizophrenia. Another historical link to WFMH is the fact that he first tried his ideas about the combined social and psychotherapeutic treatment of paranoid schizophrenic young men in the late 1920s at the Sheppard Pratt Hospital in Baltimore, where my offices have been located since 1986. During that period he also gave some lectures and supervised the psychotherapy of the University of Maryland's Department of Psychiatry, which I headed from 1957 to 1977.

There is no suggestion that, like Beers or Dorothea Dix, any of the Federation founders were motivated by the experience of personal suffering. Some biographers have suggested that Sullivan might have suffered a psychotic episode earlier in his life, and that this could account for what appears to have been his exceptional empathy with schizophrenic young men, thought in that era to be defending themselves from repressed (unconscious) homosexuality. It has also been suggested that he might have been a problem drinker. In the mid-1980s, for example, during a meeting of the International Social Science Council in Paris, I asked Otto Klineberg, one of the WFMH founders (and President, 1966-1967), to tell me about Sullivan's participation in the Roffey Park discussions. He responded without elaboration: "Oh, Harry? He was always in the bar!"

Despite these hints, there is no evidence that Sullivan's participation in the Federation's founding group was colored by his having had problems of his own. In fact the written record indicates that while his absences from Roffey Park, noted by Klineberg, were indeed in a bar, they were at a nearby Inn where he retreated with one or two colleagues to work on issues brought up in the general discussions (MM/LC; Saxton, 1995). He brought a finely honed, discriminating clinical intelligence and intuition to the process. His sympathy for the universality of the document produced by the IPC (the Manifesto), and his acceptance of diversity are suggested in his well-known comment about schizophrenic patients: "they are more simply human than anything else" (Sullivan, 1964). It is evident that he had a significant influence on the ideas which, mediated by Rees and others, shaped the Federation's initial program. Almost alone among the professional clinicians of his day he believed that such issues as racial and ethnic prejudice, the avoidance of nuclear war, the reduction of poverty and of international tensions were proper subjects for practitioners of psychiatry and psychology. Two years earlier, in 1946, in an introduction to Brock Chisholm's published lectures, he had proposed a "cultural revolution to end war" to be led by psychotherapists and social scientists (Sullivan, 1946; Cushman, 1995). Professor Adolf Meyer at Johns Hopkins, who had been an early supporter of Clifford Beers, was also intrigued by these ideas and had been an influence on Sullivan during his early years at Sheppard Pratt. These ideas and his interest in a fusion of psychiatry and social science, germinated in his early associations with anthropologist Edward Sapir and (psychoanalyzed) political scientist Harold Lasswell, were nearly identical with much of the thinking contained in *Mental Health and World Citizenship*. He was, in fact, a co-author of that statement's summary, which received wide circulation and was the basis for journalistic abbreviations.

Sullivan, who had a history of chronic heart disease and had predicted his age of death years earlier, died at the age of 56 in a Paris hotel on 14 January 1949 while attending a UNESCO meeting on his way back to the United States from the WFMH executive board meeting in Amsterdam. Soddy, then honorary secretary of the board, wrote to the group on 27 January

1949: "We shall miss the impetus given by his single minded devotion to the promotion of harmonious living." His friend, colleague,and fellow idealist, Brock Chisholm, attributed his premature death to his unceasing efforts for world peace and to educate people for worldmindedness (Chisholm, 1949a).

Evolving Psychiatry and Mental Health

Rees and Sullivan were alike in recognizing the role of social context in relation to health. They both had great faith in the potential contributions of social science to international and intercultural harmony, expressing the wish that more social scientists could be involved. While Rees first referred to this in relation to the IPC, the idea recurred repeatedly in later years. With a few exceptions, however, this wish has not been fulfilled. During the 1950s and 1960s, psychiatrists, especially academicians, remained prominent in most of the world's developing national mental health movements. Although in the industrial democracies their role was shifting from one of direct leadership to that of consultant, they were not replaced or supplemented by social scientists but by nonprofessional citizen volunteers, some of whom shared a distrust for technical professional knowledge and authority. This change was associated with the voluntary associations' developing sense of autonomy and wish not to be subordinated to the historically authoritative medical profession, concerned with pathology rather than health. It has accelerated with the rise of clinical psychology, psychiatric social work, and psychiatric nursing, all of which maintain a strong interest in and support for the voluntary mental health movement. At the same time psychiatrists have withdrawn their interest from the idea of mental health and refocused it upon the idea of disease. This was in part a consequence of the systematization of cross-sectional diagnoses effected by the American Psychiatric Association's Diagnostic and Statistical Manual III of 1980 and the proliferation of psychotropic drugs. DSM III and its sequelae (DSM-III-R and DSM IV) have had a global impact. Not only have they been widely adopted, but they and the American psychiatrists who created them have had a major influence on WHO's International Classification of Diseases (ICD-10). These developments accelerated a loss of psychiatric interest in previously prominent aspects of the field bearing directly on the concerns of WFMH: context in relation to behavior, individual life histories, psychotherapy, consumer participation in their own health care, and especially the social problems requiring attention in pursuit of the primary prevention of mental illness or ill health and less than optimal function. Official psychiatry has increasingly adopted the standard model of medical practice more attuned to dealing with mental disease as a biological entity, and less to mental health.

In many parts of the world, particularly those less industrialized and lacking a well-developed middle class, psychiatrists continue to dominate the voluntary mental health movement. This is apparent, despite continuing change, in Latin America and the Middle East. In Asia and Africa the Western model of voluntarism by nonprofessionals has been an important, though geographically limited, influence on mental health association development, but in many settings psychiatrists still dominate the leadership roles. Other volunteers have included educators, lawyers, judges, and planners in addition to clinicians. Their vision has been closer to that of Brock Chisholm and Jack Rees than to the hospital reformers who followed Clifford Beers. Improving standards of mental hospital care was not incompatible with the ideal of global mental health, but it was not central. Perhaps this global aim reflected an inflated view of the capacities of psychiatry. At the same time the founders were convinced of the importance of bringing the social sciences together with psychiatry in order to reduce "the toll of human waste and suffering and [promote] social well-being." WHO's Chisholm and the distinguished British biologist, Julian Huxley, first Director General of UNESCO, expected WFMH to work toward this goal through collaboration with them and other agencies of the new UN, founded only three years earlier.

THE IPC PROCESS AND THE FOUNDING DOCUMENT

The IPC theme which became the title of the WFMH founding document, *Mental Health and World Citizenship,* was suggested by the Congress Programme Committee headed by Professor Flugel. Rees felt that this theme "gave promise of widening the mental hygiene frame of reference in a practical way" (Rees, 1966, p. 74).

The document was written by the participants in the IPC meeting at Roffey Park prior to the 1948 London Congress and published afterward without substantive change. The meeting began with each member of the new IPC being given a set of volumes containing the carefully edited work of the preparatory commissions. The account in the official history is bland: it notes that after reviewing the volumes person each was asked to write a statement on "What is Mental Health," "What Constitutes a Good Society," and "What is World Citizenship" and, gradually, through the process of discussion, writing and re-writing, the sections of the final report, i.e., the founding document, emerged.

Lawrence Frank and Margaret Mead, writing in volume I of the Proceedings (Flugel et al., 1948b, pp. 74–89) noted that when the group assembled only a few had met before. They had to deal with the problems of coming from different frames of reference and not knowing each other's ways of working. They were favorably impressed though, noting that even "when personalities have once embodied a cultural form they exhibit stubborn resistance to change...human behavior is more plastic than heretofore recognized." Mead (1949) in a more personal account wrote that IPC began with a "rattling around period" while her group argued "about nothing for a while." She credited Sullivan with finding the solution: "One of the most interesting experiments was proposed by...Sullivan. Without any warning, in the middle of a session which looked as if it were not going to be good at all, he suddenly proposed that each person bring in his or her definition of mental health and world citizenship and read it. It sounded absolutely appalling.... [A]ll of us knew that it was going to wreck the meeting; at least I was sure it was. But it did not because the form of the commission was different.... [W]e were able to act as individuals, everybody worked to try to communicate with the others instead of trying...to cover themselves for the folks back home."

In fact, the organization of the IPC was described by Mead as "a new experiment...based on mental health principles.... [N]ever before in the history of conferences and congresses has so informal, so simple, and so fruitful an organizational scheme been tried...[with] individuals from different countries and of different statuses, ranging from [those] with international reputations to much less known workers, and from the revered and aged to the young and aspiring, without regard to status, representing no organization, no country, no profession—in the sense that they could compromise or involve others when they spoke—drawing fully on their nationality, their philosophy and their disciplines." She was especially impressed by the fact that after two weeks they were able to arrive at a consensus with a report presented to the Congress where after review in 30 discussion groups it was accepted by acclamation. This was in sharp contrast to her experience 14 years earlier when the same Lawrence Frank who moderated the Roffey Park commission had chaired another meeting of 14 Americans for one month to try to reach a frame of reference in which a multidisciplined group could talk together. At the end of a month they had not even finished the outline of an agreement.

The document produced by the IPC, *World Citizenship and Mental Health,* was regarded by Rees as the Federation's "Bible" (Rees, 1966, p. xi). It reflected the Roffey Park group's idealism and moral vision. It also reflected the anxieties and hopes of the immediate post-World War II era. Thus, it began with such questions as: "Can the catastrophe of a third world war be averted?" "Can the people of the world learn to co-operate for the good of all?" "On what basis is there hope for enduring peace?" The significance accorded the concept of human relations was evident throughout. Thus, recognizing "the central position of the family and the importance of human development in the unfolding of all human relationships," a section on human development was the first to be considered.

This did not imply a negation of ICMH's earlier concern with reforming mental hospital care, but rather a deliberate expansion of the mental health vision to society as a whole with special reference to reducing the incidence of mental ill health and of disability following mental illness. The document ended with concrete recommendations, both to the new WFMH and to the UN and its specialized agencies. Repeated emphases were upon the reduction of international tensions, ways of dealing with institutional change through "group techniques," and public education including the role of the media. There were also immediate recommendations for dealing with the "human aftermath of war" such as "the mental health problems of displaced persons, transferred and migrating populations, homeless children." However, many recommendations were more clinical, as they encouraged the establishment of community-based mental health services, including attention to the workplace. Some, such as the importance for mental health of systematic attention to pregnancy and the perinatal period, combined broadly social and narrowly medical concerns. Mead, on an inspirational note, regarded the Congress as having "given birth" to "a multidisciplinary, cross-national approach to the problems of a better world and a more widely responsible world...a platform on which people of all these disciplines with this common interest can work together to give a kind of moral impetus to the formation of the...world federation" (Mead, 1949). Flugel et al. (1948a, pp. 273–280) in a post-Congress commentary spoke of the enlargement of the concept of mental health emerging from the Congress as one that could only be possible in a world community in which "one society cannot permanently prosper at the expense of another." The members of the IPC, sensitive to their global purview, defined mental health as "a condition which permits the optimal development, physical, intellectual and emotional, of the individual, so far as this is compatible with that of other individuals." This takes place in "a good society...one that ensures this to its members, while at the same time ensuring its own development and being tolerant towards other societies [its 'goodness' thus being manifested on three separate planes—to its members, to itself and to other groups]." Finally, "world citizenship implies good society on a world scale."

The overall goal of mental health, then, was broadly conceived as peaceful coexistence—international collaboration in place of destruction. The guiding theme of the new Federation was to be world citizenship with mental health reflected in an extra-national allegiance to humankind as a whole. In the founding document's terms, "World citizenship means an informed, reflective, responsible allegiance to mankind as a whole...a world community built on free consent and on the respect for individual and cultural differences." "The ultimate goal of mental health" it concluded "is to help [people] live with their fellows in one world." Although the authors did not complete their translation of these ideals to the personal level, the interpersonal corollaries seem apparent. They are the ability to empathize, relate, and collaborate. The failure of empathy, the ability to see the world through one's neighbor's eyes, is revealed in prejudice, stereotyping, discrimination and, perhaps, in hostile and destructive acts. A person's individuality is replaced by a perception of him or her as a member of a feared, hated, despised, or ignored social group. The target is, in effect, dehumanized. The implied emphasis on empathy is compatible with Freud's definition of individual mental health as the capacity to love, work, and play. It is consistent with Brock Chisholm's initial conception of the role of psychiatry as a peacemaker, and a view of health as the capacity for optimal function (Brody, 1987).

Overlapping the concerns of human rights activists in many fields, the founders planned in terms of a broadly inclusive humanism embracing the ideals of universal brotherhood and sisterhood. These ideals remain congruent with evolving Federation goals for groups of people conceived as vulnerable to illness or disability. They are couched in terms of values relevant to optimal function and positive mental health or well-being rather than to mental illness or acute distress.

The more clinically oriented statement of mission, "to promote among all people and nations the highest possible level of mental health in its broadest biological, medical, educational and social aspects," permitted broad social and idealistic aims to be translated into concrete goals and projects. Over the life of the Federation these have covered such a large area of human existence that some members have been concerned that they might result in a loss of advocacy leverage for projects with more apparent and direct mental health significance.

Are WFMH Standards Universally Applicable?

The question of the possibly culture-bound nature of the IPC document arose on several occasions. Margaret Mead (1949), for example, recognized "the extent to which the mental hygiene movement is tied down to our own particular Western European cultural forms." The IPC members were aware that their conclusions reflected a particular set of values. As stated in the document itself "the pursuit of mental health cannot but be part of a system of values" (Flugel et al., 1948d).

Some of the ideals expressed through the Federation's goals and projects are globally acceptable. Others reflect the value systems of the Western industrial states with their emphases on individual autonomy and self-realization rather than the interdependency and community prized in the East and in many of the world's low income populations. Indeed, Rees (1966) recognized that the "effort to reach a high degree of mental health is, in some respect, an expression of Western cultural achievement." However, he added that "this by no means implies that mental health as understood in Western countries is in any sense…at variance with the sense in which it is understood in other countries. On the contrary…here might be found a basis for common human inspiration."

A similar commitment to a cross-cultural, universal standard was revealed in the IPC's agreement that in every civilization human beings can learn by applying their intelligence to alter themselves and their institutions. Indeed, the new Federation's unique feature was its focus on the possibility of improving the social and psychological health of humankind as a whole, regardless of sociocultural context.

As the WFMH grows toward increasingly genuine regional participation, especially in the non-European and non-North American world, some of the views of its founders may be regarded as culturally ethnocentric, but the motivating force of idealism persists. This is also reflected in the fact that the WFMH has no economically bound constituency and, unlike the international trade unions for psychiatry, psychology, social work, and nursing, is not concerned with the well-being of any particular profession. The Federation at age 50 has not become unsympathetic to "world citizenship" as a guiding Federation concept. It is true that in the years since the atmosphere of idealism and hope which informed the IPC, its member associations have continued a major focus on advocating for improved delivery of mental health services and higher standards of patient care. On the other hand, the global activities of the WFMH, including its committees and collaborating centers, have closely approximated the vision of the founders. These two faces of Federation activity come together in the importance it accords to sustaining a universal standard of competent, dignified, humane mental health care in the face of local standards of acceptability and concepts of right and wrong. The need to reconcile universal with particular standards of care and ethical behavior has been most evident when service delivery impinges on local values concerning the status of women, reproductive behavior, and the roles of ethnic, racial, religious, or national minorities.

Postscript

Once the IPC document was completed some controversy and uncertainty remained regarding its final editing and distribution. Mead, in a 16 September 1948 letter to Rees, recommended that it should be issued with a list of participating countries and disciplines, but with the names of individual participants omitted. She also recommended an editorial subcommittee to produce an abbreviated version, to include "at least minimally Frank, O'Dougherty, Sullivan, and Dicks." This suggestion was submitted to the Committee members and overruled. Plans were made for its publication to sell in Great Britain for one shilling. Rees, on 6 October 1948, proposed that "on the last page of the newbound copy of the statement there should be a very brief, dignified reference to the World Federation." However, even before an official copy was prepared, Sullivan published it in his journal, *Psychiatry* (1948b).

Despite the harmony and generally good feelings about the IPC deliberations there were some critical reactions. Some felt that interpersonal tensions within the group went unexamined (Saxton, 1995, p. 32). A letter of 1 November 1948 from Querido to Soddy noted: "I must warn against leaving too much to spontaneous activity. Too little guidance was the weak point of Roffey Park and also of the group work before the Congress. The recommendations of the Statement are for the larger part too vague to serve as starting points." He felt that it would have been better to offer a set of mental health problems classified as to urgency, local or general interest, and character (research, clinical, organizational) to WFMH working groups. They should have been encouraged to select a subject for study and WFMH could then have coordinated the groups in different countries and kept them informed of parallel efforts. It would also, he felt, have been desirable, but not essential for each WFMH working group to be in contact with the national mental health association in its country. A follow-up letter of 8 November from Querido amplified this initial criticism: "At present there is marked resentment in some groups which feel their work neglected by the Congress."

Sullivan, writing to Soddy on 27 December 1948, agreed with the idea of listing issues by priority. He felt that the greatest mental health need was for postdoctoral training and recommended the immediate organization of training projects, especially bringing psychiatrists and social scientists together so that they might be "capable of multi-disciplined thinking and collaboration on transnational problems."

THE FOUNDING MOMENT
The Third International Congress on Mental Hygiene

The Congress during which this founding moment occurred attracted approximately 2500 delegates representing 60 countries, with the notable exception of the Soviet Union. As recorded by Flugel et al. (1948b) there were 806 psychiatrists, the largest group of professionals in attendance. There were 161 other physicians, 300 psychologists of varying definition, 300 psychiatric social workers, 100 general social workers, and 168 administrators. Only 21 attendees identified themselves as social scientists.

The Congress encompassed, as noted above, three meetings: those of the International Committee on Child Psychiatry, the International Federation for Medical Psychotherapy, and the International Conference on Mental Health. Rees initially regarded the agreement to operate the first two along with the mental health conference as a mistake, but in retrospect felt that "on the whole all were quite profitable" (Rees, 1966, p. 75).

The meetings were held in Central Hall, Westminster. The unpublished account of a psychiatric social worker (M. Elvin, MM/LC) who attended the three conferences making up the Congress, suggests the difference between them: "For half of the first week there weren't as many members present as there were for the second half. Every one came out full-force from all the countries for the Conference on Mental Hygiene...The whole idea was for [them] to contribute their knowledge of human behavior and with their understanding to determine how to have a better and peaceful world, a good world where people could live in harmony...the main emphasis was on the study of group relationships in the community, industry and between nations." She reported that "One of the recommendations made was that an international vocabulary be formulated in order that a common understanding of ideas could be expressed in such a way as to be understood by all...some of the translations were not quite what the speakers had said. On the whole, however, the language differences were skillfully handled." This was enhanced by distributing copies of the main speech for the day so that the audience could read while listening. After each paper despite discussants from the heterogeneous audience there was still an expressed need for more intensive interdisciplinary comment.

The Congress mornings were devoted to lectures and many afternoons to visits to hospitals and clinics as well as places of touristic interest. However, the most intense interest was in the opportunity to meet with one's peers and colleagues from strange places and to learn about their training and their work. As Elvin wrote: "It was a really wonderful experience to be there and to talk to people from so many different countries and different disciplines."

Flugel et al. (1948b, p. iv) noted that since their texts were not received from some of the French-speaking chairmen of sessions, their summaries were not included in the proceedings. Elvin confirmed the existence of language problems observing that, although most papers were read in English, only a few of the large, non-English speaking, French delegation were supplied with earphones for simultaneous translation. Winifred Overholser, M.D., superintendent of St. Elizabeth's Hospital in Washington, DC who headed an official United States delegation of government mental health specialists, evidently noted the same phenomena, but interpreted it in the opposite way. He wrote in his official report: "It was highly noticeable that at no time were the headphones provided for the French speaking delegates all in use. There would seem to be no question that English is now the international language!" Overholser, in his 9 December 1948 letter to the U.S. State Department was also careful to note that attendance at the Congress did not imply a role in the formation of the WFMH, which was a separate activity by delegates previously appointed by the mental health associations of their countries: "The official delegation of the United States did not participate or make any commitments on behalf of the United States."

A final note suggests the reactions of many who attended this world congress. They were inevitably interested in the personalities as well as the ideas on display. Thus Elvin observed that among the "very famous people from the United States," anthropologist Margaret Mead was "one of the most popular speakers" with "a radiant personality which just charmed her audience" (MM/LC). Sullivan, who felt that the conference had gotten off to a slow and discouraged start, described Mead's report on the second day as "practically the kick-off for the Congress...greatly illuminating and immensely inspiring" (Sullivan, 1948; Saxton, 1995).

The closing session was addressed by Huxley and Chisholm, both of whom expressed the hope that, as a result of the meeting, a permanent World Federation for Mental Health would be established to act as a continuing source of information and advice to WHO and UNESCO on matters relating to mental hygiene. The articles of association were formed in accordance with the Swiss Civil Code, establishing a corporation designated as the World Federation for Mental Health with its "principal office and seat in the care of the law firm of MMes. Borel and Paul Lachenal" in Geneva. It was noted that the WFMH Assembly reserves the right "at any time and from time to time to change the principal office and seat of the Federation."

The purposes for which the Federation was formed were: "To promote among all peoples and nations the highest possible level of mental health (which term wherever used in these Articles shall be deemed to include mental health in its broadest biological, medical, educational and social aspects)." In furtherance of this purpose there was listed a series of subpurposes ranging from cooperation with UN agencies to fostering "the ability to live harmoniously in a changing environment." The founding members were defined as "the national mental health associations from countries eligible for membership in the United Nations (approximately 22 in number at the time of the organisational meeting to adopt these articles) known to and to be certified by The International Committee for Mental

Hygiene, Incorporated, together with such organizations as shall be approved by a vote of a majority of the aforesaid members present at the first annual meeting of the Mental Health Assembly which shall be held without notice immediately following the adoption of these Articles."

A New Organization, the World Federation for Mental Health

The resolution to found the WFMH, begun with a meeting in the British Ministry of Health building during the London Congress on the night of 18 August and completed on the night of 19 August 1948, was announced by Rees at a plenary session on the 20th. It was ratified by the official delegates to the London Congress in a plenary session on the following day, 21 August 1948 attended by ministry level officials of the British government. The approximately 133 delegates who voted unanimously to establish the new organization were members of mental hygiene societies that had belonged to the ICMH. There were evidently some dissenting opinions, if not votes, from people who were not convinced that the ICMH needed to be changed, because Rees had to defend the process. At the 20 August 1948 plenary session he was compelled to state: "Some people have felt with regard to this Federation that something was being engineered…well, if one comes to think of it, everything has been engineered…but this has been engineered democratically as far as we were able. More than a year ago we sent suggested draft articles of association to mental health associations in every country in the world and asked for delegates. We did all we humanly could to get a representative group of people from different countries" (Flugel et al, 1948b, p. 210).

The countries represented by voting delegates were Argentina, Australia, Austria, Belgium, Brazil, British Guiana, Bulgaria, Canada, Chile, China, Cuba, Czechoslovakia, Denmark, Egypt, Eire, Finland, France, Great Britain, Greece, Holland, Hong Kong, Hungary, Iceland, India, Iran, Italy, Luxembourg, Malta, Mexico, Netherlands East Indies, New Zealand, Norway, Pakistan, Palestine, Poland, Portugal, Puerto Rico, Siam, Sweden, Switzerland, Syria, Turkey, Union of South Africa, United States of America, Uruguay, and Venezuela. These delegates elected an executive board from among themselves. Most were psychiatrists: E. Eduardo Krapf, M.D., Professor of Medical Psychology at the University of Buenos Aires, Argentina; Henrique Roxo, M.D., Professor Emeritus at the University of Brazil and president, Brazilian League of Mental Hygiene (representing the continent of South America); J. D. Griffin, M.D., of the Canadian Mental Health Association; J. Stuchlik, M.D., of Czechoslovakia, who also served at that time on the executive board of WHO; M. L. el Kholy, M.D., of Egypt, at that time head of the Mental Health Services of his country; Yves Porc'her, M.D., of France, then secretary of the Ligue Francaise d'Hygiene Mental; Doris Odlum, M.D., of Great Britain, a pioneer in mental health and medicine in relation to social welfare; H. C. Rumke, M.D., Professor of Psychiatry at the University of Utrecht, who was elected board chairman; Keki Masani, M.D., president of the Indian Council for Mental Hygiene (representing the continent of Asia); Dr. J. Russell of New Zealand, director of the Mental Hygiene Division of his country's Ministry of Health; and George Stevenson, M.D., of the United States. The sole nonphysician was Miss Kerstin Hesselgren of Sweden, a social worker and the first Swedish woman member of Parliament who was president of the Swedish Association for Mental Hygiene.

The officers, including Rees, who was to be President for the first year, were all psychiatrists: Andre Repond, M.D., president of the European Committee for Mental Hygiene and the Swiss National Committee for Mental Hygiene (representing the continent of Europe), as Vice-president; Frank Fremont-Smith, M.D., of the United States as Treasurer; and Kenneth Soddy, M.D., of Great Britain as honorary secretary. Everyone who had been at Roffey Park was immediately placed on the advisory interprofessional committee to WFMH, at first designated AIC, then IPC, the same initials as those for the International Preparatory Commission.

All delegates to the foundation meetings, even those counted in the unanimous vote, did not later signify their desire to join the new Federation and two had to be refused membership on the grounds that they were not truly "national" in the sense that the areas in which they lived were not recognized as independent nations by the United Nations organization. These were Scotland—which had not actually been present at the foundation meetings—and Palestine. The contemporary sensitivity to UN acceptability was indicated later when in December 1948 Sullivan, Stevenson, and Griffin questioned the wisdom of having an executive board meeting in the Netherlands where there were pending Security Council charges of a UN truce violation. In a telegram of 23 December 1948 to other board members Sullivan wrote: "this event which could entail explosion from United Nations cannot faithfully be ignored by volunteer organizations cooperating with international agencies."

The 21 August 1948 announcement was the culmination of a process begun with the Canadian Brock Chisholm's suggestion in George Stevenson's New York office of the U.S. National Committee for Mental Hygiene more than two years earlier. It was historically apposite that two psychiatrists of an older generation who had been close to Clifford Beers during the germination of the International Committee on Mental Hygiene were also there with Chisholm: his fellow Canadian Clarence Hincks, M.D., who was inspired by Beers to form what became the Canadian Mental Health Association and then join with the U.S. Committee to form the first international association of its kind; and American Arthur Ruggles, M.D., a prominent supporter of the concept, and then a colleague and friend of Beers.

A Review of the Organizing Process

Jack Rees, in the aftermath of the Third World Congress on Mental Hygiene, enthusiastically promoted the establishment of a new organization to succeed the ICMH. The first step had been his 1946 acceptance of the presidency of ICMH in order to facilitate the hoped for transition. Within a year, in 1947, he and his organizing colleagues—especially Frank Fremont-Smith, the ICMH's former president and now vice-president who maintained the office in New York—had already made the initial moves toward a preliminary infrastructure for the new WFMH. They sent draft articles of association to all of the ICMH member mental hygiene societies asking for the nominations of delegates to attend the forthcoming Congress and establish a new organization to succeed ICMH. The new Federation was to be "not a membership of individuals nor of countries, but of societies" (Flugel et al., 1948b, pp. 210–211). Its initial voting members, therefore, were members of the existing societies. Later, letters of invitation were sent to persons occupying mental hygiene or (now) health-relevant posts in all of the world's countries, including those with no existing mental hygiene societies. The first circular letter of WFMH went out on 12 November 1948 from its temporary address, 12 Manchester St., London. But the old ICMH from which it was formed had what might be called its posthumous last board meeting for administrative purposes on 16 December 1948 (MM/LC).

The official hope, voiced by Rees, was "to bring into real cooperation all the societies which are concerned with mental health, alike on the educational, the psychological, the anthropological, and the sociological side" (Flugel et al, 1948b, p. 211). At the time of this writing that hope is still not realized. The WFMH has not become the truly multiprofessional, social science oriented organization of which he had dreamed, one capable of promoting international harmony. However, it has evolved in another direction, which has also proved itself capable of international bridge building. This is the increasingly decisive involvement, beginning in 1981 after the era of working presidents, of citizen volunteers who have, to a significant degree, replaced professionals as active members of national mental health associations. 1982 saw the beginning inclusion of those who have learned about mental illness and psychological distress at first hand: survivors of illness and trauma, users of psychiatric and psychosocial services. Members of the user's movement have become increasingly vocal and constructive elements in forming the Federation's international mental health agenda. The 1990s have seen for the first time the inclusion, especially in world congresses, of members of organizations of relatives of mentally ill persons. The involvement of these active and dedicated members— mental health association volunteers, users and survivors, relatives—does not presage a diminished Federation interest in the contributions of professionally trained persons who are also volunteers in the mental health cause. It emphasizes, rather, the ecumenical nature of the voluntary, global, inclusive mental health movement that the WFMH was founded to lead.

Chapter 3

The Rees Era and Beyond: 1948–1966

OVERVIEW
John Rawlings "Jack" Rees

John R. Rees, familiarly known as "J. R." or, certainly in the United States, as "Jack," was asked in 1946 by the United Kingdom's National Association for Mental Health to take the lead in organizing a Third International Congress of Mental Hygiene. His background and the phase of this work, which began with forming the Congress Preparatory Commissions, are described in Chapter 2.

The Rees era of the World Federation for Mental Health began with his being named president of the Federation's predecessor, the International Committee for Mental Hygiene (ICMH), and his forming the national preparatory commissions for the London Congress on Mental Hygiene. Federation life proper began with its founding during the Congress and Rees' election as its first president. His vision for the new organization was global, with a perception of mental health influenced by all of the socioeconomic and cultural factors involved in the relationships of human beings with each other and their world. In his "Address by the Retiring President" on 22 August 1949 at the beginning of the Federation's second annual meeting in Geneva, he cautioned the audience: "Whatever the difficulties and the obstructions and indifference that we have to meet, we must neither be cynical nor disillusioned in the face of the massive world-wide problems, nor on the other hand must we be naively enthusiastic" (WFMH, 1948–1949, p. 22).

During his tenure as the World Federation for Mental Health (WFMH) Director from 1949 through 1961 he was constantly on the move, visiting countries all over the world, frequently the United States. There he kept in touch with the New York fundraisers, American international thinkers such as Frank Fremont-Smith, Margaret Mead, and others, and the United Nations (UN) headquarters. In retrospect he called the period of his active leadership of the Federation "the most enjoyable and one of the most strenuous tasks I have ever attempted in my life" (Rees, 1966, p. 84).

He announced his impending resignation several times, beginning in the mid-1950s (see Chapter 4), but it was not until the autumn of 1961 that he announced that he would definitely leave the post by the end of that year. He attributed this decision to age and health. However, neither health nor age kept him from continuing Federation activity after January 1962 when his successor, Francois Cloutier, M.D., took office. He continued to be involved in various activities, particularly in the Caribbean, after Cloutier's resignation in late 1965 when Dr. Pierre Visseur took charge of the Geneva Secretariat, until its final closure at the end of November 1967. His continuing involvement lends credence to the view that he was "simply fed up" with the never ending tasks of raising money to keep the operation going, including his own salary (Beaty, 1995).

After Rees' resignation, as of the end of 1961, the reflections of his continuing influence in the role of consultant were most apparent in the Caribbean. This extended aspects of his era until approximately 1966. The Federation's Caribbean involvements in this period are described in Chapter 9, dealing with regional issues. Its later Caribbean resurgence, from 1972 to 1974, during the presidency of Michael Beaubrun, M.D., professor and chairman of psychiatry at the University of the West Indies in Jamaica, is described in Chapter 5, dealing with organizational issues.

Much that could be included in a chapter on the Rees era is dealt with elsewhere. For example, finances occupy a prominent place in this chapter. However, much of the constant concern with financing, and the continuing efforts to reorganize or reinvent the Federation's structure characterizing Rees' tenure are described in later chapters, especially 5 and 6. The substantive achievements of the era, related to what I have come to call the Federation's "international mental health agenda," are described in Part III of this volume. Much of the organizational work of the Cloutier period, covered in Chapter 4, had its roots in the Rees era. Chapter 8, dealing with the UN, is a continuation of the account of Rees' work with the UN included in this chapter.

THE LONDON SECRETARIAT 1948–1961

Establishing a Central Office

Within weeks of its founding the leaders of the new WFMH agreed that in order to function the organization required a central office, a secretariat, to be headed by a person who could fulfill the duties of a chief executive. According to William "Bill" Beaty II (1995), whose role is described below, the names initially considered for chief executive included three Americans, all of whom had been involved in the International Preparatory Commission (IPC) and were active founders of the Federation. They were Margaret Mead, then a senior curator at the American Museum of Natural History and a world figure in her field; Frank Fremont-Smith of the Josiah Macy, Jr. Foundation of New York; and George C. Stevenson, then medical director of the U.S. National Committee for Mental Hygiene, later to become the U.S. National Mental Health Association. However, none of their names appear in the Board minutes as actual nominees for the post. It seems likely that if they had been asked to consider it each would have declined, since each already occupied a responsible and rewarding post. Beaty felt that they were ruled out because they were Americans—the founders felt, he said, that since some of the initiative and most of the funds for the new organization came from the United States, it would not be perceived by other countries as genuinely international if its secretariat were also in that country. In any event Jack Rees, by virtue of his immensely successful organizing work and his continuing leadership as the first WFMH president during 1948–1949, was the logical candidate for the post.

At the Amsterdam meeting of 5–9 January 1949, its first as an operational body, the Board applauded a gift from an anonymous donor for 3 years' salary for the director and a nationwide funding campaign being planned for the United States. However, it "was seriously perturbed" to learn that no other substantive steps had been taken to fund the director. Believing that "it would be an unhealthy situation if the Federation had to depend almost wholly on the US and Britain" for funds, member associations in other countries were urged to contribute (WFMH Bulletin, 1948, 1, p. 11). It was in this context that Rees recommended that the new director "should preferably be under the age of 45 [Rees was 58] and because of the great activity of the

British on the organizational side...we should at first look elsewhere than among British candidates." There was general agreement that the candidate should have "a broad background of psychiatric experience which should include as many as possible of the various fields of mental health work...some administrative experience, and ability to write and to speak...facility in more than one language would be an important extra...ability to plan boldly but wisely and to foster good international relationships" would be essential.

Kenneth Soddy, M.D., a child psychiatrist and medical director of the U.K. NAMH worked with Rees during his presidency as an unpaid volunteer in the capacity of WFMH honorary secretary. A letter of 27 January 1949 from him to the Executive Board and the Interprofessional Advisory Committee (successor to the IPC) described Rees' situation. Rees had been approached about taking the post, but remained uncertain. As reported by Soddy, he urged the Board to continue looking for "likely candidates for the new post of Director or Secretary General of the Federation when it moves its Headquarters to Geneva." A few days earlier, on 24 January 1949, Rees had written to Rumke, to be copied to everyone else, that it had never occurred to him to take on the job, he was too old, and an appointment in Geneva would "mean terminating my professional work as a consultant which has always been my method of earning my livelihood." He had also, for more than twenty years, given considerable time to Tavistock, then the war, and the Congress. So he concluded, "I really need to get down to paying my way and saving some money against a possible retirement...I have not been able to save, and have never had a pensionable job." Deciding that he could not take on the job of director for less than £4000 a year he stipulated: "We must have some clear indication that funds are going to be made available and are coming in from various countries as a demonstration that the member societies really do want such an organization and are prepared to raise funds for it. If the Director or Secretary General had to devote his time to raising his own salary it would be rather disastrous, and if he were burdened with, as the Americans say, 'living on a shoestring' with regard to overhead expenses, travel etc., that would limit very much the usefulness of the central office." (Rees, letter to Rumke, 24 January 1949) (MM/LC).

There were varied reactions to Rees' views, some contained in another letter from Soddy to the board (MM/LC). On 11 February 1949 Fremont-Smith expressed two convictions: first, the post should not be filled from the United States and second, that Rees was the best fitted for the job. Mitrany thought that Rees should not allow himself to be absorbed by administrative tasks. Stuchlic felt that an administrative assistant would be essential.

The situation remained unresolved by the 11–13 March 1949 board meeting in Geneva. Andre Repond, M.D., of Switzerland, already elected president for 1949–1950 to begin in August 1949, noted that the Federation member associations were not even able to support the travel of their members to meetings, let alone support a central office. He did not comment directly on Rees' position, but said that the WFMH should be certain of at least one year's income before moving to Geneva, and that it should stay in London—implying that Rees, if he felt himself able, could more easily assume directorial duties.

The final decision was not made until Rees approached the end of his term as president. It was at the third meeting of the executive board, 18–20 August 1949 in Geneva. Professor Rumke was the Chair and Repond was preparing to become president. Twelve nominations are noted in the minutes, including that of Rees. All were psychiatrists except for a sociologist, Dr. J. Seeley, nominated by John ("Jack") Griffin, M.D., general director of the Canadian Mental Health Association. As Rees' presidency was about to end he did not withdraw his name from candidacy; as there were no viable competitors he was appointed as the Federation's chief executive, to take charge of its central office or secretariat, which would be the focal point for its global activities. The appointment was for three years on a half-time salaried basis, pending the acquisition of sufficient funds to make it full-time, with the office remaining in London, "for the present." From the very beginning it was expected that it would, in due course, be transferred to Geneva.

Initially there was some uncertainty about the best title for the new chief executive. The titles of medical director and secretary general (following UN usage) were considered, but unadorned "director" was chosen, almost by default. Soddy was given the title of secretary general, reporting to the director on a one-day-weekly salaried basis. Within a year he became the assistant director and his involvement as an organizer, reporter, and convener of groups progressively increased. Later he became the Federation's scientific director. In this role he was more involved in policy making and served as senior editor of the proceedings of the international study group, which met in 1961 to assess future directions for the Federation.

After Soddy's move to assistant director, Esther Thornton, a former director in the wartime British nursing service, and an outstanding administrator and organizer, was appointed secretary general. She functioned as a combination supersecretary, office manager, and agency executive director, preparing reports for foundation grantors, keeping minutes, looking after salaries, and managing the details of the office. She was in every way the effective administrative director of the London secretariat, freeing Jack Rees' time for programmatic matters.

This office or secretariat remained in London during Rees' tenure from 1948 through 1961, and continued there until his successor, Francois Cloutier, M.D., moved it to Geneva in 1963. However, it depended heavily upon the New York-based U.S. Committee for WFMH, Inc. for financial support.

FUNDING THE REES ERA

ICMH Transformed into the WFMH: U.S. National Committee Inc.

The organization technically responsible for the Third International Congress on Mental Hygiene was the United States-based ICMH. With the emergence of the new Federation it prepared itself for dissolution. However, the process was halting and, despite hopes for an earlier transformation into the WFMH, this was delayed in order not to forfeit any gifts or bequests that might be made to it. Thus, while it held what was called its final meeting at the end of the 1948 Congress and no longer conducted international mental health projects, ICMH remained intact as an entity incorporated in Delaware and held the yearly administrative meetings required for its continued legal existence. In order to accomplish this, membership was reduced to five people who elected themselves as a governing board. All of the other members submitted their written resignations and the bylaws were amended to reflect the change. Operational responsibility remained in the hands of its secretary, William Beaty II. Through him gifts to it were transferred to WFMH (WFMH: U.S. National Committee Inc., 1966).

In 1952, a decision was made to change the ICMH name to the "U.S. Committee for WFMH" with Beaty as its executive director (Beaty, 1995). However, its final dissolution as a legal entity (despite the fact that it had had a different operational designation for five years) was again delayed. It was not until 1957 that it formally changed its name to World Federation for Mental Health: United States Committee Inc. (WFMH: U.S. Committee Inc., 1966). In 1958 the Committee was incorporated in the state of Delaware, as the ICMH had been.

Thus, while the WFMH had its central office in London, and was registered as an international non-governmental organization (NGO) in Geneva, its existence and capacity for achievement between 1948 and 1965 were, at first, dependent upon the ICMH, and later upon the entity into which ICMH was transformed: the World Federation for Mental Health: United States Committee, Inc. Its gifts and grants, as the earlier ones to the ICMH for transfer to the WFMH, came largely from enthusiastic people of good will in the United States, mainly in New York City. These included sympathetic foundation executives like Fremont-Smith of the Josiah Macy, Jr. Foundation (WFMH President, 1954) who had been involved with the Federation since its founding.

Beaty, Keeper of the Keys in the Rees Era and Beyond

As indicated above, Beaty, a part of Federation life during the Rees and Cloutier administrations, had been a key player from the point of its founding in 1948. As secretary of the ICMH, and then executive director of its successor, the WFMH: United States Committee Inc., he was involved in every aspect of their work. As noted in Chapter 4 the U.S. Committee ceased operations at the end of 1966, approximately one year after Cloutier's 1965 resignation. In 1967, when the Geneva secretariat finally closed its doors, the Federation was, for the moment, as Beaty put it, "dead in the water." He deposited his records at Cornell in the archives named after Oskar Diethelm, its professor and chairman of psychiatry during those years. After a time, the Oskar Diethelm Library, as it was known, was moved to the New York Academy of Medicine where the papers are available for study.

Bill Beaty moved gracefully in his varied roles. A socially adept, mannerly and gently accented North Carolinian, he reinforced that status by referring from time to time to a farm that had been in his family for nine generations. Well-connected in the New York foundation world, he knew the foundation heads and wealthy individual donors whose gifts supplied most of the Federation's early funding. To these credentials he added those of a graduate of the New York School of Social Work with a specialization in community organization. He also knew most of the significant mental health figures of the time including such seminal Federation achievers as Mead, Fremont-Smith, and Stevenson. He credited Marion E. Kenworthy, M.D., a child guidance pioneer and professor at the New York School of Social Work with starting him in mental health work.

When I interviewed Bill Beaty in New York City on 20 November 1995 he was 72 years old, being treated for cancer with chemotherapy, and still suffering some memory loss from a mild stroke six months earlier. However, his observations were sharp, and marked by irreverent humor. He retained his ability to describe the atmosphere of New York fundraising for the Federation in that era as well as the political context in which the new world organization had developed. As he recalled, when the 1948 founding document "Mental Health and World Citizenship" became known to the American press, "it branded us all as communists... we had a terrible time with that. The U.S. National Committee for Mental Health [forerunner of NMHA] wanted to endorse the international thing, but didn't want it in-house. They had too many problems of their own."

Once the WFMH: U.S. Committee Inc. was named in 1957 and formally incorporated in Delaware as a United States organization in 1958 with Beaty as its executive director, it had to formulate a mission statement. Its chief purposes, according to its archives were: "To engage in charitable, scientific, literary and educational activities, with particular reference to the promotion and conservation of the mental health of the people of all nations; to the study, treatment and prevention of nervous and mental disorders and mental defect; and in general to the promotion of the welfare of man" (WFMH: U.S. Committee Inc., 1966). However, the introduction to the archives notes, less elaborately, that its "major function...was to fund raise in the United States for the goals" of the European office. As Beaty put it even more bluntly, the Committee was formed as a "purely financial device," necessary because the WFMH, registered in Geneva from the beginning, had no official United States status to recommend it to the fund givers, who resided almost exclusively (if not entirely) within the United States. Potential donors and foundations were reluctant to send money overseas. Not only were there no tax advantages, they were also sensitive to the possibility of U.S. Congressional investigation by legislators who saw them as possibly un-American and exploitative or subversive. Once the U.S. Committee was established, American foundations and other donors were able to give money to it. Then, acting as a conduit, it made regular grants to the London secretariat. According to Beaty, Jack Rees was sufficiently impressed to ask him to work under him as executive director of the Federation. He had no wish to move to London, however, and instead agreed to serve, simultaneously with his U.S. Committee post, as the WFMH regional director for an ill-defined region including, besides the United States "anything contiguous with it, like Mexico." More formally stated, the Committee was "the New York Regional Office of the WFMH for North, Central and South America and the Caribbean." Regional Office functions included sending newsletters, periodicals, and annual reports to individual and organizational members in the Americas. The office asked for renewals of these members and "organized regional meetings on various topics of interest." (The archives contain no records of any regional meetings in these areas). Another function was to supply administrative backup for the WFMH representatives to the UN in New York. This included typing, office space, and sending reports to the WFMH board. (WFMH: U.S. Committee Inc., 1966).

After the Committee was formed it recruited, in the tradition of glamorous charities, affluent, socially prominent people including some psychiatrists, psychoanalysts, and psychologists, or their wives. Some individuals gave $1000 yearly, and several hundred WFMH members gave smaller amounts yearly. The Committee board was large, with one-third being elected or re-elected every year. One leader was Mrs. George Stern whose father, associated with the banking house of Lazard Freres, had perished on the Titanic. Jane Stern was a prominent fundraising party giver. As Beaty reported the process: "The ladies said we should do special events so we started having an annual dinner dance." The theme would reflect the country scheduled to host the next WFMH annual meeting. According to Beaty, most of the evenings cleared at least $50,000 net. This New York group, the nucleus of the Committee incorporated in 1958, supplied from 75 percent to 100 percent of Federation funds from 1948 until it ended its work in 1966. It included people such as the actress Celeste Holm and others whom Beaty described as being "in the Larry Kubie crowd." Kubie, a dean of American-born psychoanalysts in those years, was in fact the therapist for many well-known personalities, including some in the entertainment world. He was also a leader in bringing foreign-born analysts, refugees from Hitler, to the United States. As noted in Chapter 2, he was a friend and admirer of Jack Rees and wrote his obituary for the WFMH Bulletin.

CONTINUING ORGANIZATIONAL DEVELOPMENT DURING THE REES YEARS

Membership and Other Recurrent Themes

The Federation's continuing struggle to define itself administratively and organizationally, and its various attempts to reinvent its mission, are detailed in Chapter 5. However, the annual reports for the Rees years reveal additional issues, never solved to the satisfaction of everyone during its first half century of existence.

The report for 1948–1949, including the second annual meeting held in Geneva in August 1949, lists 62 member associations in 33 countries, with the largest number in the United States. The plethora of associations from a few of the industrial democracies of the global north, coupled with the small number from elsewhere, especially in the less developed southern world, was remarked upon. There was some fear that this might make it difficult to recruit associations from the less developed nations. This was conceptualized as a problem in "the art of the international conference." A goal was for the WFMH to provide a model of constructive international collaboration: "It is a vital matter for international relations that we should seek better methods of understanding each other." This included ways of protecting associations that were the sole representatives from small or nonindustrial nations from being overwhelmed by the large number of associations from industrial nations. It was decided, therefore, that "on issues which demand a vote, the delegates from each country, (not each member society), collectively exercise one vote" (WFMH, 1948–1949, p. 7).

A related problem in that immediate postwar era was the limitation of WFMH membership to organizations in countries eligible for membership in the UN. This appeared to some to be "contrary to the best mental health principles" (p. 10). In the last years of the century this problem arose again in relation to the WFMH membership of Taiwan, which was not permitted by the People's Republic of China (PRC) to be a member of the UN or an observer at its related agencies, such as the WHO. The mental health association of that island had been a long-term member of the WFMH which, by keeping it, ran the risk of losing its accreditation as a consultant to the WHO and other agencies. After much discussion, including correspondence with representatives of the PRC, which regarded Taiwan as a renegade province, it remained in the WFMH as the "Mental Health Association in Taiwan." However, the PRC did not allow official representatives from its country to attend WFMH meetings or to join the Federation.

Another concern emerging at this early stage and recurring since then has been with intra-Federation communication. Rees, confronting various complaints, stated that, "the Secretariat considers that the main problems of how to achieve real inward and mutual communication with our members still remain to be solved in the future" (p. 14).

By the time of the third annual meeting in Paris, 30 August—7 September 1950, the membership had decreased slightly to 59 associations (in the same 33 countries), but three transnational associations had been added. Two of these, the International Association for Child Psychiatry and the International Council of Nurses, remained for many years. But Rees had to acknowledge, in his Director's Report, that "our contact by correspondence with member associations is, with some notable exceptions, not good" (WFMH, 1950, p. 10). The proposed solution, dependent upon financial support, was to arrange for personal visits by members of the executive board or secretariat "to get to know their organization work and local problems." Other problems had become familiar: insufficient technical staff to examine various proposals for work, "enormous" pressure on the secretariat from correspondence and documents from the UN and other sources, preparations for WFMH administrative meetings, and the need to produce a Bulletin.

The 1951 annual report, listing 66 associations in 37 countries and two transnational associations, included a complete list of individual members or "associates" with by far the largest number coming from the United States. There were also criticisms from professional organizations. Psychiatrists in particular felt that colleagues should not become preoccupied with the broad issues addressed by the Federation, but should stick with the clinical tasks for which they had been trained. Rees called, for the first time, for some evaluation of the outcome of the Federation's efforts—a call which nearly 50 years later has not been satisfactorily answered.

At the fourth annual meeting held on 12 December 1951 during the Fourth International Congress of Mental Health in Mexico City, a complaint about voting procedures arose, foreshadowing similar recurrent complaints during the balance of the century. Although requests for nominations for the Executive Board had gone to all member associations in October, several voting representatives stated that "they had not personally been aware" of them, and had therefore "not fully exercised their right to nominate." This had to be resolved by a special meeting called by president William Line of Canada.

By the 1952 annual report, the WFMH had 72 member associations in 38 countries and four transnational associations, including the European League for Mental Hygiene and (a consequence of the Mexico City Congress), the Latin American Society for Mental Health. Most of the director's report was devoted to programmatic issues, but it noted poignantly that the Federation's Bulletin "is produced as a rule under considerable stress" and, because of limited funds, had not yet been able to have separate language additions." Communications in a Federation of many languages, cultures, and countries was an issue then as it is now: "The Executive Board is very conscious of the fact that in this, as in all other ways, the Federation should as soon as possible be multi-lingual and truly a world organization" (WFMH, 1952, p. 16).

By the sixth annual meeting, held at the University of Vienna 16–22 August 1953, membership had expanded to 80 associations in 41 countries and four transnational associations. The president for 1952–1953, psychiatrist M. K. el Kholy, M.D. of Egypt, identified two organizational concerns. One was that it had not yet been possible to move the secretariat to "a more neutral and convenient location, in Geneva." The other was the secretariat's effort—which he congratulated while acknowledging the problems of "a very limited staff"—to serve as a clearing house for relevant information to member associations. He exhorted the members as well as other groups to send information to the secretariat. Rees, confirming el Kholy, and sounding a theme recurring throughout the Federation's life, reported that "some of our members, indeed, give us little cause for pride; they are inert and do not even answer letters."

The failure of the membership to communicate also came up in another context. Dr. Eduardo Krapf of Argentina, chairman of the Executive Board, spoke of the lack of financial support from member organizations in countries other than the United States and the United Kingdom, saying that "too many people are members in name only" and unless new support is mobilized "the survival of the Federation will be in danger" (p. 37). Noting in this respect that the question is constantly being asked "What does the Federation do for us?" Rees said that one could also inquire, "What do you do for the Federation," or "Do you feel you need a Federation for which to do something?"

THE REES AGENDA

Conferences, Consultations, and "Parish Visits"

Rees' salary, although it was not what he considered "full time," and the fact that he could delegate management of the secretariat, allowed him to devote himself mainly to the extramural work of the Federation. From 1949 through 1961, as the single continuing WFMH officer through a parade of distinguished presidents elected for one year each, and Board chairmen whose tenure lasted for two to three years, he initiated, coordinated, or directed most of its substantive activity. Some presidents were deeply involved; others were mainly figureheads. He was often away from London, sometimes 30 to 40 times yearly, en route on Federation business to farflung corners of the globe or to European capitals.

Most Federation advocacy consisted of Rees' informal conversations with influential people able to insert mental health concerns into the agendas of government departments they led. His ability to do this stemmed from his personal relationships with government and World Health Organization leaders whom he had previously known in his position of medical psychiatric leadership in the British armed forces. His stature in this immediate post-World War II era, and the still small size of many governments, especially their health, education, and welfare agencies, made it easy for him to meet with the heads of national ministries relevant to mental health. Thus, his accounts of WFMH advocacy are sprinkled with phrases such as, "I met and had a long discussion with" or "the Federation was asked if it could do something," concerning the Caribbean, or a region in Africa, or elsewhere. He notes, for example, in *Reflections* that "some years ago the Federation was asked if it could do something in central Africa to help combat the massive increase in neurotic difficulties resulting from mechanisation and industrialisation in the developing countries" (Rees, 1966, p. 121). In consequence the secretariat spent two years developing contacts with professionals working in the region. This eventuated in a 1958 conference in Bukavu, the Congo, on "Mental Health in Africa South of the Sahara." WHO's regional committee and an intergovernmental commission for technical cooperation were involved and continued to work without Federation participation in the year after the meeting.

Reflections makes it clear that when "the Federation was asked" it usually meant that Jack Rees, in his role as director, was asked; sometimes he, himself, had stimulated the question. The broad base for Federation activities was not achieved through the Board, but through involving local groups in the conduct of conferences initiated by the secretariat, often consequent to questions and suggestions from organizations in the region.

Central among these conferences were the Federation's annual meetings, which usually attracted some 300 to 400 participants. They were held each year in different countries, affording the opportunity to discuss locally and regionally important issues and to win government support. They were also useful in stimulating the organization of local mental health associations, but most were in Europe at the sites of already established groups: Geneva, Paris, Brussels, Vienna, Berlin, Copenhagen, Vienna, Barcelona, Edinburgh, and again in Paris. Three were held outside of Europe: in Mexico, Toronto, and Istanbul. Three were adjuncts to world congresses, following the one in 1948 in London. The three world congresses of the Rees era were in Mexico in 1951, Toronto in 1954, and Paris in 1961. These attracted larger crowds than the annual meetings and were viewed as opportunities to foster interest in the organization and its goals.

The conferences, congresses, and seminars listed in *Reflections*, some of which took place during Cloutier's tenure, are included in Appendix I. The topics were eclectic, most reflecting the human relations approach to mental health. One topic, that of refugees, anticipated the Federation's later focus on clinical care. Aside from the annual meetings and congresses, the Federation sponsored a number of special conferences. Among them were one on health and human relations in Germany soon after the war, a meeting on student mental health in 1956, and in 1959, two meetings on migrants and refugees. After the 1961 world congress in Paris there was an international meeting on plans for community mental health attended by officials from a number of countries.

Rees attached particular importance to his "visiting program." This involved meetings with mental health associations ("parish work") as well as with government leaders in different parts of the world. He felt that the visits exerted an important influence not only on the new mental health associations but on public opinion and the opinions of ministers of health, education, and social welfare in the countries visited. During several of them he and other members of the Executive Board organized teaching seminars for local officials and professionals. Two major examples were "Mental Health and Infant Development" in Chichester, England in 1952 and "Mental Health and Family Life" in the Philippines in 1958. In keeping with the Federation ethos of the period these were academic, scholarly, research-oriented study groups. Under Rees, there were consistent efforts to bring more scientists, especially social scientists, into the organization.

A small Scientific Committee composed mainly of psychiatrists with special research experience met in connection with the annual meetings under the chairmanship of H.C. Rumke, M.D., professor of psychiatry at the University of Utrecht in the Netherlands (WFMH president, 1953–1954). Financial difficulties brought the work of this committee to a close. However, in addition to the work with UN agencies, a number of conferences and publications (see References and Appendix I) took place, ranging from problems of infant development to the rehabilitation of head injuries.

Rees also credited academic psychiatry with effecting changes in the attitudes of governments and institutions to such issues as the prevention of mental ill health and illness: "a steady increase in awareness amongst the academic institutions of North America and Europe has led to a great deal of educational interchange in psychiatry and the development of prophylactic ideas. Much more international interest in public health has been aroused as the result of joint meetings, increased travel, the use of sabbatical leaves, or teaching fellowships...." (Rees, 1966, p. 119).

The most ambitious project of this era was suggested to the Executive Board by Frank Fremont-Smith, who had been one of its founders and then president in 1954. This was the organization of a World Mental Health Year for 1960. Its initial goal was to carry out several projects extending through Federation contacts to all of the world's countries which might yield comparative data on which to base future activities. The topics to be undertaken were conceived in academic and research terms. They included childhood mental health, attitudes toward mental disorder, mental health teaching in professional education, and mental health and industrialization. They also included two issues of contemporary interest: psychological problems of migration and mental health problems of aging.

The board was unsuccessful in finding financial and organizational support to carry out this set of projects. However, a second goal did not require special funding. This was to have member associations survey the special needs of their countries or areas in order "to make greater inroads on the problems of mental health in these localities" (Rees, 1966, p. 109). The idea was welcomed in many countries and brought their mental health needs to the attention of their governments and public. However, unlike the practical thrust of the World Mental Health Day of the 1990s, with its nonspecific, consciousness-raising emphasis on reforming inadequate clinical services, these projects were predominantly of a data-gathering nature. Of the more than 350 new or amplified projects initiated in over 50 countries, the majority, 230, were of a research or "scientific" nature.

Rees and the UN

Rees was very pleased by what he saw as the Federation's role, effected by several years of close contact, in changing the attitudes of WHO officials—and hence those of national governments—toward mental health. The opposition of one of the regional offices of the WHO, and of the chief medical officers of some countries, to spending time and money on mental health seemed to him to have vanished in the years between 1948 and the early 1960s. He was also impressed by the spread of interest in mental health within the secretariats of agencies other than the WHO. He attributed both changes to the efforts of Ronald Hargreaves, M.D., the first chief of the WHO's mental health section.

The era saw a number of collaborative projects and conferences with the range of UN-affiliated agencies. One close to the heart of both Rees and longtime board member Otto Klineberg (WFMH president 1966-1967) concerned the intramural processes of international conferences funded by UNESCO as part of its general interest in reducing international tensions. A major event was UNESCO's grant of $10,000 for a study by Margaret Mead of the socioeconomic and cultural problems arising from industrialization in the less developed countries (Mead, 1953). A later UNESCO grant through the WFMH to Marie Jahoda (1960) resulted in a study of race relations and mental health. A conference on "Uprooting and Resettlement," including representatives of both donor and host governments, was organized parallel to the Vienna annual meeting in 1958. It was one of the influences that led the UN High Commissioner for Refugees to obtain psychiatric help in dealing with the refugee camp populations. The WFMH also organized a conference on malnutrition and food habits in Mexico in 1960 at the request of the Pan-American Health Organization (PAHO), the hemispheric arm of WHO, with the cooperation of the WHO, Unicef, and FAO, the UN's Food and Agriculture Organization.

As the Federation's involvements grew, the need for representation at the several UN headquarters became increasingly important. Initially Rees, himself, as the trusted intimate of many of the first directors of UN agencies, was the primary linking person. From time to time others assumed these tasks. These were mainly university professors and other scholars with international reputations and friends spanning many different cultures, people whom he described as having "vast experience and stature." As he wrote, "probably nothing that the Federation has done has had greater significance than the establishment of friendly personal relations between the government administrators who represent their countries in the UN and the wise and experienced representatives of the Federation...." (Rees, 1966, p. 103).

However, with time, UN agencies and NGOs were becoming increasingly aware of the WFMH. Many of the new demands no longer required the "wise and experienced" volunteer statesmen who could be effective stand-ins for Jack Rees. In New York the task of representing the WFMH at a variety of meetings, and transmitting messages and impressions to its leaders, was initially handled by a secretary of the U.S. NMHA. As the work load grew, responsibility was assumed first by Mrs. Helen Ascher, who carried it as a full-time volunteer until her death, when she was succeeded by Elizabeth (Mrs. Myer) Cohen. Mrs. Cohen's husband had been a senior official with the U.S. Relief and Rehabilitation agency after World War II and they both were personally and organizationally connected with a large network of influential people. She was still present, but in the process of giving up her WFMH tasks, when I became president in 1981 and my brief contacts with her and her husband revealed them as immensely knowledgeable and effective people, in the Rees "wise and experienced" tradition. Elizabeth's main contacts as the WFMH representative to UN headquarters, New York, were mainly with Unicef, which was then called the Social Commission, and to a lesser extent with the Division of Social Defence, concerned with delinquency and criminology.

In Geneva the representative was Professor E. E. Krapf, originally of Argentina, a member of the WFMH Executive Board and its president for a time in 1956 before he was recruited by the WHO to become director of its section on mental health. He visited with the WHO, the European offices of the Social Commission, the International Labor Organization (ILO), other branches of the UN, and other international organizations. He was succeeded by Dr. Audeoud-Naville.

At UNESCO in Paris the representative was Mlle. Jeanne Duron of the French League of Mental Health. Rees himself was elected chairman of the conference of all NGOs in official relationship to UNESCO. This kind of recognition was immensely satisfying. It gave concrete form to much that was difficult to pin down since it involved stimulating positive and constructive awareness where none (or even hostility) had existed before, and working through others to accomplish goals the Federation alone had neither the manpower nor the money to achieve. Rees must have had this on his mind when he summarized his years of active leadership beginning with the preparatory commission in 1946, through his presidency from 1948 to 1949, and as director until January 1962, in characteristically optimistic fashion: "looking back I am conscious that [WFMH] has achieved far more than I could ever have visualised in the way of kindling interest in matters where none existed previously and of creating active organizations and enlisting more active government support than ever before." (Rees, 1966, p. 134).

Chapter 4

The Geneva Secretariat: 1962–1967

THE DEPARTURE OF JACK REES

Rees, progressively aware of his own diminishing capacities, began reminding various members of the board as early as the middle to late 1950s that they should begin thinking about his successor. The minutes of the 2 February 1959 finance and general purposes committee (the entire board less six members of a credentials committee) note: "The Director reminded the Committee that his resignation would have to take effect soon." Two and a half years later, at the 22–28 August 1961 meeting of the Executive Board in Paris, it had not yet taken effect, but he said that, although he had continued to fill the post of director, he had actually "retired, on account of age, some six years before." The problem was that "financial considerations had stood in the way of appointing a successor." Now, however, "it was absolutely necessary to take action."

In recent years the post of Director had been discussed with some 15 to 20 men, none of whom had wished to present himself as a candidate. But now two psychiatrists, Francois Cloutier, M.D., of Montreal and Peter Berner, M.D., of Vienna, were available for interviews. They would come as observers later in the meeting so the Board could meet them informally, and perhaps come to a decision.

There was a great deal of discussion within the Board about financial arrangements and administrative aspects of the new appointment, and a general feeling that it would be a mistake to act too quickly. It was also felt that there must be available candidates aside from the two in question. Particular emphasis was placed on the importance of appointing "younger men" to the nominating committee, rather than limiting it to former presidents. As Andre Repond (WFMH president 1949-1950), put it: "Former Presidents knew Dr. Rees' qualities so well that they might have difficulty in believing that any candidate was capable of replacing him." However, the five person nominating committee eventually appointed was made up of veteran Federation officers. Its composition suggests the board's preoccupation with salary. Sir Geoffrey Vickers, treasurer, was chairman, and James Mitchell, also concerned with board finances, was a member. The other members were all senior psychiatrists. They included Tsung-yi Lin, M.D., Professor and Chairman of Psychiatry of the National University of Taiwan (vice-chairman of the board, 1960-1961, and later president, 1974–1979); Paul Sivadon, M.D., of France, then a professor at Brussels (president, 1959–1960); and Brock Chisholm, M.D. (president, 1957–1958).

Other factors conspired to precipitate a rapid decision. Beyond the questions of his own age and health, Rees sincerely believed that it was time for new leadership. There was also a general consensus within the Board that in order to reach its full potential, the organization should move away from what some felt was the parochial atmosphere of English-speaking Britain, a view shared by the French Sivadon. The right place in their view, influenced especially by Montreal-born and Paris-based Professor Otto Klineberg, was the European world of French speaking Geneva, with its concentration of UN agencies, particularly the WHO.

The Board, bowing to Rees' wishes, accepted his resignation as WFMH director to become effective four months later, at the end of 1961. In keeping with his desire to remain associated with the Federation at a reduced level of responsibility, as well as to maintain some influence on its future course, it appointed him a "special consultant" as of 1 January 1962, when his successor was to take office. Arrangements were made for a supplemental pension and a contract "making his services available to the Federation as may be required for general consultation and special assignments." Later, while maintaining his consultant status, he became, along with Lady Priscilla Norman and Otto Klineberg, an "Honorary President."

THE APPOINTMENT OF FRANCOIS CLOUTIER

Despite the board's fear of premature action, the nominating committee moved with dispatch to appoint Rees' successor. He was psychiatrist Francois Cloutier, M.D., a bilingual resident of Montreal in the French-speaking Canadian province of Quebec. Cloutier was named Director-designate so quickly that he was able to continue as an observer later in the same executive board meeting where he had presented himself as a candidate 22–28 August 1961. His appointment was formally announced approximately one week later at the 14th annual meeting of the Federation in Paris on 2 September 1961. Much of his inaugural address to the annual meeting was in English, lauding Rees as the man who could not be replaced. But his last comments were in French: the announcement of his appointment "in the land of [his] culture and mother tongue," he proclaimed, augured well for the future. The Viennese Berner, the other potential candidate, later became Mental Health Advisor to the Office of the United Nations High Commissioner for Refugees in Geneva, and a member of the WFMH scientific committee.

Cloutier's primary sponsor, Otto Klineberg, was also born in Quebec and was multilingual. He felt that Cloutier, fluent in French and English, known as a "dynamic personality," sartorially impeccable and a charmer, would be the "golden boy" to take the Federation out of London into the truly international world of the UN and WHO. "It was to be a new day" (H. David, interview, 1996).

WFMH Presidents and the Role of Otto Klineberg

The process of recruiting and confirming the new Director went on with minimal involvement by the WFMH presidents who were members of the Executive Board. Nonetheless, they agreed unanimously to the recommendations of the nominating committee, supported by Director Rees and by Klineberg, who had been named Executive Board chairman at the September 1961 annual meeting. All expressed enthusiasm about the possible benefits of the move to Geneva.

President during the beginning of the search for Rees' replacement in 1960–1961 was French-speaking A. C. Pacheco e Silva, M.D., Professor of Psychiatry at the University of Sao Paulo in Brazil. He was grandly optimistic about the change, stating that with the appointment of Cloutier, "WFMH is…established as a mature entity with experience of mental health throughout the world" (Silva, 1961).

President for the 1961–1962 term, which spanned Rees' actual retirement, Cloutier's actual appointment, and his first six months as Director, was George S. Stevenson, who had been Medical Director and Consultant for the U.S. National Mental Health Association and, at the time, was much occupied with NMHA affairs.

The most influential and interested member of the Board, its chairman from 1961 to 1966 and then WFMH President for 1966–1967 was Klineberg. A medical doctor by training who later took a Ph.D., he was not a practicing clinician but a career social scientist who had taught at Columbia University, at the University of Paris as professor of social psychology, and in Latin America and Asia. Because of his work, and his engaging personality, he was sufficiently known by 1948 to be appointed a member of the Roffey Park group, which wrote the Federation's founding document "Mental Health and World Citizenship." Its philosophy fitted his own views. A Quaker and a pacifist, he was "deep in his heart, a citizen of the world" (Visseur, 1995). In the early 1950s he had taken a leave of absence from Columbia to accept a UNESC0 appointment as director of its Paris-based project on the reduction of international tensions. There he tried to translate into action his conviction that improving the mental health of national populations would reduce the likelihood of conflict between them.

As a much respected figure and one of the WFMH founders, Klineberg's recommendation carried great weight. Thus, with Rees urgently asking to be replaced, Cloutier was appointed without the thorough international search that might have been expected for such a sensitive and demanding post. Jack Rees, too, felt along with Klineberg that since they were both of retirement age this could be the beginning of a new and more youthful era. However, while agreeing with the importance attributed by European Board members to Cloutier's command of French, he also supported the nomination on social and political grounds. He felt that Cloutier's Canadian background would give him some of the "solidity and rationality" considered characteristic of American professionals. At the same time he could not be labelled as "American" by European Federation members endemically hostile to the idea of "domination" by the United States. As Beaty put it: "Jack thought that he was a perfect compromise" (Beaty, 1995). Beaty also commented that the potential insecurity of the job may have made it less attractive for many applicants.

No one seems to have paid much attention to the fundamental differences between the old and new Director. They were occupied mainly with losing Rees and the secretariat's forthcoming move to Geneva. Thus, the Federation was fated to experience an abrupt change of leadership from an older person of international stature with global connections, accustomed to dealing as an equal with the world's most influential health leaders, to a younger, less experienced, less well-connected, individual of modest reputation.

CLOUTIER AS DIRECTOR GENERAL: 1962–1965

Opening the Geneva Secretariat

Cloutier disliked London and the British domination of the secretariat. He was also eager on personal grounds to move the secretariat to Geneva. This would allow him and his French-born physician wife, Solange, to live and work in a French-speaking environment, more comparable than London to their native Montreal, and more congenial. Officially, the move would emphasize the Federation's status as an authentically European-based organization, as well as bring it closer to UN offices and the headquarters of other international non-governmental organizations (NGOs). Unhappily, there were delays in the availability of office space and the move was delayed for another year and a half, until mid-1963.

Organizational Development and Administration

Much of Cloutier's first year, 1962, was devoted to learning about the organization. It was at his first Executive Board meeting in London in February that the decision was made to move the headquarters from London to Geneva at some time in 1963. One of his expressed goals

(WFMH, 1962) was to "produce more publications in different languages" and "to establish more than occasional contacts with Eastern European countries." The annual meeting, scheduled for August in Peru, had to be canceled because of political unrest in the country, so it was postponed until late October in conjunction with a meeting of the European League for Mental Hygiene in Florence, Italy. In Florence the decision was made to raise the fees of the three classes of members: individual, local or state (affiliated), and national or transnational (voting). It was decided to retain the principle "that no one should be kept out of the Federation for financial reasons."

Significant time was devoted to making personal contacts. Cloutier was asked by the Caribbean Federation for Mental Health (described in the annual report for 1962 as "under the leadership of Dr. Bertram Schaffner"—see Chapter 3) to serve as a consultant in Jamaica to discuss founding a chair of psychiatry at the University of the West Indies. Several visits were made to the offices of UN-related agencies, especially the WHO in Geneva and UNESCO in Paris, and to various meetings. But aside from arranging published reports of earlier meetings there were no major advances in the Federation's international mental health agenda.

The most important organizational events of 1963 were the administrative headquarters' move to Geneva, the creation of the two new posts of associate director for administration and for the information center (see below), and the establishment of the WFMH legal headquarters in the United States, i.e., the formation of a corporation with the same purposes and objectives as "the World Federation for Mental Health an organization registered in Geneva, Switzerland." Its purpose was to "facilitate our contacts with our New York office" (WFMH, 1963).

During 1964 Cloutier was almost constantly on the road visiting member associations in the various countries of Asia, North America, and Europe ("studying the mental health situation") and attending meetings of NGOs and UN agencies. The main Federation-wide event of the year was the 17th annual meeting held from 3–7 August in Berne, Switzerland. It was largely concerned with administrative issues.

The Problem of Fundraising

A special committee led by Executive Board chairman Klineberg was convened in London in February 1963 to review the tasks of the new Director, now in the post for 13 months, in preparation for the long-delayed move to Geneva. Having executive powers, the committee was able to make decisions ordinarily reserved for the entire Board. One such decision was to approve Cloutier's request that his title be inflated to "Director General." Another concerned an addition to the new director general's staff. He was Dr. Pierre Visseur, a semi-retired political scientist also recommended by Klineberg, who was impressed by his work on projects for peace promotion for an organization known as World Brotherhood. He was to be employed as Associate Director as of 1 May 1963 with the assignment of moving the secretariat to Geneva. He soon acquired another task the Executive Board had not anticipated. Although the board had specifically requested Cloutier to assume the role of chief fundraiser for the Federation, he immediately assigned this responsibility to Visseur. Visseur was also given primary responsibility for administration, the organization of meetings and conferences, and relations with WFMH members.

Cloutier's wish not to be involved in fundraising might have reflected a legitimate pessimism about the likelihood of success in this area. In 1962, not long after his appointment, he had notified the Board that prospects for foundation and other support were not bright: "Present-day Foundations do not like to provide money to supply the general expenses of any organization's bureaucracy," and when such grants are made it is usually "in the earliest stages of the organization's existence." Cloutier continued that after 15 years of life "the Federation appears to have reached its limits in the help that can be expected" (WFMH, 1966).

Of course he was correct. In retrospect his awareness of his new organization's financial fragility, and his decision not to engage in fundraising, suggest that the rapid depletion of

Federation resources during his administration could not have come as a surprise to him. At the 1963 annual meeting in Amsterdam the treasurer, Sir Geoffrey Vickers, regretted that he could not "more confidently forecast the Federation's financial future…[its] reserves are still insufficient to bridge any large or persistent gap between revenue and expenditures and great efforts may well be needed to secure minimum revenue requirements during the next year or two.…" However, he ended on a note of optimism: "I believe that it has a better chance than ever before of securing increasingly reliable and adequate support for its work" (WFMH, 1963).

Looking back, Pierre Visseur acknowledged the fundraising burden Cloutier had shifted to him. He described himself as having been responsible for the "legal, fiscal, administrative and organizational needs" of the Federation (Visseur, 1995). Initially, though, the need to find money was not as pressing as it later became. During the first year in Geneva, 1963–1964, approximately 80 percent of the WFMH budget was still supplied by the U.S. Committee for the WFMH. But Cloutier and Beaty, the committee's executive director, had different perspectives on fundraising. Although the New York Committee received grants from a number of U.S. foundations for transmittal to the WFMH, many of its members, as described in Chapter 3, viewed the Federation as a good cause for which it would raise money through dinners and balls. Its board included some of the city's leading psychiatrists, but it was dominated by socially prominent women who enjoyed it as a socially worthwhile and internationally significant activity with a touch of glamour.

Cloutier did attend many of the social affairs and "charmed the ladies, but he made fun of them" feeling that the Committee's activities did not provide an appropriate financial basis for an international organization (David, 1996).

Again, Cloutier was correct in his perception of financial fragility. At the same time, though, he greatly "oversold the capacities and capabilities of the Federation claiming to have resources far beyond those which actually existed" (David, 1996). This had repercussions even in relatively minor aspects of office operation. Thus, he issued a memorandum saying that if any staff person took a visitor to lunch it would be at his/her own expense. He also suggested that in order to show good will staff members should pay for some of their own travel, even on official business. However, he did not observe his own dicta, spending large amounts of WFMH resources on entertainment and, particularly, on travel. As one source put it, he "was more interested in promoting his own career, living well and travelling well, than in the well-being of the Federation."

As time went on the U.S. Committee, which had taken Jack Rees to its heart, became disenchanted with Cloutier. Its leaders had found him incapable of succeeding Rees, "very brusque," a "total loss," and his appointment a "terrible mistake" (Beaty, 1995). By 1964, just a few months after the move to Geneva, the Committee's financial contributions were diminishing, a prelude to the eventual dissolution of the Geneva secretariat.

Henry David and the Information Center

The most successful WFMH activity during this period was the Information Center, which functioned between 1963 and 1965. Its roots were in a conversation between Jack Rees and Otto Klineberg in late 1962, toward the end of Cloutier's first year in office. Klineberg knew that the newly established Clearing House for Mental Health Information within the U.S. National Institute of Mental Health (NIMH) was interested in making international connections, and he thought the WFMH might be able to obtain a contract with it. He telephoned psychologist Henry David, Ph.D., asking him to explore the possibility of obtaining the hoped-for NIMH contract. At that time David was chief psychologist for the state of New Jersey, Department of Institutions and Agencies, and already held several NIMH contracts. He was also an ideal choice for international work. Born in Germany and fluent in that language, he had been sent to America by his parents to escape the Nazis. Most important were his strong personal ties to

Klineberg. As a member of the U.S. Army Air Corps U.S. Strategic Bombing Survey in Europe, he had been jeep driver, body guard, and note taker for Otto Klineberg while the latter was interviewing leading German officials during and immediately after World War II on the psychological aspects of the air war. The conversations with Klineberg sparked his interest in psychology and initiated a life-long friendship. Klineberg served on his doctoral committee at Columbia and was, in many ways, his mentor. After completing his doctoral work David became active in international psychological and other nongovernmental organizations, espousing the principles of individual integrity and freedom. He accepted Klineberg's unexpected telephone call as a possible bridge to further international involvement and agreed to write a proposal to NIMH on behalf of the WFMH.

David was successful in obtaining a one-year contract for the WFMH with the NIMH. The NIMH Clearing House wanted an organization to which it could address questions about mental health anywhere in the world and receive answers within 24 hours. Since this was manifestly impossible, its director, Dr. Lorraine Bouthelet, concurred with his idea that the new Center should prepare a series of reports about mental health activities and institutions in particular countries. It would also develop a network of correspondents and other sources of continuing information. With the contract arranged and informal agreements in place between David and Bouthelet, the WFMH Executive Board moved to bring him onto its staff. In early February 1963 Cloutier, on behalf of the Board, offered him the post of Associate Director (for Information) and invited him to attend the Executive Board meeting during the 1963 annual meeting scheduled for Amsterdam in mid-July. That was to be an important opportunity to build connections with major information-disseminating institutions since it would be attended by Eduardo Krapf, M.D. (WFMH president, 1956), retiring Director of the WHO's Mental Health Section and his successor Pieter Baan, M.D., as well as Stanley Yolles, M.D., director of the U.S. NIMH, which was to fund the WFMH information operation.

The time and place of the Amsterdam meeting had been planned prior to Rees' retirement. Its theme, "Population and Mental Health," came from a declaration by the WFMH Executive Board convened in January 1962 in the moment between directors. That declaration stated that the most important international problems of the 20th century include "the very considerable acceleration of population growth…and the fact that some of the most marked increases are coinciding with the poorest natural resources." So it happened that Henry David was offered two proposals by the WFMH. One was to become its Associate Director and Director of its new information center, officially beginning 1 October 1963. He was to be directly responsible to Cloutier for scientific matters, and to Visseur for administrative matters. The other proposal was to edit the Amsterdam proceedings. This too he accomplished, and the published proceedings are an important record of the Federation's international mental health agenda (David, 1964).

The NIMH contract also included funds for an assistant (a technically qualified reference analyst) and a secretary. However, hiring the assistant did not proceed smoothly. David, who had been promised a free hand in recruiting, was unpleasantly surprised by an 11 June 1963 letter from Cloutier that he had "an excellent assistant" for him, already working for the WHO. The *fait accompli* was confirmed by a 5 August letter informing him that the candidate to become his assistant was Cloutier's wife. Prior to coming to Switzerland she had been a medical officer in a Canadian provincial department of welfare. Cloutier pointed out that she had had experience in information gathering, that her status as a physician would be helpful, and that a precedent existed in that Jack Rees' wife (also a physician) had been heavily involved in Federation affairs. Furthermore, Swiss law stipulated that she could only work for an international organization. Yet, he noted: "Of course, you have to feel free to choose your immediate collaborator."

The situation was extremely difficult for David to accept. He told Cloutier that he did not feel that the appointment was wise "because of the delicacies" in working with the Director's wife, and he complained by phone to Otto Klineberg. However, the process had begun and in a letter of 29 August 29 1963 Cloutier informed him that "Solange's nomination has been extremely well accepted by everybody, especially in WHO circles." Finally, despite serious misgivings about the future of his relationship with Cloutier, David decided to make peace with the situation, but to resign at the end of the contract year. It is apparent that Cloutier had some sense of his discomfort as, in a letter of September 1963, he emphasized the advantages of his wife's status as a physician: "I have the impression that in many instances the kind of information we are expected to furnish under contract might only be given by one medical doctor to another, this being due to regulations concerning professional etiquette." This attempted reassurance, unfortunately, revealed a complete lack of understanding of the nature of the information expected by NIMH. In a letter written the next day he took a different, more threatening tone, telling "Dear Henry" that "If there are any queries in your mind I strongly suggest that you keep them for yourself until we meet."

Despite these difficulties David established the Center, work progressed, the country reports (see WFMH publication list) were produced and, when questions were asked that couldn't be answered, he telephoned a colleague in another country for the answer—as did the Secretary General's office after 1983. He became known to the Geneva community as a scholarly contributor to mental health knowledge, and was active in building and maintaining Federation relationships with other Geneva-based NGOs, UN agencies, and institutions. In short, the operation was sufficiently successful to warrant a grant renewal for a second year, with him as its moving spirit, and he remained.

Cloutier's Directorship Comes to an End

The information center was an oasis of stability in the increasingly turbulent and adversarial context of the Geneva secretariat. By 1964 office doors that had originally been open were closed (David, 1996). This was partly due to Cloutier's autocratic administrative style. He was especially concerned about staff comments that might be critical of his administration, and tried to control them by having all incoming and outgoing mail monitored in his office. This caused some embarrassment, as occasional letters addressed to particular individuals never reached them. He also issued memoranda about how to manage windows, electrical apparatus, smoking, and other matters.

The most difficult and continuing problem was money. Pierre Visseur, in pursuit of his assigned fundraising responsibilities, obtained some small grants for congresses, but no more. Executive Board members, mostly distinguished mental health professionals, stated their willingness to open doors and make connections through which money could be raised, but they did not act. For most of them, Board membership was "a reaffirmation of their international standing…they were less interested in actually giving time to this endeavor" (David, 1996). There were no members representing business who had mental illness in their families and might have been motivated to get corporate money. As funds were expended at a rate far exceeding income, deficits of nearly $30,000 each were incurred for the 1963/64 and 1964/65 years (WFMH, 1966).

As time went on both Jack Rees and Otto Klineberg came to regret Cloutier's appointment, "but they were stuck" (David, 1996). A tense meeting of the Bureau (predecessor of the executive committee) on 2 March 1965 focused on the Federation's rapidly diminishing financial resources. Henry David offered to resign. On 22 April 1965 he did submit his resignation in writing to Cloutier, to become effective at the end of the second year of the NIMH contract on 31 October of the same year. In that letter, though, he made it clear that he did not intend to terminate his association with the Federation.

After his return to the United States he continued for a time as a consultant and attended an occasional Federation meeting. In 1979, together we presented a symposium on mental health and unwanted pregnancy to the Salzburg World Congress (see Part III of this volume). In 1983, after his organization of a workshop on responsible parenthood at the Washington, DC World Congress for Mental Health, I appointed him chairman of a new WFMH committee dealing with that topic. From 1991 to 1995 he was an elected member-at-large of the Board, the only person to have served both as a staff member and a Board member.

Available records show that following David's resignation at the end of October 1965, the Executive Board instructed Cloutier, still Director General, to "conduct formal contract renewal negotiations" with NIMH for the information center contract. Peter Berner agreed to become its new director, but NIMH had lost confidence in the Federation's capacity to perform the work and announced that it would not renew the contract until a permanent WFMH Director was appointed—an eventuality which did not occur until my appointment as Secretary General in 1983, nearly 20 years later. However, NIMH did offer sufficient support for Berner to devote part of his time to the country surveys until it finally terminated its relationship with the WFMH on 30 November 1966, a year after Cloutier's departure.

The final decision to push for Cloutier's resignation was difficult for the Executive Board. WFMH presidents were reluctant to become involved. The three presidents during the Cloutier regime had all been administrative psychiatrists, fully occupied elsewhere. The mid-1962 to mid-1963 presidency was filled by Phon Sangsingkeo, M.D., Under-Secretary of State for Public Health, Director General, Department of Medical Services, and Professor of Psychiatry at the University of Bangkok in Thailand. In 1963-1964 the president was Professor G. P. Alivasatos, Emeritus Professor of Hygiene at the University of Athens. Two presidents covered the time during which Cloutier was visibly declining and then was discharged by the board. Alan Stoller, M.D., of the Mental Health Authority of Victoria, Australia occupied the position in 1964-1965. Chief Sir Samuel Manuwa, Federal Public Service Commissioner of Nigeria, became president in 1965, remaining until 1966, after Cloutier had resigned and the Federation's future was in doubt. Manuwa was succeeded for the 1966-1967 term by Otto Klineberg. All were capable individuals, very interested in the goals and operations of the Federation. No one, however, was ready to take the initiative to remove Cloutier and undertake yet another change of administration.

The major pressure for Cloutier's removal came, finally, from Board member George Morrison Carstairs, M.D., Professor of Psychiatry at Edinburgh. Morris, as he was known to his friends, was frugal and reserved, the opposite of Cloutier, dedicated to the goals of the Federation and rather stern and serious. He expressed his deep concern for the future of the organization and its need for an effective and sympathetic central office, and was able to persuade Klineberg, as Executive Board chairman, to see that Cloutier was removed. The decision to request his resignation was taken at an Executive Board meeting in June 1965. Cloutier could have finished out the year, but he chose not to do so. The archives contain a handwritten note from him to Visseur, dated the 6 June, just after the board meeting: "For medical reasons I have to take a few days off. I'll be back in the office on the 21st." Visseur replied, "you will need some sunshine after that much rain!" Cloutier returned to submit his resignation. He did not, however, take official leave from the WFMH until nearly five months later. That was in the course of the general assembly at the Federation's 18th annual meeting held in Bangkok, Thailand from 15 to 19 November 1965. The general assembly took place on 16 November from 5 PM to 7 PM under the chairmanship of president Alan Stoller, M.D., of Australia. Out of a total of 152 WFMH member associations (national and local), 77 from 33 countries and two transnational associations were represented.

This Bangkok meeting was the first not attended by Jack Rees, "on doctor's orders." The incoming president, Chief Manuwa, occupied elsewhere, was inducted in absentia by Dr. Stoller, who noted that this election brought for the first time "a distinguished representative of Africa to the Presidency of the Federation." The Executive Board did not muster a quorum for its regular annual session because of distance and the costs involved, but as this was the first annual meeting held in Asia, "participants left Bangkok with the conviction that [it] had been a significant milestone in the Federation's development towards extended global responsibilities" (WFMH, 1965).

In his last report as Director General (WFMH, 1965) Cloutier pointed to the Information Center as the most important scientific project of the year. He described his time with the WFMH as "stimulating," expressed his appreciation to the membership for their support during "four of the most productive years of [his] professional life," and referred to the images and emotions associated with providing "inspiration and guidance" in the course of "influencing, even modestly, the…mental health services" in many places. Finally, he noted that he had hoped to be able to present his successor (who would have the title of Secretary General) to the group. The official report of the 18th annual meeting prepared by Pierre Visseur noted that Dr. Cloutier's final statement was "received with applause" and that Dr. Klineberg, who as vice-president was in the chair in Chief Manuwa's absence, "expressed the gratitude of the organization to Dr. Cloutier for his manifold contributions towards the promotion of mental health through the channels of the Federation." This was within the Federation's tradition of courtly civility.

At the time of Cloutier's resignation, Pierre Visseur tendered his own resignation, which was not accepted. After the Bangkok meeting he became Acting Director. Just two weeks later, in December 1965, the proviso of "acting" was removed and he was appointed Director. Everyone expected the job to be temporary.

1965–1967: DIRECTOR PIERRE VISSEUR

Visseur has been described as "a splendid man" who "held WFMH together" during this difficult moment in its history (Beaty, 1995). He appears to have been especially good at repairing the tense relationships within the secretariat and building the personal associations essential to maintaining the Federation's collaboration with the WHO and other Geneva institutions. The success of his efforts is suggested in his note about the WHO Mental Health Office representative, Maria Pfister, M.D., "whom we saw often at WFMH headquarters as a valuable contributor to seminars and projects." Visseur's warmth was also reflected in his cordial relations with her husband, Hans Pfister, M.D., Professor of Psychiatry at the University of Zurich and head of the city's health services. Pfister allowed his patients free access to the university hospital's surrounding park. During the annual visit of a city government delegation a patient, seeing them walk through the park en route to lunch, shouted, "There they are again, those bastards, coming to gobble and guzzle." "Somewhat shocked," as Visseur put it, "the dignitaries asked Professor Pfister what was wrong with the man and why he was so hostile to them. Nothing seriously wrong," assured Professor Pfister, "he has only had a lucid interval!" (Visseur, 1995).

The Federation's annual report for 1965 reveals Visseur's futile attempts to stave off incipient financial disaster. He had been functioning since 1963 in the same manner as the executive director of any voluntary organization. This involved working "in close consultation with the WFMH Treasurer and Auditors," meeting with business leaders "in connection with the development of the Federation's financial structure," organizing periodic membership and fundraising campaigns, and consulting with several European member associations on problems of "organization, fund-raising, mental health information and coordination." He also arranged the annual meetings, assemblies of voting members, meetings of the board and various committees, and cooperated with Henry David in a European study of mental health legislation. With time he also became a personality in his own right. Thus, as Cloutier was preoccupied with his own approaching change of jobs and residence, Visseur began to serve as a general spokesman for the Federation, visiting WFMH member groups in Middle Eastern Islamic countries as well as Israel. The Annual Report records his officially "assuming the WFMH Directorship in December 1965, in consultation with then WFMH Vice-President Otto Klineberg."

Visseur's first full year as director, 1966, was at least as difficult. The rapidly eroding financial reserve forced a 45 percent budget reduction reflected in an 80 percent WFMH staff reduction as compared with 1965, when support was already diminishing. In order to save money the

Board closed the WFMH Regional Office in New York. The U.S. Committee had not recovered from the alienation of the Cloutier era; by 1965 its support for the WFMH was already minimal and it remained alive only on paper. As of 31 December 1966 it discontinued its support completely, ceasing what it called its "fund sharing" arrangement with the secretariat.

Despite these trials the Federation did not disappear. Its high visibility created by Rees and the allure of belonging to an international organization continued to attract additional member associations whose dues produced a basic income necessary for survival. Its mental health agenda was reduced largely to sending individual representatives to "represent" it at a range of professional and UN meetings. There is no record of their input, if any, at these gatherings, but their presence was made officially known. The year's highlight was the annual meeting held in Prague in July 1966. While the Executive Board discussions were dominated by administrative and financial issues, the meeting itself attracted 320 participants from 31 nations for substantive discussions.

In 1966 Czechoslovakia was still in the grip of the Soviet Union. Preparations for the meeting there had begun the year before. Since Henry David had visited Prague several times to develop a country report for the information center, he gave Visseur some advice: "Beware of the State Blonde. She may get you into trouble." Visseur regarded this as the usual joke between parting colleagues and, after arriving in Prague, plunged into work. When, at the end of a wearing day, a Czech colleague invited him to attend a concert, he gladly accepted. However, he arrived to find that the colleague had not come and that his seat was occupied by an attractive blonde woman. She engaged him in conversation, and after the concert took him to a wine cellar where, over drinks, she told him that her divorced husband lived abroad with their daughter. Then she invited him to visit her apartment and look at some of her pictures. It was only then, Visseur recalled, that "Henry's warning flashed through my mind: Beware of the State Blonde. She may get you into trouble!" At that point, according to Visseur's memory, he said, "Dear Lady, I know who you are and what you are after. Let us part as friends." Two men, obviously members of the police who were watching from a nearby table, understood that "the failure to recruit a new agent was not the Lady's fault. The candidate had apparently been warned by a friend. The friend was Henry" (Visseur, 1995).

Nineteen sixty-six saw the induction of Otto Klineberg as president for the 1966–1967 term and the election of Morris Carstairs as vice-president to become president for 1967–1968. Under Klineberg's sympathetic leadership Visseur did his best to hold the Geneva office together. He found Klineberg congenial and enjoyed working with him. Klineberg's sense of humor was especially appealing. Visseur recalled a dinner in Amsterdam with the board and dignitaries of the host country. Klineberg, as was his habit, preceded an after dinner speech with what was intended to be a humorous story. He emphasized the great contributions of the Dutch to world civilization and, by way of illustration, recalled the American practice of referring to a dinner at which each person pays his own way a "Dutch Treat." But while the joke was greeted with grateful hilarity by board members, the Dutch dignitaries observed "stiff silence." "Fortunately," as Visseur observed, "the incident had no negative international consequences" (Visseur, 1995).

Nineteen sixty-seven was another deficit year. This prompted the Board to adopt additional austerity measures, involving further reduction of activities and staff. Beyond this, the year was one of "rethinking and of reorientation" (WFMH, 1967). Central was a "Committee on the Aims, Methods and Structure of WFMH," including Klineberg, Carstairs, and Rees. It reviewed ways of keeping the Federation alive, first discussed at meetings in Edinburgh in Carstairs' university in April 1967, later in the year in Washington DC, and finally at the 19–23 November board meetings in Lima, Peru prior to the annual meeting under the leadership of President Klineberg and Dr. T. L. Pilkington, chairman of the board. Faced with the real threat of Federation dissolution, the Committee recommended greater concentration of authority in the person of a strong figure. That figure was Morris Carstairs. He assumed office as the WFMH president at the 50th meeting of the Executive Board on 1 December 1967 in Lima, after the annual meeting. At the same time he embraced the duties of chairman of the Board.

The Lima annual meeting, the Federation's 20th, was held from 26 November to 1 December 1967. The first ever held in South America, it was the last major educational event organized with the help of the Geneva office, drawing 450 participants from 32 countries. This high point of Federation activity in South America was not approached again until the end of the century. Much of its success was due to the advice and assistance of the WHO's Mental Health Unit in Geneva headed by Pieter Baan, M.D., and the WHO Regional Office for the Americas, the Pan-American Health Organization (PAHO), with Rene Gonzales, M.D. as its Mental Health Advisor.

The Lima meeting also inadvertently introduced me to the Federation. I happened to sit next to Henry David on the plane going to Lima where I had some consulting responsibilities. As we met and talked I learned that he was attending a WFMH annual meeting organized by Baltazar Caravedo Carranza, M.D., whom I had known in earlier visits to Lima in my roles as a consultant for PAHO and a founding member of the Inter-American Council of Psychiatric Associations. This chance encounter with Henry David proved the beginning of a long friendship, during which it was my privilege to consult for him in the late 1960s and early 1970s on his research on psychosocial aspects of reproductive behavior in Budapest and Prague.

The annual meeting was sponsored by the Peruvian League for Mental Hygiene, the Peruvian Psychiatric Association, of which I had become an honorary member in 1965, and the Peruvian League Against Epilepsy. At that time I was unfamiliar with the Federation, but acquainted with Dr. Caravedo, one of his nation's and his continent's most distinguished mental health leaders, having held high positions in clinical and educational institutions and at the national ministerial level. He was a member of the WFMH Executive Board, serving during the Rees Era from 1957 to 1961, and during the Geneva secretariat from 1963 to 1967. At his death in 1990 at the age of 75 his obituary in Peru's leading psychiatric journal noted his involvement with the WFMH.

Baltazar Caravedo was a graduate of the San Fernando Faculty of Medicine of the National University of San Marcos in Lima, where the professor of psychiatry was another and even closer friend whom I much admired as a scholar and social scientist. This was Professor Carlos Alberto Seguin, M.D., one of the world's pioneers in the study of culture and behavior. Alberto Seguin, who died in 1994, chose the 1967 WFMH meeting as the occasion for the formal opening of his Institute of Social Psychiatry, of which I later became an advisory board member.

Nineteen sixty-seven marked the end of Pierre Visseur's directorship of the Geneva secretariat and of Otto Klineberg's active leadership of the Federation. Beginning in 1968, in the office of President Morris Carstairs in Edinburgh, each successive secretariat for the next 11 years, until 1979, would be in the office of the president, in whose person administrative and executive power and responsibility would be concentrated.

Chapter 5

Internal Organization and Administration: Fifty Years of Recurrent Themes, 1948–1997

THE EVOLVING ORGANIZATION: AN OVERVIEW
Phases of Federation Life

WFMH leaders have ruminated about its mission, structure and governance, operating methods, and financial insolvency since its inception. Jack Rees, looking back, remarked that during his 1948 through 1961 tenure, first as president and then Director, there had been "much healthy self-criticism of the Federation and its methods of operation—a phenomenon which has continued" (Rees, 1966, p. 105). In response to this internal criticism, the organization has made repeated efforts to re-invent or improve itself.

Some of the concern about the WFMH mission and a structure designed to accomplish it is rooted in its prenatal period described in Chapter 2. This phase began with George Brock Chisholm's lectures in 1945 after the end of World War II and with the beginnings of UNESCO's project on reducing international tensions. Sociologist Hadley Cantril was the first UNESCO project leader, succeeded by social psychologist Otto Klineberg. Their idealistic visions of mental health as a route to world peace were translated into actual plans by Chisholm and his friend and colleague, Harry Stack Sullivan, and into operations by Jack Rees, dedicated to what was considered a new "science of human relations." The new world organization, aimed at keeping the peace through the promotion of mental hygiene, began to take form in 1946 with Chisholm's suggestion of its name and function, and Rees' acceptance of the organizing role for the Third International Congress on Mental Hygiene in London in August 1948.

The second phase of Federation life began with its formal founding during the London Congress and lasted through the dissolution of the Geneva secretariat at the end of 1967. Chapters 3 and 4 indicate the obstacles faced and overcome by Rees, and the events after the arrival of Francois Cloutier at the beginning of 1962. However, they do not indicate the briefer ups and downs in attitude and perspective expressed by various Federation leaders. The 1953-1954 president and former Executive Board chairman, Utrecht Professor of Psychiatry H. C. Rumke was pessimistic as he outlined the work of the WFMH in its sixth year of existence. Noting that "many people confess openly that they do not know what mental health really is"

(WFMH, 1954, p. 10), he advocated an intensified scientific approach, but "through lack of funds," he said, "it is impossible for the Federation to realize its legitimate aims...to employ the full-time, experienced administrators and scientists that it needs in order to extend its scope." The Federation's task, as he saw it, was "to transfer a...rather uncritical, naive enthusiasm into a strong, unflinching and patient attempt to find, in a responsible scientific way, the roots of mental health, however diverse they may be." This view of research and practice-oriented Federation goals, widely shared at that time, is quite different from those of the service delivery-oriented mental health associations supplying a significant number of Board members in the 1980s and 1990s.

But Rumke was also concerned with the broader, idealistic aims voiced by the founders: "We are at present in a trend of decreasing enthusiasm. The great impetus born of idealism and of the consciousness of the bitter necessity to preserve the world from great calamities and fostered by the conviction that we mental health workers had a duty to make a contribution with such capacities as we have developed, has diminished a great deal" (p. 9) He went on to note that the1954 Toronto World Congress had lost the Federation's initial vision: "We heard nothing about 'world citizenship'or about 'prevention of war.' Our aims have become more concrete" (p. 10).

The third phase of Federation life, its era of "working presidents," began at the end of 1967 and encompassed the presidencies of three professors of psychiatry: George Morrison Carstairs, M.D. of Edinburgh, who remained in office through 1971; Michael Beaubrun, M.D. of Jamaica, who held office from 1972 to mid-1974; and Tsung-yi Lin, M.D. of Vancouver, who served from 1974 to 1979. Their organizational roles vis-a-vis the global Federation are noted here and in Chapter 6. Their impact on Federation development in their own regions is considered in Chapters 9–11. From 1979 to 1981, the presidency of Vancouver lawyer and businessman Gowan Guest could no longer be considered "working" since an independent secretariat headed by Mrs. Roberta Beiser had been established under Lin's direction at the University of British Columbia, and the president was relieved of many of the tasks that had burdened his predecessors.

The fourth phase of Federation life can be fairly said to have begun with my 1981–1983 presidency. It was during this period that the transition to a new "permanent" secretariat was initiated. It opened its two sets of doors, in Baltimore, Maryland and Arlington, Virginia in the autumn of 1983, when I resigned my post as past president to become the organization's unsalaried chief executive officer, known after some other trial designations as its Secretary General.

This is also the story of Richard C. Hunter, "Dick" as I soon came to know him; more precisely, perhaps, it is the story of our working relationship. In fact, the fourth phase of Federation life could accurately be called the Brody-Hunter phase. During the years beginning in 1981, Dick was my chief associate, first as chairman of arrangements for the 1983 Washington, DC World Congress, in effect, the operational manager representing its official sponsor the U.S. National Mental Health Association (NMHA), which otherwise contributed only its name. After that, he was my unsalaried Deputy Secretary General. Without the two of us working together—communicating more often by telephone and fax than face-to-face—the Federation could not have had the nearly two decades of growth and development that brought it to its 50th year. From 1983 to 1997, when we passed that half-century mark, we provided the international office and communication center, and the continuing glue to hold the organization together, for seven presidents and a host of other Board members representing a range of countries, cultures, personalities, and administrative styles. The differing nature of the subcultures from which the two of us had emerged, of voluntary mental health agencies for Dick, and academic psychiatry for me, is revealed in a comment Dick made around the time of his 80th birthday. He said that I was the first physician with whom he had been able to maintain a long-term friendship, and that his apprehensions about the difficulties in relating to a doctor over time had not come to pass.

In the formal sense, I recruited Dick as a fellow volunteer immediately after my first Board meeting as president in Manila in 1981. However, although the process required several days of intense conversation and he was not thoroughly convinced about what he wanted to do, the interest was mutual. Our skills and backgrounds were complementary. As a career medical school professor, administrator, and scientific journal editor I knew the academic and professional world. As a law school graduate and conscientious objector assigned to mental hospital duty during World War II, and then career voluntary mental health association executive, he knew the voluntary agency world. He had organizational competence, interests, and knowledge which he wanted to use and we both knew would be essential to building the WFMH. The fact that we were both no longer youthful—Dick was approximately eight years my senior—contributed to our collaborative ease with each other. Our private humor as the years passed, referring to ourselves as a "gerontocracy," made it easier to view some of the potentially distressing urgencies of younger Board members with a degree of tolerance. We also discovered that we were both midwesterners, he from Minnesota, I from Missouri. More surprising was the fact that we had both been Eagle Scouts—perhaps not so unexpected considering the nature of the voluntary tasks we had assumed!

Dick's first Federation experience had been at the 1979 Salzburg Congress where we had had our first brief meeting, introduced by Hilda Robbins, a recent NMHA president. There, observing the participation of other officers of the U.S. NMHA, he was "captivated" by the idea of a worldwide voluntary mental health association. This expanded to a sense of the challenge which it offered when he attended a 1981 pre-Congress meeting on rehabilitation in the Philippine countryside outside of Manila and later, with U.S. NMHA leaders, attended a dinner given by outgoing president Gowan Guest. Our agreements to work together, first from 1981 to 1983 and then from 1983 forward, emerged with the pressure of events described below.

From Simplicity to Diversity

A major organizational difference between the WFMH which, in 1948, succeeded the International Committee for Mental Hygiene and the years after 1981–1983, lay in the complexity and diversity of its internal processes and projects, programs, and sources of financial support. Despite an ambitious program of conferences and publications, and the many meetings of its governing structures, relative organizational simplicity persisted from 1948 through 1961. This reflected, in part, the easy agreements between members of the Executive Board and its various committees and subgroups.

The 1949–1950 Board with Rees as Director (see Chapter 3), included Andre Repond, M.D., a Swiss mental hospital director, as president, and University of Toronto Professor of Psychology William Line, Ph.D., as vice-president. One new person, psychiatrist Alan Stoller, M.D. of Australia was added. All others who had been members of the International Preparatory Commission at Roffey Park were now members of an Inter-Professional Advisory Committee (IPAC, later called IPC) which had equal status with the Board in the respect accorded to its opinions. This IPC continued through 1954 when it was replaced by a Scientific Committee again, including several of the same individuals. Even though the Scientific Committee was a source of highly respected opinion, it did not survive due to insufficient funds to support its meetings.

The early Federation Executive Board members and their successors through 1967 resembled each other in values and interests. Most had academic ties, all belonged to the small group of idealistic and socially inclined clinicians and behavioral scientists of the era; most in that early postwar period, had known each other, or known of each other's work; all shared the fundamental beliefs expressed in the Federation's founding document. With few exceptions they had participated in the London Congress, had been among the Federation's founders, and had played active roles in the Roffey Park Preparatory Commission. Even though their plans were complex and ambitious, they were consistent with the Federation's guiding principles. The Roffey Park Commission had conceived the goal of mental health as humankind's ability to survive in peace in one world with itself. It had accorded high value to scientific research as a path to the effective prevention of mental ill health and the promotion of positive good mental health.

Another factor maintaining unity of purpose and relative simplicity in pursuing Federation goals was the central role of the single Director, Jack Rees. Taking office after his 1948–1949 term as the organization's first president, he remained largely responsible for everything that happened during his tenure. The succeeding presidents, with their single-year terms, followed his lead. Most of what was accomplished at the UN prior to 1962 emerged from Rees' personal relationship with medical leaders at the WHO. Many of the Federation's topic-oriented conferences and annual meeting themes reflected his interests in human relations and group dynamics stemming from his Tavistock days. The persisting influence of the Tavistock ethos was reflected in a note from Rees written on Margaret Mead's copy of his 27 August 1948 memorandum to members of the Preparatory Commission asking them all to become members of the IPAC. In it he congratulated her on her speech to the London Congress, saying "how close your attitude is to ours at the Tavvy" (MM/LC).

Geography also contributed to a certain homogeneity of attitudes and interests. With few exceptions the annual meetings, administrative Board and Committee meetings, and intermittent World Congresses were held in Europe, easily accessible to London and later Geneva. The same was true for the special conferences, many of which were financed by United States-based philanthropic groups (see Appendix II). The participants tended to share Western European values and, despite differences in language, communication was relatively conflict-free.

Finally, much of the Federation funding, as described below and in Chapters 3, 4, and 6, was funneled through a single channel, the U.S. Committee for WFMH, Inc. This may have facilitated the Board's tendency to ignore the Federation's financial fragility. This despite Rees' frquent reminder, noted in his 24 January 1949 letter to Rumke, copied to the Board and IPAC, of "a constant mild anxiety that always tends to pervade voluntary organizations with rather uncertain finance" (MM/LC). This was the same letter in which he wrote that it would be "disastrous" if the Federation's new Director would have to raise his own salary: "If he were burdened with, as the Americans say, 'living on a shoestring'with regard to overhead expenses, travel, etc., it would limit very much the usefulness of the central office" (MM/LC).

The Board's unanimity and unity of purpose began to dissolve with Rees' retirement at the end of 1961 and the directorship of Francois Cloutier. Cloutier travelled extensively in the pattern of Rees' "parish-work," which involved visiting the far-flung WFMH member organizations. However, the funds required for this expensive activity were not replenished and by late 1965, only 3½ years into his term of office, it was impossible to continue his salary. He was replaced on a part-time basis by his associate director, Pierre Visseur, and for the first time effective leadership passed into the hands of a president, now Otto Klineberg, and his Board.

Lack of funds forced the final closure of the Geneva secretariat two years later in 1967. Since no money was available to maintain an independent central office, the solution between 1968 and 1983, with the single exception of 1979-1981, was a series of "working presidents." All, as indicated above, were university professors of psychiatry who could count on their institutions to support their WFMH work.

The first "working president," George Morrison Carstairs, M.D. of Edinburgh, assumed the office during the Lima, Peru Annual Meeting at the end of November 1967 and it was he who took the major role in devising a survival strategy for the WFMH. His term, originally expected to last for a single year, was extended to four years until 1972. His activities are described below, in Chapter 6, focusing on finances, and in Chapter 11, on the WFMH in Europe.

Carstairs' successor, as described mainly in Chapter 9, was Michael Beaubrun, M.D. Professor and Chairman of Psychiatry at the University of the West Indies in Jamaica. Beaubrun did not complete his anticipated four-year term, announcing his resignation in 1973 to become effective in 1974.

The next president, whose 1974–1979 tenure just surpassed that of Carstairs to become the longest in Federation history, was Tsung-yi Lin, M.D., originally of Taiwan (Formosa), now Professor of Psychiatry at the University of British Columbia in Vancouver, Canada. The work of his term is noted below, in Chapter 6 on finances, in Chapter 10 on regions, and in Chapter 11 on the WFMH in Europe.

The roles of appointed Director and elected president were combined in these men. All were able to maintain the secretariats in their own universities. During the Edinburgh and Jamaica periods Federation administrative and agenda activities were at a minimum and there was little move toward establishing a broad base for global action. Each president had only limited time to devote to the organization as each remained officially responsible to his university on a full-time basis.

The major revitalizing event, 10 years after the Geneva closure, was the 1977 World Congress for Mental Health in Vancouver led by President Lin. This helped move WFMH back to the world stage. But while it accumulated some funds, those not utilized by Lin were expended by his 1979–1981 successor as president. He was Gowan Guest, a Vancouver lawyer and businessman, who engaged in extensive travel aimed at "exploring WFMH to find out who it really was and where they were" (Guest, letter to the author, 22 November 1995). This "search," accompanied by insufficient attention to fund raising, exhausted most of the WFMH funds accumulated from the 1977 Congress.

The first significant organizational changes after the Geneva closure were also initiated by President Lin. They were in the form of new bylaws along with a "New Design," proposed in 1977, adopted in 1979, and described below. These provided sufficient stability so that after 1981 it was possible to initiate a number of international, self-starting working groups (initially called committees) to carry on programmatic initiatives. This development was continued after 1983 with the establishment of the new permanent secretariat.

The years after 1983 when the secretariat moved from Canada to the United States saw the progressive development of new sources of independent power and initiative. I did not want the Federation's direction to be contained within the office of the Director—after 1983 the Secretary General—or within the Board with its president and other officers. With this in mind my agenda included the establishment of topic-oriented committees, university-based collaborating centers, regional councils, and increased representation to the UN, especially its New York headquarters. All of these developments, as well as an acceleration in the work of stimulating new member associations, created a new need for communication and compromise in the interest of maintaining the global enterprise.

A major structural development was the Board's endorsement during the 1983 World Congress in Washington, DC of the concept of regional WFMH councils, organizations of member associations in particular parts of the world. They were expected to provide increased opportunities for local leadership, expand the influence of the Federation in its particular localities, and carry out overall policy in a locally acceptable manner. They began to phase in, variably and with long lacunae, after 1984, adding a new set of structures to the Federation's operating capacity. The concept and reality of regionalization are reviewed in Chapter 9. A major unforeseen consequence was that the development of a council, even its possibility, transformed the regional vice-president from an individual officer of the WFMH Board to the head of a regional constituency with its own political and other demands.

By 1990 the success of the European Regional Council of the WFMH (ERC/WFMH) as the primary organization to which European members and associations affiliated (rather than the global WFMH) led to questions about WFMH's future identity as a centralized, global entity with regional arms. Could the regions become primary with the global WFMH Board and secretariat acting as a central point for communication and occasional coordination? A contrasting alternative was Rees' earlier view that the important connections should be between voting member organizations on one hand and the Federation's governance (secretariat, Board, committees) on the other. While he as Director was the primary link between the member organizations and the governance structure, he also favored organizations within a region forming loose cooperative relations with others in pursuit of particular projects. The need of individual associations for their own autonomy—in contrast to being part of a regional council—was recognized during a discussion in the mid-1950s. When it was suggested that representatives of the Board should meet with responsible officers of national mental health associations to enhance mutual communication, a North American representative noted that United States member associations (including state mental health associations and professional associations) would like a WFMH link "independent of the U.S. National Mental Health Association." In the same vein, at the spring 1996 Executive Committee meeting in Alexandria, vigorous doubts were expressed about ERC's suitability as a model because of the marked geopolitical and sociocultural differences between regions. These issues are addressed at length in Chapter 9 on regionalization. Developments in particular regions are described in Chapters 9–11.

Concern with ERC autonomy emerged in 1989 in discussions about its financial accountability between Deputy Secretary General Dick Hunter and then Regional Vice-President Josee van Remoortel. It was voiced most explicitly at the annual Board meeting in Madrid in 1994 in the context of discussion about the ERC's desire to retain a percentage of the WFMH dues from members resident in its region. Regional Vice-President John Henderson, M.D., and then ERC executive director van Remoortel predicted that regional dues-sharing would lead to an increase in membership recruitment. The speaker, in his capacity as a board member-at-large, was psychologist Henry David. An experienced international mediator, he questioned, in the gentlest terms, the impact upon the secretariat of a diminution in its already meager source of support from the dues. Henderson denounced the implication that ERC did not have a primary loyalty to WFMH. David then proposed a trial run of dues-sharing at a 25 percent level, and the day was saved. After a year's trial, the new procedure did not result in significantly more ERC members, but the dues sharing continued.

REVISING THE ORGANIZATION: THE BOARD OF DIRECTORS

In the Beginning

The WFMH governing body, originally designated the Executive Board, was elected by a vote of the annual meeting of member associations from nominations which they and Board members submitted. Its size was indeterminate, recognizing that not many people would be able to afford travel to meetings. It included six vice-presidents and it was expected that each of the world's major regions would eventually have at least one representative. However, the position of regional vice-president was not established until 1971.

In an early summation Rees described the Executive Board as a "working party representing generally about ten countries including representatives from each of the continents and a number of professions." From 1949 to 1965 it met twice yearly, usually in Europe, with variable attendance, and worked "extremely hard for five to seven days" overcoming language difficulties with simultaneous translation. By 1952 its members had travelled to meetings "approximately 164,000 miles at the Federation's cost and 412,000 miles under their own arrangements," not counting consultants or the secretariat, whose travel was supported (WFMH, 1953a). One of the yearly meetings was held at the time of the Federation's annual meeting, which lasted for six days and usually was attended by representatives from member societies in 27 to 33 countries in addition to nonmembers. From 1967 to 1977, Board meetings were truncated and irregular, sometimes being replaced by meetings of an administrative committee. After the adoption of new bylaws in 1979 they took place yearly.

From 1948 to 1967 the WFMH president, who changed yearly, was the overall elected leader of the Federation, but the leadership was nominal. The brevity of the term and the limited opportunities it afforded to initiate change were obvious, and until 1962, Rees was recognized as the effective leader. As one president (Fremont-Smith) put it, "The President of the Federation may be likened to a member of a relay team. His position is honorary, symbolic and temporary. He grasps the flaming torch from the hand of his predecessor, carries it for a brief year, and passes it on, hopefully undimmed, to his successor" (WFMH 1955a, p. 5). The Executive Board's elected chairman, who moderated its meetings, could remain in the post for several meetings to add to the continuity supplied by the Director, for whom no exact term of office was specified. The scope of his functions varied with the individual filling the post.

The initial meeting of the first Executive Board, elected by the first assembly of member associations, took place at the end of the Third International Congress in London in August 1948. As noted earlier, Rees was the first president and Rumke the first Board chairman, serving for five years from 1948 until 1953. In that capacity he was more influential in regard to the Federation's internal affairs and its scientific emphases than its presidents, with their yearly terms and major concerns with external affairs. He did become WFMH president for 1953–1954. Serving after Rees, as noted earlier, were Repond (1949–1950), Line (1950–1951), Alfonso Millan, M.D., a leading Mexican psychiatrist (1951–1952), and El Kholy (1952–1953).

The Executive Board's second meeting took place from 5 to 9 January 1949 in Amsterdam, chaired by Rumke. There it was reported in a letter dated 24 December 1948 that WFMH had been incorporated in Switzerland, after the London Congress. (The Articles of Incorporation are noted in Chapter 2). In fact Rees, as president, had expressed the hope that the secretariat could be moved from London to Geneva by mid-summer 1949. This hope, not realized until 15 years later in 1963, re-emerged in various contexts during the ensuing decade. At the Board's 27–28 August 1950 meeting in Paris the idea of a move to Geneva was again introduced by Rees, who remarked that the Federation was "more or less living from hand to mouth" and that a relocation of its headquarters should be considered. Arguments in favor of and against moving to Geneva were discussed, including the possibility of less expensive premises. However, living expenses and the scale of salaries were lower in London; in addition, Geneva nongovernmental organizations "were constantly in danger of having their workers attracted away by the higher salaries paid by the UN agencies." In consequence the Board agreed that "for the next three years or until the financial position of the Federation was more secure," the secretariat should remain in London.

This 1950 meeting of the Board, devoting at least as much time to programmatic as to administrative issues, occupied nine sessions totalling 27 hours spread over four days. The still infant, idealistic, and globally optimistic group assessed the Federation's potential joint projects with the WHO and UNESCO, the latter represented by one of the Roffey Park founders, Otto Klineberg. Several years later, after a period as Executive Board chairman, he became president in 1967. The volume of proposed projects was large, and funds and personnel to carry them out were doubtful, but although it seemed unlikely that many would be accomplished, there were no pessimistic voices.

From the organizational standpoint, the Board was largely occupied with housekeeping, reports of donations to cover staff salaries, leasing quarters, and developing committees. A prolonged discussion about the appointment of a treasurer and the raising and disbursement of funds foreshadowed the continuing concern with finances. In this respect eyes turned toward the New World: It was "the general opinion...that there were many advantages in having a Treasurer...resident in the USA." Another possible adumbration of the future was the formation of a short-lived credentials committee, in retrospect the forerunner of regional representatives, with six members each representing one of the WHO continental regions: Africa, North and Central America, South America, Asia, Australia, and Europe. Its chairman was Eduardo E. Krapf, M.D. of Argentina, who became WFMH president in 1956. The rest of the Board formed the Finance and General Purposes Committee.

Board committees, conceived as ad hoc working groups, were already active. Many of the issues with which they dealt at this meeting were those typically encountered in the initial stages of any organization's life. Board membership was often a concern. Within the initial four years it was agreed that elected substitutes could attend meetings when members were unable to attend, that the vice-president would become president at the beginning of an annual meeting, and terms of office were reviewed. Dr. Porc'Her of France recommended the naming each year of a president-elect as well as a vice-president, chosen because his place of residence would make it easy for him to attend meetings of the Bureau (the administrative-executive group). However, Rees thought the designation confusing and no action was taken. It was decided that an article of the initial WFMH constitution requiring prior attendance at the Assembly as a condition for election to the Executive Board was too rigid and should be amended to permit exceptions.

At that 1950 Board meeting discussion was also begun about the potential usefulness of issuing an annual report (brief, in French as well as English, with no attempt to reach "every member of every member-association") "to help people raise funds in their own countries." Annual reports were prepared by the secretariat for the years through 1967. However, there was a hiatus of 22 years until I revived them in the form of a Secretary General's Report beginning with 1989–1990. For some years we were limited by finances to distributing it in typed form only to the Board, Committees, UN representatives, and collaborating centers. After I obtained a grant from a private foundation beginning in 1992, they were printed and distributed to the entire membership.

The practice was initiated of designating colleagues as consultants who in the course of their own work might carry the WFMH banner and viewpoint, and report back. As noted in the minutes of the 20–23 August 1952 Executive Board in Brussels, "This is a development of the principle which, as you know, we have followed for some time, whereby we try to make use of the services of those who are paying visits either for the UN agencies or the programmes of other national or international groups, for the benefit of mental health work.… It would be of great value if those going to countries other than their own could inform us in advance, so that we could try to make use of their presence in these countries."

Finally, the 1952 Board reached agreement on a schedule of meetings. An annual meeting would be held each year, with the proviso that "until the financial state of the Federation be more secure, in every alternate year the Annual Meeting…be restricted to a consideration of administrative affairs." In the intervening years the meetings would be of "wider and more scientific scope." Approximately every four years the annual meeting would be accompanied by an International Congress. By 1952 there was already Board discussion about "revitalizing" the annual meetings.

By 1953 awareness of the new Federation's existence had become so widespread that it generated an increasing number of invitations for its representation at conferences. It was agreed in principle that a member living in the area where the conference was taking place should represent the Federation, but that hopefully he would be briefed on Federation policy regarding the topic under discussion. There was, however, no discussion of the possible advocacy or educational responsibility of these representatives to other organizations. While the Federation's mission determined that its representative would offer a generally humane and socially sensitive point of view, it formulated no specific position in relation to most issues.

The Interpersonal Dynamics of the Board

The group process characterizing Board meetings varied as procedures became institutionalized and ways of working together more familiar. It also varied with participants and topic. In the early days much interaction seemed to be aimed at privacy and establishing the limits of discussion. Thus, at an 11–14 August 1953 meeting in Vienna, Assistant Director Soddy objected to sending reports of the "confidential meetings of the Executive Board" to consultants, many of whom "were not in close touch" and "could not get the correct perspective on the discussion which was often highly controversial and sometimes contained matter which might be injurious to international relations."

At the meeting of 23–24 August 1953 in Vienna there was a debate, dominated by members from non-English-speaking countries, on "the disadvantages of having too many English speaking members." This was carried forward in anticipation of the forthcoming 1954 Congress in Toronto by a psychiatrist, Professor Carlos Alberto Seguin, M.D., of Lima who had become a Board member in 1952. He expressed concern about the difficulties that would be faced by delegates who could speak neither English nor French and asked for a special effort for Spanish in simultaneous translation, noting that group discussions were of no value unless actively carried on in a language that all could speak. In 1996, 44 years later, an almost identical concern was expressed by Past President Federico Puente S., M.D. of Mexico, pointing out that the Federation leadership had become almost exclusively "Anglo-Saxon."

In his memoirs, Jack Rees recalled that a "cooperative team sense" was, as a rule, passed on quickly to new members. However, he remembered at least three "non-cooperative and rather silent" European members of the Board who, probably, "were not wisely chosen." Inevitably, Board meetings were not always characterized by a "cooperative team sense"; nor, as Rees wished, was it possible to arrive at all decisions by consensus (Rees, 1966). In later years some members pursuing their own agendas or disagreeing with proposals on the floor have been silent. One or two have been aggressively talkative, rising to object, sometimes loudly, to almost every point made. This reached a peak at the Post-Dublin Congress Board meeting in 1995 when several female members from widely dispersed areas of the globe accused a male European colleague of being culturally insensitive and intimidating. Following this confrontation he made his points in a less strident manner.

Rees reported disagreements between Board members that reflected essentially chauvinistic preoccupations: "In some cases newly elected members would…begin their Board careers by overemphasizing the needs of their own particular association or country. But soon they began to see that there were other more important matters…." In a manner akin to that of the WHO, Board members had to realize that they were not appointed to represent the special interests of their own countries. Instead they were to have responsibility for "the widest possible view of world problems" (Rees, 1966, pp. 112–113).

THE FIRST COMMISSION TO EVALUATE THE FEDERATION

What is the WFMH?

Nineteen fifty-three, only five years after the founding moment, saw the first proposal for a Commission to Study the General Purposes of the Federation. It convened at the Fifth International Congress on Mental Hygiene in Toronto in 1954. Discussion there revealed problems of definition and communication that still persist, although in varying form, as the WFMH approaches its 50th anniversary. Thus, Repond "deplored the difficulty of explaining WFMH and its objects to the public," noting that "there is great confusion in Switzerland, even among psychiatrists, between WHO and WFMH."

Membership and Voting

The Federation was originally conceived as an organization of organizations, but its original articles of organization stated that one vote should be given to each national delegation rather than each member association (so as to counterbalance the fact that some countries had many associations and others few). Another category was added when an ad hoc committee meeting on 5 September 1950 recommended that "transnational" member organizations, to a maximum of five, should have voting privileges, the limitation in order not to "disturb the balance of votes" of national associations at the Annual Meeting. The 1979 bylaws did not make the issue less opaque by permitting up to five votes per country.

Much discussion by the 1954 Toronto Commission centered on the idea that only national organizations should have a direct link with the WFMH and that local or state groups should not have such direct contact. However, at Rees' advice, seconded by Soddy, it was agreed that the principle of direct membership in the Federation would be upheld. The question of organizational membership criteria also emerged. At first both specialized scholarly, including social science and professional, as well as voluntary mental health associations were deemed eligible. Related to this issue was the matter of membership-derived income. The first suggestion for increasing it had come at an Executive Board meeting on 20 February 1950 in London. That was to charge higher dues to federations of associations that joined as a unit than to single-member associations.

On 29 August 1950 Rees recommended yet another category of membership. In order to increase its income, the Federation should admit individual members. Called Associates, they would not have the vote. Although the Board was not optimistic about the increase in revenues this would bring, it favored the idea as having "missionary value" and helping many people "become world citizens." The regionally oriented Credentials Committee, noted above, constantly reviewed well-known figures in mental health (almost exclusively psychiatrists) who might be recruited to become Board members capable of contributing new ideas and adding luster to the infant organization.

In this era of still-occupied Germany, credentialing touched on another concern, especially sensitive for an organization devoted to "world citizenship." That was the admission of German observers into Federation discussion groups. Related to this was a resolution to be submitted to the 1950 Assembly that it would no longer be necessary to restrict Federation membership to organizations in countries eligible for membership in the United Nations. The most prominent example nearly 50 years later was Taiwan, expelled from the UN in 1971 at the request of the mainland People's Republic of China. The island was not restored even to observer status at the UN, but the Mental Health Association in Taiwan was one of the oldest and most active WFMH member associations. In December 1996, as described in Chapter 10, in a period marked by military threats against it from the People's Republic, it hosted a meeting for individual and organizational members of our Western Pacific region. It was important for them to make sure that Kunihiko Asai, M.D, our Honorary Secretary from Japan, Shimpei Inoue, M.D., Regional Vice-President, also from Japan, Professor Lin and I were all present in prominent roles.

THE BOARD AND ITS COMMITTEES: 1948–1997

The Bureau and Administrative Committee

Much of the initial work of the Board was carried out by a steering committee called the Bureau. Its members were the chairman of the Board, the president, vice-president, Director, Assistant Director, and secretary with past presidents serving ex officio for one year after the end of their terms of office. It met two or more times yearly in Europe between 1948 and 1955 and approximately yearly after that until the closure of the Geneva secretariat. There was always concern about the members' ability to attend, and sometimes they or substitutes were chosen because of geographical convenience. Other groups were formed, meeting on several occasions each, sometimes for several years, and then dissolved. One was the IPAC, which had its name changed for convenience to IPC.

From time to time, depending upon the availability of funds and the time of interested colleagues who continued in their other careers, the secretariat acquired additional members for varying lengths of time. In 1957 Soddy, formerly designated as Assistant Director, became the combined Deputy Director and Scientific Director. His replacement as Assistant Director was United States psychiatrist Mottram Torre, who had been a clinical consultant for psychiatrically disturbed U.S. State Department personnel. (During this time his wife assisted Helen Ascher in her representation of the WFMH to the UN in New York). Both Soddy and Torre retained these posts on a part-time basis through 1961, when the Rees directorship came to an end. Afterward, Soddy continued as Secretary to the Scientific Committee (still headed by Rumke) and Scientific Advisor to Director General Cloutier. During the Geneva era, as described in Chapter 4, Pierre Visseur was Cloutier's Associate Director for Administration and Henry David, salaried by a U.S. NIMH grant, was Associate Director for Information.

Between 1972 and 1979 executive power was invested in the Administrative Committee. This was due partly to the unwieldy nature of the Board, partly to the financial impossibility of bringing it frequently together, and partly to the distaste of most of its members for activity between annual meetings. Its membership was opportunistic including, besides the president, treasurer, and vice-president, whomever else was available and seemed to the president able to add something to its deliberations.

The Executive Committee

The Administrative Committee was succeeded, following the 1979 bylaws, by an executive committee composed of the Federation president, president-elect, past president, treasurer, and honorary secretary including, after 1983, the Secretary General as a nonvoting member. The Executive Committee was empowered to carry out the functions of the full Board in the interval between meetings. For years it did so uneventfully, confining itself mainly to non-controversial issues. However, the 1990 Board, meeting at WHO headquarters in Geneva under the presidency of Stanislas Flache, M.D. (1989–1991), voted that no significant decision would be taken by the Committee without ratification by the full Board. This vote, intended to reduce its autonomous power, was a consequence of concern by ERC officers about its approval of WFMH co-sponsorship of events in Europe and its role in accepting European organizations into membership.

In 1991, though, incoming president, psychologist Max Abbott, Ph.D., who had been executive director of the Mental Health Foundation of New Zealand for several years, moved in the opposite direction. He increased the power and autonomy of the Executive Committee by insisting that it have at least yearly or twice yearly meetings. Although there was some resistance, he carried the day by threatening to resign before even beginning his presidency if this could not be arranged. Regular yearly meetings of the Executive Committee quickly became a tradition, as successive presidents found them a convenient mechanism for exercising influence. An unintended consequence was that Executive Committee meetings tended to duplicate the agendas of full Board meetings, adding a sometimes wearing burden of redundancy to the proceedings.

The secretariat was less enthusiastic about these additional meetings because of the extra time and work required to arrange agendas, minutes, and other reporting. There was also another concern, relevant because of our limited budget. Even though many people paid for their own travel, some from distant, less developed countries, needed help. We were also expected to arrange for housing and meals, placing another burden on the Federation's fragile exchequer. Dick Hunter and I dealt with this by having the meetings as often as possible in Baltimore at the Sheppard Pratt Hospital or at the WFMH Secretariat in the NMHA headquarters, now in Alexandria, Virginia.

The administrative emphasis initiated by Abbott was continued by President Federico Puente Silva of Mexico, who took office during the 1993 Tokyo World Congress. He was proud of having "modernized" the Federation by introducing the practice of bimonthly telephone conference calls in order to facilitate the conduct of Federation business. Unfortunately, the use of conference calls for planning purposes, with its emphasis on administration, tended at first to reduce rather than increase attention to the Federation's international mental health agenda, its reason for existence. After a year, the calls were reduced to approximately quarterly because of their cost. This was a consequence of their unexpected duration, with calls planned for 45 minutes sometimes extending to up to two hours. An unintended consequence of the Puente decision was the increased cohesiveness of the Executive Committee, leading to sometimes casual decision-making bypassing the Board. This predictably led to protests, particularly by ERC representatives who felt, legitimately, that some decisions were not being adequately ratified by the Board in the spirit of the bylaws or the 1990 Geneva Board decision. The protests were ignored and when the issue came up once or twice for discussion it centered around the definition of "significant" as a criterion for full Board involvement. In time the concerns of the regional vice-presidents were met by their being invited to elect one of their number to represent them at meetings of the Executive Committee (see Chapter 9). This move, like others in the period, was carried out without changes in the bylaws, as a major revision was anticipated at some time in the near future.

The Administrative Process

The Puente presidency, 1993–1995, was marked by an increase in Board time, both during meetings and conference calls, devoted to administrative and procedural issues. However, it did increase the feeling of participants that they were personally involved in the administrative process. The growth of a developing Board-centered bureaucracy was formalized during the 1994 Board meeting in Madrid when Puente asked then past president Abbott to form a committee "to review all aspects of Federation functioning, including the status of the developing regional councils." Abbott, ever a conscientious administrator, took the request seriously and embarked on the development of what was to become a Policy and Procedures Manual. This became a major focus during the 1995 Board meetings before and after the Dublin World Congress. The Manual was intended to provide standard operating procedures to reduce the time required for certain types of decision making. In recognition of the need for the "P and P," as it became known, Abbott was appointed at the 1995 post-congress Board meeting in Dublin by incoming President Beverly Long of the United States, to the new post of Deputy Secretary General for Special Projects.

The Interprofessional Advisory Committee, IPAC

The 1949 Board meetings in the first year of Federation life were noteworthy for the presence of the Advisory Interprofessional Committee (the AIC), later to become the Interprofessional Advisory Committee (IPAC). This interdisciplinary group, the main standing committee of the first Executive Board, was conceived as a link between the ideas of professional mental health workers and the Board. It was also regarded as a source of research and discussion topics from an interdisciplinary viewpoint. At that time, although there was no reservation about the WFMH devoting attention to research, and it was dominated by psychiatrists, questions about the organization's relationship to the professions were already emerging. One was elaborated by psychiatrist Ronald Hargreaves, representing mental health interests in the WHO (which did not yet have a formal mental health section; see Chapter 8). It arose in relation to the question of WFMH participation in a forthcoming international congress of psychiatry. Hargreaves made the point that the WHO's general policy was preventive, different from the curative outlook of medicine, and that its policy in mental health would probably follow similar lines. This did not inhibit agreement about the value of the WFMH sponsoring lectures or symposia at scientific meetings. Professor Rumke, later to chair the WFMH scientific committee, described AIC as "the brains and soul trust" of the Federation, which would formulate its suggestions to the WHO and other international bodies. At Harry Stack Sullivan's suggestion it was agreed that the journal *Psychiatry*, of which he was editor, might be used as a vehicle for scientific communications from AIC members.

Discussions about the role, functions, and membership of IPAC were prominent in later meetings of the Board and influenced the Federation's evolving mental health agenda. The existing Committee originally recommended enlarging itself according to profession, including people in anthropology, psychology, social work, and psychiatry. Some members from the less-industrialized world, however, favored "outstanding personalities in mental health" rather than representation according to field. They also objected that proposed members so far were "exclusively Anglo-Saxon."

At the 1951 Board meeting in Mexico City psychiatrist Alan Stoller of Australia presented a scheme involving the IPAC at the supranational, regional, subregional, and local levels. At the top level it would relate to the WFMH executive board and secretariat as well as other supranational agencies. At successive levels there would be regional and working IPACs, culminating in "community multidisciplinary research projects." This was the first of several proposals for direct scientific and educational work by the WFMH which did not materialize because of lack of resources and an inadequate infrastructure.

IPAC, initially intended as a core WFMH body in association with the Executive Board, was never able to translate its ideas into action and gradually faded into obscurity. It was succeeded after 1956 by Rumke's scientific committee. In time this too was discontinued, in part because of difficulty in funding meetings. Its disappearance, like that of the IPAC, also reflected the Board's increasing sense that while the WFMH should advocate research it did not have the capability to carry it out. Perhaps as important was a general change in attitude toward science, which began at the end of the Rees era and became most marked after 1982 with the involvement of consumer/user/survivors of mental illness. This change was accompanied by a growing tendency among nonmedical European leaders, such as Edith Morgan, to emphasize the role of volunteers and diminish the dominance of psychiatrists and other professionals. Corollary was distrust of research as a major function of a consumer-oriented voluntary mental health associations. The intramural politics of this issue led psychiatrist and research administrator Gaston Harnois of Montreal, after his 1979 election as honorary secretary, to be concerned with the organization's changing relationship to the WHO with its major focus on research. In early 1980, noting the concern of some members with possible Federation dominance by professionals, he wrote: "As far as I am concerned the future of the Federation lies in the capacity of both lay and professional members to respect each other's competence and work together toward the achievement of agreed-upon goals." He described the issue of whether or not the WFMH should engage in "scientific activities" as "delicate." His proposed solution, "a standing scientific committee" to recommend particular projects for at least "some tangible support" (Harnois, letter from the secretary of the Executive Board to Gowan Guest, 6 February 1980.) No such committee was established. However, beginning in 1986, I was able to approach the need for WFMH-science collaboration by recruiting university groups concerned with issues of interest to the WFMH to become our collaborating centers. We also recognized the necessary basis of practical mental health work in scientific research in the theme of the 1991 World Congress in Mexico. A year prior to the Congress Puente, the Congress organizer, Virginia Gonzalez Torres, founder of the Mexican Institute of Rehabilitation, and I tried to formulate a theme that would articulate a Federation position. Our joint idea, which became the official Congress theme, was "People and Science: Together for Mental Health." The 1991 Congress was, in fact, outstanding for its many "tracks" devoted to such applied science issues as refugee mental health and mental health and population.

These efforts were applauded by most Federation leaders. However, the idea that Federation advocacy should be based on scientific knowledge met with pockets of resistance which, though limited, were vigorous. Their main expression came in an 11 May 1990 letter from Josee van Remoortel, then vice-president for the WFMH European region and chair of the ERC for the WFMH. She was particularly concerned about a pending agreement to establish a WFMH collaborating center headed by Professor of Social Psychiatry Marten de Vries at the University of Limburg in Maastricht, and about the formation of an International Honorary Scientific Advisory Committee for the 1991 World Congress scheduled for Mexico. Apparently reflecting the views of her Regional Board, she wrote: "The ERC does not wish to be involved in bio/medical/scientific research and does not therefore need advice on it."

The increasing demands of Federation administration and the increasing number of its own conferences drained much of the energy that had been invested in liaison with professional societies. In consequence the earlier practice of having Federation-sponsored symposia at professional psychology and psychiatry meetings went into abeyance except for co-sponsorship of meetings organized by other groups. It was revived in August 1996 when de Vries, who had been voted in as president-elect during the 1995 Dublin Assembly, organized a WFMH-sponsored symposium on mental health and public policy at the World Psychiatric Association convention in Madrid.

THE ERA OF WORKING PRESIDENTS: 1967–1979

Reorganization for Survival

The difficult period in Federation history following the 1967 closure of the Geneva secretariat was marked by repeated rethinking of how best to ensure the organization's survival. Attention to reorganization actually began in 1967 while Pierre Visseur was still in place as WFMH Director managing the (much reduced) Geneva operation. A special committee of the Chairman of the Executive Board, T. L. Pilkington, M.D. of Great Britain, prepared a series of amendments to the bylaws that had been adopted in 1963. It recommended greater concentration of authority in the person of the WFMH president, who would also assume the responsibilities of chairman of the Board and, in addition, remain in office for an extended period of time. Other recommendations favored greater regionalization of WFMH meetings since annual intercontinental meetings imposed such heavy demands on WFMH staff time and budget. These proposals were discussed in Edinburgh in April 1967, by the full Board in Washington, DC in November 1967, and again by the general assembly at the annual meeting in Lima, Peru later in November 1967. However, the situation was urgent and Carstairs assumed the post of "working president" before the new arrangements were formalized by Executive Board action. The survival mode adopted by informal agreement in these emergency circumstances resembled that of many international academic or professional organizations. The president would combine in himself (except for Margaret Mead, all to this point had been male) the functions of chief executive and chief operating officer (neither term was then used), and his institution, with WFMH support for a senior secretary, would supply the secretariat. Thus, no one could be president who did not belong to an institution willing and competent to meet the administrative requirements and expenses of the office. In this way the organization survived its first life-threatening crisis through the efforts of research- and teaching-oriented university professors of psychiatry. They differed both from their treatment-oriented clinician colleagues and their community-oriented Federation colleagues in their shared belief that improving world mental health at the international and intercultural level required the kind of growing evidentiary base that could only be achieved by systematic research combining clinical and social science elements. They also echoed the belief of Rees and his colleagues in the value of education.

A final decision about the 1967 revisions of the 1963 recommendations was slow in coming. It was not made until 1968 during the WFMH 20th Anniversary Congress in London over which Carstairs presided, and it was not publicized until the Federation's Winter 1970/71 Bulletin. It covered five general points, some elements of which have recurred since then in modified form.

The first recommendation was aimed at increasing "democratic participation" by member associations in the affairs of the Federation. This would be accomplished by creating national committees for mental health representing all of the member associations in a particular country and serving a coordinating function for that country. Each national committee, as well as each transnational member association, would designate a representative to sit on the Federation's Board of Directors. This last decision, a major contributor to the Board's rapid growth to unmanageable size, led to no discernible increase in the "democratic" nature of its proceedings. It remained in effect until the 1979 "new design" initiated in 1977 during the Lin presidency (see below).

The second point concerned the locus of decision-making about WFMH affairs. This involved redefinitions of the presidential functions and term and that of the Executive Board, now functioning more as a committee differentiated from the newly enlarged Board of Directors. The president, now a "working president," would be elected by the directors for a period of two years, renewable once (i.e., he could have a four-year term). Assisted by a secretary (never formally defined as a Board-level officer) he would make the day-to-day executive decisions. The next level would be the reconstituted Executive Board (now comparable to the former administrative committee), which would deal with developmental and policy issues. It would include the president and two directors appointed by him plus four others elected by the directors, each for four-year staggered terms. Finally, major policy decisions would be taken by the full Board of Directors, including members-at-large elected by the Board itself; the number of these at-large members would not to exceed 25 percent of the nations represented. The overall Board of Directors would meet every two years at a biennial international meeting.

A third level of governance would be the General Assembly, including representatives of all member associations, affiliated organizations, and individual members. Again, this was modified by the 1979 bylaws to limit it to representatives of voting member, i.e., national or transnational associations.

Fourth, it was recommended that a biennial international meeting should replace the annual meeting. After 1979 the biennial meeting became the World Congress for Mental Health, but the Board of Directors and Assembly continued to meet, by statute, annually. It was recognized that the Assembly in non-Congress years would have limited attendance, mainly from the region in which it was meeting.

Fifth, it was proposed that "regional activities involving a number of adjacent countries" should be encouraged, and to promote these it was proposed that there should be six regional vice-presidents. These would cover the Americas, Europe, Eastern Mediterranean, Africa, Southeast Asia, and the Western Pacific. They would not be elected by constituents from their own regions, but by the directors. Rather than acting as "representatives" for the interests of their regions they would act as agents of the Board in promoting mental health projects in them.

These recommendations were finally acted upon during the annual meeting in Hong Kong in 1971, as the term of the first "working president" Carstairs was coming to an end.

THE WORKING PRESIDENTS

George Morrison Carstairs, M.D., 1967–1971: Edinburgh, Scotland

After the permanent closure of its Geneva office at the end of 1967, the WFMH could have sunk into oblivion. In fact the people who constituted its executive group, including then Vice-

President Carstairs, who expected to become president for the 1967-1968 term, were divided about the wisdom of trying to rescue it. Optimists prevailed and he accepted the burden of leading the effort at revival from his office as Chairman of Psychiatry at the University of Edinburgh. The Board understood that the previous system of one-year presidential terms was no longer feasible since there was no longer a central secretariat to manage routine Federation affairs or to act as a continuing point for the formulation and execution of policy. Four years seemed about right, and Carstairs assented to his election for an additional three-year term, which would carry his tenure through 1971. Succeeding presidential terms were also expected to last for four years and the concept of "working president" was implemented.

Morris Carstairs was a brilliant man with a strong interest in the relation of cultural context to behavior, a capacity for deep thought, and an aptitude for writing. Although possessed of a natural reserve and dignity, he was an activist as well as a theorist and, unlike many colleagues, was willing to assume the leadership tasks of furthering causes in which he believed. In these leadership tasks he was not shy and could be direct, even blunt. This extended to the written word. His editorial in the Spring/Summer 1972 Bulletin, for example, referred to associations "nominally dedicated to mental health" which "have expended a disproportionate amount of their energies in mutually denouncing each other, or in frankly regressive tantrums and sulks."

An obituary by Norman Kreitman published in the London Independent on 23 April 1991 gave an idea of his life story. Carstairs came from a family which had for centuries been associated with Edinburgh. Born on 18 June 1916 in India where his father was a Church of Scotland missionary, he spent much of his childhood there and throughout his life continued to be bilingual in Hindi and English. He was educated in Edinburgh, where he also held the Scottish three-mile record in distance running for several years and was elected to run for Great Britain in the Olympics.

After graduating from medical school in Edinburgh he trained in psychiatry and also completed a degree in anthropology at Cambridge, subsequently working for a time with Margaret Mead, later to become one of the Federation founders and its president (1956–1957). His interests in individual psychopathology within a closely defined social context, first expressed in the stay in a village in northern India reported in his book, was to mark the rest of his life's work. All of this was a prelude to a distinguished academic and administrative career, beginning with the chairmanship of psychiatry in Edinburgh in 1963 and at the same time directorship of the Medical Research Council Unit. He held the post of Vice-Chancellor of York University from 1973 to 1978, and later returned to research and writing, again spending some time in India.

I knew Morris first through his classic work on Hindu believers in reincarnation, *The Twice Born*, published in 1957, and admired him greatly. He was responsible for my initial affiliation with the Federation. We talked about it in 1966 during the World Psychiatric Association meeting in Honolulu, and then after he became president he appointed me, although the procedure had not been formally adopted, as a director-at-large for a four-year term, 1969–1973. The informal nature of the proceeding is reflected in the fact that I received no official notification of the appointment, did not attend a Federation Congress until that in Vancouver in 1977, and did not become a dues-paying member until 1979, when I was elected to the Board under the new bylaws inaugurated by President Tsung-yi Lin (1974–1979). Nonetheless, I represented the WFMH at a meeting on family planning at WHO headquarters, Geneva, in April 1970 (see Chapter 13); the minutes of the 8-9 August 1970 Executive Board in Jerusalem indicate that I was active in a drive for new individual members (Associates); as noted in Chapter 9, I served as Carstairs' WFMH representative to the Caribbean Federation for Mental Health in 1971; and, as described below, was a member of President Michael Beaubrun's (1972–1974) Administrative Committee. Morris and I lost touch after the 1979 World Congress for Mental Health in Salzburg when he tried, unsuccessfully, to persuade me to become a candidate for WFMH president. We had a brief encounter in Washington, DC in 1981 and he attended and wrote me a laudatory note about the 1983 Washington, DC World Congress. But, when we saw each other next at the time of the 1985 World Congress in Brighton, he was unable to recall some of our earlier shared experiences. He died in Edinburgh, not quite six years later, on 18 April 1991.

The WFMH was fortunate to attract this unusual man to its ranks, and then to its presidency, in a time of crisis. He was able to bring a multidisciplinary view with an emphasis on social process to the problems of mental illness in a range of developing countries. But it was painful for him to solicit the money necessary to keep the organization together. Nonetheless, despite his reluctance and in the face of setbacks, he persisted in what he once described to me as distasteful begging, and obtained a considerable gift from a private United States donor (see Chapter 6). This allowed the Federation to observe its 20th anniversary with a major congress in London in 1968. Then, with the help of the U.S. NMHA he saw to it that the 1969 annual meeting was in the United States, where there were better opportunities to recruit members and raise money than in Europe. He also outlined a way of working based on biennial world congresses plus a number of smaller, task-oriented meetings covering as much as possible each of the six WHO-designated geographical regions of the world, now adopted by the WFMH as its regions.

In May 1971, in preparation for the November meeting in Hong Kong when a new president would be named, Carstairs summarized the state of the Federation as he saw it in a letter to the Board. Due to "austerity budgeting" there was a balance of $70,000 to cover administrative costs for the following year. He considered it vital to create a small administrative committee that could meet at least yearly at minimal expense to "share with the Working President the tasks of fund-raising, planning and carrying out future activities."

Most significant in terms of the Federation's formal global focus with a major emphasis on the United Nations, he wrote: "If WFMH is to thrive it will have to be nourished at the grassroots level.... WFMH activities [must] form part of the programme of the mental health associations and allied organizations of every country." In the same vein he noted: "We have found in Edinburgh that one does not need to wait for an ambitious Regional or International meeting in order to promote a WFMH sponsored International Forum—interested and motivated participants are already here in our midst, and respond readily whenever we invite them to join in discussing one of the many challenges to mental health with which we are confronted both in the developing and in the richer countries."

Even before this a search had begun for a new working president to support the Federation after Carstairs retired. There were no immediate applicants for this potentially overwhelming responsibility. The 8–9 and 12 August 1970 Jerusalem Board minutes indicate some of the efforts made by the nominating committee. Drs. Jack Griffin, Kurt Palsvig, and Khunying Meesook, old Federation hands and former Executive Board members, were all approached and declined. Dr. Allan Stoller of Australia, a former president, reflected a bit longer and also declined. The Committee, meanwhile, had decided to look outside the Federation and suggested Professor Michael Beaubrun, who had attended WFMH meetings in Lima, Edinburgh, London, and Montreal. Prepared to take on the office and provide premises in the University of the West Indies (UWI) in Jamaica, he accepted the nomination, which was tantamount to election, and was named president at the November 1971 meeting in Hong Kong. The secretariat moved to Jamaica at the beginning of 1972.

Michael Beaubrun, M.D., 1972-1974: Kingston, Jamaica

With Michael Beaubrun the Federation acquired the support of one of the Caribbean's outstanding citizens. Born on 29 December 1924 in Grenada in the British Windward Islands, he grew up in Grenada and Trinidad. At the age of 17 he won a scholarship, which took him to Edinburgh University to study medicine after a preliminary period of premedical science at McGill University in Montreal. We met when we both spoke at a meeting of the Inter-American Council of Psychiatric Associations in San Jose, Costa Rica in 1970. By that time, as described in

Chapter 9, he was Professor and Chairman of Psychiatry at UWI, serving 14 Caribbean countries. It was there that he extended an invitation for me to be a visiting professor on his faculty at some future date. The focus was to be on race relations. We met again through Morris Carstairs. Because of my work in South America as well as Mexico during the 1960s, Morris asked me to represent the WFMH at a meeting of the Caribbean Federation for Mental Health (CFMH) in August 1971 in Paramaribo, Surinam. Michael was there as the meeting's chairman in his multiple capacities as vice-president of the WFMH, past president of CFMH, and president of the Association of Caribbean Psychiatrists, which he had founded. At the Paramaribo meeting he renewed his invitation, this time for February 1972, when he would have WHO funds to support me at UWI for two months in order to establish a training program leading to a diploma in psychotherapy in accordance with the British tradition. I accepted this opportunity to visit and work in a new environment. Thus, I was present at the outset of his WFMH presidency. He was an excellent fit for the post. A tall, dignified man, his sense of ceremony imparted an air of significance to all of the activities in which he took part. To his British Commonwealth experiences in Canada and Britain, congenial to Jamaicans who identified themselves as Commonwealth members, were added extensive and influential associations throughout the Caribbean. This and his academic status in the multinational UWI facilitated acceptance of the Federation throughout the region.

Michael, as I soon came to know him, attributed his nomination to the WFMH presidency to his having met with Jack Rees, but his close association with his immediate predecessor, Carstairs, could have been a factor. He had been a medical student in Edinburgh where D. K. Henderson, M.D., then professor of psychiatry, had influenced him to enter his field and then to become his assistant in the psychiatric hospital. Some years later, after a brief return to the Caribbean, he came back to Europe where he met Carstairs, who by that time occupied the Edinburgh chair of psychiatry.

I continued as an intermittent visiting professor at UWI during Michael's tenure, and through 1975 after his departure for Trinidad. In addition to some teaching I was supported by the Smithsonian Institution of Washington to investigate the social and cultural obstacles to the use of contraception on the island, whose leaders were concerned with its rapidly increasing population and large numbers of children born to parents unable to care for them. The research involved a consulting appointment with the National Family Planning Board in order to work with the Jamaican Family Planning Association on a study of why local women did not use the contraceptives which were abundantly available to them. It led to collaboration with several members of Michael's staff, resulting in several papers and finally a book entitled *Sex, Contraception and Motherhood in Jamaica* (Brody, 1981).

Since I was going to be on the scene periodically and required no travel assistance, Michael co-opted me to become a member of what was then called, following Carstairs' recommendation, the Administrative Committee. Its first meeting was in February 1972, shortly after my arrival on the island, the secretariat having moved from Edinburgh to the UWI just one month earlier. This body, successor to the Bureau and precursor of the Executive Committee, met whenever its members could be present, at least once and sometimes twice yearly. Aside from Beaubrun and Carstairs, it included Tsung-yi Lin, another friend and colleague of long standing. He was a WFMH veteran, having served intermittently in various capacities on its Executive Board, as a member for 1958–1959, in 1959–1960 as chairman, and for two years thereafter as vice-chairman under Otto Klineberg. Paul-Marcel Gelinas, executive director of the mental health association in Quebec, and Treasurer Samuel Steinwurtzel of the United States, a banker, completed the active group. Mrs. Irma Tobing of Suriname, representing her mental health association, was usually unable to attend. The first meeting of the Committee was scheduled so that we could all speak at a public meeting co-sponsored by the Jamaica Association for Mental Health and the UWI. The topic, Mental Health in a World of Change, gave us each the opportunity to discuss issues of personal interest. The papers were well-received and the atmosphere encouraging.

This was the beginning of a period from early 1972 until spring 1974 when the WFMH became a prominent entity in the Caribbean. Beaubrun, as its president, was much in evidence at ceremonial occasions and meetings of local mental health associations in Jamaica and other islands of the region. He also carried the Federation banner to events in other parts of the world. These included, thanks to Gelinas, the annual meeting of the Quebec division of the Canadian Mental Health Association; an anniversary celebration at the Institute of Living, a private hospital in Connecticut, where Clifford Beers had had a brief, second (and voluntary) hospitalization; African psychiatric meetings in Khartoum; and a symposium at a private mental health center in Arizona. Carstairs arranged an international WFMH forum in Edinburgh on Psychiatric Services in the Developing World, and the Federation was represented at other international gatherings by members of the Board who happened to be conveniently located. There were also several important initiatives. One was a joint meeting, proposed by Beaubrun, between the leaders of the WFMH and the European League for Mental Health in Geneva on 11 March 1974. This is described in Chapter 11. Another, in keeping with his expertise on drug addiction, took place later in the same month when the WFMH joined with the International Council on Alcohol and Addictions and the Bahamian government in sponsoring a conference on strategies to prevent drug abuse in developing countries.

Despite these activities and my personal admiration for Michael I found it increasingly difficult to grasp the central thrust of the organization, and its reason for being, aside from its emblematic function and sponsoring or co-sponsoring occasional meetings. The appellation "paper tiger" came inevitably to mind. It did not live up to the grand expectations or even the actual accomplishments of Jack Rees and the Roffey Park founders. I did understand, though, that as a body affiliated with the UN it could lend stature as a co-sponsor or participant to events and programs, particularly in the smaller or less developed countries. It also facilitated travel for WFMH officers and through them had an international educational function. I realized this when Michael asked me if I would like to join him as a speaker at the Arizona meeting. Another opportunity arose in 1972, through a travel agency specializing in educational travel for American physicians, to arrange a teaching seminar lasting several days at the University of Nairobi in collaboration with the Kenyan Ministry of Health. Michael gave the go-ahead to my inquiry about possible WFMH sponsorship, and the activity was launched. The seminar was successful, we contributed to the education of the Nairobi mental hospital staffs with which we spoke, and the safari that followed was exciting. However, I remained burdened with the feeling that the Federation, despite its distinguished antecedents and emblematic significance for international mental health, was not doing much more than any other group of peripatetic psychiatrists.

After the initial meeting, most Administrative Committee dicussions concerned organizational issues and the lack of money. Finally, boredom overtook me. When I was offered a trip to Australia for the WFMH's annual meeting in 1973, billed as its 25th Anniversary World Congress, I decided that it was not worth my time or the Federation's money and tendered my resignation. After that 8–13 October 1973 meeting in Sydney Michael, citing his advancing glaucoma, resigned his positions, first with the WFMH and then at UWI, to return to Trinidad.

Meanwhile, the WFMH Board had been growing. By 1972, six years after the closure of the Geneva secretariat, it had more than quadrupled in size. The first WFMH annual report, issued from Beaubrun's office in Jamaica (WFMH, 1972a) listed some 70 officers and Executive Board members. These included (with some individuals serving in more than one capacity): President Beaubrun, Past President Carstairs, Treasurer Steinwurtzel, six regional vice-presidents, the administrative committee, an Executive Board-at-Large with 15 members, and the three WFMH representatives of the UN—at UN New York, WHO Geneva, and UNESCO, Paris. A concern with regional representation was reflected in a National Executive Board composed of 36 representatives of national member organizations, and a Transnational Executive Board on which I found myself listed as well as on the Administrative Committee. A full-time staff secretary was assigned from Beaubrun's department. There was little expectation that this unwieldy body, with its inevitable absentees, could make decisions in an expeditious or effective way. Despite the presence of a number of able and experienced people who were eager to work, it appeared to exist largely to afford the appearance of representation and whatever local honor that might bring the incumbent at home. It also offered a reservoir of potential helpers in times of need.

Only a few members of that Board of a quarter-century ago, in addition to myself, remained affiliated with the WFMH as it approached its 50th anniversary: Edith Morgan of London, later to become a WFMH president (1985–1987), and founding president of ERC/WFMH; Dr. Henry David of Maryland, former board member-at-large, and chairman of the WFMH Committee on Responsible Parenthood; and J. L. Armand-Laroche, M.D. of Paris, who continued as a WFMH representative to UNESCO, Paris. Professor Lin was a past president and honorary president. Dr. Khunying Ambhorn Meesook of Bangkok, former Vice-President for Southeast Asia, was an individual WFMH member, active in the mental health association in Thailand.

Tsung-yi Lin, M.D., 1974–1979: Vancouver, British Columbia, Canada

At the WFMH Executive Board meeting in Sydney, Australia, 13 October 1973, Beaubrun, who had been expected to remain as president at least through 1974, announced that he would be leaving Jamaica to return to Trinidad in June of that year. In view of this he suggested that it might not be in the interest of the Federation to move the secretariat to Trinidad for only 1½ years. It was therefore agreed that while Lin would take office upon Beaubrun's departure from Jamaica the secretariat would remain at UWI, moving to Vancouver in January 1975. Lin, as a former chairman of the WFMH Executive Board, a Federation vice-president in 1969–1971, and a sometime visitor to Beaubrun's Jamaica headquarters as part of the Administrative Committee, was able to manage from a distance. This was aided by his thorough familiarity both with the Federation's distinguished history and its currently depleted state. In office for much of 1974 until mid-1979, he became the longest-serving WFMH president.

Lin was able to undertake the demanding tasks of a working presidency while continuing his professorial responsibilities because his department at UBC was headed by a mutual friend, Professor Milton Miller, M.D. Miller, who related to him with admiration and affection, was an idealistic, ebullient man who had spent some time in China and, like Lin, could speak Mandarin. He understood that he and his department would have to assume significant financial and organizational responsibility for the WFMH when its secretariat was transferred to the Vancouver campus, but accepted that in good humor in the interest of doing something about world mental health. Looking back at his encounter with the Federation's unmet needs he had no illusions about its strength and capacity for independent existence. He described Beaubrun's resignation on grounds of failing eyesight in skeptical terms: "Actually his vision was 20/20 or better and what he saw he didn't like. So, on a rainy day, I'm sure, the files of the WFMH arrived in Vancouver…. [Its] treasury was broke(n)" (Miller, 1996). In a similar spirit he wrote: "Tsung-yi and I did pull the creature from the sea as it was submerging for the third time back in 1972, provided CPR (cardio-pulmonary resuscitation), celebrated briefly, put a little money into its pocket, but then…went in separate directions."

Miller was not alone in his skepticism about the Federation's capabilities. Questions continued as to whether or not it was competent to carry out any functions besides the operation of Congresses and, perhaps, some regional meetings. Its value and very survival were in doubt. Gowan Guest, later to become the WFMH treasurer and then its president, described the process of self-assessment accompanying its transfer to Vancouver as he encountered it: "endless and essentially fruitless organizational introspection…about who, what and where the Federation could and should be…navel gazing…." (Guest, 1995). But that evaluation's implication of inactivity was not totally accurate. With Guest's professional help Lin achieved corporate status for the WFMH under the Canada Corporations Act along with a charitable tax classification under the Canadian Income Tax Act. It was also quickly decided that the only way to do something about the question of money was, in Miller's words, to "have a show!" So in 1972 planning began for a 1977 World Congress, as Miller put it, "the big party," to be held on the UBC campus, with available dormitory housing and university meeting facilities. The Canadian Association for Mental Health in the person of George Rohn, its general director and a new member of the WFMH Executive Board, shocked President Lin by declining to co-sponsor the Congress or offer financial support. However, the Canadian government provided $100,000 in start-up money, and the likelihood of success seemed high.

The 1977 Carstairs Task Force: A Third Evaluation of the WFMH

Despite the success of early planning for the Congress, the renewed vigor of the Newsletter, and other signs of anchoring in its new environment, doubts about the organization's future and ultimate value continued. In 1976, a year after its transfer to UBC, President Lin called for a third evaluation of the WFMH: its past, present and future. With a certain sense of deja vu, Morris Carstairs agreed to head a task force on The Future of the WFMH. There had, after all, been similar evaluations at Toronto in 1955 and, in London, the Soddy Task Force of 1961. Other current task force members—all on the Executive Board—were (despite his lack of support) George Rohn; Mary Chase Pell, a recent president of the U.S. National Association for Mental Health and WFMH Vice-President for North America; Member-at-Large Gaston Harnois, later to become WFMH Honorary Secretary; and Edith Morgan, WFMH Vice-President for Europe, later to become the WFMH president (1985–1987). Professor Tolani Asuni, M.D., Vice-President for Africa, and Brian O'Connell, the executive director of the U.S. NMHA, had also been asked to serve but declined.

The Task Force's charge, as stated by Lin, initially included a reconsideration of the wisdom and feasibility of "relocating the Secretariat every 3 or 4 years with the working presidents, the increasing need for regionalization of WFMH programs and activities, and the increasing reliance on member associations and individual members for financial support," all of which made it important to "review and to search for better structure, organization and functioning of the Secretariat" (WFMH, 1977). As time went on, though, the essential question became whether or not the Federation should survive at all. There are no available minutes of the task force's deliberations, but anecdotal fragments suggest that there were arguments on both sides of the survival issue. It submitted its recommendations in time for presentation to the Executive Board prior to the 1977 Vancouver World Congress. The conclusion was that the Federation was worth saving. However, this was stated in unenthusiastic terms of minimal activity, recommending that the WFMH "should continue to play its role on a modest scale, commensurate with its income, as an international, non-governmental voluntary organization in a complex and changing environment" (WFMH, 1979a). A major continuing activity, the only one if straightened circumstances demanded it, would be sponsoring international meetings, especially of regional scope. In this respect the recommendations were similar to those of Carstairs' initial review a decade earlier when he had become the first incumbent in the era of "working presidents." Among other recommendations foreshadowing future developments was that for a stable location for the secretariat.

A "New Design" for the WFMH

An important determinant of my return to the Federation was Tsung-yi Lin's invitation to review his proposal for a major revision of its bylaws, the basis of what he termed the New Design for the WFMH. It was composed after the task force's decision that the Federation should live. I agreed and when I first looked at the copy of the bylaws sent to me by mail before the Congress realized that their adoption would change much that had concerned me about the organization. Upon receipt of this draft document I immediately sat down at my typewriter and produced several pages of notes for Tsung-yi to consider. Then, upon my arrival in Vancouver he invited me to attend a meeting of a group from the Executive Board to review what by now had become a semi-final version; it was nearly ready for presentation to the 1979 Board in Salzburg, who would be responsible for finally passing or rejecting it. The intensity of the group's discussion, especially some of the objections to proposed changes, took me aback. Again, I was reminded that the WFMH was an umbrella organization. While its members shared the common goals of promoting positive mental health, preventing illness, and improving the lot of those defined as mentally ill, they often had quite different points of view about how to accomplish them. Among the most apparent tensions surfacing in that small group of experienced, long-time voluntary mental health workers were those I was to encounter repeatedly in later years: the citizen volunteers' distrust of professionals; the conflict between favoring the organization of voting member associations by country (with power concentrated in an all-inclusive national mental health association) versus an understanding of member associations as semiautonomous entities entitled to express themselves individually or within coalitions of their own making; views favoring a smaller Board structure so as to maximize the possibility of effective action versus a preference for a larger Board including more people and organizations in order to ensure a more "democratic" form of decision-making.

The major features of the New Design for WFMH supported by President Lin (WFMH, 1979a) included the recommendation that the president should function essentially as a chief executive officer responsible for all of the financial, legal, and programmatic actions of the organization. His or her primary colleague in this work would be a chairman elected by the Board who would lead in formulating policy decisions and translating policy into action. An executive director would be responsible for the day-to-day administration of the secretariat. The debate about this last person's qualifications centered on the degree of policy and public relations involvement required. The job could be a narrow one filled by an efficient executive secretary or a broad one requiring knowledge and experience in the mental health field. It was also recommended that the regions represented by WFMH vice-presidents (since 1971) should be changed to smaller, more manageable units, with the responsibilities and powers of the vice-presidents strengthened. This brought up the question of WFMH dues paid by individuals and organizations residing within particular regions. Foreshadowing issues prominent in the 1990s, President Lin noted that while it was desirable for revenues collected in particular regions to be shared between the regions and the central secretariat, any such distribution should be "carefully defined" (WFMH, 1979a).

The New Design drastically reduced the overall size of the swollen Board in the interest of encouraging meaningful discussion at meetings. The total number would be similar to that of the Rees years. It would include only the members of a newly created Executive Committee (president-elect, president, past president, honorary secretary, and treasurer), plus four members-at-large and the regional vice-presidents. Significant was the specification of two-year term limits for all elected officers, permitted to succeed themselves once, so each could serve a maximum of four consecutive years in the same position.

The new bylaws also specified that only national and international member associations, professional or volunteer, were to have a vote. As dictated in new articles of incorporation in Canada, they would be represented in a newly created Assembly of Voting Members meeting annually at the time of the Board meetings. Elections would be held biennially at the time of the World Congresses. Thus, the new bylaws undid the practice, intensely supported by European Board members, of permitting a vote only to a single national voluntary mental health association in each country. This had been a chronic source of conceptual confusion in light of the original idea of the WFMH as a federation of associations, not of political entities. It was impossible, however, to get completely away from this representational problem: in order to remedy the disparity between numbers of voting associations in various countries, no more than five votes were to be permitted per country. Among other changes, the revision removed any doubt that professional associations were to be full voting members on the same basis as national mental health associations.

The 1977 Vancouver World Congress for Mental Health

It is important to note that with the Federation in Vancouver President Lin received maximum support from his wife, social worker Mei-chen Lin. This was emphasized in Miller's recollections: "As we came closer to the moment of our BIG PARTY...in the history of man and womankind no couple ever worked harder than Tsung-yi and Mei-chen," both of whom he characterized as "heroes" (Miller, 1996).

The Vancouver Congress of 1977 was sufficiently successful to revive the Federation's fortunes and facilitate its re-entrance onto the world mental health stage. With 2000 participants, rather than the expected 800, and the patronage of then United States First Lady Rosalynn Carter, a long-time mental health volunteer, it was the largest and most influential World Congress for Mental Health since 1948, producing a cash surplus sufficient to support presidential travel as well as expenses of the new secretariat not covered by UBC. This was due to Lin's long experience, numerous international connections and energy, as well as the Congress site, itself a drawing point for many attendees. The meetings of the Executive Board immediately prior to the Congress were "the best attended in memory" (WFMH, 1978a).

Tsung-yi and I had known each other for many years and collaborated in regard to the welfare of foreign medical graduates in the United States, so his success came as no surprise to me. But a basic requirement was the commitment and devoted work of Milton Miller. Milton combined clinical, investigative, and administrative talent with intense social awareness, passion, and a capacity for writing elegant prose. The continuing United States military involvement in Indochina had led him to the difficult decision to leave his post as professor and chairman of psychiatry at the University of Wisconsin and move to Canada. Seeing the WFMH as a way to contribute to world mental health and a possible reduction of international tensions, he engineered the basic support of UBC for the new secretariat, the Congress enterprise and its sequelae. He was pleased with the outcome: "In Vancouver we clearly had returned WFMH to the world map." (Miller, 1996).

My own significant involvement with the Federation (after representing it to the CFMH in Surinam in 1971, and the fundamentally insignificant participation in the Jamaican Administrative Committee in 1972–1973) had begun with Lin's invitation to attend the pre-Congress Executive Committee review of the New Design. More attractive was the accompanying invitation, including paid travel, to speak at that 1977 Congress. The assigned topic, "Health by the People: Right Here, Right Now", seemed a difficult nucleus around which to organize a coherent lecture. It came as a relief, therefore, on the evening before the Congress opening at a party at the Miller's home, when the late, great family therapist and group worker Virginia Satir, my co-speaker, proposed an alternative. She would blindfold me and tie me up on the stage while I free-associated out loud. My free associations would continue, with her interpretations, as she removed the blindfold and ties. In this way she hoped to give the audience a feeling about the subjective experience of entering and recovering from a psychotic experience. The experiment worked. Miller, in retrospect, noted, "I loved that moment when Virginia tied you up and asked how you felt, and you said, 'Dependent, Virginia'." My visibility in front of the large crowd, newspaper photographs, and publication of the taped record of the event (Satir, Brody 1978) gave me enough instant recognizability to allow election to the Executive Board at its 1979 Pre-Congress meeting in Salzburg, Austria.

The Vancouver Secretariat

Miller, looking back, recalled the constant, recurrent pre-1977 efforts to keep the Federation alive. He described them, including his diversion of his department's funds to the WFMH operation, in terms of "that ancient Chinese responsibility of needing to care (for the rest of your days) for the person (or organization) that you save from drowning" (Miller, 1996). While Lin was able to discharge his WFMH presidential responsibilities with funds acquired through the 1977 World Congress, he still depended on support from Miller's budget.

The first secretary for Lin's WFMH office was Roberta "Bertie" Beiser (Mrs. Morton) with an M.A. in Counselling and Guidance. By the end of the Vancouver Congress, in which she had been deeply involved, she was familiar with the Federation's style of operating and was promoted to the title of Administrative Assistant to Lin. In 1979 Guest, with Lin's approval, promoted her to the position of Executive Director of the WFMH, understanding that the post might be temporary. In that capacity her office became the Federation's secretariat, she was an important worker for the 1979 Salzburg congress, and worked with Lin in Manila on publicity for the 1981 World Congress scheduled for that city. At the same time, as a Federation spokesperson, she participated with him in the effort to forge new links with "heretofore somewhat neglected" associations in Australia, New Zealand, and Southeast Asia (Lin, letter to the author, 21 May 1980). I was also in the region in February and March 1981, when I was a visiting professor for a short time with cultural psychiatrist John Cawte, M.D. at the University of New South Wales in Sydney, Australia, and for several weeks with Professor Basil James at the University of Otago in New Zealand. Thus, as president-elect, I was able to hear Bertie represent the Federation in Australia where she visited after being in Manila. She was a good speaker with a pleasant manner, and I could see that she was an appropriate person for the job of Executive Director as it had been envisaged by the New Design with supervision from the president and a board chairman.

1979: World Congress, Salzburg

During the discussion of the New Design conflicting views had emerged around the issue of World Congresses. While only a few of the annual meetings between 1948 and 1977 had been associated with World Congresses, Executive Board discussions prior to the 1973 Australian meeting had favored them on a biennial basis. Regular congresses on a predictable schedule, rotating among different regions, were regarded by those who favored them as important bases for regional as well as national mental health education and advocacy. Arguing against this view were some long-time European members, led by Edith Morgan, who felt that congresses occupied too much time and energy and favored more modest annual meetings instead. It was decided that a test case would be the next biennial World Congress scheduled for 1979. Its success or failure would determine the future course of such gatherings. The question of its location was felt to be important. After the two preceding World Congresses in Australia and Canada, Europe was the logical venue and, within Europe, Austria was regarded as most accessible for mental health activists hoping to attend from Eastern Europe. Since Vienna was deemed too costly, suggestions from several interested parties, including Norman Sartorius, M.D., recently appointed director of WHO's Mental Health Division, led Lin and his Vancouver colleagues to select Salzburg as the site.

I attended this, my second Federation world meeting, in part because the Pathfinder Fund had awarded me a grant to organize a symposium on the prevention of unwanted pregnancies—a sequel to the Jamaica family planning research (see Chapter 13). More immediately, however, Tsung-yi had asked me, in Vancouver, to become a candidate for Executive Board membership, with candidacy regarded as tantamount to election. I was favorably inclined as my interest in the Federation had been rekindled by participation in the Vancouver Congress, and the new bylaws seemed a sound basis for the continuing revival of the WFMH as an international force. Furthermore, the projected Salzburg program reflecting the International Year of the Child seemed to be of very high quality (see Chapter 11). However, the actual speeches and discussions, along with a comparatively small attendance, were anticlimactic after the triumph of Vancouver. More dispiriting, a psychiatrist friend in a senior administrative United States government position commented on what he perceived as the Congress' disorganization and hoped that I wasn't going to desert psychiatry for this ambiguous and not very effective group. But the gathering, with paid attendance by 728 people from 51 countries, was pronounced a success by Federation leaders (WFMH, 1979b).

I was duly elected to the Board at its pre-Congress session, so I could participate in the post-Congress Board's debate about adopting the new bylaws. This was my first such meeting and I was not prepared for the atmosphere. With President Lin seated at the distant end of a long table, and perhaps 50 to 60 people vying for speaking time, the scene was, at least superficially, contentious. There was much resistance to the new bylaws, and its opponents, led by Edith Morgan, were distinctly negative in their views.

Finally a vote was taken and the motion to adopt the new bylaws carried. Only the recommendation for a Board chairman was not followed, leaving the president without this close colleague. The question of the Executive Director's qualifications and responsibilities was held in abeyance, leaving the secretariat to function, as it had since 1968, with a single secretary in the office of the president, but the vote was not unanimous. A number of advocates of the old order made no secret of their unhappiness. I was taken aback to be told *sotto vocce* by one veteran European member that President Lin "represented the worst in international psychiatry," which was inherently antithetical to the mental health aims of the Federation. This was especially surprising since my own status as a psychiatrist who had worked internationally was well known to the critic. However, I had already realized that schisms existed within the Board and listened without responding. The distrust of professionals by long-time mental health association volunteers, and the fear that admitting too many professional, especially medical psychiatric, associations to voting status would dilute the voice of the nonprofessional sector were prominent. The animus stemmed largely from Europe. In other parts of the world, in the Philippines, for example, where professionals associated with the WFMH included educators, lawyers, judges, and others, there was no evident hostility against psychiatry.

GOVERNANCE AND ITS VICISSITUDES

The Board of Directors: Volunteers and Professionals

As indicated in Chapters 3 and 4, the Board during the years leading to the 1967 closure of the Geneva secretariat was dominated by professionally trained persons with shared interests in science and research. Under the leadership of Morris Carstairs, the first of the "working presidents" (see above), the 1968, 20th Anniversary, World Congress was scheduled for London. Responsibility for arrangements was assumed by MIND, the Mental Health Association of England and Wales, which assigned them to Edith Morgan, at the time a key member of its staff. Whether or not this Congress marked the early beginning of a new period of nonprofessional volunteer and mental health association staff involvement in the Federation is unclear. But it may be significant that in 1971, the last year of the Carstairs presidency, MIND leaders felt it necessary to have a meeting on the professional/volunteer relationship—the first time that this particular relationship became an issue for the Federation.

In the autumn of 1979 after the Salzburg Congress, a meeting on Volunteers in Mental Health again stirred feelings about professional/volunteer relations, bringing some 40 delegates, including professionals, to London. With Edith Morgan, then European vice-president of the WFMH, as coordinator, it was sponsored by the Federation's not yet formally organized European region in cooperation with the two organizations for which she had been a staff member and project leader: MIND and the International Hospital Federation (IHF). The possible hostility between professionals and volunteers implied by the repeated organization of meetings on the topic puzzled me since I had not encountered it in my years of service to the New Haven, Connecticut, Metropolitan Baltimore, Maryland, and U.S. National Mental Health Associations in the 1960s. Nor, of course, was it an issue in other areas of the world such as Latin America, where most volunteers, aside from charitable religious organizations, were the professionals themselves.

Another concern of the same European leaders was for greater representation in the Assembly and other decision-making arenas by local and state or provincial rather than national volunteers. This was justified in terms of achieving greater "democracy" and giving people a feeling of belonging. Nearly 10 years later, at the 1986 Board meeting at Cumberland Lodge outside of London, then-president Edith Morgan proposed that the method of voting by organization adopted in 1979 be modified in favor of some form of individual voting. This proposal was rejected, but she did find support for another move to increase the number of board members-at-large from 4 to 5, including a discretionary appointment by the president. The question of increasing the number of Board members, to include representatives of particular constituencies such as ex-patients and users of mental health services, surfaced with increasing frequency during ensuing years. Intermittent calls, mainly from the ERC, for more individual voting and broader opportunity for Board membership continued into the 1990s.

Regional Vice-Presidents

A continuing factor in the nature and growth of the Board, almost from its inception, was recognition of the importance of regional development (see Chapter 9). However, it was not until the 1971 Annual Meeting in Hong Kong that the concept of a single vice-president preparing to succeed to the presidency was abandoned in favor of a group of regional vice-presidents. The vice-presidential positions were conceived as two-way conduits, bringing regional information to the Board and simultaneously acting on behalf of the Board to encourage the development of mental health associations and programs within a region. The initial designations followed that of the 1950 Credentials Committee with six vice-presidents representing different WFMH regions of the world. Based on WHO classifications these were the Americas, the Western Pacific, Southeast Asia, Africa, the Eastern Mediterranean, and Europe. Succeeding presidents influenced further regional divisions. After the 1951 Millan presidency in Mexico, and throughout Michael Beaubrun's 1972–1974 presidency in Jamaica, the Caribbean was identified as a region to be taken into account in the rotation of officers and meetings.

In 1979, with the secretariat still in Vancouver, the all-encompassing Americas Region was divided into North America (including the United States, Canada, and Bermuda) and Latin America. In 1980 New Zealand, Australia, and Pacific Islands were separated from the Western Pacific Region to become a new WFMH Oceania Region (see Chapter 10).

In 1983 the Board's assignment of a high priority to the development of regional councils changed the dynamics of the situation. The position of regional vice-president was no longer dependent for its status and potential power upon the global WFMH and its Board. Instead it became the head of a regional constituency with immense potential power at the grass-roots level.

At the 1986 Board meeting President Edith Morgan called a meeting of the regional vice-presidents to consider their functions. At her request the Vice-President for Oceania, Dr. Max Abbott of New Zealand, chaired the group which produced a "job description" later published in the Newsletter. But the problem of regional vice-presidents kept recurring, and reviewing the "job description" became a frequent feature of later Board meetings. Part of the problem lay in the ambiguity of their relationship with member organizations in their regions and the lack of a Federation infrastructure or funds to support their participation with them. The only regional vice-president with a clearly defined program was that for the European Region which by now was well launched on the development of its Council. The vice-president chaired the Council, which by 1996 was rapidly becoming a quasi-dependency of the European Union into which it became progressively integrated (see Chapter 11). As other Councils developed (see Chapters 9 and 10) the demands of regional needs and loyalties tended to dilute in some measure the allegiances of regional vice-presidents to the global WFMH (see also Chapter 6).

In 1991 the Board, meeting in Mexico City prior to the World Congress, decided on a further reorganization combining the essentially Hispanic Middle America with the multicultural Caribbean Region. This became the Caribbean/Central America/Mexico Region (see Chapter 9). At the same time the Latin American designation was abandoned, and the South American continent was recognized as a separate region of its own. This did not, however, yield the active representation for which the Board hoped. When at the end of his WFMH presidency (1993-1995), Federico Puente S. of Mexico decided unilaterally to form a Latin American Council of the WFMH (LAC/WFMH) encompassing both the Caribbean/Central America/Mexico and the South American regions, the Board passively acquiesced without significant discussion of the ramifications of a supraregional Council. There was no opposition from the vice-president of the first encompassed region, psychoanalyst Dr. Andreas Gaitan of Mexico or psychiatrist Benjamin Vicente, M.D., of Concepcion, Chile, who filled the post of vice-president for South America. It was generally expected that LAC/WFMH would be a short-lived, transitional entity, not persisting past the World Congress scheduled for Chile in 1999. A South American Council was formed by Vicente during the December 1996 Board meeting in Concepcion, Chile. At that time the LAC/WFMH dissolved in favor of CACMC/WFMH (see Chapter 9).

In the 1995 Board meeting in Dublin, European Vice-President John Henderson, a former WHO Regional Mental Health Advisor in Europe and in Southeast Asia, stimulated the regional vice-presidents to request specific representation on the Executive Committee. Although the possible consequences of this move were not explored, incoming president Beverly Long invited him to participate in the 15 March 1996 Executive Committee conference call as a representative of the regional vice-presidents. There he complained that the vice-presidents were effectively disenfranchised from the central WFMH decision-making process because the Executive Committee made decisions without having them ratified by the Board. He also asserted that the regional subdivisions according to which vice-presidents were named were geographically inequitable and recommended, in keeping with his former WHO experience, a return to that organization's regions as a basis for representation. Their subregions would then determine the actual number of representatives per region. A specific example drawing his criticism was the allocation of three vice-presidents for the Americas (South America, Mexico/Central America/Caribbean, and North America) even though all of the Americas constituted a single region for WHO. As noted in Chapter 9 on regionalization, he continued his campaign to revise the regions at the 3–4 May 1996 Executive Committee meeting in Alexandria and at a Strategic Planning Retreat outside of Washington, DC in May 1997. However, while the number, status, and functions of regional vice-presidents remained a significant organizational concern for the Board, the prevailing view after 50 years was that the regions should be smaller rather than larger as in the WHO classification.

Electing the President and the Advent of a President-Elect

From the outset WFMH elections for president and a vice-president to succeed him were conducted during the annual meetings. While the Federation was conceived as an organization of associations, the nation rather than the member association was the accountable unit in the election: each country in which member associations existed was limited to a single vote, preferably cast by a national mental health association that would speak for the entire national constituency. This changed, as noted above, with the new 1979 bylaws after which the dependence upon a single national voice was abandoned, and individual associations, professional as well as voluntary, cast their own votes. Each country, however, was limited to a total of five votes regardless of the number of those cast. This led to some fractional votes being recorded.

During the years from 1948 to the closing of the Geneva secretariat at the end of 1967, as noted earlier, the president had been limited to a single term of one year. Appendix II lists these early presidents and their countries.

After 1967 the situation changed drastically. There were no funds and no administrative structure to support a Director. Survival would depend upon the capacities and institutional support of people willing to serve as president. As noted above, the logical candidates with the requisite support from their institutions were the three professors of psychiatry: Carstairs, Beaubrun, and Lin, with Carstairs serving for approximately 4½ years and Lin for approximately 5 years. The nominating process was highly informal. Lin's choice as his successor to be elected at Salzburg for the 1979-1981 term was Gowan Guest, who had been treasurer of the 1977 World Congress. Guest was the first nominee for WFMH president who was not a professional mental health worker. Perhaps this explains Morris Carstairs' refusal to support him for the presidency as reported by Guest: "You have no vested interest in it" (Guest, 1995). Despite this warning Guest informed Lin that he could put forward his name: "The Board was far from unanimous, but when 'they'had no other nominee at hand, 50% plus one would determine the issue" (Guest, 1995, p. 6). The nomination had been made public so I was surprised to receive a delegation led by Carstairs and Morton Beiser, the North American vice-president. They asked me if I would become a candidate for president at the elections to be held during that very Congress in Salzburg. I answered that I was honored, but knew too little about the organization to accept the candidacy. Also, I did not want to compete with Tsung-yi's nominee, whom I had not yet met. The issues for me were my own lack of knowledge and my desire to go along with Tsung-yi rather than any reservations I might have had about the apparent candidate.

The election was held and Guest, the only candidate, became president for 1979–1981. Then, much to my surprise, Tsung-yi asked me at lunch on the day after the Congress if, following the new bylaws, I would consider being a candidate to become the Federation's first president-elect, succeeding to the presidency in 1981. There had never been a formally elected president-elect before, and it was planned to organize the election before the end of the year. I agreed with some misgivings, but at the same time with excitement about the possibilities of doing something for that ill-defined entity, "world mental health."

Although the election was a long way off, and it was by no means sure that I would become president-elect, Gowan Guest was quick to take advantage of my becoming his potential successor. I agreed to go to Vancouver soon after the Salzburg Congress in order to consult about the future of the WFMH. The visit was pleasant and gave me a chance to know the small WFMH secretariat located at UBC. However, it added little to my understanding of the WFMH's organizational strengths and weaknesses. It was presented as an NGO which advocated mental health-relevant good causes by trying to influence the UN, holding its own Congresses, and co-sponsoring other worthy meetings. It appealed to my interests in international bridge-building and the view that much mental ill health and inability to function optimally were rooted in the remediable social circumstances of development and adult functioning, but the possibilities for action it offered were ambiguous. When I expressed my misgivings to Gowan he told me not to worry because he and Tsung-yi, "like two elephants," would be "propping [me] up on either side."

An early letter (Guest, letter to the author 25 September 1979) brought up the need to alert the newly formed nominating committee about my candidacy and the forthcoming election. The committee, aside from Guest and Immediate Past President Lin, included Canadian Mental Health Association General Director George Rohn, then vice-presidents for North America, Chasey Pell and, for Europe, Edith Morgan and Tolani Asuni, from Nigeria, now posted with the UN Social Defence office in Rome. Guest wrote that he had spoken about the election with Pell and Morgan indicating that my name had been suggested: "It was apparent," he reported, that "they both wondered at the suggestion of yet another North American." In time the Committee nominated one of its own members, Dr. Asuni, so there were two candidates for the post. The election was held on 22 November 1980 with the results tabulated in Vancouver. Besides the Canadians only Edith Morgan and I were present. I was not told how many ballots had been mailed, nor the exact results, only that I had become the Federation's first president-elect, the first ever to be chosen by an open vote of all the member associations, and that I would function in that role, rather than as a Board member-at-large for the next half year until I took office as president during the Manila WFMH World Congress in the summer of 1981.

Lin's New Design did not specify all of the procedural issues required for orderly elections. Even when they were detailed they did not obviate the interpersonal and human factors in the electoral (as well as other) processes that have remained significant throughout the Federation's first half-century. I had learned as much in Salzburg. Now, before I had even come to terms with the idea of my new organizational status, I was faced with the need to think about my successor, who would be named president-elect during the same Manila Assembly at which I would succeed to the WFMH presidency. There was no apparent consensus about a potential leader for the 1983–1985 term so when Lin suggested an old friend of his as president-elect I took it seriously. She was Estafania Aldaba-Lim, a distinguished Philippine citizen who had been a member of the Marcos cabinet but resigned in protest over policies with which she disagreed. Although she had devoted most of her career to public service and volunteer work she had been trained as a psychologist with a doctorate in 1942 from the University of Michigan at Ann Arbor. I had seen her on the stage at Salzburg where she represented the United Nations 1979 Year of the Child. At Tsung-yi's suggestion I visited her just prior to the 1981 Congress in her Manila home where we talked at length. I learned, among other things, that she had been a member of the WFMH Executive Board from 1956 to 1958 in her capacity as president of the Philippine Mental Health Association, continuing from 1958 to 1960 while she was Director of the Institute for Human Relations of the Philippine Women's University in Manila. She and Tsung-yi were on the Federation Executive Board together for much of this period. It was evident that she was an experienced international worker, already familiar with the WFMH, and I asked her to become a candidate. She accepted, but made it clear that it would be difficult from her base in Manila to be an active manager, and she would have to depend on the assistance of a secretariat—either that in Vancouver or one that might be developed at the Philippine Mental Health Association. That was fine with me. I duly reported my interview to Tsung-yi, he nominated her, and she was elected.

After my return to Baltimore, the work toward institutionalizing the electoral process continued. The 1982 Board meeting held in Washington, DC, established the immediate past president as chair of the nominating committee. The 1984 Board meeting at Sheppard Pratt Hospital in Baltimore approved a series of instructions for nominations and voting prepared by Honorary Secretary, Professor Basil James of New Zealand. These worked well for several years, largely because the details of the procedure were often ignored in favor of facilitating the overall outcome. However, this informality was coming to an end in the move toward bureaucratization initiated during Max Abbott's 1991–1993 presidency and accelerating during Puente's 1993-1995 presidency. This may have been an inevitable aspect of the Federation's growing complexity and the need to institutionalize procedures for new Board members and member organizations. It was also driven by the rapid movement of the ERC/WFMH toward a tight, rather rigid model of organization. In consequence of this atmospheric shift the decision was taken in 1995 to develop the Policy and Procedures Manual. Its status was reviewed, with special reference to nomination and election procedures, at the December 1996 Board meeting in Chile. However, a quorum was barely present because of the absence of so many, including myself, at the Western Pacific Regional Meeting in Taipei. The consequently insufficient review probably contributed to the intense confusion about exact procedures within the 1997 Nominating Committee headed by now Past President Puente. It was not until April 1997 that a final version of the procedures was available to be published in the Newsletter for the instruction of potential voters at the mid-summer 1997 election in Lahti, Finland.

REESTABLISHING A PERMANENT SECRETARIAT

The Concept

The Carstairs task force had agreed after the dissolution of the Geneva secretariat that a permanent secretariat should be reestablished. It would provide a badly needed headquarters and communications center for the Federation. It would afford continuity between the terms of elected officers, and be an office to which the world mental health constituency could turn with some expectation of consistent knowledge and availability. Following the New Design it would be headed by an Executive Director responsible both to the president, elected by the voting member organizations, and to a Board chairman elected by members of the Board. This recommendation, thus, did not envisage another Director in the style of Jack Rees who, as an accomplished internationally known psychiatrist, brought the Federation the advantages of his own reputation and interpersonal network and filled the role of chief executive officer as well as spokesman and policy director. In any event it seemed unlikely that there would be sufficient money to pay for a senior person of Rees' caliber, but enough, perhaps, to pay the salary of a responsible executive secretary. The real authority would be vested in the elected president and Board chairman, advised by the board of directors.

The Search for a Site, Funds, and an Executive Director

Carstairs' recommendation for a permanent secretariat required a decision about a suitable site and the identification of an appropriate executive director. This would take time, so the Board asked Tsung-yi Lin to extend his presidency for two more years. He agreed and, in the spring of 1978, began his search for a site with a visit to London. It had been suggested as a possible site for historical and geographical reasons. It was also thought to have available and experienced mental health executives who might become candidates for the post of Executive Director, as well as relatively reasonable costs in comparison with other locations, such as Geneva. Lin discussed this possibility with Morgan and others in the hope that MIND could assist in the initial stages of the secretariat's operation, perhaps with quarters and personnel (WFMH, 1978b). However, no concrete suggestions were forthcoming. Nor was he able to arrange a meeting with Tony Smythe, MIND's director at the time. Smythe, an ardent civil libertarian, was beginning to engage the British psychiatric establishment in a battle about its presumed infringements on the civil rights of patients, and this may have been a factor in his unavailability. Lin extended an invitation to him to join the next Carstairs task force meeting in Montreal on 13 June 1978, but he was unable to attend.

By the time that Guest assumed the WFMH presidency in Salzburg in July 1979 the formal search for a new secretariat site and an Executive Director was in abeyance. However, in my role as a newly elected member of the Executive Board and candidate for the post of president-elect, he pressed me into service in the search for funds to support a permanent secretariat. There was an almost immediate opportunity because I was planning a trip to London 12–21 October to consult on a research problem and to speak to the National Childbirth Trust. This was the beginning of many years of travel paid for by host organizations upon which I "piggy-backed" Federation business. Guest asked me to look for support for a permanent secretariat in London, advising me "to give an impression…of confidence and activity in WFMH," and "to attempt to persuade those connected with various organizations that organization memberships are important, not only as a gesture of support but as a vehicle of involvement." He hoped that I might do better than a British colleague who he said "looks more to the deficiencies of the past than the potential of the future."

In London I brought official greetings from the WFMH to the annual meeting of the Trust celebrating the "Year of the Child." the WFMH honorary president, the Lady Priscilla Norman, who had been close to the Federation founders, gave me the better part of an afternoon. We spoke of its mission and "what the world would miss if WFMH did not exist." She also felt that the Federation was not sufficiently visible among organizations concerned with mental health, broadly defined, rather than psychiatric illness. It was important, she believed, that WFMH stay "close" to them because "It has not made itself known sufficiently amongst groups which do not just concern themselves with psychiatric disorders but with factors, as you say, 'contributing to optimal functioning.'"

In regard to the pros and cons of a permanent secretariat, she came down firmly for permanence as "essential for growth." However, she was the first to suggest a move away from the Vancouver secretariat, which she regarded as transitory. When I suggested a possible site in the American Psychiatric Association building in Washington, DC, she felt that might jeopardize the Federation's major strength, that is, its "multidisciplinary identity." However, "a close link with an academic institution is very important and so could be an office in a National Association for Mental Health building, provided it is a strong and well respected Association, not too left or too right in its political views and has support in the medical, psychological and social work fraternity." She was prescient: our United States secretariat managed by Dick Hunter was eventually located in the National Mental Health Association building in Alexandria, Virginia.

I was also fortunate in being able to arrange a long talk with Dr. Richard Thompson, head of the United Kingdom Mental Health Foundation. It was facilitated by two members of his advisory board, Professors John Wing and Julian Leff of the Maudsley, with whom I had spent a day consulting about a problem in the epidemiology of schizophrenia. Thompson was already reported to be negative toward the Federation, having expressed the feeling that few foundations would be willing to fund an organization "which seemed to many to be a travel club for its Board." However, he turned out to be a candid, energetic, and interested advocate of mental health who was friendly at the same time that he expressed his misgivings about the precise goal and mission of the WFMH.

Edith Morgan was out of town, but I was able to talk at length with Miles Hardie, director general of the IHF, of which she was a staff member. In contrast to Thompson his attitude toward the Federation was unreservedly supportive. He suggested having the next WFMH Board meeting at the end of March in Belgium at the time of IHF's conference on Alternatives to Mental Hospitalization, which listed the WFMH as a co-sponsor.

Upon my return from London I sent the Board a report of relevant contacts from my trip (Brody, letter to the WFMH Board, 1 November 1979). Chasey Pell responded with enthusiasm to Hardie's suggestion for the WFMH Board meeting in Belgium, especially if IHF would give us a place on its program (Pell, 1979). Edith Morgan, however, was doubtful and concerned about the possibly negative impact of non-European Board members on IHF proceedings: "I'm sure that any WFMH representation would be welcome though I suppose we shall have to bear in mind that this is a European regional meeting so the organisers will probably want to keep the emphasis fairly strongly European" (Morgan, letter to the author, 8 November 1979).

This response to my outreach efforts was disappointing. I discussed it in a letter dated 20 November 1979 addressed to Pell, Guest, and Rohn: "Although Edith indicates that we should not interfere with the European orientation of the IHF meeting I would not hesitate to suggest a WFMH panel or some other relevant contribution which would add perspective and effectiveness. [Having our Board] meeting there would give us a chance to support the European activities, 'show the flag,' enhance the viability of WFMH etc." Guest's response was negative as he very much wanted to have the Board meeting in Mexico—a prospect I strongly opposed because of the factions within Mexican psychiatry which I thought would make it very difficult for us to gain a foothold there (see Chapter 9). Guest, as president, however, carried the day and we had our Board meeting in Mexico City on 12–13 April 1980. As predicted it did place us squarely in the midst of the chronic feud between psychiatric leaders and organizations. When, 11 years later in 1991, we were finally able to have a World Congress in Mexico City the feud still continued and our identification with one of the warring parties led the other to effectively boycott the Congress.

Building Bridges to Other Organizations

My main reason for suggesting that the 1980 Board meeting be held in conjunction with the IHF meeting in Belgium was that I wanted to realize the new possibilities opened up by the revised bylaws for communication between the WFMH and the professional organizations that had been among my major international bridges. When, for example, Peter Berner of Vienna, then Secretary General of the World Psychiatric Association (WPA) wrote on 2 August 1979 to remind me that I was still the liaison from WPA to PAHO, I suggested that we think about possible ways in which WPA and WFMH might collaborate. He responded affirmatively, but perhaps because of the differences in outlook and goals of the two organizations, nothing significant evolved. In May 1980 Tsung-yi Lin, after speaking with officers of the American Psychiatric Association (APA) during the 2nd Pacific Congress of Psychiatry in Manila, asked me to do whatever possible to strengthen ties with them (Lin, letter to the author, 21 May 1980). Over the next several years, despite generous support from the American Psychiatric and Psychological Associations, I reluctantly realized the fundamental differences between the goals and capacities of the WFMH and the professional organizations. The former, with an ecumenical membership, was dedicated solely to achieving mental health goals. The latter, with economically bound guild memberships, were in fact trade unions whose ultimate goals were the welfare of their professional members whose high dues provided their large budgets. This did not, of course, mean that they could not be valuable allies.

Non-mental health agencies and organizations also required attention. Like Priscilla Norman, Chasey Pell agreed about the importance of influencing general health agencies and organizations to consider mental health in all of their work. She was especially interested in my suggestion that the WFMH might consider co-sponsoring the 1980 Berlin Congress of the International Society for Psychosomatic Obstetrics and Gynecology (ISPOG). I was on its Board at the time and regarded its work as having a particular bearing on the mental health of pregnant women and new mothers and their infants. Although our Executive Committee did not agree to the co-sponsorship at the time, it was possible to bring our interests together in our later concerns with women's mental health and the prevention of ill-health (see Chapters 8, 10, 11, 13). In 1980 I attempted, without success, to interest the International College of Pediatrics, of which I was a Senate member, to join the WFMH. An early co-sponsorship was the April 1982 meeting of the Association for Behavioral Sciences and Medical Education (of which I had been president in 1970) in Taos, New Mexico on Training Clinicians for Work in Multi-Ethnic Societies. But its relationship with the WFMH was transitory. As its 50th anniversary approached the WFMH Board agreed to our co-sponsorship, along with UNHCR and several other agencies, of the October 1997 meeting of the Society for the Study of Psychiatry and Culture on migration.

In April 1980, again in London for professional reasons, I encountered distinctly negative feelings about MIND in the psychiatric community. Some colleagues with whom I spoke, including those at the Royal College of Psychiatrists, regarded it as hostile to the practice of psychiatry. This followed continued accusations from MIND, led by Smythe, that psychiatrists were depriving patients of their civil rights. The central villain in question turned out to be a professor of psychiatry whom I had known well in the past. I went to see him and discovered that he had instituted intravenous feeding in a semicomatose anorectic patient in danger of death. There was some uncertainty, given her mental state, about whether or not he had obtained proper informed consent from her for the procedure. He was quite firm in his opinion: "I refused to let her die on my service. If her family wanted to have her transferred to another hospital that would be alright with me." I didn't learn all of the details of this and other cases, but the accusations were sufficiently serious and insufficiently supported so that MIND was threatened not only with the loss of support by British psychiatry, but with the loss of its government subsidies. Smythe was subsequently replaced by another MIND director.

THE WFMH SECRETARIAT IN BALTIMORE AND WASHINGTON: 1981–1997

The Transitional Baltimore Secretariat: 1981–1983

The question of moving the secretariat from Vancouver arose again immediately after I became president in Manila in July 1981. Bertie Beiser reminded me that the Executive Director served at the pleasure of the president and that now, at the beginning of my term, I should confirm her appointment for the next two years. It was impossible for me to make an informed decision, and I was not ready to deal with the confusion and added work for my university office the Vancouver secretariat's dissolution would entail. Furthermore, I was favorably impressed by the work she did for the Federation, including the publication of the regular Newsletters which constituted the main communicative link among the far-flung membership, the Board, and the secretariat. Therefore, I indicated that we would maintain the status quo for my term in office. At the same time it was becoming evident that many required decisions and initiatives were beyond the capacity of a nonprofessional executive, however competent. This was true even for the recruitment of professional organizations as new voting members. For example, I regarded it as important to the growing strength of the WFMH that the American Psychiatric Association should become part of our umbrella Federation (Brody, letter to Melvin Sabshin, M.D., 11 October 1979). Rather than ask Bertie to handle this, I personally got in touch with the APA Medical Director, my old friend Melvin Sabshin, M.D.

It gradually became necessary for me, even with the help of the Vancouver office, to act as yet another working president. My University of Maryland office, capably managed by Eileen Potocki until 1983 and then by Kathy McKnight, M.Ed., gradually took over many functions of a Federation secretariat. This was made possible through the support of Professor Russell R. Monroe, who in 1977 had succeeded me as chairman of the University's Department of Psychiatry and Director of its Institute of Psychiatry and Human Behavior. My intent at the time was simply to survive my two years of presidency, work with Dick Hunter—already deep into its preliminary organization—on the 1983 World Congress, and let my successor as WFMH president, "Fanny" Aldaba-Lim as I now knew her, decide whether or not to disband the Vancouver office. But after discussions with her, Dick, and some key members of the Board I decided that this was a decision that could not be taken without adequate preparation. Therefore, before the end of my first six months in office, and with the cooperation of Bertie Beiser, Tsung-yi Lin, and others, I appointed two committees to illuminate the situation. First, I asked Aldaba-Lim to chair a new committee on the structure, function, and location of the secretariat (including its cost). Second, I asked our honorary secretary, Professor Basil James, in whose University of Otago, New Zealand Department of Psychiatry I had been a visiting professor earlier that year, to review the WFMH committee structures and the functions of the various officers in relation to the Executive Director. On the basis of their preliminary findings the Board, in Washington, DC in mid-1982, voted, contingent upon resources, to consider at its post-Congress meeting in 1983 a transfer of the secretariat from Vancouver to the United States. In time, both Aldaba-Lim and James came up with the same recommendation: that if quarters and professional help could be arranged with a promise of stability for several years the Federation would be best served with a secretariat on the eastern seaboard of the United States. Among the advantages would be its ready accessibility to NGO and UN offices in Washington, DC and/or New York City and the presumed greater ease of fundraising in the United States than in Canada.

Decisions: Toward a Permanent Baltimore-Washington Secretariat and a Secretary General

The final recommendations of Aldaba-Lim and James did not come until early 1983. The first hint that I might have to make the decision about a new secretariat myself had come earlier, on an autumn afternoon in 1982 in London, a bit over a year into my presidential term. Edith Morgan and I were waiting for the train to take us to visit Lady Juliet Bingley, who then chaired the Board of MIND. Edith mentioned that she and Gaston Harnois, then the WFMH honorary secretary, had wondered if I would be willing to take on the tasks of directing the Federation, perhaps for five years or so after the completion of my term as president. She made it clear that I would not be an "executive director," but would function in a manner analogous to the way in which Jack Rees managed the organization. A retrospective letter from Harnois recalls his feeling that as a veteran fundraiser for my university institute and an administrator relating to several professional schools I might be asked to stay on to help in the Federation's organizational and financial development. As he wrote: "I recall that this is when your name came about as being a potential leader in this process. This was also tied to the idea that, whereas previous to that the secretariat had moved with each president, maybe then the time had come to establish a permanent secretariat, more than likely in the United States since this was judged as being the country from which eventual financial support was most likely to come" (Harnois, letter to the author, 15 November 1995).

In the ensuing months other colleagues weighed in with their own opinions. Thus was initiated a period of intense introspection and organizational discussion about the idea of establishing a permanent WFMH secretariat on the eastern seaboard of the United States. I was concerned about the impact of such a commitment upon my personal career, including a potential loss of professional status. Accepting the WFMH post, requiring up to two-thirds of my time, would mean abandoning other activities and a dilution of my identification with the field of psychiatry, which had been my major source of professional and personal support. I also had to consider the loss of earning capacity. The post would occupy much of my working time and the major part of my energy. The WFMH was no longer able to afford a salaried director, as it had with Jack Rees, and it would be necessary to work as a volunteer. Finally, I continued to have doubts about the Federation's capacity to evolve into a genuinely viable organization, able to make an impact on that elusive and somewhat grandiose entity, "world mental health." However, the concept was appealing, and like other optimistic persons, I felt that I might make a difference. Most compelling, in retrospect, was the feeling that it "fit" my life course and personal interests, and that at the end of the road I would have a greater feeling of fulfillment than if I continued a career as a professional psychiatrist. At that time I was, after all, 61 years old, already disengaging from career goals, and able to commit much of my physical and emotional energy to a volunteer job.

Unavoidably, the issue of accepting leadership for a new secretariat became intertwined with preparations for the 1983 World Congress scheduled for Washington, DC and, especially, the role of Dick Hunter as its operational manager representing the U.S. NMHA. He was on the brink of retirement from his post as NHMA Deputy Director and, for a short time, as Acting Director. Now we added to our discussions about the financing and planning of the World Congress a year-long dialogue about the future of the secretariat and our possible roles in it. It was obvious to both of us that I could be overwhelmed by the job of WFMH organizational development. Months of working together had resolved his doubts about our compatibility, and had given me great confidence in his organizational and managerial ability as well as his dedication to Federation goals. After much reflection I decided that without his close collaboration I could not accept the challenge of continued Federation leadership after 1983. His agreement to become my most senior associate (later formalized in the role of Deputy Secretary General) was the major factor in my decision to accept the job of succeeding Jack Rees. It wasn't exactly that, since Rees was salaried, and supported by a significant infrastructure, while I was to be part-time, unsalaried, and had to create my own infrastructure. But Rees' post provided the model for the role I had in mind.

As discussions progressed and included more people, President-Elect Aldaba-Lim began to play a central role. With the informal agreement of the Executive Committee, she prepared to put a motion to the post-1983 World Congress Board to establish a permanent WFMH secretariat somewhere "on the Eastern seaboard of the United States." This would be done with the understanding that, on a nonsalaried basis, I would accept a part-time post equivalent to that of Director with functions analogous to those of Jack Rees, and that Dick Hunter, also nonsalaried but full-time, would be my primary associate. At first there was some uncertainty about my new title. Director General, the title used by Rees' successor, Francois Cloutier, was proposed, but after trying it briefly I decided against it, since there was no budget and no staff to "direct." The job was more that of a policy and program initiator, coordinator, and communicator, as well as an organizational chief executive. Dick and I would have to set the Federation on a new organizational and programmatic course, and do it with minimal resources. Finally, in keeping with the practices of many international organizations we reached an agreement that the title of Secretary General would be most appropriate for the position of chief executive.

The proposed location "on the Eastern seaboard of the United States" was sufficiently ambiguous to allow reflection as how best to organize the physical aspects of the new secretariat. However, the basic choices had already been made. I continued in my University of Maryland office, which had been the WFMH president's office between 1981 and 1983. With little difficulty it became, between 1983 and 1987, the secretary general's office. When I retired completely from the University in 1987 the groundwork for another move had already been laid. A few years earlier I had moved my editorial offices for the *Journal of Nervous and Mental Disease* to the Sheppard and Enoch Pratt Hospital in Baltimore. Now the hospital's president, Robert Gibson, M.D., strongly supportive of our organizational efforts and ready to accept a nomination as WFMH treasurer, agreed to add another office to the *Journal* suite to house my Federation secretary. He also agreed to charge our basic WFMH expenses, mainly for telephone, fax, and mail, to the hospital budget. In effect, except for the secretarial salary, Sheppard totally supported the office from 1987 to 1996, when financial difficulties made it necessary to reduce its support. Its contribution to the WFMH, first through Bob Gibson and later through his successor as president, Steven Sharfstein, M.D., are inestimable. The offer of a free chief executive's office along with two unsalaried senior executives to keep the Federation going were important in the Board's acceptance of the proposal to establish a new secretariat.

Meanwhile, Dick Hunter had begun to function as, in essence, the Federation's senior administrator—what I came to think of some years later as our chief operating officer. He rented space in the headquarters building of his long-time employer, the U.S. NMHA, where he would be in charge of the main office of the new secretariat when his imminent retirement from the association became effective. These arrangements were supported by the Board.

Organizational Consequences of a Stable Secretariat

After 1983 a stable, professionally well-connected and knowledgeable secretariat was able to provide successive presidents with a central office to aid in the formulation and implementation of their ideas and free them from routine organizational maintenance tasks. This made it possible to increasingly involve them and other Board members in the tasks of leadership. It also made it possible for the first time since the end of the Geneva secretariat to have presidents who did not have their own institutional bases capable of supporting a Federation office. Thus, we were able to have such presidents as Estafania Aldaba-Lim, Ph.D. (1983–1985), Edith Morgan (1985–1987), Gamal Abou El Azayem, M.D. (1987–1989), Stanislas Flache, M.D. (1989–1991), Federico Puente Silva, M.D. (1993–1995), and Beverly Long (1995–1997). Only Max Abbott, Ph.D. (1991–1993), then Director of the Mental Health Foundation of New Zealand, had the institutional support as well as experience and capability to have done it independently in the fashion of a "working president." Marten de Vries, M.D. (1997–1999) with the institutional as well as personal capacity, probably would not have accepted the nomination if his institute and university had been required to support a WFMH secretariat.

In keeping with the Carstairs task force report of 1977, a gradual shift of decision-making, and the initiation of projects and programs, away from the Secretariat and to the elected officers was one of my eventual goals from 1983 on. It was a goal that required a secretariat capable of independent supportive action. Some elected leaders, however, especially those at a considerable geographic and cultural distance, relied heavily on the Secretariat not only for management, but for programmatic and policy decisions. In these instances I used the authority of my role as Secretary General to make policy-related decisions without prior consultation either with the Board or the Executive Committee. Most significant were recruiting and establishing topic oriented committees and collaborating centers, and deciding on WFMH co-sponsorship of conferences. I also recruited, appointed, and monitored the work of our representatives to UN headquarters in New York, Paris, Geneva, and London, with three exceptions. The exceptions were Stanislas Flache, M.D., appointed to Geneva by President Aldaba Lim; Elena Millan-Game, appointed to Paris by President Morgan; and after Millan-Game's resignation two years later, Madeleine Riviere, M.D., appointed by President Puente Silva.

The Secretariat's Role in Organizational Development

In 1992, in anticipation of some additional funding, Dick and I began to discuss how, with the addition of new staff, our respective offices might best foster the Federation's organizational development. Since we wanted to be sure that the Board understood what we had in mind, we scheduled discussion time for the 1993 Tokyo post-Congress Board meeting chaired by incoming President Puente Silva. We briefly described the possible development of professional staff people to work with us in "program development, regional development, and resource development, understanding that all responsibilities are overlapping and interdependent." We tried to make it clear that "all three of these basic activities involve a dual orientation: both to process and management (most evident in resource development), and to the substantive issues with which process and management are concerned (most evident in program development)." The Board approved our general perspective on organizational development, but the press of other business made it impossible to have a detailed discussion. Therefore, I inserted a separate sheet into the August/September 1993 Newsletter describing an enhanced role for the secretariat. It was entitled Post-Congress Board Discussion in Japan; Organizational Development: the Role of the Secretariat. I thought that this might stimulate Board members to respond with positive or negative suggestions, or even with disapproval. But, as was all too frequently the case, there was no response at all.

Dick and I decided to interpret approval at the Board meeting and the lack of response to the Newsletter insert as encouragement to proceed in a systematic organizational development effort. In this role he initiated World Mental Health Day, described in the sections on the international mental health agenda. As described in Chapter 6, he successfully solicited funds from Eli Lilly and Company, which allowed him to employ a competent full-time staff person, first

Christine Skennion, and then Catherine Gray, in the role of Associate Director for Development. Although he had employed other part-time people as fundraisers in the past, none had produced the hoped-for results. This was to be "the big push," enabling him to leave as his legacy an endowed Federation. It also permitted him to plan for other developments, most prominently the acquisition of a staff person to maintain contact with the WFMH regions, especially Africa. In this last respect I thought that if we were able to acquire funds they might be better spent to build up the offices of the regional vice-presidents in the three unsupported regions: Africa, Eastern Mediterranean, and Latin America. This grass roots-oriented policy, I thought, might take precedence over building the central office.

As far as my office was concerned the change was mainly titular. Earlier in 1992, Kathy McKnight had moved to become Managing Editor of *The Journal of Nervous and Mental Disease* which, since it was located just across the corridor from our WFMH offices, allowed her to continue as an informal consultant to the WFMH, with which she had been so closely involved for over 10 years. I was fortunate to be able to fill her Federation post with Elena Berger, who had a doctorate in economic history from Oxford. Dr. Berger combined secretarial with administrative and policy-related functions (I continued, as always, to write most of my own letters) and I had called her an executive assistant. Now, at Dick's suggestion, her title was changed, in a manner parallel with that of Dick's assistant, to Associate Director for Programs. The new title did not change her responsibilities, which were already enlarging to include basic communication with UN representatives, work on some committee projects as indicated in Chapter 13, and related issues. The main point was that she was more alert than before to programmatic possibilities that might be explored.

In 1993 I was fortunate enough to obtain, through Richard Mollica's good offices, grant support from a private foundation to pay for Berger's salary, publication of the Newsletter and Annual Report, and the installation of an Internet system including a web page and e-mail capability. This last was conceived as the nucleus of a mental health information clearing house. However, the funds were not sufficient to hire the additional personnel that would be necessary to develop it as a project. We began to activate it at a minimum level in 1995, at which time McKnight was able to give us some time as a publications and Internet consultant. I was proud of having put the WFMH on the Internet, but this new development elicited no significant comment from the Board, which seemed to take it as a matter of course.

AS THE FIRST HALF CENTURY AND THE FOURTH PHASE OF FEDERATION LIFE ENDS

By the 1990s, along with increasing Board attention to administrative procedures, the era of single-handed decision making by the Secretary General was drawing to an end. There was another factor to be taken into account. Dick and I were growing older. At the time of the 1992 Board meeting in Sydney, we formally directed the Board's attention to the need to prepare for a succession when one or both of us were no longer able to continue in our volunteer jobs. This stimulated President-Elect Puente to action. During the first Board meeting of his presidency a year later in Tokyo after the 1993 WFMH World Congress, he announced that he was going to move the Federation from Model A, in which it was effectively run by the Secretary General with the support of the Deputy, to Model B, in which decisions, particularly of a policy nature, were to be in the hands of the president and Board. Unfortunately, he did not include the essential fundraising activities as a Board responsibility, and he was so occupied with the administrative process that he made little impact on the international mental health agenda. He also initiated a new controversy within the Board with a series of proposals intended to keep ex-presidents in active positions of power. These stimulated prolonged and sometimes vehement discussions extending to his last Board meeting as president, prior to the July 1995 World

Congress in Dublin. By then agreement had been reached that the WFMH should have a council of former presidents but not, as he had wished, that the immediate past president should chair it, and emphatically not that the Council's chairperson would sit on the Board—which would have extended his period as a Board member by two more years.

Nonetheless, I decided to assist in the move from plans A to B. Beverly Long, who assumed the presidency at the 1995 post-Congress Board meeting in Dublin, was an experienced voluntary organization leader, the former president of the U.S. NMHA and someone in whom I had had sufficient confidence to suggest her nomination for president. She accepted the mandate to deal seriously with policy issues. Her obvious competence allowed me to feel comfortable in turning over much of my formal responsibility as chief executive officer to her, and she embraced it with enthusiasm. The idea was to encourage her as incoming president to do more, and I knew that she had the background, interest, and time to do just that. Indeed, she did demonstrate that, given knowledge and ability, sufficient time and assistance, the WFMH president might be able to take over from the Secretary General as the organization's chief executive—that is, to function in the manner envisaged by the 1979 bylaw changes. Among other activities, she defined the advocacy role of the Federation, focused attention on prevention activities, and devoted special attention to developing programs to raise the priority level of mental health concerns in national health ministries, utilizing, in particular—as noted in Chapters 8 and 13—the support of the WHO. She was also active in building bridges with various regional groupings, and an ardent user of conference calls. Finally, she pushed with enthusiasm the development of the "P and P" Manual under Max Abbott's aegis.

After the Dublin Congress, I withdrew my investment in organizational development and leadership from approximately 66 to 45 or 50 percent of my time, and, as I spent more time writing this memoir and history, turned over more of my responsibilities to Elena Berger. Her accurate title, reflecting a gradual development since I recruited her in 1992, would have been "assistant secretary general." Her scholarly and international background and analytical mind allowed her to become a key figure for a number of the projects initiated by or monitored by my office, as well as the maintenance of the Federation's communications center.

By mid-1996, halfway into Long's term, it was clear that the new arrangement was working well. I felt that I had done what I could for the Federation, and that in any event Mother Nature would sooner rather than later require Dick and me to step aside. I proposed to the 4–6 May 1996 Executive Committee meeting at the Alexandria secretariat that the Board meeting after the 1997 WFMH World Congress in Finland should include a full-dress discussion of possible new ways of organizing the functions of the secretariat and the Federation's general manner of doing business. I also pointed out that Dick had been functioning very much in the fashion of many executive directors of voluntary agencies, and proposed (as he and I had discussed earlier) that our discussions include the status, role, and functions of a chief operating officer who might replace both the Secretary and Deputy Secretary General. I thought we might be able to find a salary for such a person, and that if the post of Secretary General were maintained, it could be filled by another semiretired professional who would bring his or her network and status to the task. These ideas and others about the WFMH future were included in my Message from the Secretary General sent to the Board prior to its December 1996 meeting in Concepcion, Chile, which I did not attend because of my prior commitment to our Western Pacific Regional Conference in Taiwan (see Chapter 10). As it happened, no major discussion of this issue took place in Concepcion. This reflected the failure to reach a quorum until the second day of the meeting, partly because no Asian board member was present: Kunihiko Asai and Shimpei Inoue were both involved in Taipei. Beverly Long accepted my suggestion and plans were made for a total review of our mission, operations, and bylaws with the Board and some selected others acting as a committee of the whole in preparation for the Finland Board. This was to begin with a strategic planning retreat in May 1997. Treasurer J. David Robinson, in collaboration with Dick, obtained essential assistance on a pro bono basis from Andersen Consulting, one of the world's largest management firms. The process began with a series of conference calls to small groups of colleagues from different regions asking four questions: (1) What mental health problems are appropriately addressed through international advocacy? (2) What are our current activities and capabilities? (3) Which organizations compete with or complement us? (4) What do our constituents need and want from us? Meanwhile, I was on the phone with a follow-up letter to the president of the foundation that supported my office activities. After an approximately one-hour telephone conversation, she indicated her willingness to make a grant to cover travel and retreat expenses for Board members from distant parts of the world, saying, "Dr. Brody, I trust you." This left me with a mild feeling of uneasiness and obligation, but I felt that our cause was just and this was an opportunity to clarify our view of the future.

The actual retreat was held from 2 to 4 May 1997 at Airlie House just outside of Washington, where the four issues noted below were the focus of discussion about our *unique* mission. After that we discussed issues of governance, infrastructure, succession plans, and sources of funding. It was anticipated that by July a draft of a plan would be ready to present to the Board and Assembly in Finland. The final outcome of the process was in the process of being sifted and analyzed as mid-1997 approached. Some things were clear, however. First, despite the looseness of our Federation organization, and our status as a community of committed individuals rather than a strong, tightly structured institution, we were resilient and able to take advantage of opportunities for constructive mental health work as they arose.

Second, the need for greater Board involvement in both the organizational and substantive work of the Federation was compelling. Members-at-large should be elected to fill particular portfolios.

Third, the WFMH would not progress without a more adequate infrastructure. The tendency remained to suggest additional tasks and functions for the Secretariat without assuming responsibility for adding the staff necessary for them to be carried out.

Fourth, there was no question of a regional versus a central organizational focus. The WFMH must remain a global organization with regional arms rather than a network of regional Councils with a coordinating central office. A problem was recognized in the potential rigidity and inhibiting effects of some models of regional Council organization evident mainly in the ERC/WFMH, which some participants felt was losing its ability to function independently of its quasi-dependent relation with the European Union. It was important for the Secretariat and Board to feel free to communicate with WFMH member organizations within a region as well as with the Council itself—and vice versa. This was part of a general feeling that the center, i.e., the Board and Secretariat should, as in the early days, reestablish closer contact with member organizations.

In 1997, the Federation's longest-lived international Secretariat has been in the Baltimore-Washington region of the United States. Beginning with my 1981–1983 presidential office it has endured for 16 years. In this period it has been rebuilt and revised, and has surpassed the capacity for influencing mental health on a global basis, which distinguished it during the Rees era. However, it has not succeeded in accumulating the endowment necessary to ensure its full potential and survival.

Chapter 6

The Unending Search for Money: Where is the Pot of Gold?

OVERVIEW

Variations in the governance and programs of the Federation have reflected the interests and energies of the volunteers who constitute its most important resource. More obviously, they have reflected its chronically fragile financial state and consequent lack of infrastructure. This was true for the abandonment of the Interprofessional Advisory Committee and its subsequent Scientific Committee, the curtailment of projects such as the 1960 World Mental Health Year, and the wandering Federation headquarters in the years after the collapse of its Geneva secretariat in 1967. In the period after 1981 and the establishment of a new "permanent" secretariat in 1983, donated office space and volunteered time from its senior executives made it, again, a significant international force for mental health. However, lack of resources kept it from realizing the full potential of the new structures formed in this era: topic-oriented committees, university-based collaborating centers, regional councils, and enlarged and more active WFMH representative teams at UN offices in New York, Geneva, Paris, and Vienna. Lack of resources has also prevented the full development of projects such as World Mental Health Day, initiated in 1992.

In fact, finances have preoccupied WFMH leaders since the organization was first conceived. Although they succeeded—especially during the Rees era—in obtaining significant sums of money from gifts and grants as well as dues, the funds have never been sufficient to ensure continuity, either of the central operation or of particular programs. Seventeen years after the organization was founded, and 4 years after Rees had retired as Director, he was still ruminating about his inability to establish a secure financial base for it: "A fundamental shortcoming at the time of the Federation's founding was inadequate planning for the financing of its work" (Rees, 1966, pp. 133–134).

Despite difficulties and scarcity, however, there was steady—although slow and insufficient—growth in resource accumulation between 1948 and Rees' retirement at the end of 1961. Between January 1962 and autumn 1965, during the administration of Rees' successor, psychiatrist Francois Cloutier, who assumed the title of Director General, spending outstripped funding. This became most severe with the 1963 transfer of the Secretariat from London to Geneva.

The eventual result was its financial collapse, leading to Cloutier's resignation at the end of 1965 and the Secretariat's final closure at the end of 1967. These events are described in detail in Chapter 4. By mid-1968 the Secretariat had moved to the offices of then-President Carstairs, supported by his Department of Psychiatry at the University of Edinburgh. Thus began the era, described in Chapter 5, when the Secretariat moved with the office of successive presidents. The loss of a stable central office for the Federation was a source of great concern. Rees' final message dealt with the financial basis for this instability. In the Summer 1968 number of the WFMH Bulletin, precursor of the Newsletter, he wrote: "Lack of finance has been the bogey throughout and still is. You and I and our friends must make a determined effort to change this. The right people and the proper knowledge are available to carry out this work, if we can ensure the financial backing."

As described in Chapter 5 Carstairs assumed the presidency under most inauspicious circumstances. The Federation was in a state of financial collapse and without a Secretariat. At first, writing in the Spring 1968 WFMH Bulletin, he avoided confrontation with financial issues by appealing to voluntarism: "WFMH is not a wealthy body and in my opinion it has no need to become one, because its riches consist in the experience, the expertise and above all the good will of its members in over sixty countries." His reference to localities was deliberate as he considered it essential to increase the number of regional meetings, which might have greater access to funding than global activities. Later, however, he accepted the importance of reviving a strong central office. He was able to overcome his intense dislike for fundraising and to obtain funds from an American donor, Mr. Clement Stone of Chicago, which along with Edinburgh University's support for basic Federation office expenses helped keep the organization afloat.

The 20th Anniversary 1968 World Congress in London was financed by sources outside of the Federation's central budget (see Chapter 11). At its final session Carstairs launched a special fundraising campaign—called the WFMH President's Appeal—in order to eliminate the accumulating WFMH deficit. He announced an offer by Mr. Stone to match all contributions received up to 31 December 1968 with an equivalent sum in dollars up to a maximum of $40,000. However, the matching effort was unsuccessful. Consequently, the Federation was able to sustain only a minimal program, holding its annual meetings and co-sponsoring some others. This state of affairs continued through the Beaubrun presidency from 1972 to 1974 with the central office at the University of the West Indies in Kingston, Jamaica.

It was not until 1977 that the organization regained a measure of solvency sufficient for it to again become an active player on the world stage. This was due to support from the University of British Columbia and especially the 1977 World Congress for Mental Health in Vancouver, Canada led by WFMH President Tsung-yi Lin, who held the office from 1974 to 1979 (see Chapters 5 and 10). That World Congress, the largest and most impressive in Federation history to date with 2000 participants, was an international event. It also produced a financial surplus. But Lin's presidency was followed by two more years of renewed spending without systematic fundraising. His successor, Vancouver lawyer-businessman Gowan Guest, WFMH president from 1979 to 1981, realized what was happening and his own role in the process. He was aware of the heavy expenditures during that period, especially on travel, knew that little money was coming in, and that the organization could again regress to its 1967 condition. He wrote in the first quarterly number of the 1981 WFMH Newsletter: "At the current rate of encroachment on reserves…[they] are likely to be exhausted in about three years." This fitted his first view of the WFMH in 1974-1975 when it moved to Vancouver. He described it as an nongovernmental organization "with no visible means of support and no marketable program to solicit public and corporate support" (Guest, letter to the author, 22 November 1995). But because of his stature as a lawyer and financier and his previous service as president of the Canadian Mental Health Association (in 1967), Lin overcame his skepticism and recruited him in 1976 to help with finances for the Vancouver Congress. The preparatory work for that Congress confirmed his earlier perception of a WFMH suffering from "chronic impecuniosity" (Guest, letter to the author,

22 November 1995). Despite these insights he used the remaining reserves to support his presidential travel and other activities and did not take the active steps necessary to halt the slide into insolvency. However,the ensuing threat of bankruptcy that led to his abrupt resignation from the Board in 1982 (see below) could not have come as a surprise.

Another Federation leader during the Lin presidency, Gaston Harnois also expressed his concern, summarized in a retrospective account. "In those days," he wrote, "one of the key concerns of the Federation was of course financial and we were very much looking for ways in which to ensure a greater financial stability to the Federation." He believed that the time had come to once more establish a permanent secretariat, "more than likely in the United States since this was judged as being the country from which eventual financial support was most likely to come" (Harnois, letter to the author, 15 November 1995).

1948–1981

Raising Money: 1948–1967

Although organizational dues were recognized as a source of funds the prevailing perspective was one of dependence upon gifts and grants. Both hope and dependence were reinforced in the Federation's first Christmas season. In a letter of 28 December 1948 to WFMH President Rees, Fremont-Smith, the first treasurer (then called honorary treasurer as the basic accounting was done by Miss W. H. Duncan, Financial Officer in Rees' office), announced an anonymous gift of $7500 to meet the salary of a Federation executive for three years. This became the core of the first Director's salary. An additional $7500 came from the International Committee for Mental Hygiene (ICMH), still functioning, but as described in Chapters 3 and 4, only as a fund receiving and dispensing entity. However, the ICMH gift was not available to support operations since it was earmarked for United States organizations to use in a fundraising drive. Any money received would be divided between the U.S. National Association for Mental Health, the National Mental Health Foundation (of which Dick Hunter was then executive secretary), and the WFMH. Between $2000 and $2500 were also expected through the ICMH from the London 1948 World Congress, including receipts from the sale of published proceedings. The estimated ongoing expenses of approximately $3000 yearly were met by a bank loan secured by the anonymous gift noted above. With these receipts the Federation's Annual Report for 1949 notes that despite beginning the year with a deficit, it ended with an operating balance that permitted planning with some confidence. However, it still functioned "at a marginal level."

At the earliest Executive Board meetings, beginning in Amsterdam 5–9 January 1949, discussion concerned the financial requirements for the Federation's survival and its justifications for fundraising. Most comments reflected the perception that the United States was the most likely source of money and a nationwide fundraising campaign was, indeed, being contemplated for the United States. Thus, nominees for the post of treasurer were considered in light of the opinion noted earlier, "that there were many advantages in having a treasurer of the World Federation resident in the USA." At the same time member associations in other countries were urged to contribute. Rees felt that funding from other countries would be "a demonstration that the member societies really do want such an organization and are prepared to raise funds for it" (Rees, letter of 24 January 1949). Already considering the post of Federation Director, he was so concerned with its Board's uncertain efforts at fundraising that he made it clear that he would not become responsible for finding the money to pay his own salary and support the central office. He stated unequivocally that "the central Secretariat should not be responsible for raising funds…the members of the Executive Board should, themselves, do their utmost to raise or stimulate the raising of funds." There was no definitive response to this assertion; it was the first of recurrent, mainly futile, appeals to members of the Board to finance the work of the Federation for which they had accepted responsibility.

Board members Otto Klineberg and George Stevenson (see Chapters 1–5) did report inquiries by well-meaning United States citizens who wished to contribute money to "some project concerned with peace and mental hygiene," but there is no record of these inquiries having led to action. The question of funding by UN agencies was also raised with particular reference to UNESCO, which had given $17,000 toward the 1948 Congress expenses. However, Klineberg, part of UNESCO's international tensions project (see Chapter 2), explained that "it would be difficult for an organization such as the Federation to obtain a financial subsidy from UNESCO to support its general operations." A specific project that fitted in with its social science department might receive support "to a limited extent." But no project was forthcoming, and although a few possible projects for submission to the WHO were reviewed, none were deemed suitable. Both UNESCO and WHO were abandoned as funding sources for the time being.

By the 18–20 August 1949 Executive Board meeting at the end of the Rees presidency, when he began his duties as WFMH Director, a deficit already existed. However, Treasurer Fremont-Smith was able to arrange a generous multi-year grant from the Josiah Macy, Jr. Foundation, of which he was medical director. He realized that Macy had made exceptional contributions to the Federation's support, but acknowledged its importance in "this critical period of [WFMH's] existence," and referred to the successful beginning of the American fundraising campaign by the U.S. National Committee for Mental Hygiene and the National Mental Health Foundation. After its hopeful start the campaign was postponed pending a possible merger of these two bodies with the U.S. Psychiatric Foundation.

By the following year, 1950, Director Rees remarked that the organization was "more or less living from hand to mouth." Individual membership dues alone were not sufficient to maintain it. The annual cost of organizing the members and sending out literature "at no time left very much of a balance accruing from their fees for the general work of the Federation.... [I]ndividual fees have not been of any help in solving the continuously harassing problem of financing Federation activity" (Rees, 1966, p. 106). The need for a finance committee was considered so pressing that the Executive Board decided to act as a committee of the whole in pursuit of funding. But despite their resolve they took no action and the problems of financial planning and fundraising remained in the hands of the Director and United States colleagues.

An unforeseen factor was the apparent inability of national member associations to form the identification with the global organization essential to its support. Successive treasurer's reports in the 1950s indicate that national associations were often in arrears in their dues, largely because they "did not have the money," although currency restrictions affected some. Stevenson's report for 1952, for example, noted that of 76 member associations nearly one-quarter were in arrears. Of these, eight had never paid their dues and 10 others had not paid for the current year. Two hundred sixty-five individual members had allowed their memberships to lapse, leaving 982 in the individual category. In order to encourage more generous giving the title of Life Associate was granted to persons making gifts of $100 or more.

Rees had also thought about this matter, touching on a theme that was to recur with greater intensity after 1984 with the development of regional councils: "Certain member associations were afraid to allow appeals for funds in their own countries, since any money that could be got from the relatively few people who would finance work for mental health was needed for their own service projects" (Rees, 1966, p. 107). Raymond Prince, a well-known Canadian specialist in cultural psychiatry who reviewed Rees' book and the Soddy report (1961) was impressed by this problem. As he put it, the WFMH was ailing because "The organism does not supply its brain with blood!...As the world evolves towards an international community, more and more local organizations will be faced with the problem of support of an international 'brain'.... [T]here can be no effective supranational organization without a small portion of national funds being diverted for support of the integrating principle" (Prince, 1969, pp. 277–278).

The United States Fundraising Group

As detailed in Chapter 3 the United States group, which constituted the New York Regional Office of the WFMH, decided to convert the ICMH, still existing on paper as a fund receiving and disbursing organization, into the U.S. Committee for WFMH, with William Beaty II as its executive director (Beaty, 1995). In 1958 it was finally incorporated in Delaware as the World Federation for Mental Health: U.S. Committee Inc., permitting tax deductions for United States contributors and accelerating the flow of funds. Long before this, however, beginning in 1948, with Rees as its new president, the ICMH had sent out constant appeals for money to United States foundations, corporations, and individuals. In response, a growing list of corporate and foundation donors continued to keep the organization afloat. Among them were the Josiah Macy, Jr. Foundation, the New York Foundation, the Ford Foundation, the Commonwealth Fund, the Grant Foundation, the Field Foundation, the American Mental Health Foundation, the Milbank Memorial Fund, the Ittleson Family Foundation, the Old Dominion Foundation, and others. Beaty estimated that from 1948 until its dissolution in 1966 the New York group supplied from 75 to 100 percent of Federation funds. After 1958, in addition to the corporate and foundation grants funneled through the U.S. Committee for WFMH Inc., the group also raised significant sums through social events in New York City. Many foundations were helpful, as Beaty noted, by "providing general support funds longer than was customary under their policies."

Although the early United States treasurers, including Fremont-Smith, Stevenson, social worker Mildred Scoville, and Jonathan Bingham did excellent work under difficult circumstances, Rees and other Board members wanted "an international business man with understanding and knowledge of our objectives" (WFMH 1957a, p. 8). In 1956 Erwin Schuller of Toronto, an Austrian by birth who was familiar with Europe, accepted the appointment. Unfortunately, he resigned after a year because of the "pressure of business" (WFMH 1958b, p. 11). Stevenson took up the job once more, and 1957 turned out to be a good year. With receipts of $69,593 from individuals as well as foundations, not including funds for special projects, there was a surplus of $1651. The new World Federation for Mental Health: U.S. Committee would soon be incorporated and was expected to attract tax-deductible gifts from the United States donors.

More money did come in, but by the end of fiscal year 1958 there was a deficit of $15,016. Both Rees' Director's Report and Stevenson's Treasurer's Report referred to the increasing numbers of people making demands on the Federation without contributing to its support. Increased staff and space had become necessary in both London and New York, and the donated space for the New York office in the U.S. National Mental Health Association (NMHA) headquarters was terminated, making it necessary to pay for rented space there. Another significant increase in expenditures came in 1958 when Rees, who had been paid on a part-time basis, began receiving a full-time salary. The Grant Foundation was now paying for most of Soddy's work as scientific director, and the Macy Foundation paid the salary of a full-time administrative planner for a World Mental Health Year projected for 1960. Stevenson said that it was to be expected that most WFMH financial support would come from the United States, but he made a strong plea for funding from other countries.

Stevenson's Treasurer's Report for the year ending 30 September 1959 sounded a similar note. He characterized "the struggle for funds" as "a hand-to-mouth affair" in which in some years "we have just been saved by the sympathetic generosity of some Foundation" (WFMH, 1960p. 22). In 1958–1959, because of "a generous life-line thrown out by the Taconic and Aaron E. Norman Foundations," the preceding year's deficit was overcome and a small positive balance remained. But, as Stevenson put it, the WFMH was "certainly still on the edge of the water."

In 1959 the new WFMH Committee in the United States increased its activity as a conduit for gifts and grants. Mr. Lewis Cullman of New York became chairman of a National Appeal for World Mental Health under its auspices, launching a more systematic fundraising campaign. In

1960 the last-minute rescue scenario was repeated. A $7445 deficit at the end of fiscal year 1959-1960 was recouped by a gift from the Alfred P. Sloan Foundation of New York, which further promised $25,000 yearly for three years for general expenses. Another gift given special notice came from Smith, Kline, and French pharmaceuticals. Despite this welcome assistance the Executive Board decided that, unless there was an unexpected improvement in the financial situation, it would save money by canceling its usual winter meeting.

Stevenson retired from his long service as treasurer on 30 June 1960. He felt that part of the Federation's financial problem was because members of local mental health associations who did not attend its meetings did not understand their value. It was important, he believed, for those who had participated to "interpret them on their return home so it might become evident that the Federation and its Annual Meetings were not just a good excuse for a visit to another country, but that without them there would be an actual deficiency in the programmes of the member-associations" (WFMH, 1960, p. 38). The solution was not just to increase memberships, but to make the Federation known to potential donors who might not yet have heard of it.

The incoming treasurer, Sir Geoffrey Vickers of the United Kingdom, made a case for a specific fundraising operation that would not claim "an undue share of the time and energy of those also engaged in the directly productive work of the Federation" (Annual Report, 1960, p. 25). Among the basic sources of support he stressed increased membership and higher dues, and special projects carrying an allowance for general overhead expenses. Vickers' tenure as treasurer coincided with increased activity of the U.S. Committee and major continuing grants from the three New York foundations, Sloan, Grant, and Avalon, as well as an increase in memberships. The overall trend of increasing revenues and increasing expenses evident since 1950 continued, and there were no deficits. He felt justified in saying in his final Treasurer's Report that the Federation "has a better chance than ever before of securing increasingly reliable and adequate support for its work" (WFMH, 1963, p. 35).

The Financial Consequences and Fate of the Geneva Secretariat

With Rees' retirement at the end of 1961 and the employment of his successor, Francois Cloutier, in January 1962 it was decided that the original 1949 decision to locate the Secretariat in Geneva should now be implemented. More than a year was required to organize the funding for the move, which was accomplished in several stages in the late spring and early summer of 1963. The expenses of this operation and its sequelae interrupted what had been an inadequate, but orderly and continuing, improvement in the Federation's financial position. Among other new costs were an additional pension for Rees, who was now to serve as a Special Consultant; the salaries of new Associate Director Dr. Pierre Visseur and his supporting office staff; the expenses of maintaining the office in Geneva, which were considerably greater than they had been in London; and Cloutier's heavy travel schedule. Another factor, as noted in Chapter 4, was the total disenchantment of the U.S. Committee with Cloutier (Beaty, 1995). The Committee had been motivated by Rees, and with his departure its enthusiasm waned.

The Board had been aware that costs would be higher in Geneva than in London, that Cloutier expected to travel, and that he wanted additional staff. With that in mind they had requested him to be in charge of fundraising. But as described in Chapter 4, he immediately assigned this responsibility, along with that for most other administrative issues, to Visseur. Shortly thereafter he notified the Board that in his view prospects for foundation support, especially for the "organization's bureaucracy," were not good, and that after 15 years of existence the Federation appeared "to have reached its limits in the help that can be expected" (WFMH, 1966). By 1964 its financial health was indeed declining. The contributions of the U.S. Committee were beginning to diminish and overall income could not keep up with expenditures. Nor had there been any deposits into the World Mental Health Fund, which the WFMH had authorized as an endowment from which interest would provide for general operations. The Fund died an unnoticed death.

The Federation's inability to pay his salary or support his office forced Cloutier to resign from his WFMH directorship in late 1965. Visseur was able to keep the Secretariat open, but on a greatly reduced basis. In the autumn of 1966 the U.S. Committee, again interested because of Cloutier's departure, considered the possibility of a major campaign for funds to revive the Federation and save the Geneva office. A 31 August 1966 memorandum to its Board from Executive Director Beaty described the problem: "The critical financial situation which faced WFMH [since late 1965] has been accentuated since that time. The books of the Geneva office presently carry a deficit of approximately $27,000 in the form of debts and loans.... Eighty percent of the salaries of the directors of the Geneva [Visseur] and New York [Beaty] offices have of necessity been deferred for the months of August, September and October."

As the basis for a possible fundraising effort he sent the Board a list of 17 United States foundations that had given in the past, noting again that they "had been providing general support funds longer than was customary under their policies." He also offered an analysis of the outlook. On the positive side the goals of the WFMH remained valid; its activities were "of unquestionable value"; its membership list was "impressive" with 146 associations in 53 countries and approximately 4000 individual members; its leaders had been "among the most distinguished persons in their fields"; UN statements "attest to the need for and value of WFMH"; and it "has demonstrated its value through many pioneering activities in the international mental health field."

On the negative side most donors who give seed money to establish an organization expect it to become self-supporting in time, and few if any are interested in funding the operations of a central office. Beyond this Beaty noted generic problems, which continued in later years. Fundraising for mental health is less successful than for other causes; it is less successful for organizations that do not render direct services to individuals; it is difficult to raise money for international organizations; the organizational structure of a federation limits the financial support that may be obtained from member groups; in many countries outside the United States fundraising is difficult because of the level of economic development, the lack of a voluntary tradition, and features of the tax structure. And, as suggested above, most donors prefer to support specific projects rather than general operating costs, including the bureaucratic structure, which any organization develops as it grows and matures. Both the positive evaluations of the Federation and the obstacles to obtaining adequate support have been as valid in the late 1990s as in 1966.

More specific to the Federation of that time were the factors that led to overspending: the Secretariat's move from London to Geneva, the change in administration, and the organization's financial overextension in its effort to broaden the base of its support to countries other than the United States. Beaty observed that attempts to raise funds in other countries, "particularly Western Europe, have not yielded results of any consequence to date." At the same time he concluded that the Federation's financial security could not depend upon general operating support from United States foundations. In the same vein as some early treasurers he recommended drives for expanded membership, particularly of individuals.

Financing Federation Travel

The Federation's lack of financial capacity created particular difficulties in regard to travel for Executive Board members. It was necessary for them and committee members to meet with some regularity in order to maintain the Federation's organizational integrity. Initially, individual members, with some exceptions, financed their own travel or had it paid for by their own institutions; some were able to "piggy-back" Federation activities on trips supported by academic and other groups which invited them to lecture or consult. In his report for 1949 Treasurer El Kholy of Cairo noted that while regular meetings of the Executive Board and Inter-Professional Advisory Committee (IPAC) are essential, it would be "a completely impossible strain on individuals to provide their own travelling and maintenance costs." He added that under the circumstances the task of making a budget becomes "somewhat confusing." In his 1950 report, presented in 1951, he was cautiously more optimistic. Some expenses had diminished as secretarial support for United States Executive Board members and WFMH representatives to UN New York was supplied by the Division of World Affairs of the U.S. National Association for Mental Health. The director of that division, Mrs. Grace O'Neill, was officially named as executive officer of the WFMH in the United States, and remained so until the U.S. Committee was formed in 1957. Additionally, foundation funds had been obtained to pay for Board and IPAC travel for their spring meetings. However, these were not sufficient for all required travel. At the time of the 1951 World Congress for Mental Health in Mexico Mrs. O'Neill and her co-workers arranged lectures at American universities for European Board members on their way to Mexico. This so-called "Flying Seminar" involved 16 members of the Board and secretariat and was regarded as an exemplary way for the Federation to manage some of its travel.

Stevenson, who succeeded El Kholy as treasurer, noted in his report for 1952 that the WFMH had "to throw back the tremendous burden of finding their own travel costs on to individual members of the Executive Board." This remained a matter of concern and occasionally of contention. While some presidents and occasional Board members expected Federation support for their travel, mainly to annual and executive meetings, many paid for themselves or had their universities or other institutions pay for them. Stevenson estimated that an ideal budget, allowing a systematic increase in Federation work, including travel support, would begin at $200,000, advancing to $600,000 yearly over a period of five years. His immediate aim, however, was to exceed the minimal budget of $64,352 on which the Executive Board had worked during 1951.

An important concern for Rees was the financial limitation on his travel for organizational consulting and what he called his "parish work"—visits to member associations around the globe. These occasionally involved other WFMH representatives and he sometimes asked WHO friends and other professional experts, mostly from the United States, to represent the WFMH in their travels and consultations. He noted, however, that the bulk of the visiting, especially to member associations, fell to him as the only salaried professional in the Secretariat. During his tenure as Director he was able to visit between 60 and 70 countries, where he spoke with professional and lay groups, and often with government officials. While some member associations, especially in Latin America and Asia, covered major elements of his travel and subsistence expenses, he said that the visiting and consulting function that "should be undertaken by the Federation" cannot be effectively carried out unless the Federation becomes "more free than it is now from financial problems" (Rees, 1966, p.99).

The Problem of Language: Interpretation and Translation

The lack of funds had special significance for an international, multilingual body needing the expensive services of interpreters and translators. Rees was particularly troubled by the unfilled need for simultaneous interpretation so people from different language groups could understand each other during Board meetings as well as conferences and congresses. There was also the issue, given special importance by members from Francophone countries, of publishing translations and summaries of conference papers in French, the second official language of the WFMH after English. The WFMH was "overwhelmed by financial difficulties and the cost of getting translations made prevented our publishing to any extent in more than one language"

(Rees, 1966, p. 91). Although there was no comparable pressure for translation into Spanish, Arabic, or other official UN languages, the dominance of English was mentioned by Latin American colleagues at some early meetings (see Chapter 9). At the 8–13 August 1960 Annual Meeting in Edinburgh, professor of psychiatry Ramon Sarro of Barcelona suggested the formation of "regional leagues of mental health associations" whose meetings would "overcome the language difficulties…and make it easier to draw into the mental health movement those countries where English was not understood. WFMH should promote the formation of such groups on the basis of a similar culture, or of language" (WFMH, 1960, p. 43).

It was expected that multilingual communication would become possible once the Secretariat had moved to Geneva in 1963, but this did not materialize. After the 1967 closing of the Geneva secretariat most discussions and publications were presented in English. As time passed and English became more widely used as the language of international exchange, most Board members and attendees at congresses became more comfortable using it.

Achieving the Organization's Potential

Inadequate financing was recognized as limiting not only essential travel and communication, but the overall achievement of the Federation's potential. H.C. Rumke put it succinctly in his foreword to the 1954 Annual Report: "Because of lack of funds the Secretariat and the Board are not adequately equipped to give leadership, and the same lack of reserves prevents IPAC (the International Professional Advisory Committee) from working in an effective way." The report of the 1961 International Study Group planning future initiatives (Soddy and Ahrenfeldt, 1967) described the organization as so hampered by lack of funds as to make the likelihood of ambitious future activities uncertain.

Frank Fremont-Smith, who as its medical director had been able to facilitate generous grants from the Josiah Macy, Jr. Foundation of New York, expressed his concern in his 1954-1955 Presidential Foreword to the 1955 Annual Report: "…both the current work of the Federation and the development of its potentialities continue to be severely hampered by lack of adequate financial support. The Federation cannot hope to fulfil its responsibilities on a basis of year to year financing…without assurance of income for our basic activities, each new project becomes an undue burden upon the Secretariat and a threat to our financial security" (WFMH, 1955a, p. 9).

1981–1983

An Introduction to Federation Finances

My personal introduction to the Federation's chronic insolvency came, as described in Chapter 5, in my first Board meetings as president-elect and then as president before and after the World Congress in Manila at the end of July and the beginning of August 1981. It was unexpected and disturbing to hear grave doubt expressed by longtime members more knowledgeable than I about the Federation's financial capacity to survive as more than an interactive post box. The pre-Congress Board chaired by outgoing President Guest repeated concerns of earlier years and foreshadowed those of the 1990s, resolving that "in view of WFMH's precarious financial situation" member organizations having dues in arrears for the preceding calendar year would lose their right to vote. After two years of non-payment they would lose their membership unless special consideration was granted by the Board." In her own report to the Board, Executive Director Beiser, who had been appointed with a modest salary by Guest upon his 1979 accession to the presidency, stated: "Unless our income is increased we will be 'out of business' within the next few years. Simple as that" (WFMH, 1981a).

A mood of gloom pervaded this post-Congress Board, the first I had chaired as president, as we contemplated a future without financial support. Isaac Mwendapole, of Zambia, already on the Board, advocated defensive, conserving inaction: "There is nothing to do but hunker down!" However, Past President Lin, who had been responsible for my assuming an active Federation role (and whom I now realized had said nothing about funding) espoused the opposite point of view. He said that if the Federation remained inactive it would die. The only solution was to have a 1983 Congress in Washington, DC. His view carried the day, but my acceptance of the challenge was contingent upon finding appropriate help. That help, as noted in Chapter 5, did arrive in the person of Richard C. Hunter, but it required several days of discussion. The organization of the Congress, especially its funding, made the period 1981–1983 the most stressful of our years with the Federation. The U.S. NMHA, of which Dick was the official representative, was the Congress' primary sponsor, but it contributed no financial support. However, with the help of my university, the American psychiatric, psychological, and other professional associations, and because of the interest of President Robert Gibson, M.D. of the Sheppard and Enoch Pratt Hospital of Baltimore, we accumulated the necessary "up front" money, and were able to pay our bills when it was all over. The 1981–1983 effort, not only for the Congress but in rebuilding our network of potential advocacy partners, initiated the new phase of Federation existence described in Chapter 5.

The fact that the Federation's financial situation came to me as a surprise reveals my naive failure to have investigated it before, or even after, accepting the nomination as president-elect. By the time I was able to examine the books it was apparent that the most immediate cause of insolvency after the Lin surplus was due to the drain of funds during the Guest presidency. More fundamentally it was part of the chronic pattern of insufficient funding that had plagued the WFMH since its founding. Among other factors I realized that its Board, in contrast to that of most other voluntary organizations, had never assumed significant responsibility for fundraising. Part of the problem was that it kept perpetuating itself with the addition of other professional people and volunteers. It did not make a significant effort to add business people, financial leaders, or even popular figures who might have been able to attract donors. The sole exception was the brief incumbency of Colleen (Mrs. Sam) Nunn, wife of the influential U.S. Senator.

The situation was worsened by the absolute default of such responsibility during the 1968–1979 period to whoever was president and supported the Federation in his university office. Not unexpectedly, it was left to me, with Dick's invaluable collaboration, to raise the money needed to start the Congress organizing process. In that period, as described in Chapter 5, my Federation work was totally supported by the University of Maryland. This included the salary of my longtime secretary Eileen Potocki, who had managed my office and was the source of advice and counsel for 26 other secretarial personnel during my years as a department chairman, institute director, and sometime dean. Although by 1981 I had retired as an administrator I was still a professor, but devoted major energies to the tasks of being WFMH president. This involved both preparations for the Congress and reviving the Federation in general, including the institutionalization of many procedures long carried out on an ad hoc basis. I called in the numerous IOUs from friends and organizations for which I had done favors in the past. Dick called on his own network and I found his competence most reassuring, although we both speculated about what might happen if we incurred bills we couldn't pay.

I was also comforted by Gowan Guest's promise to be a stabilizing force on the Board, providing me with advice and support. This comfort was rudely shattered during the 1982 Board meeting in Washington, the first opportunity to work with Board members to prepare for the 1983 Congress and reconstitute our agenda. Guest was not present. He was to have been at the Board helping, as he had promised in his own words, to "shore up" my efforts at this difficult moment of Federation history. I expected a message that he had been delayed and would be arriving at any minute. Instead there was silence during most of the first day and, finally, a telephone call from Vancouver. He had chosen this means of telling me—insulated from face-to-face contact—that he was resigning not only from the Board, but from the corporation in Canada where we were still a corporate entity prior to our later incorporation in the United States. His reason was not reassuring: he was afraid, he said, that the Federation would have to declare bankruptcy and he did not wish, as a Board and corporation member, to be held responsible by debtors—a fate he implied might lie in store for those of us who remained with what he saw as a sinking ship. He recommended, as a money saving move, the emergency closure of the Vancouver secretariat and the immediate termination of Roberta Beiser from the Executive Director's post to which he had appointed her. With diminished support from the University of British Columbia, he perceived even her relatively small part-time salary (supplemented by her contribution of significant volunteer time) as a potentially disastrous expense. Guest's unexpected announcement by long-distance telephone was bad news and a harsh blow. After consultation with Dick, I decided not to follow this advice, but to keep Vancouver open for the rest of my presidential term. First, it would not have been fair to Beiser. Second, we were already in the process of a gradual transfer of responsibilities to Baltimore. In any event we needed her good will and that of her husband, UBC psychiatrist Morton Beiser, M.D., program chairman for the 1983 Congress. An abrupt closure of the Vancouver office seemed to be both a political and operational mistake.

The destructive impact of Guest's withdrawl is revealed in letters to the Board around that time. My letter of 29 September 1982 to Western Pacific Vice President Akira Hoshino of Tokyo who, not present at the Board meeting, had written about initiating a new project, stated: "At last the tumult of the last three weeks or so is dying out. The defection of a leader whose affiliation with the Federation long antedated mine, and who was treasurer from 1975 to 1979 and then President from 1979 to 1981 was a severe shock. Now, though, I believe that we are getting ourselves reorganized."

After Guest's resignation Dick and I, already stretched to the limit by the demands of setting up the Congress, added the fear of bankruptcy to our concerns. This turned out to be unnecessary, but at the time we were very apprehensive about the future. The Congress turned out to be a great success in terms of promoting our substantive concerns. We were left without demanding creditors and, indeed, a tiny surplus. This was due largely to Dick Hunter's knowledge and wise and meticulous management. It was also due to his steadfast refusal to pay a hotel bill for meeting rooms that did not conform to our original contract.

The Congress ended with a gala reception at Blair House, the residence for visiting presidents, which I had been able to arrange through the kindness of Ed Brandt, M.D., then the United States Assistant Secretary for Health who was to become dean of the University of Maryland Medical School. It was attended by former United States First Lady and longtime mental health advocate Mrs. Rosalynn Carter, who joined me in the receiving line with United States Secretary for Health, Education and Welfare Margaret Heckler, and WFMH President-Elect Aldaba-Lim. The reception was underwritten by the Sheppard and Enoch Pratt Hospital through the good offices of Bob Gibson. In my final report to the Board as president I tried to put the best face on our fiscal fragility: "The events of these past two years reflect the spirit and mission of the World Federation for Mental Health.… [T]hey also mirror the organizational and financial problems arising from its broad-based and geographically extensive nature.… [I]nadequate financial support has been recurrent during the Federation's life" (Brody, 1983a).

AFTER 1983

Establishing the New Secretariat with Volunteer and In-Kind Support

As Dick and I were establishing the new Baltimore-Washington Secretariat in 1983 we inadvertently became responsible for reinforcing the Board's passivity, especially in regards to obtaining financial support. First was our agreement to work as volunteers, which made it unnecessary for it to obtain salaries for their two senior executives. Since then Dick has devoted 100 percent of his time to the Federation. From 1983 to 1990, I gave approximately 66 percent (⅔ time) depending upon the need for travel, reports, and the regular Newsletter deadlines. Later, I reduced this to approximately 50 percent.

A second element reinforcing the Board's insulation from reality was the fact that my office operation was carried out at almost no cost to the WFMH. During my presidency, 1981-1983, and for four years after I became Secretary General in 1983, as noted in the previous chapter, my office, including all services and secretarial help, was totally supported by the University of Maryland. My successor as chairman of psychiatry during those years was an old friend, Professor Russell R. Monroe, M.D. Not only did he support my Federation work, he also contributed department funds to the success of the 1983 Washington, DC World Congress.

After 1987, when I retired completely from the University, my WFMH office in the Sheppard Pratt Hospital was established in space which had been part of my *Journal of Nervous and Mental Disease* offices already supported by the hospital in return for publicity and its name on the *Journal's* masthead. WFMH expenses, except for the salary of my assistant, were charged to the *Journal* cost center. For this, as noted previously, we owe thanks to the two Sheppard presidents during this period, Robert Gibson, M.D. from 1986 until 1991 and, after that, Steven Sharfstein, M.D.

We depended on Federation funds to pay rent and service charges for the Secretariat, managed by Dick Hunter, to the U.S. NMHA in whose headquarters building in Alexandria, Virginia, it is located. However, because of Dick's long previous service as an NMHA executive, the Association was accommodating in regard to the late payment of bills.

A graphic indication of our lack of funds is contained in a letter of 8 September 1983 to a hopeful entrepreneur who wanted to edit a Newsletter for us. At that time the Vancouver-based Newsletter had ceased publication. I wrote to the hopeful editor: "For the moment…the Federation's financial status is such that we are quite unable to consider anything more than the briefest newsletter, perhaps in the form of a personal missive." My June 1985 Message in the Newsletter, which had been revived as of March 1984, was less drastic but continued the same theme. After enumerating the major gains achieved since 1983 I had to say: "We do not yet have sufficient membership to ensure continuity, and fund raising so far has been able to maintain only a limited momentum. In order for the WFMH to realize its potential its officers and members during 1985–1987 must utilize the stable organizational platform which has been created as a springboard for major membership and financial expansion." The appeal to the Board was not answered, and our need to cope with enforced frugality continued. At each yearly meeting Dick and I issued dire warnings about what could happen when, inevitably, health or other factors would force one or both of us to leave our volunteer positions. However, the intrinsic rewards of the work and the appeal of its goals were such that we continued to give the Federation an effective international central office without its having to be concerned with its support.

The Board as Fundraiser

The passivity of most Board members in this respect probably reflected their status as mental health professionals and volunteers rather than financiers and business people, but it may also have had its origins in the fact that they carried little real financial responsibility from the very beginning. For some, the local honor attached to being an officer of an international NGO in official relations with the UN seemed a sufficient reason for accepting nomination. Their main interests were domestic, and while international recognition was important for status at home, they had no desire to spend excessive time working to support the international organization.

After a stable Washington-Baltimore Secretariat was established in 1983 there were repeated discussions by Board members of sometimes grandiose ways of obtaining funds. There were also promises at the end of several meetings that they would set themselves financial quotas. A discussion at the 5–6 July 1990 Board meeting in Geneva, chaired by President Stanislas Flache, M.D., exemplified this approach. Dick and I spoke of the importance of the Board assuming greater responsibility for fundraising, membership, and overall development. This was taken up by Board members emphasizing the importance of their having sufficient status and influence in their own regions, if not internationally, to do the job. Being effective in fundraising meant attracting new individual and organizational members, and raising the regional status and visibility of the Federation. The key point was emphasized by Board Member-at-Large Hilda Robbins, a former president of the U.S. NMHA and former vice-president of the WFMH North American region. She stated it unequivocally: "Accepting membership on the WFMH Board means accepting its responsibilities and opportunities," including the financial ones, "as primary over regional and other concerns." Again, promises and commitments were made. However, none were ever achieved and, typically, were forgotten by the time of the next meeting. The situation was exacerbated by the not totally unreasonable perspective of some regional vice-presidents in resource-poor countries that "the Federation" should be prepared to finance their activities.

Dick Hunter introduced several devices to encourage dues payments including membership cards, the ability to pay with credit cards, and in the mid-1990s a reduced membership fee if dues for two years were paid at the same time. In May 1996, however, members of the Executive Committee meeting at the Alexandria Secretariat were dismayed to learn that nearly 50 percent of all organizational and individual members were in arrears in their dues. This finding, eerily reminiscent of the Federation's earliest days, prompted a recommendation that the Secretariat, now supplied with a computer program adequate to the task, monitor the dues situation more meticulously. No attention was paid to the possible reasons why so many members were in arrears.

The early attempt at a finance committee of the Board in the Rees era had long been forgotten, but the idea was implemented once more in 1996 under the leadership of President Beverly Long. She was encouraged to do this by the advent of a new incoming treasurer, J. David Robinson, the Freddy Mac Corporation's Vice-President for Community Affairs who had been recruited by Dick. But even with the close collaboration of a new development director (see below) the financial campaign headquarters remained in the Secretariat and, except for the president and treasurer, the Board remained uninvolved in the effort.

Corporate Gifts and Membership Recruitment

We were able, in this early phase of the new Secretariat, 1983–1989, to obtain significant gifts from corporations, including private hospitals, drug firms, professional associations, and others to help the WFMH Secretariat become reestablished in its new locations, and for specific purposes such as obtaining word processing capability in the Alexandria office, printing a membership brochure or supporting fundraising Embassy Receptions (see below).

The WFMH Newsletter published in Vancouver had been discontinued with the Secretariat's move to the United States. The last number emerging from Vancouver was in 1982. I was able to revive it, with the first number appearing in March 1984, with the assistance of my university-supported Federation executive assistant Kathy McKnight, M.Ed., who had succeeded Eileen Potocki upon the latter's retirement. I did most of the writing and Kathy the layout. Almost every number carried reports of new financial contributions. By July 1984 I was able to arrange a small yearly grant from the International Social Science Council (ISSC) to help support the Newsletter. We could also pay our ISSC dues from it. This continued until mid-1996 when UNESCO, which had been the ISSC's main source of support, revised its funding practices.

During these years our rapidly increasing international visibility confronted us with increasing demands on our time and facilities at the same time that we were concerned with long-term funding to support a growing operation. A message from me in the June 1984 Newsletter noted: "Our needs are becoming greater as our activities widen…." This was only the first of repeated exhortations in the Newsletters over the ensuing years. My September 1985 message, for example, highlighted the need "to make progress in the tasks essential to the Federation's survival as a functional entity," including the identification of "new sources of non-membership funding." Six years later, in September 1991 I wrote: "Since 1981 we have [developed] a momentum which we cannot afford to lose. However, we remain underfunded and unable to take advantage of the opportunities increasingly available to us." The following April 1992 then-president Max Abbott of New Zealand wrote, immediately after that year's Board meeting: "The Federation is going through a phase of expansion. However our financial situation remains precarious and organizationally, growth has created strains."

Like others before us, Dick and I concluded that the WFMH had to act like a membership organization in order to give it the minimum financial basis for survival. That meant that unlike previous Federation administrations, we would plan for repeated recruiting campaigns. Professional leaders who knew us were usually willing to allow their names to be listed as fundraising sponsors. The fact that I had once belonged to the American Psychological Association, and was a Life Fellow of the American Psychiatric Association and a Life Member of the American Psychoanalytic Association, made it easier to encourage professional colleagues to join. The Medical Director of the Psychiatric Association (Melvin Sabshin, M.D.) and the Executive Director of the Psychological Association (Mike Pallak, Ph.D.) had both accepted my presidential discretionary appointments to membership on our Board in 1981, and they were very helpful. Their two associations continued during the 1990s to give us by far the largest numbers of new individual members. The first major membership campaign, aimed at the American Psychological Association with the collaboration of its officers and the support of Otto Klineberg, was planned under Dick's leadership in February 1986. In preparation a survey of 577 United States WFMH members was carried out. The results indicated that 75 percent of them were aged 50 years or older, 39 percent were psychiatrists, about 25 percent psychologists, and only 6 percent defined themselves as "non-professional." In 1986, the combined Psychological and Psychiatric Association drives yielded 1200 new individual members, including several who joined as Life Members.

By this time the Federation's increased visibility had already brought it a small but steady increase in both individual and organizational volunteer membership from other world areas. Membership dues had been changed in January 1986 (through a vote of the post-Congress Board in Brighton in July 1985) setting different levels for individual members according to the economic development of their regions. The cumulative dues of organizational as well as individual members increased from 1983 to the early 1990s to the point where they could provide a minimum level of support for some of the functions of the Secretariat and Board. But after the mid-1990s, while worldwide organizational membership continued to grow at approximately the same pace, the rate of new individual member acquisition, especially in the United States, diminished. This may have reflected the increasingly drug-oriented perspective of younger psychiatrists, and their narrower, more clinically oriented interests, in contrast to those of the post-World War II generation. We also noticed that while World Congresses typically attracted a number of single or two-year memberships, the intervening years tended to see significant attrition.

In 1997 individual membership was 3225 (almost the same as in the late 1950s); there were 157 voting member organizations of national or transnational scope and 142 nonvoting affiliate organizations of local, state, or provincial scope.

Regional Competition for Funds

A chronic issue noted by Rees and others in the Federation's earliest days was that of the local/regional versus global identifications of Board members. It was captured by Raymond Prince's pithy comment about the WFMH's financial ill health: "The organism does not supply its brain with blood!…There can be no effective supranational organization without a small portion of national funds being diverted for support of the integrating principle" (Prince, 1969, pp. 277–278).

The "brain-body problem" was intensified with the gradual rise of regional councils (discussed in Chapters 5 and 9), led by that in Europe. One debate became especially prominent in the 1980s and 1990s with recruitment activities in Eastern Europe and the less industrialized world. It concerned fixing organizational dues according to the number of members in an association and reducing them for worthy groups, especially in low-income countries that could not afford it.

The early reluctance of national member associations to contribute to the parent body was succeeded after 1983 by competition between the needs of the Federation as a global entity and those of its developing regional components. This issue, noted in Chapter 5 on governance and detailed in Chapter 9 on regionalization, became intense after the mid-1980s with the development of the European Regional Council of the WFMH (ERC/WFMH) and the growth of regional interests elsewhere. The conflict became overt in 1989 in the interventions of the new WFMH Vice-President for Europe (and head of ERC/WFMH) Ms. Josee van Remoortel, a former executive director of the Flanders Mental Health Association. Muted controversy about financing, expressed mainly through correspondence, emerged almost immediately with her reluctance to submit ERC financial records for review by the WFMH auditors. This contravened the bylaws, which clearly stated that component parts of the Federation are considered elements of the same corporate body, and that their financial records are subject to central office scrutiny.

DICK HUNTER, TREASURER AND OPERATIONS OFFICER DE FACTO

A Financial Legacy

Dick said on several occasions that he wanted his legacy to the Federation to be a financial base adequate to ensure the survival of the Secretariat. It might have seemed more logical for this to be a goal of a president or a treasurer. Indeed, the treasurers appointed by the president with our advice did their best as individuals (and in the case of Robert Gibson, M.D., President of Sheppard Pratt Hospital, made significant institutional gifts). However, no contemporary president until Beverly Long in 1996 established a systematic fundraising committee, and the treasurers were not sufficiently stimulated to initiate one on their own. Dick had no competitors in his ambition to provide a WFMH legacy. His role soon came to include that of effective obtainer, manager, and dispenser of WFMH funds.

His protective attitude and assumption of personal responsibility were revealed in his often carrying large Federation bills on his own credit card, sometimes for months. When I chided him for this, saying that the Board would never be forced to confront reality, he replied that there "was nothing to gain by trying to force them to do what they didn't want to do," and it was, after all, his own choice. There was another factor: he wanted to avoid obtaining a corporate credit card with the likelihood that we would end up carrying a large balance putting our credit rating at risk. It was less dangerous, in this respect, to use his personal credit card for Federation purposes. I thus became an accomplice, since Dick was my deputy and I could have made an issue of it. However, that would have impaired our cordial working arrangement and, in the absence of a sufficient cash flow, might have paralyzed the capacities we did have. It also might have made it necessary for me to become more personally involved in financial management. I had devoted much energy as an academic administrator to finding financial support for my institute and didn't want to get into the business of looking for money and disbursing it again, so I was glad to let Dick take on both of these tasks.

My own efforts began with obtaining our free offices at the University of Maryland and Sheppard and Enoch Pratt Hospital. Later, a small grant for our Newsletter was paid yearly from 1984 through 1996 by the ISSC. In the fall of 1989, through professional connections, I began to obtain some project grant funds from foundations or agencies to be disbursed through Dick's office. This permitted some allotment of overhead, or interest, to Federation operating expenses. In 1993, through the advice of Richard Mollica, M.D., director of our Collaborating Center, the Harvard Program in Refugee Trauma, I found substantial funding from a private foundation that has chosen to remain anonymous. This was used first for the Newsletter, then the Annual Report, the project to put the WFMH on the Internet, this Federation history, and, most significantly, the support of my primary assistant, Elena Berger, D.Phil., who had succeeded Kathy McKnight when Kathy became Managing Editor of the *Journal of Nervous and Mental Disease*. The private foundation funds also allowed a small consulting retainer to Kathy to function as a publications consultant for the WFMH Newsletter and Annual Report, and most significantly for our Internet project, which involved the purchase of computers for my office (and one for that in Alexandria), the development of our WFMH web site, and e-mail capacity. In this way the Federation had, without direct cost, a whole new system of communicative capacities and two people in my office, both familiar with the organization's nature and way of operating. While the Board was pleased to learn of this new outside support and the new computers and Internet capacity, they were not moved to greater fundraising efforts. Nor was there any reaction when, at Dick's request, Catherine Gray was entitled Associate Director for Development and Elena Berger was designated Associate Director for Programs.

The Embassy Receptions

Dick, as a former voluntary agency executive, was familiar with many approaches to fundraising from private sources and he used all of them. One was through receptions to which corporate executives were invited for a price. Each was held at a Washington, DC embassy with a prominent list of hosts from the U.S. Congress—headed for the first few years while Mrs. Nunn was the WFMH Treasurer by Senator and Mrs. Sam Nunn—and the basic costs covered by a corporate gift obtained by Dick. This marked the beginning of a new tradition and a new and time-consuming burden for Dick and his assistants in the Alexandria office. As the years passed it became evident that the financial yield from these events was considerably less than hoped for. They were, however, occasions to invite friends and supporters. The social and public relations gain made the receptions ultimately worthwhile. Dick worked out a program to ensure that some significant information as well as our good will was transmitted. It required that we interrupt the eating and drinking of the guests for a brief review by me of Federation activities during the preceding year, a task I resisted at first, but which Dick persuaded me was essential. An important presence at most receptions, again arranged by Dick, was Rosalynn Carter. Although she usually wasn't able to stay for the bulk of the festivities, she joined the receiving line with the Ambassador as host, the current president and I representing the Federation, and occasional others. In 1995 Mrs. Carter and Tipper Gore, the wife of Vice-President Al Gore, did the speaking, and in 1996 WFMH President Beverly Long reviewed some of her concerns and presented an award for good citizenship to one of our old friends, Professor Arthur Kleinman, a Harvard psychiatrist and anthropologist whose initiative was behind a volume on world mental health used by the WHO as a basis for some of its work.

The first reception, with then WFMH president Edith Morgan of London in attendance, was held in 1987 at the residence of the Ambassador of Great Britain with the British as hosts. The second, with President Gamal El Azayem of Cairo in attendance, billed as a 40th anniversary celebration, was held in 1988 at the Embassy of Turkey with the support of Bristol Myers. The 1989 reception, with the presence of President Stanislas Flache, a French national living in

Geneva, was held at the French Ambassador's residence, supported by a grant from Occidental Petroleum. The 1990 reception, underwritten by Merck & Co., Inc. at the residence of the Japanese Ambassador, was graced by the presence of the Honorary Chairperson of our Host Committee for the occasion, the Honorable Mike Mansfield, a distinguished former Senator from Montana who until recently had been the much-respected United States Ambassador to Japan. Dr. Louis Sullivan, the United States Secretary of Health and Human Services, also made an appearance. The 1991 reception, looking forward to the WFMH World Congress in Mexico later in the year, took place in the Mexican House of Culture without a corporate underwriter. Federico Puente, the Congress chairman, and several of his colleagues were present. A sixth Fund Raising Reception in 1992 saw the advent of Rosalynn Carter as Honorary Chairperson, a post she retained for future receptions. This one was held at the Australian Embassy with Health and Human Services Secretary Sullivan's participation and financial sponsorship from several pharmaceutical/chemical firms: Eli Lilly and Company, Merck & Co., Inc., The Upjohn Company, and Sandoz Pharmaceuticals, Inc. In 1993 the reception site was the Embassy of the Russian Federation. Financial support came from The Upjohn Company, Gannett publishers, Abbott Laboratories, and Sandoz Pharmaceuticals.

The 1994 reception was in the residence of the Ambassador of the Republic of Indonesia supported by the Gannett Company, the Institute for Mental Health Initiatives, Eli Lilly and Company, and Sandoz Pharma Ltd. At the 1995 reception at the Embassy of the Argentine Republic Mrs. Carter was joined by Mrs. Tipper Gore, also a prominent advocate for mental health issues. This was also the first time that the Executive Committee's meeting—joined by the organizers for the 1995 WFMH Congress in Dublin—was scheduled at the Alexandria secretariat prior to the reception, permitting additional WFMH representation at the gathering. On this occasion the event was underwritten by the Gannett Company with additional support from the Coca-Cola Company and Eli Lilly and Company. In 1996, anticipating the 1997 World Congress in Finland, the reception was held at the Embassy of Finland, again with the attendance of the Executive Committee, the organizers of the Finnish Congress, and support from Gannett and Lilly. The 1997 reception at the residency of the Panamanian Ambassador was supported by Gannett and Eli Lilly and marked by the presentation of an award, in absentia, for mental health work to the wife of Panama's President.

Toward a Resource Development Office: The Capital Fund Campaign

Dick's push for a development office was a revival nearly 40 years later of the 1948-1949 plan to use a $7500 gift from the ICMH for a fundraising drive with some of the proceeds going to the U.S. National Mental Health Foundation, of which he was then executive secretary. During the late 1980s and early 1990s, under a succession of WFMH presidents, he borrowed against a bequest that had come in the Vancouver days and utilized several small corporate gifts to hire a possible WFMH fundraiser. The receipts from these efforts, however, did not surpass the costs.

The social success of receptions, the intermittent receipt of gifts, and the steady though low-level income from dues nurtured Dick's belief that the WFMH would achieve its vast potential if it could obtain an endowment. We needed an assured source of salaries for the staff we did have and we needed more staff, if only to give adequate attention to the growing volume of routine matters. The volume of UN material alone was sufficient to overwhelm a single staff person. Regional development could occupy several, although there was some question about the relative merits of funding the offices of regional vice-presidents or a staff position in the Secretariat first. Similarly, the offices of the WFMH presidents and the various committees needed support. Finally, there were the needs for travel, translation, the Newsletter, Annual Report, and other communications. Behind all other considerations was the undeniable fact that Dick and I would not be there to provide unpaid services indefinitely. The best approach seemed to be through using the money we could collect to develop a full-time development office. This approach fitted Dick's perspective and he set about accumulating funds to build a development office through the launching of a Federation Capital Fund Campaign.

Most of the gifts came from my fellow psychiatrists. The first, specifically designated for a WFMH resource development office, was a check for $5000 from the Sheppard and Enoch Pratt Hospital donated by Robert Gibson in honor of former United States First Lady Rosalynn Carter. Bob Gibson presented it to Mrs. Carter, who passed it on to me at the dedication of the hospital's new Education Center on 14 April 1988. Other early contributions came mainly from psychiatric organizations in the United States, Japan, and the Middle East. It was disappointing to note that almost nothing came from the voluntary mental health sector. In 1989 the Resource Development Fund, as it was then designated, received a total of $30,500 from several contributors, including private hospitals: six from Japan and two in the United States. However, the campaign languished and despite a few people hired by Dick on a part-time basis, the development office awaited a major gift. I was still distressed at the non-participation of the Board in the Campaign. My Newsletter message of September 1989 noted that "it is essential that the Board become more active in this endeavor if it is to succeed."

Support from Pharmaceutical Manufacturers: A Source of Controversy

In time, professional psychiatry became a less dependable source of contributions. The Capital Fund Campaign died a quiet death. However, Dick, through his long representation of NMHA in Washington, had a number of friends among drug company representatives. From the beginning of his WFMH affiliation he began to discuss the possibility of their funding some Federation activities. This led to the gifts for the support of Embassy receptions. In 1993 these relationships led to a financial breakthrough. After long negotiation he was able to obtain a significant grant from Eli Lilly and Company. In the next year a much more substantial sum from the same company, with a promise for three years of support, went to pay the salary and expenses of a professional fundraiser in his office. The position was filled at first by Christine Skennion, who also relieved him of many tasks associated with the Embassy receptions and World Mental Health Day (see Chapter 13). Unfortunately, her talents were in great demand and she departed for another job in 1995, to be replaced by another competent person, Catherine Gray, who additionally had useful computer skills.

The addition of this new staff member was essential for the expanded functioning of Dick's office, especially in regard to financial development. It became, however, the occasion for continued recriminations from European members of the Board conveying the vows of the ERC/WFMH, "never" to accept "drug company money." They alleged that accepting such support would result in a loss of autonomy, making the WFMH an agent of the pharmaceutical manufacturers. Board members with opposing views argued that no more "autonomy" would be lost in this way than through the acceptance by most European mental health associations, and many elsewhere in the world, of governmental money in return for which they provided services as though they were a branch of government. The ERC was cited as an example of an independent NGO in danger of becoming a captive of the European intergovernmental system. Under these circumstances NGO policies are inevitably influenced by government policies, and the issue of freedom from outside influence may be moot.

The hostility of ERC Board members toward pharmaceutical firm contributions ("drug money"), and their attacks on Dick (and the Secretariat in general) for having accepted them were not shared by Latin American, Asian, and African colleagues, mainly psychiatrists accustomed to receiving funds from industry sources. North Americans had a pragmatic view. Nor had the negative attitude been present in the Rees era. In fact, for some time pharmaceutical companies could obtain Federation membership. Thus, the 1954 Annual Report lists six well-known firms with Swiss bases as affiliated members. Of four other affiliated Swiss member organizations, two were private psychiatric clinics and two appear to have been businesses, although their exact products are not clear. However, in 1977 several Board members had opposed accepting financial assistance from pharmaceutical companies for the WFMH World Congress in Vancouver; this despite the fact that the Canadian Mental Health Association (which did not contribute to the Vancouver Congress) had accepted major funding from a company allowing it to participate in Canada's 1967 Centennial Expo in Montreal.

Federation concern about drug company contributions seems to have been influenced by the consumer/user movement and the strong British reactions, at the time, to the possibly adverse effects of benzodiazepines. Many ex-patients and current service users had intensely negative feelings about neuroleptic drugs, with their often disturbing side effects, as well as about psychiatry in general, which they experienced as an oppressive force (see Chapter 7). Objections to pharmaceutical contributions also reflected negative feelings about the well-publicized donations of pharmaceutical manufacturers to psychiatric organizations. They have constituted a tangible presence at psychiatric meetings throughout the world and been generous contributors to the profession's education and research endeavors. They are also major contributors to research-oriented voluntary associations of patient relatives such as the United States National Alliance for the Mentally Ill (NAMI), concerned in some measure with what they see as the deleterious consequences of lack of parental or medical control over the behavior of chronically ill people at risk for hurting themselves or simply deteriorating without treatment. The U.S. NMHA, more oriented to patient autonomy and the avoidance of involuntary hospital admission, has not been so close to the industry, nor has the WFMH. This has been intertwined with concern about the antitherapeutic effect of exclusive dependence upon pharmacological treatment. On the other hand, the notion of such exclusive dependence was seen by many Board members, even some from Europe, as a straw man. Notable, as described in Chapter 7, was America's Hilda Robbins' unequivocal statement on the value of psychopharmaceuticals in treating her own episodes of depression. Since the 1980s research findings have moved North American psychiatry, particularly in the United States, toward more rational combinations of psychosocial and pharmacological treatment for disabling mental disorder.

The issue first surfaced for general WFMH discussion at the Assembly meeting during the 1987 World Congress for Mental Health in Cairo, Egypt. Many Federation members were annoyed because the psychiatrist Egyptian Congress organizers had allowed ubiquitous advertising exhibits from both pharmaceutical companies and firms manufacturing electroencephalographic equipment in the corridors and public areas. Strong objections to accepting "drug money" were raised during the Assembly by several ex-mental hospital patients and current users, supported by some Board members. However, Robert Gibson, then WFMH treasurer, made a strong case for accepting some funds under certain conditions. First, there would be no pharmaceutical advertising at future Congresses. Second, and most important, such money would be accepted only if it did not compromise the Federation's advocacy positions.

A consensus was reached and for several years the issue did not re-emerge, largely because no significant funds became available to us from these sources. But the tension was kept alive as the ERC became increasingly involved with survivor/user groups, for many of whom neuroleptic drugs represented everything they feared and disliked about psychiatry. The ERC was also influenced in part by the antipsychiatry movement in the United Kingdom and northern Europe. There was no real equivalent of this in the United States where, despite continued wariness, most consumers or ex-patients (the term "user" did not become the preferred designation) recognized the advantage of maintaining relationships with psychiatrists and others who could be helpful in times of stress or during exacerbations of illness. Perhaps this was due to the fact that United States psychiatry, unlike that in Europe and the United Kingdom, depended rather little on the use of such treatments as electroshock therapy and had a long tradition of egalitarian communication between doctor and patient. Many of the issues important to ERC leaders, such as the use of restraint and seclusion in mental hospitals, were no longer relevant in North America and were accepted without comment in the less developed world. Possibly more important, United States investigators were seriously concerned with developing combinations of minimal dose techniques and psychosocial therapies in order to reduce the undesirable side effects of antipsychotic medication and make it more acceptable to those who would sometimes prefer their illness.

This was the organizationally divided context in which Dick Hunter, after several years of trying, was finally successful in 1993 in obtaining a grant from Eli Lilly and Company to support the first World Mental Health Day telecast. Some European Board members reacted bitterly, fearing that the WFMH's status as a voluntary organization would be impaired. They suggested that ERC members would begin to regard the WFMH as a financial dependent of the drug industry. Further negative reactions rather than plaudits followed his 1994 success in obtaining a significant sum from the same corporation to be devoted to the support of a person to lead the fundraising effort for the WFMH. Despite their negative feelings, however, they recognized the Federation's need for money and did not attempt to block Dick's acceptance of the gift. This recognition foreshadowed a gradual, but not explicated, change of heart. Before that, however, a distressing error intensified the ERC attacks. In mid-1994 a notice was mailed from the Deputy Secretary General's office, without consultation with me or the Board, to all WFMH member associations inviting them to participate in the third World Mental Health Day (10 October 1994). The problem lay in its announcement that the Day would be presented jointly by the WFMH and Eli Lilly. The ERC and mental health associations in Europe reacted with outrage. Some said that they would have nothing to do with World Mental Health Day. It was necessary for me to tell the ERC assembly at their Belfast annual meeting in August 1994 that it had all been a mistake. When I joined the ERC Board at dinner that evening, most accepted the explanation. One or two others, however, remained hostile and inclined to place the worst interpretation on it. Upon returning to the States I reported my experience to Dick who, after some introspection, sent letters of apology for his error to the ERC Board. The fact was that he had never intended that World Mental Health Day, already co-sponsored with the WHO, would in any way become the property of an organization that helped to support it. After prolonged discussion the WFMH Board agreed that, beyond assurances already made, no drug company or any other corporate donor would ever again be listed as a "partner" or "co-sponsor" of events such as World Mental Health Day. The issue seemed to have been settled and there was no reason to expect further divisive action. However, the next number of the ERC bulletin carried a highly visible, and potentially inflammatory, box on its front page reminding readers that its Council had voted unanimously to refuse any financial support from drug companies.

At a late spring 1995 meeting in Alexandria, Virginia the Executive Committee, joined by both NMHA and drug company representatives, met at Dick's initiative to explore the possibilities of a conference focused on "the ethical distribution of neuroleptic drugs." This followed a suggestion made by Marten de Vries, professor of social psychiatry and director of a University of Limburg (Maastricht, Holland) WFMH Collaborating Center, who was also our treasurer. There was general agreement that the ethical "distribution" of neuroleptic or psychoactive drugs required attention to their ethical "use." It was apparent that the Federation was in a position to make a significant contribution to the education of clinicians and users, and to the acceptable use of psychoactive drugs in psychiatric treatment. No conclusion was reached as to whether or not drug companies should be asked to finance the conference. Within the framework of the discussion about funding it was again noted that accepting support from other types of corporations, as well as governments or intergovernmental organizations such as the European Union, also risked a loss of independence. There was general agreement that organizations accustomed to government support are not, in fact, independent in that their donors may limit or stop funding if the organization's policies are deemed not to fit the interest of the particular governmental or intergovernmental entity involved. In contrast, voluntary associations which do not receive government subsidies are free to criticize or operate independently of government policy if that is what they judge best.

While there was general agreement about the value of the proposed drug distribution conference, no systematic effort was made to find funds to support it. As of 1997, when de Vries became president, it was still in the category of potential projects.

"Drug Money" and the Politically Incorrect Use of Diagnostic Labels

With the rise of the user movement the anti-drug money position became associated with the avoidance of terms like "mental illness." A few of the European Board members began to refer instead to "serious emotional distress." This fitted the self-perceptions of many, although not all, users. It was reminiscent of the 1985 World Congress in Brighton, England where users circulated a petition asserting that "mental illness" did not exist and was the social construction of power-seeking psychiatrists. Although no Board member signed the Brighton petition, it marked the beginning, for many, of increasing caution in expressing views that were potentially unpopular with the mental health consumer community as well as with some Board colleagues. The courageous stands at that time and later of Hilda Robbins, then Vice-President for North America, as someone who had benefited vastly from effective medication for serious depressions, seemed to have little effect on the thinking of the anti-drug medication school. In fact, accepting the value of pharmacological treatments, like being in favor of accepting pharmaceutical company money, became equated by some European members with lack of support for the user movement. Corollary was an implication that the psychiatrists who are empowered to prescribe drugs behave in a less morally desirable fashion than nonprofessional volunteers or mental health association staffs.

The major departure from an ideology combining a reluctance to acknowledge the existence of mental illness, an anti-drug money position, and reluctance to work with patients' families came during the 1995 Dublin Congress. Psychologist Dr. Maria Simon, former Dean of the University of Vienna School of Social Work and the WFMH representative to UN Vienna, spoke forcefully in favor of medication when necessary, as well as the need in some instances for involuntary hospitalization (Simon, 1995). Writing from the perspective of a "carer," the mother of a 20-year-old son with schizophrenia, she accused some Federation leaders of resorting to euphemisms to avoid using such terms as "illness," implying that a certain amount of self-deception might be involved. At the same time she regretted that many clinicians do not take the time to educate patients and families or to build the trusting relationship which usually makes it unnecessary to resort to coercion. She noted, as had others, that the anti-medication and anti-"illness" attitude of some European WFMH leaders, implicitly agreed with the proposition of many "users" that there was no such thing as mental "illness." Its extreme emphasis on patient autonomy made it difficult to collaborate closely with such family-centered organizations as the Schizophrenia Fellowship and the Alliance for the Mentally Ill. Their goals overlapped with those of the WFMH, but because of their energetic support of research and their interest in the treatment possibilities offered by advancing neuroscience and pharmacology they, especially the Alliance, had far outstripped the Federation in acquiring resources.

Realism Prevails

By 1997, as funds were increasingly difficult to acquire even for the ERC, with its subsidies from the European Community, the Europeans became less vociferous in their objection to money from pharmaceutical companies. Dick arranged for an Eli Lilly representative to meet with ERC representatives so that each could understand the other's point of view. Some ERC member associations did accept industry funding for particular conferences or activities. The event that most impressed and surprised volunteer observers was WHO's acceptance of two million dollars from Eli Lilly, announced in mid-1996, to support what it called its Nations for Mental Health Initiative (NMH). With this image before them the ERC leadership's negative utterances were muted, although not completely extinguished. The May 1996 Executive Committee meeting in Alexandria, Virginia with NMH leader Benedetto Saraceno, M.D., and WHO Mental Health Division Director Jorge Alberto Costa e Silva, M.D., accepted WHO's invitation to submit a project based on the potential availability of this money (see Chapter 8). ERC members of the Committee reminded President Long that in 1995, she had agreed to "canvas" the WFMH membershipabout its views on this score. In response, she published a statement about "fund raising policy" in the first quarter's Newsletter for 1997. It reiterated the Federation's freedom to raise money from whatever source seemed appropriate as long as it did not require any compromise in our advocacy positions. It also invited comment from readers. None was forthcoming.

In late 1996 the WFMH finance committee, headed by Treasurer Robinson, was systematically canvassing a number of corporations, mainly in the United States, with international interests. These included but were not limited to pharmaceutical firms. As 1996 ended a mood of cautious optimism regarding fundraising possibilities began to emerge. Although no major gifts had been obtained, relationships were being forged among Dick Hunter, Catherine Gray, David Robinson and possible corporate givers. An important donation of time and energy, as described in Chapter 5, came from Andersen Consulting. This too fueled the optimistic mood and an expectation that a systematic review and analysis of the WFMH mission, structure, and functions would lead to success in fundraising.

Counterbalancing factors were also emerging. The Lilly grant that paid Gray's salary was coming to an end. While my office expected its funding to continue, that required renewal on a yearly basis and it was not rational to expect renewals to continue indefinitely. By the time of the 2–4 May 1997 Strategic Planning Retreat led by an Andersen Consulting person, Robinson had submitted his resignation as treasurer in order to accept a position elsewhere in the country. This was an unexpected blow, which required rapid action. Although European Vice-President Henderson had strongly advocated that future Federation treasurers should be elected rather than appointed, incoming president Marten de Vries followed the still valid bylaws and appointed a treasurer to replace Robinson in time for sufficient overlap to permit an adequate transmission of knowledge about the work involved. In keeping with the traditional belief that the United States was the best source of funds and the desire of the Secretariat to have the treasurer close at hand, de Vries appointed Dr. John Gates of the Carter Center in Atlanta, Georgia to fill that post, effective during the Finland World Congress in July 1997. Still, it was difficult to digest the fact that the treasurer and finance committee chair, in whom so many hopes were invested, was going to disappear! Then, by the end of 2½ days of intensive discussion during the Airlie House retreat,the inflated mood of magic expectation began to evaporate. The deflating pinprick was renewed confrontation with the gross inadequacy and fragility of our infrastructure and continuing uncertainty about how Dick Hunter and I could be replaced when we finally felt free to resign our volunteer jobs. Even Dick, ordinarily upbeat, could not help saying that a major result of the consulting process so far was a lot more work, which the participants expected the Secretariat to handle.

Chapter 7

The WFMH and Consumer/Survivor/User Movements

HISTORICAL ANTECEDENTS
North America: Dix and Beers

The 19th and early 20th century American concern with participation by citizens in decisions affecting their own futures presaged what, in the later 20th century, became the self-help and social advocacy organizations of those with similar experiences of illness or distress. The early organizing efforts of Dorothea Dix and Clifford Beers, both survivors of disabling mental pain, struck a responsive cord in United States legislators and social leaders who wished to treat society's less fortunate (and often less privileged) members in a manner congruent with their own professed moral standards. Beers, in particular, who had experienced a punishing hospitalization, created the Connecticut, United States, and International Committees on Mental Hygiene as organizations that would include survivors as well as other volunteers in the cause of mental hospital reform. His biographer, Norman Dain, has identified earlier struggles of United States ex-patients to change the laws permitting involuntary hospitalization, especially the commitment of wives by their husbands (Dain, 1989). But as noted in Chapter 1 Beers, despite some continuing distrust, eventually found his major allies not among other former patients, but among the professional leaders of his era.

The Context of Consumer, Self-Help, and Ex-Patient Liberation Movements

Users of psychiatric services were latecomers to the self-help and advocacy world. It required the post-World War II social climate to transform them into a collectivity, a group of people committed to action on the basis of a shared value system (Parsons, 1952). This climate fostered self-awareness and collective efforts at self-realization by a number of minority populations: those with inadequate channels to sources of societal power who suffered discrimination at the hands of the dominant culture because of their membership in a devalued or frightening group. Prominent among them were members of socially visible ethnic groups, particularly people of color and recent immigrants, practitioners of religions other than that of the majority, and in some instances homosexuals. Major efforts at achieving social and legal equality were embodied in the black power and gay rights movements. Women, the elderly, and the physically handicapped (especially those depending on wheelchairs), also developed their own advocacy movements (Brody, 1968). In this context people who had suffered mental illness began to understand themselves as right-seeking minorities trying to claim the social power essential to survival (Brody, 1983b). The more militant claimants sought political action aimed at social system change. The less militant, including both the medically ill and emotionally distressed people called patients—in traditionally paternalistic relationships with their physicians—took two not incompatible routes. The most conservative was that of consumerism, involving continuing, though modified, dependence upon professionals. The second was the self-help movement.

CONSUMER AND SELF-HELP MOVEMENTS

Consumerism in Medicine

The initial, more conservative, change began with medical patients' efforts to achieve a more egalitarian relationship with their professional helpers. In the second half of the 20th century those who were better educated, politically liberal, and did not wish to be blindly dependent on their physicians' prescriptions increasingly designated themselves as "consumers" of health services. They attached high importance to sharing whatever was known about the goods and services for which they paid. They felt that participation in decisions about their own care was a fundamental right.

The consumer philosophy has been widely embraced by the medical profession, especially as advancing technology has presented physicians and patients with moral as well as technical choices requiring joint decision-making (Brody, 1993b). It has not, however, been easily applicable to people defined by mental health professionals as having serious mental illness, regarded by them and the general public as cognitively impaired, and therefore incapable of making rational or helpful decisions about their own care.

Self-Help for Emotionally Distressed Persons

Self-help groups depending on social support, and sometimes the guidance of a professional, have proliferated since World War II. By the 1980s and 1990s they covered the range of human difficulties and disabilities including such psychiatrically diagnosed conditions as obsessive-compulsive disorder and the varieties of anxiety states. Some have referred to themselves as ex-patients. Others preferred the term, "survivor," not only of illness, but of the trauma of hospitalization. The most significant contribution of these groups is mutual support between peers who have experienced similar difficulties and do not relate to each other on the basis of status or academic knowledge. Their encounters take place in a range of settings: in each others' homes, drop-in centers, or small user-run businesses. For some, the self-help movement offers a compromise between an attempt to achieve total autonomy and continuing dependence upon trained professionals, both in dealing with distressing or incapacitating symptoms, and making major life decisions. However, as O'Hagan pointed out, this compromise is not always feasible. In her view, authentic self-help services must be totally directed and run by survivors. She contrasts "the overriding value" of choice and autonomy in such settings with services where "removal of symptoms has paramount value," justifying the treatment of people "against their will" (O'Hagan, 1995b, p. 4).

A major example of a self-help group for people diagnosed with severe mental illness is Fountain House, with its origins in New York state. The concept is that of a club with participants called members rather than patients. Some Fountain House clubhouses are residential;

others operate on a day visiting basis. Most have at least one senior staff member, typically a social worker, with some part-time helpers. Ideally the clubhouse functions not only as a social center, but as a prejob training site, a transitional employment place (comparable in some ways to a sheltered workshop), and a referral source for jobs and housing. In some areas members are able to hold jobs in the larger community, returning to the clubhouse only at night. Those who require medication or counseling obtain the needed help, independently, at clinics unrelated to the club. A recent account of one club member's experience with chronic auditory hallucinations responsive to medication indicates the point of view of a member who depends both on the self-help possibilities offered by the clubhouse and the support available at a clinic: "Today I fight a battle daily to take the miracle medicine which stopped them [the voices]…the choice is now finally mine…all I need to do is take my medicine, side-effects and all…one day at a time; one pill at a time…one way I resist the temptation of not taking [it] and returning myself to the company of those voices is by doing things like writing about my experience…." (Steele, 1996).

The 1983 World Congress for Mental Health in Washington, DC, was the first at which survivor/users and self-help representatives were invited to be on the program. I was eager to include them because my own experience with people diagnosed as mentally ill had made it clear that they had much to contribute to the organization and operation of treatment programs. I was especially pleased to welcome the Director of Fountain House in Stockholm, Kerstin Nilsson. Two months earlier, in May 1983, she arranged an international WFMH co-sponsored meeting bringing together mental health workers from 17 countires to examine the applicability of the social club model for chronic mental patients in a variety of cultural settings. My wife and I attended, along with several other WFMH members. Notable was the attendance of three representatives of our local organizations in the Arabic/Islamic world, all of whom came to the 1983 Congress in Washington. Osama Al Radi, M.D., the first Director of Mental Health in Saudi Arabia, was there with his daughter, the first woman in the Kingdom to be trained as a psychiatric nurse. (This was the first time, she confessed to my wife, that she appeared in public unveiled—although her hair was convered—and she felt quite uncomfortable). From Pakistan came Mohammud Rashid Chaudry, M.D., Professor at the King Edward University in Lahore. And from Egypt came our Board member, later to be the WFMH President (1987–1989) Gamal M. Abou El Azayem, M.D., of Cairo. These last two, inspired by the visit, established Fountain House organizations in their own countries, each with a distinctive cultural stamp. Part of this cultural stamp was reflected in the continued retention of paternalistic control by psychiatrists, facilitated by the socioeconomic gulf between doctors and patients. Fourteen years later, in 1996, it was my privilege to visit a Fountain House club in Johannesburg accompanied by Lage Vitus, national director of our member organization in South Africa, and one in Capetown in company with Toni Ticknor, director of the Cape Mental Health Society (a local branch) which participated in its support and oversight. At this time, shortly after the abolition of apartheid, the club members were largely, but no longer exclusively, white. They were impressively frank in discussing their psychotic episodes and the tension between a wish to be free of dependence upon medicines and the need to continue with them in order to be free of distressing feelings and experiences such as hallucinations. All felt that the open atmosphere of the clubhouses and the opportunity for close communication with all kinds of people supported their hope of someday being free of medication.

SURVIVORS AND EX-PATIENTS' LIBERATION

As pointed out by O'Hagan, the designation "consumer" has been rejected by most former mental hospital patients because it implies a choice (as "in the marketplace where the customer is king"), which they did not always have. This included both the choice to use services at all or which services they would use. (O'Hagan, personal communication, 1996). Mental hospital patients and ex-patients thus tended to identify themselves not as consumers, but as users of mental health services, or survivors of mental illness, and in some instances as survivors of "psychiatric oppression." Some who supported this last perspective, feeling themselves victims of organized psychiatry, became advocates of the "anti-psychiatry" idea embodied in the writings of critical observers such as Michel Foucault and psychiatrists such as Thomas Szasz (Szasz, 1961). Szasz was the leading anti-psychiatry theoretician with his view of mental illness as a myth constructed to maintain the social dominance of psychiatrists. The debate he fostered was mainly an intellectual exchange between professionals that included no practical efforts to involve the increasingly active ex-patients. However, some of its ideas and perspectives, for example his critique of the patients' rights movement led by attorneys and professionals, have been useful to ex-patients in formulating their own goals. These include maintaining their absolute freedom of choice, especially in regard to attempted psychiatric intervention, which might lead to involuntary hospitalization or the administration of drugs or procedures defined as "treatment."

Judi Chamberlin, a survivor of hospitalization, has produced a brief history of the ex-patient's movement in the United States. While recognizing the self-help aspect of the movement, she concentrates on advocacy or working for political change, addressing problems that "go beyond the individual" (Chamberlin, 1990, p. 331). "The mental patients' liberation movement," as she described it, is a political activity started in the early 1970s by people who had experienced psychiatric treatment and hospitalization. Its major goals were "developing self-help alternatives to medically based psychiatric treatment and securing full citizenship rights for people labelled 'mentally ill'" (Chamberlin, 1990, p. 323). The first Conference in which Psychiatric Oppression was linked to human rights took place in 1973 at the University of Detroit. It was sponsored jointly by academic psychologists and the Mental Patients Liberation Project, which was founded in New York City in 1971.

"Ex-patients" do not constitute the only group with an interest in avoiding the threat of involuntary detention in mental hospitals. Perhaps the majority of those experiencing distress and illness have not had the benefit of psychiatric services. They avoid professionals and deal with their difficulties with their own resources, the help of friends, families, and such readily available listeners as ministers and bartenders. Still others, having perceived hospitalization as a battle with oppressive jailers, eschew the term "user," preferring to regard themselves simply as "survivors" of illness or psychological and emotional distress, or punishment at the hands of doctors and hospitals. Yet others, whom professional clinicians might define as mentally ill, prefer to be perceived simply as having special and desirable characteristics. As O'Hagan put it: "How different would our experience of madness be if it was valued and given status?" (O'Hagan, 1995b, p. 5). Some with depressed or elated mood swings, for example, have described themselves in terms of greater than usual capacity to experience and express feelings (O'Hagan, 1995a). Nearly a century earlier Sigmund Freud (1901) described the paranoid person as particularly sensitive to cues about the feelings of others of which "normal" individuals are typically unaware: "...he recognizes something that escapes the normal person: he sees more clearly" (Freud, 1901, p. 255). However, while recognizing an element of truth in the paranoid person's interpretations of the behavior of others, Freud regarded them as essentially "worthless" because they were so significantly determined by projection "onto the mental life of other people of what is unconsciously present in his own" (p. 255). Despite Freud's denials, some contemporary psychiatrists have paid special attention to the poetic sensitivity and perceptiveness of talented people who have been diagnosed as schizophrenic. Many, stimulated by user/survivor associations, have become more sensitive to how their power to classify and commit people to mental hospitals might reflect their own culture-bound values. As former patients articulated their experiences of unwilling hospitalization, and made their psychotic behavior more intelligible in terms of their particular environments, their accounts have been studied with greater seriousness by students of culture and mental illness. They reinforce doubts about whether or not the seemingly objective "diagnostic" criteria used by organized psychiatry are in fact, equally valid for persons of all social classes and cultures in all settings (Brody, 1994).

THE INVOLVEMENT OF THE WFMH
1981–1983

National mental health associations have traditionally been the primary preserve of the affluent upper middle class, which has regarded them as a charity; only a few have been sensitive to the potential contributions of ex-patients. The WFMH did not take formal notice of the possible contributions of users or survivors until the early 1980s. When I became WFMH president in 1981, I began to receive literature and correspondence from people active in a variety of self-help movements for people with emotional and psychological difficulties, including the still embryonic ex-psychiatric patients' movement in the United States. I was receptive to these messages, since a long career as a psychiatrist had made me realize that most of my colleagues found it difficult to empathize with those who sought their help—to see the world through their eyes. The professional emphasis on "objective" findings, and since the 1970s on psychopharmacological agents, had led to a devaluation of patients' subjective reports.

My sensitivity to the wishes and claims of illness survivors was also heightened because I had grown up in close contact with a mentally ill relative whose high intelligence and advanced education permitted life in the community despite continuing auditory hallucinations and a well-defined set of delusions. It was exciting, therefore, to realize the potential of the WFMH as a link between the survivor/user/consumer movement, traditional volunteers, and professionals. With this in mind I got in touch with our Board member, Edith Morgan of London, who I knew was concerned about the interaction of professionals and volunteers in the mental health movement in Europe. I suggested the possibility of an Atlantic Basin Meeting including both European and North American participation on the role of self-help and ex-patient groups in formulating and implementing the goals of the Federation. She responded enthusiastically and, in the name of the WFMH, organized a seminar held in London 21–23 July 1982. In keeping with her own concerns of that time, however, she did not place people with psychological and emotional difficulties at the center of our deliberations. Instead, she entitled the meeting Professionals and Volunteers: Partners or Rivals, and it was more focused on traditional citizen volunteers than on consumers. Dick Hunter and I, though, were reluctant to give up the initial concept and asked for help in achieving it from several of our United States member associations. They responded. The American Psychiatric and Psychological Associations, along with the National Mental Health Association, supported the London travel of American user/survivor Judi Chamberlin, who had already published a volume describing her own experiences and philosophy (Chamberlin, 1978a). For this we owe thanks to Melvin Sabshin, M.D., Medical Director of the American Psychiatric Association (my discretionary Presidential appointment to the WFMH Board in 1981), and Mike Pallak, Ph.D., Executive Director of the American Psychological Association. This was a first for these two professional associations, as well as a milestone in Chamberlin's development as a consumer advocate. We were able to make that London meeting the first time that the Federation "explicitly confronted the issues of paternalism and elitism" in patient care. It asked, for the first time, "which group writes the rules upon which the social contract between help-seeker and help-giver is based?" (Brody, 1982). This question made it clear that it could no longer be taken for granted that the rules of therapeutic interaction would be laid down by society's designated helpers without a dialog with the help-seekers. It provided a basis for transforming the status of help-seekers by granting them previously unobtainable elements of power and autonomy.

Partly in consequence of this developing interest of the WFMH, the newer mental health associations, especially in Europe, began to encourage membership by people with direct personal or family experience of mental illness. In contrast, members of long-established mental health associations tended, with occasional notable exceptions, to share the major orientations of organized psychiatry (Carstairs and Morgan, 1983). Within the WFMH, Hilda Robbins of Philadelphia, a former president of the U.S. National Mental Health Association, was an important catalyst for recognizing the contributions of survivors of mental illness. Her identification of her own recurrent episodes of depression, and the benefit she had gained from appropriate medication, increased the sensitivity of WFMH leaders to the valuable insights of people with personal illness experience.

The World Congresses of the past had provided a place for what Priscilla Norman had called "a parliament" of mental health association representatives. However, this was not formalized, nor was it institutionalized. It surprised me to learn that the WFMH, while it realized the membership of mental health associations as central to its existence, had offered them no regular place in which to come together, share ideas, and gain mutual strength. Nor had we ever had a formal place for the contributions of those who had survived mental illness. We had never offered either group a preferred spot on a World Congress for Mental Health program. I therefore suggested that each Congress, beginning with that in Washington, DC in 1983, should include both a special section at which mental health associations could meet and a symposium or a section for ex-patients, survivors, or as they came to be largely known, "users" of mental health services.

After some discussion the first suggestion was incorporated in the form of Mental Health Association Day to precede the Congress proper and to be devoted solely to presentations by member associations from around the world. It was an idea whose time had come and Board members embraced it with alacrity. Dr. Estafania Aldaba-Lim, president-elect from Manila, was particularly helpful in fleshing it out, as was Hilda Robbins, who became WFMH Vice-President for North America at the 1983 elections. Hilda agreed to manage our first Mental Health Association Day during the 1983 World Congress and did such a superlative job that she became identified with the Day and supplied its essential leadership for the following decade.

Despite Hilda Robbins' ability to bridge the two ideas, a Mental Health Association Day and a special forum for ex-patients, the latter did not become institutionalized. However, the 1983 Congress did feature a symposium of self-help and ex-patient contributors for the first time in Federation history. This was the beginning of independent and vital participation by these groups, inside and outside the formal structures, in all succeeding World Congresses. It also set the stage for the eventual election of a survivor/user (Mary O'Hagan) to the Board.

The 1983 Congress also saw a decision by its European Regional Workshop to hold a meeting in 1984 on Legal Issues Concerning Commitment and Civil Rights of Mentally Ill People. Thus began the Federation's systematic interest in the human rights of people defined as mentally ill or at risk for such illness or incapacitating emotional distress.

Consequent to the 1982 London conference and the 1983 Congress, Judi Chamberlin (already in Australia at the invitation of an ex-patient group), was invited to visit WFMH member the Mental Health Foundation of New Zealand and then to become a member of the planning committee for the 1985 WFMH World Congress in Brighton, England where, following the example of the 1983 Congress, a section was to be devoted to self-help and ex-patient groups.

1984–1985

The patients' rights conference planned in 1983 took place on 12–15 August 1984 in Copenhagen with the active, informed, and influential participation of spokespersons from ex-patient associations. It was chaired by Professor Knud Jensen, President of SIND, the Danish Society for the Welfare of the Mentally Ill (and chief psychiatrist at the Odense Hospital) along with Bent Pedersen, the Society's executive director. I noted in the September 1984 number of the newly revived WFMH Newsletter that, "if WFMH is to be an authentic, global mental health coalition its members must include persons who have experienced the kinds of disturbances called mental illness and the life changes which are part of the status of being a 'patient'."

The deliberations and conclusions of the Copenhagen conference will be described in the section on human rights in Part III of this volume dealing with the international mental health agenda, but the years since that time have been marked by the emergence of survivors of mental illness with their own agendas. During the 1985 Brighton Congress activists from the newly energized user movements in the United States, Britain, the Netherlands, and other European countries met for the first time. A group of former patients, led by Chamberlin, circulated a petition to the effect that mental illness did not exist, but was a social construction, an attempt by psychiatrists to dominate distressed people by medicalizing their problems. Although the WFMH Board declined as individuals and as a whole to sign the petition, no major confrontation ensued. However, since then some WFMH European leaders have tended to avoid the terms "mental illness" or "disease" in favor of such phrases as "serious emotional distress." Conversely, some American, as well as continental, psychiatrists who were present have tended to look at the Federation as leaning toward a denial of the scientific advances that led to the concept of mental illness as a treatable entity.

After 1987: Collaboration with the Establishment

Despite these concerns as the user movement grew in subsequent years, there was increasing rapprochement among its members, psychiatric and medical leaders, and the WFMH leadership. The Secretariat successfully negotiated with the U.S. National Institute of Mental Health (NIMH) for funds to bring users to World Congresses for Mental Health beginning with that in Cairo, Egypt in 1987. NIMH and the Maryland Department of Health and Mental Hygiene, represented by its Assistant Secretary Thomas Krajewski, M.D., brought nine representatives of patients' rights and ex-patient organizations to Cairo to present a workshop on The Patient as an Important Treatment Resource. At the Assembly of 20 October 1987 during that Congress Joe Rogers, representing the National Mental Health Consumers Group (USA) offered three resolutions that were accepted as a basis for further exploration, with a follow-up report scheduled for the 1989 Auckland, New Zealand WFMH Congress. They called for greater participation of consumers in Federation activities, direct consumer-recipient representation in every national delegation to WFMH Congresses, and an advisory panel of recipients of mental health services to be consulted regarding Federation policy and activities. The Egyptian authorities' view of the consumer emphasis was, however, uncertain. The General Secretary of the WFMH Congress, psychiatrist Abdel Moniem Ashour of Ein Shams University, felt that since most candidates for self-help groups in Egypt had never been diagnosed, they would be "inviting social stigma" by coming forward.

Several other examples of the new collaborative mode emerged. One was WFMH co-sponsorship of a 26–28 September 1988 meeting organized by MIND and the Brighton, England Health Authority on User Involvement in Mental Health Services. Yet another was a new openness by empathic psychiatrists to questions about the suitability of relatives as decision-makers for people declared mentally incompetent. Some user groups favored the selection of a friend as a guardian or substitute decision-maker, sometimes as a member of a volunteer committee, rather than a "next of kin," even the most devoted "carer." The evolving WFMH position, while regarding a case-by-case approach as most desirable, is one of caution about ceding all powers of control to the patient's (or user's) family.

In 1989, during the World Congress for Mental Health in Auckland, New Zealand, special attention was paid to the follow-up from the resolutions presented two years earlier in Cairo. The main consequence was a proposal to form a new WFMH-affiliated organization, the World Federation of Mental Health Consumers, with both the Board and Assembly formally indicating their support.

In 1990 planners for the 1991 World Congress for Mental Health in Mexico, led by Hilda Robbins, Adriana Lopez, and Lourdes Quiroga, met in Houston, Texas to develop enhanced opportunities for consumer participation in the Congress. In order to gather ideas from the grass roots they mailed requests for abstracts and ideas to all available consumer addresses. They also continued to develop the groundwork for a future global organization of consumers or survivors begun in Auckland. Mary O'Hagan, then coordinator of the Astenoa Network of Psychiatric Survivors in New Zealand, compiled a master mailing list of consumers to solicit suggestions about the future organization, now tentatively re-designated as the World Federation of Psychiatric Users (WFPU). Meanwhile, with support from the European Community, the ERC was working on a collaborative project, Consumer Evaluation of Community Mental Health Care, with site visits in the United Kingdom, Ireland, Italy, and Denmark.

The 1991 World Congress in Mexico included a Subcongress on Consumers, which passed a Human Rights Bill for Hospitalized Mental Patients. Its contents will be discussed in the section on human rights. Consumers/survivors/users meeting during the Congress formally founded the new WFPU "to facilitate the development of user groups worldwide and to expose and stop violations of user rights and self-determination." Its initial membership included individuals from Mexico, Japan, New Zealand, the Netherlands, England, and the United States. Among its goals were the "support of user struggles in the Third World" yet its relationship to the WFMH was clear, as it indicated its intention "to liase with WFMH and assist the 1993 Tokyo Congress Committee to develop the consumer/user theme." O'Hagan and Paolo del Vecchio, from the United States, were elected as co-chairpersons of the new WFPU.

Because of the costs and difficulties in organizing international meetings the solution has been to coordinate them with WFMH Congresses. In 1993, during the Tokyo World Congress for Mental Health, the WFPU was beginning to come of age. O'Hagan was elected to the WFMH Board of Directors. In early 1995 she was invited by the United Nations to serve on the panel to monitor the implementation of UN Standard Rules on the Equalization of Opportunities for Persons with Disabilities.

WFPU News, in its fourth number (July 1995) accepted the idea of mental illness as it noted: "the disability movement is finally recognizing mental illness as a disability." By this time it included approximately 500 individual members in 25 countries, many of whom, along with members of the European Users and Ex-Users in Mental Health, attended the 1995 WFMH World Congress in Dublin. This was the largest attendance of survivors/users at any Congress to date and the WFPU had regular evening meetings with an attendance of approximately 100 people. O'Hagan and del Vecchio, feeling that two terms in office were sufficient, resigned from their positions, and were replaced as co-chairpersons by Leonie Manns from Australia and Gilberto Romero, a veteran of the Chicano civil rights movement, from the United States. He was already a professional "user," having hosted a local weekly radio program on mental health issues for three years, and holding the job of public relations and public education officer with the New Mexico Division of Mental Health.

During that Dublin Congress I participated with other WFMH leaders in a protest by user/survivors against press stereotypes of "mental patients" as a danger to the public and efforts to reduce support for systems of community mental health care. WFPU leaders speaking at the protest included Judi Chamberlin, Mary O'Hagan, Laura Van Tosh, and others. Among other points they stated: "WFMH must stand for the rights of people diagnosed with mental illness to live in their communities of choice with the same rights and responsibilities as other citizens of their respective countries." However, the fundamental ambivalence of user leaders toward the traditional volunteers was revealed in an editorial in the Autumn 1995 number of *The European Newsletter of Users and Ex-Users in Mental Health.* On one hand, it had kind words for WFMH participation in its demonstration, and noted the large and significant input from users and workshops and plenary sessions. On the other, it referred to "the main difference between the user movement and WFMH:...we dare to tell the truth about the dark sides of psychiatry—in this case the horrible Mental Treatment Act of Ireland. Not a word was mentioned about this at the WFMH Congress in Dublin! Of course not—WFMH had to 'be polite' to their hosts even if it means suppressing some unpleasant truths!" (Jesperson, 1995). Much of the Newsletter was devoted to the Irish law of 1945, still in effect. It described a new organization of victims of the law, Wrongly Institutionalized People (W.I.P.).

THE FUTURE OF WFMH-SURVIVOR/USER COLLABORATION

Philosophical Differences Despite Mutuality

Since 1981–1983, and with increasing acceleration since 1989, the WFMH has demonstrated the value it attaches to the mental health survivor/user movement, both in its self-help aspects and its more militant patient liberation aspects. It has supported it through publicity in its Newsletters and Annual Reports, inviting and funding its members' participation in regional and world meetings, helping to form the WFPU, and electing one of its leaders to its Board of Directors. The movement, sufficiently diverse to warrant caution in conceiving it in unitary terms, has accepted the relationship—insofar as some of its goals overlap with those of the WFMH—without giving up its essential independence. Its reservations are partly expressed in Chamberlin's commentary on the U.S. National Association of Psychiatric Survivors (NAPS) founded in 1985, promoting the same ideals as those articulated by Thomas Szasz. As she has written: "NAPS was formed specifically to counter the trend toward reformist 'consumerism' which developed as the psychiatric establishment began to fund ex-patient self-help. Ironically, the same developments which led to the movement's growth and to the operation of increasing numbers of ex-patient-run alternative programs, also weakened the radical voices within the movement and promoted the views of far more cooperative 'consumers.' The very term 'consumer' implies an equality of power which simply does not exist; mental health "consumers" are still subject to involuntary commitment and treatment, and *the defining of their experience by others*" (Chamberlin, 1990, pp. 333–334; italics mine).

Jan Dirk van Abshoven has provided an account of the first European Conference of Users and Ex-Users in Mental Health organized in Zandvoort, the Netherlands, in 1991 by the British and Dutch user movements (van Abshoven, 1994). It attracted a total of 39 delegates from 16 European countries, sufficient to decide to form an organization. September 1993 saw the founding of the European Network of Users and Ex-Users in Mental Health.

Van Abshoven's philosophy clearly differentiates his perspective as a user from that of professionals, and arguably from the bulk of non-user volunteers. That is, he conceives of mental health as a human rights rather than a health issue: "Absolute health does not exist...the person's individual dignity outweighs...health." This perspective is immediately relevant to the strongly held views for and against the use of neuroleptic medications which reveal significant differences of opinion within the user/survivor community, as well as between them, their relatives, and the psychiatrists whom society has made responsible for their care. Family members usually believe in the need for pharmacological treatment for seriously and chronically disturbed young adults; but they may also believe there are instances in which respect for patient autonomy may not be in the patient's best interest—or in theirs as responsible relatives—and that, sometimes (as in the case of patients who have stopped taking essential medications), treatment should be compelled.

The Report on the Kolding Seminar of the European Network of Users and Ex-Users in Mental Health (1994) is devoted to the self-understanding and self-definition of 30 user/survivors from 11 countries who were invited to answer questions about how they saw themselves as former patients. While there are notable differences within this small group of respondents, some commonalities are apparent. They prefer to be viewed as "just people" rather than in terms of psychiatric illness. Many regard their humiliating experience with professional psychiatry, rather than their presumed mental illness, as what differentiates them from others. Most agree that they are more sensitive or vulnerable than others to disturbing life situations, that they view the world differently, and have had special emotional, psychological, and spiritual experiences. But most would not agree that these experiences are indicative of illness or disease.

Philosophical differences between the professionals and, perhaps, most of the citizen volunteers in the WFMH and the survivor/user movement are further illustrated by the reports of Maths Jesperson of Sweden, Editor of the *Newsletter of the European Users and Ex-Users in Mental Health*. During the 1995 Dublin World Congress, Jesperson circulated materials on the user movement including his article in the Dutch magazine *Deviant* about the user organization in Sweden (Jesperson, 1995). The world's oldest national organization of its type, it is called the National Association for Social and Mental Health. It was founded in 1966 in a large mental hospital on the outskirts of Stockholm, as an outgrowth of a program intended to prepare patients for life outside the hospital. Its formal establishment at a public meeting of 62 people, including professionals and a member of parliament, in the Stockholm Civic Hall, was in January 1967. By 1995 it had 10,000 members in 26 regional divisions with 110 local clubs. Despite its "firmly antipsychiatric position," its initial governing boards included many professionals and "outsiders." But by 1995, with increasing emphasis on its being solely a user's organization, 95 percent of its members and all of its elected officers were users or ex-users. At the same time its militancy had diminished to the point that some members viewed it as "too smooth and adjusted to authorities" with its actions concentrated mainly on social and economic welfare for discharged psychiatric patients. Despite this internal criticism it has carried out a project critical of neuroleptic medications and the possibility has been raised that the European Network might "revive a more anti-psychiatric direction of its actions" (Jesperson, 1995).

Well-established user's organizations, not all of identical type, exist, as O'Hagan (1995b) has pointed out, in the democracies that "accommodate liberation politics and the pursuit of individual fulfillment." These include most notably the Nordic countries, the Netherlands, United Kingdom, United States, Canada, and New Zealand. New national organizations emerged during the 1990s in Germany, the Czech Republic, and Japan, and as the 20th century draws to a close psychiatric survivors are beginning to organize in Mexico, Nicaragua, Eastern Europe, and the former Soviet Union.

Persisting Uncertainties

The issue of compulsory treatment may never be satisfactorily resolved. On one hand, certain broad rights to refuse treatment seem ethically essential. This is unquestioned in regard to general medicine, with general agreement about a medically ill person's right to move from a state of being treated to one of being comforted, even though exercising this right forgoes the possibility of lengthening one's life (Brody, 1993b; Veatch, 1981). This is most commonly encountered in the case of prolonged, painful, ultimately incurable malignant disease. On the other hand, professionals have tended to view the right of a nonrational person to refuse treatment as problematic when treatment, itself, is designed to restore clinically defined rationality (Bonnie, 1982). This is the situation occasionally encountered in dealing with acutely disturbed individuals clinically defined as psychotic. From the conventional ethical point of view, treatment in these instances, even when it is compelled or involuntary, can be regarded as essential to restoring autonomy. But this does not take into account the inequities in status, power, and resources between patient and physician. These last suggest the value of intervention by advocacy groups—particularly of other survivor/users—whose power can balance out some of the differential in means between doctor and patient. While it is understood that the physician-patient relationship is always a fiduciary one, with the physician acting as the patient's advocate, the lay advocate, with the patient's consent, should also have sufficient authority to enable negotiation with the physician (as well as the family) regarding the definition and protection of the patient's best interest (Brody, 1985). This bears on a matter of great interest to users, that of the "psychiatric will," based on the concept of a living will to be used in case one is unable to communicate one's desire not to be forced to survive. The Psychiatric Will indicates the kind of treatment, if any, one wishes to receive in the event of an episode of acute disturbance when the capacity for rational communication is impaired. But it does not appear to have totally allayed the fear of compulsory hospitalization and treatment. Several survivor/users have told me that they had specified in their Wills that, in the event of an acute episode or relapse, they should be given no treatment at all.

The Meaning of Symptoms and Coping with Them

Those who have lived with family members whose lives revolve around a delusional system, or repeated hallucinatory experiences—especially of "voices"—are familiar with their efforts to maintain some personal equilibrium in the face of them. They are also familiar with their different meanings. In some instances they can be comforting, constituting what Norman Cameron described some 40 years ago as a "paranoid pseudo-community." At other times, under other circumstances, and for other patients they can be profoundly disturbing and life-threatening. The same is true for mood swings and other mental states. O'Hagan, who had learned "how to protect [herself] when [her] mood swings approached and how to live to the full when they subsided," eventually concluded after trials of drug therapy that "psychiatry is bad for people's mental health." Although drugs "stabilized" her mood swings she wanted "alternative ways of stabilizing them which involve me as an active participant and give my mood swings the meaning that has always been denied them" (O'Hagan, 1993, p. 51). Concluding her report of visits to movement centers in several countries, she identified a central theme that "can be condensed into the word *meaning*. What is the meaning of our madness?" (O'Hagan, 1993, p. 95). With this conclusion she has inadvertently come to partial agreement with those of us who were engaged in psychotherapy with patients defined as psychotic or seriously distressed in the pre-neuroleptic medication era. Our prolonged, intensive, and emotionally taxing efforts, often of several years' duration, were at their core searches for meaning—not only in relation to the patients' early development, but to their current social and cultural contexts and relationships (Brody and Redlich, 1952). As pharmacological treatments became available our experience, as well as systematic research, indicated that they too were most effective when combined with systematic psychotherapy and sometimes with what has come to be called "psychosocial treatment." These are lessons that appear, at least temporarily, to have been lost with the overwhelming flood of easily available pharmaceuticals, the immense pressures on the time of psychiatrists, and the virtual abandonment in many centers of systematic psychotherapeutic education.

A hopeful sign in recent years is increased attention by psychiatrists and psychologists to patients' techniques of coping with their discomforts. A historical moment was the first formal organizational expression by survivor/users of the sense of sharing a special characteristic (understood by psychiatrists as symptomatic, but by others simply as a phenomenon). It was an international meeting of "people who hear voices" in Maastricht, the Netherlands, in autumn 1995. This meeting was organized with the support of the WFMH Collaborating Center Institute for Psycho-Ecological Research of the University of Limburg, headed by then WFMH president-elect Professor Marten W. de Vries.

PREDICTING THE FUTURE

If its first 50 years are a basis for prediction, it seems likely that the WFMH will continue to be dominated during its next 50 years by professionals and citizen volunteers rather than by consumer/survivor/users. It will not be a surrogate for the user movement. Even if the WFMH were willing, it seems doubtful that the user movement could agree. Organizational relationships are vulnerable to misunderstandings. Thus, while the European Regional Council of WFMH had been, from the outset, an advocate for users, a published interview in the Newsletter of the European Network of (ex—) Users and Survivors of Psychiatry with the ERC Executive Director contained a number of points with which user movement leaders disagreed. This led to the Network's November 1996 Board meeting to suggest that she was following the "manipulative and paternalistic way of trying to control the users [which is] used by many professionals...[attempting to] destroy our network and replace it with a handful of users they chose and direct themselves" (The European Newsletter, Winter 1996). The Network's Board felt that it was important to strengthen its relationships with other international nongovernental organizations focusing on disability in general, rather than confining them to nongovernmental organizations concerned with mental health.

This episode illustrated the difficulties encountered in systematic relationships between organizations with disparate social power and different goals. While WFMH proved itself a useful ally in the movement's efforts it was apparent that in order to maintain a collaborative rather than an antagonistic stance, it could not claim to "speak for" patients, ex-patients, or other emotionally distressed persons. It must be prepared to cede some of its power to them in its attempts to defend the human rights of those at risk of psychiatric diagnosis, or already detained in mental hospitals.

Some organizational changes have taken place within the movement as WFMH's first half-century is reached. The initial pre-eminence of the World Federation of Psychiatric Users faded and the European Network has expanded from its regional base in Europe to become a global organization. At the Assembly during the 1997 World Congress in Lahti, the Network's Chair, Peter Lehmann of Germany, powerfully backed by outgoing European Vice President Henderson, moved that the expanded organization should occupy a central position on a proposed advisory committee to the WFMH Board of Directors. While the proposal received a positive vote from the post-Congress Board meeting, composed largely of newly elected members without a history of Federation work, the exact mechanism for implementing it was not specified. It was clear, however, that—with increased personal contact between Federation officers and user activists—multiple channels of communication would develop. Not long afterwards, for example, in November 1997, I received a letter from Clemens W. Huitink, Secretary of the Network's "European Desk," who had spoken at the October 1996 UNESCO-WFMH panel on human rights in Paris. He enclosed, for my comments, a draft manuscript on "Assistance in Cases of Suicide by Patients with the Psychiatric Handicap" which had been translated into English by a member of the Dutch Clients Union. This request for collaborative consideration of an important issue, one which is difficult, as Huitink noted, for the user-movement (letter to the author of 21 November 1997), may presage a constructive way for professionals and users to work together as peers.

Chapter 8

The WFMH and the United Nations

THE NONGOVERNMENTAL AND THE INTERGOVERNMENTAL

The nearly 50 years of Federation interactions with the United Nations (UN) and its specialized agencies reveal the interdependence of both sectors concerned with world affairs: the nongovermental (NGO) and the intergovernmental. They also underscore a fundamental difference between them that fuels recurrent concerns with how nongovernmental-UN relations might be made more useful. This difference is rooted in the fact that the intergovernmental UN is a creature of its member states that supply its budget and personnel and have thier own political agendas. In contrast (and unlike the commercial and professional, as well as governmental, sectors) NGOs have no *inherent obligation* to increase the power of any national or corporate entity. Unlike the international professional unions, which comprise the majority of mental health-related NGOs, WFMH is not dedicated to improving the status of a particular profession or academic discipline. Its position is ecumenical and its mission and purpose may be either facilitated or inhibited, by the UN. The Federation has continued for 50 years to be driven by the ideal of allegiance to the human family, expressed in its 1948 founding document.

In one sense the UN agencies are tools through which the Federation goals are accomplished. (From its perspective the UN could similarly say that NGOs, including the Federation, are among the means through which it accomplishes its aims.) Its search for mental health ranges from the World Health Organization's (WHO's) concerns with psychiatry and patients' rights to the broader purviews of other agencies, notably the UN Educational, Scientific and Cultural Organization (UNESCO) and the units of the Economic and Social Council (ECOSOC), concerned with the social and cultural environments into which people are born, grow, live, and work. The agencies with which the WFMH has worked, informally or in "official relations" during its 50-year history, include UNESCO and its affiliate, the International Social Science Council (ISSC); Unicef (the UN Children's Fund); ILO (the International Labor Organization); UNHCR (the office of the UN High Commissioner for Refugees); the agencies that comprise ECOSOC; UNFPA (the UN Fund for Population Activities); and UNBRO (the UN Border Relief Organization). Telling the WFMH-UN story anticipates this volume's Part III, as it details significant aspects of the Federation's international mental health agenda, and indicates some of its accomplishments.

OVERVIEW

The UN's Founding Role for the WFMH

The account of The Federation's founding in Chapter 2 begins before the founding of the UN with Clifford Beers' 1919 establishment of ICMH, the International Committee for Mental Hygiene. Dormant since the first International Congress on Mental Hygiene in 1930 in Washington, DC, it was reactivated after World War II to engage in planning for the International Conference on Mental Hygiene (part of the Third Congress) in London in 1948. In 1946 John R. "Jack" Rees was made ICMH President in order to facilitate his organization of the Congress of which the founding Conference was a part. At that moment, the agencies of the new UN established in 1945, entered the picture. George Brock Chisholm, scheduled to be the WHO's first Director General, was a prime advocate for a new organization to succeed ICMH, and it was he who suggested that it should be called the "World Federation for Mental Health."

UNESCO also contributed to founding the Federation. The ideological roots of the WFMH 1948 founding document, Mental Health and World Citizenship, lie in the 1947-1948 UNESCO project on reducing international tensions. Several authors of the International Preparatory Commission (IPC) report, which was the basis of the founding document, were active in the UNESCO "tensions project." Among them were Harry Stack Sullivan, Otto Klineberg, Margaret Mead, Henry Dicks, T. S. Simey, Chisholm, and Rees. The relationship with UNESCO was strengthened and symbolized by professor Julian Huxley, UNESCO's first Director General, and one of the world's leading biologists, when he addressed the closing session of the 1948 founding Congress in London. From the UNESCO perspective the WFMH's role in relation to the UN was the promotion of international peace and intercultural and interpersonal harmony. This was compatible with Huxley's broadly conceived interest in mental health.

A 16 May 1947 letter (MM/LC) from ICMH Secretary General H. Edmond Bullis to Margaret Mead, then a member of ICMH's governing board, describes the anticipated relationship of the new Federation to the new UN through its WHO. It is specific about the proposed exclusivity of the relationship in regard to mental health-related activities. The recommendations "on mental health matters" to come from the Conference would, in Bullis' words, be "formally presented to WHO.... It is expected that the ICMH [later to become WFMH] will be the only mental health organization accredited to the World Health Organization." Bullis also noted a WHO function, "preparing the way for individuals to become citizens of the world," which required "that activities be started at once so as to propose practical methods of action to the World Health Organization." This last goal, proposing practical mental health actions to the WHO, was enunciated by Chisholm and fostered during his term as its Director General.

The WFMH in the New World of NGOs

In the years immediately after the formation of the UN relatively few NGOs were granted "official relations" with its specialized agencies. However, an energetic NGO leader such as Jack Rees and a few of his well-placed friends could become personally known to UN officials and country representatives. This had consequences as the UN people, new in their posts, were disposed to take the views of their NGO friends into account in formulating policy and actions.

The Federation's first recommendation in 1949 for the establishment of a mental health section within the WHO was immediately accepted. Its early relations to various UN agencies, most prominently the WHO, Unicef, and UNESCO, are briefly described in Rees' *Reflections* (1966). Indicative of the closeness of the early relationship, when officers of one organization would sometimes work for the other, was the difficulty for many citizens, and even government officials, in differentiating between the assistance or influence of the WHO or other UN agencies in their countries, and that of the WFMH (Rees, 1966, p. 114). This closeness was treasured and Rees was proud of the fact that during his 1948 through 1961 tenure as WFMH Director the Federation was represented at all but two of the World Health Assemblies of the WHO. At "quite a number" (p. 136) of the WHO's annual meetings and those of its regional committees, "the personal contacts established, the help given members of the UN secretariats, and the chances of making suggestions to government delegates attending these meetings [did] a great deal to establish the Federation, to earn considerable respect from the UN secretariats, and to help change the climate of opinion about mental illness and mental health in many countries" (p. 136). He was especially pleased that the ECOSOC secretariat in New York invited the Federation to hold panel meetings in the UN headquarters on three occasions. These meetings were attended by UN secretariat personnel, some delegation members, and members of other NGOs.

With the passage of time the WFMH became only one of some 10,000 NGOs with formal relationships with the UN. Its ability to influence policy was inevitably diminished. At the same time there were increased opportunities to work in concert with other NGOs, both professional and voluntary. Over the years their combined impact heightened international concern with such overlapping issues as health, welfare, and human rights. These had been traditionally regarded as the "internal affairs" of particular states, and hence protected from oversight by other states, the intergovernmental system (the UN), or international NGOs. Almost imperceptibly the NGO community, with the WFMH as a prominent member, has contributed to an erosion of national sovereignty and greater acceptance of international intervention in dealing with victims, not only of natural disasters, but of abuse by their own governments.

The Projected and Actual Relations of the WFMH with the UN

The WFMH, according to its founders, was intended to fill a specific role in relation to the UN. That was, in the words of Brock Chisholm, to serve as "a two-way conduit between UN agencies and the grass roots" (Rees, 1966). In order to accomplish this it was granted consultative status with the WHO immediately after its 1948 founding, and with UNESCO soon thereafter. That was made easy because, as noted above, the practical idealist Chisholm, who suggested the formation of the WFMH, was also the WHO's first Director General. The Report of the IPC for the WFMH was the basis of the 1948 Congress' recommendations to the WHO, which were incorporated into the 1950 report of the WHO's first Expert Committee on Mental Health and sent to every member society of the WFMH. A list of the pre-IPC reports of the Congress' preparatory commissions was also sent to the WHO, and at its request "authoritative information" gathered by United States and United Kingdom member organizations about establishing child guidance clinics. The WHO also asked the Federation to assist in the collection of public education materials and to answer a range of other inquiries about mental health issues coming from international governmental organizations. Kenneth Soddy's review of these initial issues in his capacity as WFMH honorary secretary (later assistant director) is replete with such terms as "friendship" and "friendly" describing what appears to have been a warmly reciprocal relationship between the nongovernmental WFMH and the intergovernmental WHO at the beginning of the Rees era (WFMH, 1949).

As the WFMH reached its 10th year in 1957, Rees' summation of its activities attempted to make a bridge between the mental health-related aims of international harmony contained in its founding document and the more narrowly conceived psychiatric aims of the national mental health associations that had flourished in the following decade. An important part of the bridge was emphasis on the broader goals of prevention carried out by a "combined effort" of NGOs and UN agencies in many countries: "To ensure some steady progress in the care of the mentally sick and some advance in our comprehension of the basic facts about mental illness is important, and perhaps even more so are our efforts to ensure that the children of this generation and those who follow them will have a better chance of avoiding the handicaps and disablements of neurosis or severe mental illness." Then he went on to reaffirm the original perspective of the Federation's founders: "The critical tensions in the world situation at the present time certainly emphasize the need for better relationships and greater wisdom in the affairs of groups and nations, as well as in individuals. We in the Federation cannot ignore the challenge thus presented...it must be our responsibility...to try to add to the sum of wisdom available for those who govern" (WFMH, 1957a, p. 10).

"Those who govern" included leaders of the UN's member states and of the UN itself. In some respects the efforts of the WFMH to "add to the sum of wisdom" of national and international leaders were those of a UN lobby. Rees was sensitive to the pitfalls of this position, noting that because the WFMH was the only international NGO specifically concerned with mental health its representatives "have to avoid any appearance of being pushful or becoming lobbyists. There are many opportunities where, through friendly relationships with the secretariats of these bodies or with the delegates representing the various member countries, it is possible to discuss some mental health aspect of a particular problem which may help to affect the approach that is being taken to this matter though sometimes results may be delayed rather than immediate."(WFMH, 1957a, p.15).

Margaret Mead, as the WFMH president in 1956–1957, had a somewhat different perspective on the role of the WFMH in relation to the UN agencies. While recognizing the UN as "the organized channel through which world-wide concern can express itself," she emphasized its dependence upon "a widespread supporting interest and initiative among the citizens of its constituent nations. If this responsible concern is to make itself felt, then the people of each country who are alert to the needs of the peoples of the world must be able to trust each other, to meet and to communicate, quickly, surely, on matters of urgency and moment." In her view the Federation was building such a group of "responsible, intercommunicating persons" through its Executive Board, discussion groups and special seminars (WFMH, 1957a, p. 8).

With Rees' retirement at the end of 1961 and the January 1962 succession of Francois Cloutier to the WFMH directorship the Federation's intimate relationship with UN leaders and their agencies faded. Although the 1963 move of the Secretariat to Geneva was expected to facilitate communication with UN agencies, the major energies of the Secretariat were invested increasingly in its own survival. With the Federation approaching bankruptcy, and with Cloutier's resignation at the end of 1965, the interaction of the WFMH and the UN declined still further. As described in Chapter 5 and below, Professor of Psychiatry Morris Carstairs of Edinburgh, the Federation's first "working president" from 1968 through 1971, concentrated on WFMH revival through small working conferences in different parts of the world. These were not related to UN agencies, but to voluntary mental health and professional psychiatric organizations. He felt strongly that in order for the Federation to grow and prosper it had to be closely tied to "the grass-roots," and these were more locally significant than the UN. During the 1972–1973 presidency of Professor of Psychiatry Michael Beaubrun of Kingston, Jamaica, the Secretariat was organizationally as well as geographically remote from the WFMH representatives at the European and New York headquarters of the UN. However, a WHO-related meeting did take place in Edinburgh, and as a representative of his government to the Pan-American Health Organization (PAHO) and to WHO headquarters Beaubrun was able to maintain some WFMH visibility.

This nadir of collaborative WFMH-UN activity which began, paradoxically, with the secretariat's move to Geneva persisted through the transition from the Jamaica secretariat to that in Vancouver, Canada at the beginning of 1975. Professor of Psychiatry Tsung-yi Lin of the University of British Columbia, who succeeded Beaubrun as president in mid-1974, announced in his presidential address that his major goals included the development of closer relationships with the UN and its specialized agencies, especially the WHO and Unicef. This was not unexpected from a former WHO scientist. Lin's earlier friendship with Norman Sartorius, M.D., the new director of WHO's Mental Health Division was an important factor in the renewed closeness of the WFMH and the WHO. During 1975–1976 he was instrumental in having the department of psychiatry at the University of British Columbia (UBC) named a WHO Collaborating Center directed by the department's head, Professor Milton Miller. A number of other activities in that year helped restore the Federation's former position of influence with the UN. However, as suggested by the lack of attention paid to mental health during the Alma Ata Conference of 1978, this was never completed. Aside from Sartorius, the new leaders of the WHO were not as sensitive to the role of mental health in relation to general health and well-being as their predecessors had been. However, other UN agencies were open to collaboration.

As incoming President in 1981, and as Secretary General beginning in 1983, I was interested in our effective connections with all of the UN agencies including the WHO, UNESCO, the units of the ECOSOC, UNFPA, and UNHCR. Among other moves this required renewing my acquaintance with Norman Sartorius, whom I had first met in Geneva in 1970. A brilliant leader and investigator, he had made a point of including the broad concerns of the WFMH and other NGOs in the description of "WHO's New Mental Health Programme," published in its entirety in the July-September 1978 number of the WFMH Newsletter. However, much of his attention was focused on systematic research aimed at establishing the worldwide unity of psychiatric diagnoses, regardless of country or culture, especially as defined (after 1980) by the American Psychiatric Association system of nomenclature. This emphasis on universally acceptable classifications and interests was complicated by the fact that the agendas and publications of the specialized UN agencies are not only influenced by, but subject to scrutiny by, the member states that determine their budgets and have their own particular perspectives. One reflection of this was that the WHO Mental Health Division's Social Dimensions of Mental Health (1981), while referring to the adverse health effects of massive population growth and early childbearing, included no mention of the WFMH interests expressed at the 1979 Salzburg Congress in parental choices or professional practices influencing their children's well-being, i.e., family planning, sex education, pregnancy care, and birthing practices. These omissions suggested the political sensitivities of the agency producing this document (Brody, 1983).

Despite this concern I was sympathetic to the research orientation of the Division, and stayed in touch with Sartorius and a number of his colleagues, particularly John Orley, M.D., who had done work on mental health and psychiatric illness in Uganda. Succeeding WFMH presidents, however, who had not emerged from an academic background, were less interested in the WHO's research and more oriented to the practical work of improving patients' welfare. Britain's Edith Morgan (1985–1987), New Zealand's Dr. Max Abbott (1991–1993), and America's Beverly Long (1995–1997), emphasized the advocacy roles of the WFMH for traditional mental health association aims at the national as well as the intergovernmental level. This was compatible with their backgrounds, Morgan and Abbot as former staff leaders in their national mental health associations, and Long as the former president of the National Mental Health Association in the United States.

The major WFMH-WHO liaison beginning in 1985 was in the hands of our new senior ("permanent") representative in Geneva, Stanislas Flache, M.D. His life-long professional background culminating in the post of assistant director general of the WHO gave him a different perspective than colleagues with mental health association or academic backgrounds. The needs of his former organization, the WHO, were always prominent in his view of the issues that interested him most: the human rights of patients and those at risk for serious illness, and the delivery of mental health services in primary health care settings. He shared with Abbott and Long an interest in prevention, sometimes expressed in WHO terms as health promotion. In general, though, he recognized along with the rest of us that attempts to reduce the frequency, severity, and chronicity of mental and neurological illness bring the advocacy effort into its broadest arena as it involves the promotion of social change. This kind of change is aimed at improving the positive mental health of vulnerable segments of the world's population as well as reducing the occurrence of disabling illness. These vulnerable people include mentally ill and emotionally distressed persons and their families as well as those who are medically ill and subject to treatment with biomedical technologies; but they also include such broad population groups as the very young, children in especially stressful situations including those who have been abandoned, the elderly, women and other minorities defined on ethnic, racial, national, or religious grounds, the socioeconomically deprived, and refugees and other traumatized groups. Prevention is the broadest and most difficult to define goal, and the one most frequently attacked by governmental and other agencies because it involves intrusion into their "internal affairs."

The WFMH and the UN: Partners and Critics

Rees, reflecting on the Federation's 10-year history (WFMH, 1957a, p. 15) noted that the relationship between a voluntary association and a government department concerned with mental health may be quite difficult: "Government departments on the whole tend not to be very fond of voluntary associations which have the freedom to make suggestions and at times to be critical. It is only when the voluntary body shows that it can be helpful that it becomes accepted." This could be said for agencies of the intergovernmental body, the UN as well.

While the WFMH has valued its relationship with UN agencies, and tried whenever possible to work through them and support their initiatives, it has also valued its independence. The independence of NGOs in general became so onerous to Soviet UN representatives that in 1970 they proposed that they should be limited to responding to questions by UN bodies or member states, and not be permitted to initiate their own inquiries or to introduce topics for discussion. The Soviet proposal was not accepted by the UN General Assembly, but NGOs are still perceived as continuing threats by totalitarian and traditionally authoritative regimes. This was indicated by the attempts to stifle moves toward improved status for women at the 1993 international population congress in Cairo, and by the Peoples Republic of China's removal of the 1995 NGO forum on women to a site remote from the forum for government representatives.

The WFMH's independence in relation to the UN was formally articulated in two resolutions, both during Lin's 1974–1979 presidency. The first reflected the fact that he was born in Formosa, later to become Taiwan, which was expelled from the UN in 1971 at the request of the mainland People's Republic of China. Passed during a WFMH annual meeting in Copenhagen in 1975, it responded to the 1974 UNESCO general conference's exclusion of Israel from participation in its work. The WFMH condemned "all efforts to exclude any nation from participating in the social, cultural and educational agencies of the UN as destructive of the principles of the UN, the wellbeing of the human family, and the UN itself."

The second resolution was passed during the 1977 WFMH World Congress in Vancouver. It responded to UN concerns about objections from the People's Republic of China to the acceptance of a mental health association in Taiwan as a WFMH member. The WFMH Board asserted that "the mental health association in Taiwan represents…only Taiwan," voted that its membership in the WFMH should be maintained, and that applications from the People's Republic of China would also be welcomed. Its resolution states: "Whereas the WFMH receives with the closest attention and highest regard all recommendations and advice from UN agencies, including the WHO and UNESCO, the fact remains that the WFMH is an independent, non-political, non-governmental organization with its own constitution and rules, from which the WFMH itself cannot deviate. The WFMH, therefore, in principle cannot accept that any outside body should, merely on political grounds, tell the WFMH as a non-governmental organization, whom it should, or should not, accept as members."

Nor have the WFMH's goals always been supported by the intergovernmental system. A leading example was the September 1978 WHO-Unicef International Conference on Primary Health Care in Alma Ata, The Republic of Kazahkstan, U.S.S.R. This conference produced what was called The Declaration of Alma Ata, with the slogan Health for All by the Year 2000, intended to guide the UN's health efforts for the rest of the century. The emphasis was to be on primary health care. However, WFMH President Lin was the only representative of mental health or psychiatry among the 3000 participants. In spite of his efforts, and those of a number of others, mental health was not considered a part of primary health care, nor was it mentioned in any of the Conference documents, or the actual Declaration of Alma Ata (Lin, 1978). One possibly apocryphal explanation was that "mental health" could not be included because it was equated by the Soviet authorities with "bourgeois individualism." It was only after two years of intensive lobbying between 1978 and 1980 by WFMH representative Elizabeth Cohen at UN New York that mental health was included in the post-Alma Ata documentation (Cohen, personal communication, 1982). By the time that Health for All by the Year 2000 became the WHO's institutional rallying cry it included, almost as an article of faith, the idea that mental health services in less-developed countries that could not afford them should be delivered within the context of primary care service delivery. In practical terms this approach has involved training less expensive professionals, such as nurses, in mental status assessment and counselling. In the least-developed areas of Latin America, Asia, and Africa, where these professionals have not been available, the most intelligent and interested villagers, regardless of formal education, have been offered the basic training essential to becoming a local mental health as well as general health worker.

In part because of the Alma Ata Conference's failure to acknowledge the importance of mental health, Lin convened a special study meeting of Unicef and the WHO with the WFMH after the Salzburg World Congress on 14 July 1979. Its stated aim, congruent with the UN's proclaimed International Year of the Child, for which former Executive Board member Dr. Estafania Aldaba-Lim of Manila was the UN leader, was to discuss how to meet the health and mental health needs of the world's children. While no concrete projects emerged, there was general agreement on the importance of the UN and NGOs exchanging information about mental health problems and programs on a worldwide basis, stimulating new programs and promoting research to evaluate their effectiveness. Above all it was agreed that the WFMH should continue advocacy for mental health programs in all countries of the world (WFMH, 1979b).

After this exchange of information and good will it was completely unexpected when two months later, in September 1979, further differences and misperceptions about the WFMH emerged at a meeting of the WHO coordinating group for mental health programs, despite the fact that it included J. S. Neki, M.D., of India, WFMH vice-president for Southeast Asia, and Professor Carlos Leon, M.D. of Cali, Colombia, a former WFMH Board member. The intense continuing activity of the WFMH seemed to be unappreciated by the WHO. Dr. A. N. Costa's statement on behalf of the WHO noted that although WFMH "has had the pleasant opportunity of sharing information and fellowship with the World Health Organization on most issues concerning mental health…two impediments, as identified by the Chief of the Division of Mental Health…have stood in the way of a more intense cooperation between WHO and the intergovernmental organizations." These were "the relative inactivity of the non-governmental organizations of the type of WFMH between their periodic congresses" and "the…constitution of some of the non-governmental organizations, particularly WFMH, that admits even paraprofessionals to their membership." This statement, reflecting outdated prejudices, seemed particularly inappropriate in view of the need for paraprofessionals and volunteers to achieve the goal of "health for all by the year 2000." It convinced the WFMH leadership of the need for more intensive dialogue between the WHO and the WFMH (WFMH, 1980).

The WFMH's human rights-oriented social focus has also required it at times to proceed without the collaboration of the WHO's Mental Health Division. For example, political sensitivities may also have contributed to the division's decision not to co-sponsor a 1987 WFMH seminar on sexuality and family planning for mentally distressed and handicapped persons. Without WHO's blessing it was organized by Dr. Henry David, chair of the WFMH Committee on Responsible Parenthood, on behalf of the WFMH jointly with the Danish Family Planning Association and the Dutch Mental Health Association (Osler and David, 1987). As an NGO the Federation can operate more flexibly and with greater freedom than the UN agencies subject to the political and self-preservative concerns of the member states. (Brody, 1987)

THE WFMH AND THE UN IN THE REES ERA
Personal and Institutional Relationships

Work with the UN was relatively easy in the immediate postwar era when its agencies were small and in their infancy. Relationships were close and personal. WFMH dealings with the various specialized UN units were less insulated from each other than in later years. In retrospect it seems that the agencies were more inclined than in recent years to collaborate with each other. Sometimes they found it useful to ask the Federation to initiate projects in which they could be participants. For example, a 1958 conference on refugees was organized by the WFMH at the request of the UNHCR and one on malnutrition and food habits in Mexico at the request of the Pan-American Health Organization of WHO (PAHO) in 1960.

The most operationally effective relationships were between Jack Rees and the WHO physician leaders who, beginning with psychiatrist Ronald Hargreaves, M.D., were his old friends. Hargreaves became the first director of the WHO Mental Health Section established in 1949 at the WFMH's recommendation, but this did not keep him from functioning in a dual role. In 1949 during WHO visits he was also an "unofficial envoy" for the WFMH encouraging national mental health activities in Yugoslavia and Austria (WFMH, 1950). At the 1950 WFMH annual meeting in Paris he stated that the WFMH provides "the other channel for communication...not for governments, but for professional groups. WFMH has the role of professional watchdog regarding interests which may be neglected by governments under pressure" (WFMH, 1951b). Psychiatrist E. E. Krapf, M.D., of Argentina, also played a dual role, acting both as a member of the WFMH Executive Board and a WHO consultant in the Philippines in 1950. His network of relationships allowed Rees to arrange occasional meetings with WHO regional officers, especially those in Europe, to compare and review activities and projects which the two organizations were considering. As he noted, these meetings stimulated the development of new ideas and avoided overlap "in that certain projects can best be carried out by WHO, whilst some others are better attempted by the Federation" (WFMH, 1955a, p. 15).

In 1950 the consultative status of the Federation with UNESCO and the WHO was reviewed and confirmed. It was also placed on the Register of the Secretary General of the UN as a body which could be consulted and could send observers to the meetings of ECOSOC. This was considered significant because many of the projects of ECOSOC's Social Commission had major mental health aspects. But while this move was greeted with enthusiasm, WFMH Honorary Secretary and then assistant Director, child psychiatrist Kenneth Soddy, remained uncertain about the exact meaning of "consultation." Unlike the pragmatic and always optimistic Rees who accepted opportunities to exert influence as they arose, Soddy was still attempting to clarify the relationship between the WFMH, and the UN. In 1951 he wrote that a major advantage of NGOs is that "they represent the spontaneous efforts of concerned individuals wishing to take direct action in a field in which they are expert" and are "not content merely to follow the lead of government" (WFMH, 1951d). Rees, representing the WFMH as an observer in WHO's annual World Health Assemblies (where his major effort was to argue, usually unsuccessfully, for greater financial support for mental health work), phrased the matter in less provocative terms: "Relatively few people amongst the Public Health delegates of governments [to the WHO Assembly] have the knowledge or the special concern to initiate...a discussion about the place of mental health in the whole scheme of the Organization's [WHO's] work, and consequently it falls to us to put such a matter [in this instance, the need for financing] forward."

Changing Relationships

Over time, as particular personalities came and went, and policies in both the UN agencies and the WFMH were formed and dissolved, the relationships between the WFMH and the various agencies fluctuated in nature, intensity and warmth. 1953 was a year of change. There were new directors for UNESCO and for Unicef, the former United Nations Children's Fund (now converted from an ad hoc body to permanent status). Chisholm who had been an inspirational leader for the WFMH decided not to continue as Director General of the WHO and succeeding directors did not have his emotional and ideological investment in the WFMH. However Rees tried hard to maintain his relationships at the top level, expressing the Federation as being "delighted to act as publicists and one might say sales agents" for consultant visits and seminars arranged by the Mental Health Section in many countries (WFMH, 1953a, p. 15). At the Section level, in fact, relations remained close since its leader was still Hargreaves, Rees' close personal friend. In February 1954 several WFMH representatives spent two days discussing the mental health situation in Europe with the WHO regional office there. A feeling of optimism prevailed. WFMH observers at the May World Health Assembly reported that "the general climate of feeling with regard to mental health was improving sightly. Some of the various Government delegates who in the past had rather tended to brush aside work for mental health now showed a change in their attitude towards it" (WFMH, 1954, p. 16).

Hargreaves' 1955 departure was a major loss. A committed advocate of social approaches to prevention and treatment in psychiatry, he resigned as head of the WHO's Mental Health Section in order to become Professor of Psychiatry at the University of Leeds. This came as his perspective, and that of the WFMH, were becoming less influential in the field with the development of increasingly effective psychopharmaceuticals. However, in 1956 a good friend of the Federation,. Maria Pfister, M.D. of Zurich was appointed to the technical staff of the WHO Mental Health Section, providing another conduit to its decision-making group. She did not wield the same authority as Hargreaves, but her perspective on psychiatry was similar.

From 1953 until 1956, the major WFMH contacts in Geneva, which did not involve Rees or Hargreaves, were handled by Krapf who was simultaneously a WFMH Executive Board member and a WHO staff member. In 1956 he succeeded Hargreaves as WHO Mental Health Section Director. At the same time, having finished a year as WFMH Vice President, he became President at the Ninth Annual Meeting on 15 August 1956 in Berlin. But his new WHO post made it necessary for him to immediately resign the WFMH presidency in favor of Margaret Mead who had been elected Vice President for the 1956–1957 term. By this time the burgeoning WHO was acquiring adequate support, in contrast with the WFMH's inability to maintain the flow of funds essential to its own development. Dependent on voluntary donations, the Federation could no longer maintain its status as an equal partner of the WHO with its massive budget allotted by the world's governments. The period when the two organizations could divide up the necessary global projects between them had come to an end. The WFMH, though, continued to act as a source of ideas and materials and a stimulus to activity. And it continued to have observers at a range of WHO headquarters and regional meetings, many of which had a clinical focus, e.g., the epidemiology of mental illness. Its participation in UNESCO meetings also continued, and at UN New York, beginning in 1958, volunteer Mrs. Mottram Torre, whose husband was briefly a part-time Assistant Director for Rees, became for a time the regular WFMH representative to the NGO Committee for Unicef.

By this time Rees was deciding that he had served the Federation long enough. After he left the WFMH directorship at the end of 1961 the easy collegiality and informal decision making of the early years with UN agencies, particularly the WHO, was not re-established This reflected both the growing size and complexity of the UN and its agencies and the increasingly divergent backgrounds of the WFMH and WHO officers, no longer predominantly World War II medical colleagues.

With time, expansion and intensified requirements for budgetary accountability, the UN agencies also became more bureaucratic. By the late 1970s the informal conversations of the earlier era were replaced by requirements for collaborative work proposals necessary for the maintenance of "official relations." An excerpt from a 1980 letter from Honorary Secretary Gaston Harnois to WFMH President Gowan Guest (1979–1981) indicates the difficulty for NGOs in achieving meaningful contact with WHO: "...we will be evaluated as to our relationship with WHO approximately in January 1981 [which] should involve a close review of WHO's medium-term program to see which areas of its activities are corresponding to those of WFMH...we should rather candidly concentrate on the few areas [in which we] are capable of working effectively with WHO...how will we bring about such a coordination of views and projects in order to develop a more effective relationship with WHO? This is not an easy one to answer...I got the impression that there is a fair degree of confusion at WHO as to who the spokesmen of WFMH are: the names of [five people] were all mentioned without there being a clear notion as to what everyone is supposed to do. May I suggest that a person be designated as spokesman vis-a-vis WHO...[or] we ought to resort to the creation of a very active committee" (Harnois, 1980).

WFMH Representatives to the UN

During most of the Rees era the active and personal contact between organizational leaders, made it unnecessary to appoint specific WFMH representatives to various UN offices. But beginning in autumn 1956, WFMH President Krapf, jointly with Director Rees, appointed an official WFMH liaison person, designated as an Observer, accredited both to the WHO office in Geneva, including the World Health Assembly, and to the International Labour Organization (ILO) which had just started a list of NGOs with which it would have relationships. She was A. Audeoud-Naville, M.D., an ophthalmologist and psychoanalyst living and practicing in Geneva. Her history fitted her admirably to be not only an observer but a contributor in this international context. Born in Rumania she had been a nurse and then a mid-wife before going to medical school and becoming a physician. Prior to her association with the WFMH she had worked with the Association of Women Doctors and the World Medical Association. Although her main concerns were the public health issues which preoccupied the WHO, she also took an interest in child labor, occupational health, and the employment of vulnerable groups which occasionally came up in the ILO agenda.

The first WFMH representative to UNESCO Paris, was delegated in 1952 by the major French mental health association of the period, the French League of Mental Health. She was Mlle. Jeane Duron. However, most contacts with UNESCO were handled from the WFMH Secretariat, and, as noted in Chapter 3, and above Rees held the post of Chairman of the NGO Conference and its continuing committee for the four years beginning in 1952 and in this capacity was often at UNESCO-Paris.

In New York WHO professional concerns did not require attention, and most contacts were with ECOSOC, the Economic and Social Council, a forum (with its counterpart located in Geneva) of special commissions, units and committees concerned with specific issues such as human rights, crime prevention and aging. There, full-time volunteer, Helen (Mrs. Charles) Ascher, who was also affiliated with the U.S. Committee for WFMH, Inc. (see Chapters 3, 4, 5 and 6) became the general WFMH representative. In 1952 the formation of an Advisory Committee to the UN's Health Department in New York was undertaken at Rees' suggestion. (This is described at greater length in Chapter 9's section on the WFMH in the Caribbean). As noted above 1954 saw the WFMH granted consultative status to the UN Children's Fund (Unicef). For a time, volunteer Helen Speyer attended its meetings in New York, but was unable to continue and her tasks were taken over by Ascher who, according to Rees (WFMH 1956c, p. 12) did much to "ensure the greater acceptance of concepts of good mental health in many of the UN activities." For a time in 1957–1961, while Mottram Torre, M.D., served as a part-time assistant Director to Rees, Ascher was assisted by Mrs. Torre. In addition to Unicef, her special interest, they dealt with the social commission, NGO committees on human rights, the status of women, public information and others. Ascher, whose devoted representation of the WFMH over many years was warmly recognized by Rees, died after a long illness in March 1960. She was succeeded, as noted in Chapter 3, by Elizabeth (Mrs. Meyer) Cohen.

Consultative and Collaborative Work

WFMH advocacy with UN agencies during the Rees era was effected largely through informal consultations, teaching seminars and conferences, and supplying information more easily gathered through NGO than intergovernmental sources. For their part, beginning in 1950, UNESCO and the WHO, and occasionally other agencies, began sending representatives to WFMH annual meetings. UNESCO specialists came from its Departments of Social and Natural Sciences, Education and Mass Education. This was stimulated both by the WFMH's strong support for its continuing International Tensions Project and a series of detailed recommendations for its program. However, UNESCO was selective in its response. It did not accept WFMH recommendations to study the individual effects and the sociological implications of concentration camps, or social conditions under apartheid in South Africa. It did accept recommendations for a seminar on training teachers in mental health principles, for WFMH help in the field of mental health and human relations in Germany (expanding recent Macy supported conferences in the U.S.), and work on mental health films. Following WFMH interest in international conference processes UNESCO granted it $2500 for scientific observations of its 3rd Annual Meeting (of WFMH).

In 1951 pleasurable notice was taken of the fact that the words "mental health" appeared for the first time in one of the projects of the UNESCO work program. In that year also, largely through Ascher's efforts, four dinner conferences sponsored and financed by the Josiah Macy Jr. Foundation allowed representatives of the WFMH to meet with UN officials, particularly from the technical assistance branches. The International Refugee Organization was converted into the Office of the High Commissioner for Refugees, UNHCR, and after the 1951 WFMH Congress in Mexico the Executive Board sent UNHCR a series of resolutions concerned with better care for the mental health of refugees. While succeeding reports indicate continuing and "friendly" discussions with UNHCR there is no record of any response to these resolutions.

In July 1952 the WHO provided fellowships for 51 representatives of 30 member states, mainly mental health professionals, to participate in a three week WFMH organized Seminar on Mental Health and Infant Development in Chicester, England (WFMH, 1955). This Seminar stimulated both professional teaching and mental health service development in several of the countries from which participants had come.

The practical public-health oriented collaboration of the WFMH and the WHO was supplemented not only by occasional scholarly and research-oriented activities such as the Chichester Seminar, but by work sponsored by UNESCO. The Federation was a planner and participant in several UNESCO sponsored conferences at the end of the decade of the forties. Perhaps most prominent in that post-Nazi and post-War era was the series of meetings on "Health and Human Relations in Germany" (Conferences, 1950 and 1951). These involved four international interprofessional groups located in Germany from which interest spread to involve, by 1953, eight groups focusing on different aspects of the situation. The effort in part was to stimulate a "grass-roots" mental health movement in Germany, and it led to the revival of two societies and the formation of two new ones. In ensuing years, the WFMH was very much on the scene as a participant in the World Health Assemblies, an informal discussant of WHO programs, an advocate for mental health advisors in the WHO regions, and a publicizer of WHO recommendations to governments. In his Director's Report for 1961 Rees emphasized the importance of the Federation being represented by Observers at the Regional Committees of the WHO "so long as we could have as our Observer someone who knew the subject and knew the Federation." It was taken as a mark of successful influence that WFMH Observers were present at five of the six Regional meetings in 1961. Satisfaction was also expressed that the Technical Discussions in the 1962 World Health Assembly were to be on "Mental Health Problems in Public Health Planning." This revealed the influence of its Mental Health Section Director E. Eduardo Krapf, who had moved to that post from his presidency of the WFMH (WFMH, 1962a).

Although Rees' closest personal relationships were with his fellow physicians in the WHO, the WFMH was also involved with Unicef, ECOSOC and UNESCO during the years from 1948 through 1961. A major project was instituted in 1952 when, with UNESCO funding, WFMH sponsored a survey by Margaret Mead and co-workers resulting in the publication of *Cultural Patterns and Technical Change* (Mead, 1953).

In 1953 the WFMH became a member of the NGO Committee for Unicef acquiring consultative status with it. In the same year UNESCO's General Conference arranged meetings between members of its secretariat and representatives of the 105 NGOs in consultative status with it, focusing mainly on its Departments of Social Science, Education and Mass Communication and to a lesser degree on those responsible for technical assistance and fellowships. Rees became Chairman of the NGO Committee for UNESCO and played a leading role in these meetings which helped influence the organization's future program. He noted with pleasure that "the principle of bringing in non-governmental organizations like ourselves to discuss the general form and detailed content of the programme for the ensuing two years is an important advance in our relationships with the governmental delegations that constitute the UNESCO General Conference" (WFMH, 1954, p. 15). In association with this development UNESCO made a small grant to help with the Federation's central administration. In 1954 New York representative Helen Ascher was able to supply needed information to several of the ECOSOC units, especially its Social Commission. Through her, Rees wrote,"the influence of the Federation on the thinking of some of the secretariat of UN is undoubtedly increasing in a modest and sensible way" (WFMH,1954, p. 15).

The significance of the WFMH for the UN aside from the WHO was clearly heightened by Margaret Mead's prominence in the organization. In 1954 ECOSOC invited it to hold a meeting at UN New York with her as the main speaker on Social Implications of Technological Change. It was attended by a number of government delegations, people from the UN secretariat, and representatives of many NGOs. This was followed by an invitation from UNESCO to hold a conference on Mental Health Problems of Urbanization with Mead as an anticipated speaker. In 1956 its Social Science Department contracted with the WFMH to provide working materials and a participant for this conference.

In 1957 with the assistance of Mrs. Torre, Ascher now maintained the WFMH liaison with ECOSOC's Social Commission, Human Rights Commission and Committee on the Status of Women as well as the NGO Committee for Unicef, and the Department of Public Information. WFMH's status with ECOSOC was further reflected in its being asked to convene a third conference in the UN building, this time in 1959 on mental health in Africa. Of particular relevance to the Federation's broader aims was an NGO Conference on Prejudice and Discrimination called by the Human Rights Commission in 1959 with Past WFMH President Brock Chisholm in the chair.

In the latter part of 1959, UNHCR, although it had for years maintained "very friendly " relations with the WFMH, moved for the first time to recognize the importance of mental health for the care of refugees. As a by-product of World Refugee Year it employed psychiatrist Hans Strotzka, M.D., of Vienna, as its Mental Health Advisor for a year. As Rees noted: "He did an admirable job...in planning and starting the rehabilitation of the so-called psychopathic 'hard core' of the camps in Germany and Austria and elsewhere" (WFMH 1960, p. 13). He was succeeded in this work by psychiatrist Peter Berner, M.D., of the University of Vienna, who, as noted in Chapter 4, became a candidate to succeed Rees as WFMH Director beginning in January 1962 .

During all of this time WFMH used its own publications to reprint UN materials or to announce mental health relevant UN activities. By 1955 these had increased to the extent that the WFMH Bulletin, published quarterly though sometimes irregularly through most of the Rees era, was unable to maintain the coverage which it had intended. The items which it selected for coverage in the Bulletin reveal the eclectic interests of Kenneth Soddy its Editor. Among them were his own working paper,"Prevention of Juvenile Delinquency," submitted to the First UN Congress on the Prevention of Crime and the Treatment of Offenders; "Social Implications of Technical Assistance" describing a meeting called by the WFMH at UN headquarters in New York; a statement of the UN's International survey of Programmes of Social Development; an account of ECOSOC's Conference on the Eradication of Prejudice and Discrimination; the Report of the General Conference of Consultative Non-Governmental Organizations; Consultations on the UNESCO Programme for 1957-58; the Report of a WHO Study Group on the Child in Hospital, and of the Eighth World Health Assembly; and, finally, a series of reprints from the *WHO Chronicle*. Except for one on "A Human Approach" by Prime Minister Nehru of India, a plea for human relations and attention to the needs of children in international affairs, these last dealt exclusively clinical psychiatric problems.

THE WFMH AND THE UN: 1962–1981

Transitions

Rees' resignation as WFMH Director at the end of 1961 and the accession of Francois Cloutier to that post (renamed for his tenure as Director General) marked the beginning of the end of the era when intimate personal relationships were a major vehicle of WFMH influence on the UN. The period between 1962 and 1981 covers the directorships of Cloutier and his successor Pierre Visseur through the 1967 closure of the Geneva secretariat, and the era of working presidents until 1981.

As described in Chapter 4, the WFMH secretariat's move to Geneva in mid-1963 facilitated informal relations with the now easily accessible WHO and the UN offices located there. The proximity of the WFMH secretariat to the WHO and the Geneva based agencies led to more personal contacts, attendance at committee meetings, and explorations of possible collaboration. They did not, however, yield a renewed closeness of the kind which had marked the Rees years. Nor did repeated discussions of avenues of possible cooperation lead to action. The optimism of 1962 was not regained.

The French speaking Cloutier did make a special point of familiarizing himself, personally, with WHO personnel in Geneva. However, his attention was drawn more obviously to UNESCO headquarters, perhaps because it was located in Paris. In addition he spent time visiting UN leaders in New York. As noted in Chapter 4, Bert Schaffner remembered his presence on one or more occasions during this time when he, Schaffner, encouraged by now Consultant Jack Rees, was raising money for his WFMH affiliated mental health project in the Caribbean.

At UN New York, Elizabeth Cohen, in relative independence of the Director, the Secretariat and the Executive Board, was increasingly active and becoming better known to a range of UN officers and staff, as well as people in other NGOs. Most notably, she met with Unicef's Executive Board and ECOSOC's Social Commission. Among her new activities was acting as the WFMH observer at the UN Commission on the Status of Women, and the Social Commission. She nominated; different colleagues to represent the WFMH for the first time at the U.N. Population Commission in 1964 and 1965.

Paradoxically, 1965, the year of Cloutier's resignation and departure from the WFMH, saw a burst of activity in relation to the UN. Along with several other NGOs, the WFMH helped prepare a report for the Third UN Congress on Crime Prevention and the Treatment of Delinquents to be held in Stockholm. 1965 was also designated by the UN as "International Cooperation Year," and the shrunken WFMH secretariat, in which Pierre Visseur was playing an increasingly executive role, tried to give as much publicity as possible to this initiative designating the WFMH Bangkok annual meeting (which did not achieve a quorum) as a "special activity of international cooperation."

In 1966 Visseur, who had succeeded Cloutier in November 1965, completed a full year as Director. With a substantially reduced budget and staff he barely managed to keep the Geneva Secretariat afloat. Cohen in New York, Audeoud-Naville in Geneva and Veil in Paris continued their full schedule of attendance at relevant meetings, but with little instruction from the Board or Secretariat, and little reporting back.

1967 was the last year for Visseur and the Geneva Secretariat, now even more drastically reduced in staff and scope. With the Secretariat's 1968 move to President Carstairs' offices in Edinburgh, the reactivation of the Federation as a global force no longer focused on the UN, but on the organization of regional conferences by local associations under WFMH auspices.

The WFMH and WHO: 1962–1973

The major WHO-WFMH event of 1962, Cloutier's first year in office, was the annual World Health Assembly in Geneva with its Technical Discussions centered for the first time ever on mental health. This focus and the significant WFMH participation, however, were essentially Rees' legacy, a function of his outgoing administration. The large WFMH delegation included Rees and Dr. Claude Veil of Paris who acted as reporters for two of the eight working groups. The major background document for the Discussions was prepared by another WFMH veteran, Professor of Psychiatry, Arie Querido, M.D., of Holland, who had been a participant in the pre-1948 Congress International Preparatory Commission for the WFMH at Roffey Park. The WFMH Secretariat collaborated in assembling the material upon which his document was based, with a special contribution coming from a joint meeting of the French Ministry of Health and the WFMH in September 1961. Beyond these contributions the Discussions, had particular significance for the WFMH since they were led by its former President Krapf, now in his role as head of the WHO Mental Health Unit. It was a major success for him as a bridging personality. However, he died in the next year, on November 9, 1963.

Krapf's post was filled after his death by Professor of Psychiatry Pieter A. Baan, M.D., of Groningen in the Netherlands, who was President of one of the WFMH member associations. We already had a professional relationship beginning when I consulted at a PAHO meeting on psychiatric education in Vina del Mar, Chile in 1962 with Jorge Velasco Alzaga, M.D., of Mexico, the PAHO Mental Health Advisor. It continued after 1964 when, speaking at the City Hall in Lima, Peru, at the request of Daniel Blain, M.D., American Psychiatric Association President, I helped launch the Interamerican Council of Psychiatric Associations. Between 1966 and 1968, I saw both Baan and Velasco Alzaga on several occasions when, at the request of Blain and Howard Rome, M.D., in addition to my posts at the University of Maryland, I agreed to direct the Council's two year Interamerican Mental Health Study Program. This task entailed visits to Mexico, Argentina, Peru, Ecuador, and Chile, in addition to Brazil where I had been a Visiting Professor at the Federal University of Rio de Janeiro since 1964. These visits produced not only knowledge but friendships which were valuable for the WFMH in later years. Colleagues from Uruguay and Venezuela participated with the others in a final meeting in 1968 which was supported by the Hogg Foundation for Mental Health supported by the University of Texas. That was the first of a number of situations in which Dr. Wayne Holtzman, later to become the

Foundation's President, supported projects of WFMH interest (Brody, 1969). In 1968 Baan and I were also thrown together when we both spoke at a conference on migration in Dakar, Senegal. Along with our mutual friend, the late Leon Chertok, M.D., of Paris, we visited a village some miles into the countryside. There we were both introduced to the importance of accepting and consuming with exaggerated relish the eyes of a sheep roasted in honor of the visiting dignitaries.

The WFMH Bulletins which had lapsed under Cloutier reappeared with the removal of the Secretariat to the Edinburgh offices of Professor of Psychiatry, President Morris Carstairs (1968–1972). They regularly included news about the WHO, but none about other UN agencies, and, although there were WFMH "representatives" at occasional meetings there was no systematic feed-back or attempts to influence the UN. Nor was there any productive collaboration with the UN's specialized agencies until April 1970. At that time the Edinburgh Secretariat accredited me as the official WFMH representative to the first joint consultation of the WHO's Sections on Mental Health and Human Reproduction, co-sponsored by the International Planned Parenthood Federation. As the Rapporteur, I could depend for advice upon Dr. Henry David, Director of the Transnational Family Studies Institute of Bethesda, Maryland who was a key resource person for the consultation. It included a valuable review of mental health in relation to reproductive issues in cultural context and also highlighted some differences between the participants, especially in regard to pregnancy termination as a medical procedure. It was disappointing when the Secretariat offered no advice and asked for no report on the meeting. Because of his earlier residence in Geneva as one of Cloutier's WFMH Associate Directors (see Chapter 4) Henry was a friend of psychiatrist Norman Sartorius, then an epidemiologist with the WHO Mental Health Section. Norman and Vera Sartorius had just had their first child, and, through Henry, it was my privilege to pay them a visit. Thus began a more than 25 year relationship which facilitated later informal communication after Norman became the Director of the Mental Health Section.

With the presidency of Professor of Psychiatry Michael Beaubrun of Kingston, Jamaica, beginning in 1972 the WFMH secretariat moved to his offices in the University of the West Indies (UWI). Perhaps because of the drastic geographic shift there occurred a hiatus in reports from official Federation representatives at the various UN headquarters. However, WFMH concerns were introduced at various UN conferences by its officers who had been invited in their other (non-WFMH) capacities. Beaubrun, representing the Jamaican government, and I, as a Temporary Advisor, i.e. consultant, were invited to a PAHO/WHO meeting on the training of psychiatrists with special emphasis on residency training in the developing countries of the Americas. The meeting from 26–30 June 1972 in Bogota, Colombia, was attended by a number of friends whom I had known since the 1960s through the Interamerican Mental Health Studies Program. Among them were Rene Gonzalez, M.D., of Venezuela, the PAHO Mental Health Advisor, Alvaro Gallegos, M.D., the leading psychiatrist of Costa Rica, who later became WFMH Vice President for the Region, Humberto Rosselli, M.D., of Bogota and several other colleagues from Colombia. Although neither Beaubrun nor I had been asked as representatives of the WFMH we took advantage of the opportunity to draw attention to the Federation's work and the ways in which University training programs could collaborate with voluntary mental health associations. This was difficult in a region in which the concept of voluntarism was not well developed, but we encountered general good will and an interest in learning more. In the same year Beaubrun, also at the recommendation of the Jamaican government, had another opportunity to sponsor the NGO viewpoint in the councils of the WHO. He was appointed a member of the WHO's Expert Advisory Committee on Mental Health for a five year period. Appointees were asked to inform the WHO of mental health developments in their countries and regions.

The WHO Conference on Comprehensive Psychiatric Services and the Community, noted in Chapter 5, was held in Peebles, Scotland near Edinburgh in May 1972 during the Beaubrun presidency. While the WFMH was not a co-sponsor, ex-President Carstairs and J. D. Sutherland, M.D., of his Department of Psychiatry at the Royal Edinburgh Hospital served as its representatives. At the end of the conference, Carstairs, in keeping with his philosophy of introducing Federation themes wherever possible, organized a WFMH International Forum on psychiatric services in developing countries. During these years Audeoud-Naville also remained interested and involved in the UN meetings in Geneva and reported to the WFMH Board on meetings of ECOSOC, the Executive Council of the WHO and the World Health Assembly.

The WFMH and UNESCO: 1962–1973

WFMH relations with UNESCO had been at their high point with Rees' chairmanship of its associated NGOs. Between 1962 and 1965 Cloutier maintained a personal relationship with its officers through his visits to its Paris headquarters, but there was no formal collaboration, although Dr. Claude Veil continued to attend meetings as the WFMH observer. However, it appears that the WFMH was no longer regarded as important by UNESCO leaders. At the 8-9 and 12 August 1970 meetings of the Executive Board in Jerusalem, Veil reported that the Federation had not been invited to a UNESCO meeting of Experts on Aggression, raising a question about its role and position in relation to the agency. Other involved NGOs had also stated, according to Veil, that they were not clear about the role of the WFMH. This was a matter of considerable distress, leading him to submit his resignation as the Federation representative to UNESCO after January 1971.

In 1972, however, President Beaubrun's special interest in substance abuse, stemming from the persisting Jamaican concern with marijuana, led to the WFMH's being invited to at least one meeting sponsored by UNESCO (WFMH, 1973). Held at UNESCO headquarters in Paris, 11–20 December 1972, it concerned drug abuse prevention through education in more developed countries. David Lynton Porter who attended on behalf of the Middlesex England Health Education Council also represented the WFMH and shared his report with its Secretariat.

In the following year psychiatrist Jean Louis Armand-Laroche, M.D., of Paris, recognizing the organization's prominent position in his city, volunteered to be the regular WFMH representative to UNESCO, and Veil agreed to stay on as the Federation representative to the International Social Science Council (ISSC), affiliated with UNESCO. Armand- Laroche was a prominent institutional and academic psychiatrist with a long-time interest in the UN and mental health, and a long-time leader within French volunteer circles. He faithfully sent reports to the Board and the Bulletin/Newsletter, but operated for the most part in relative isolation from the Federation's central leadership.

The Renewal of Active WFMH-UN Collaboration: 1975–1981

The period of relative quiescence in the WFMH-UN relationship came to an end with the presidency of Professor Tsung-yi Lin and the Secretariat's move at the beginning of 1975 to the University of British Columbia (UBC) in Vancouver, Canada. As always the Federation was able to benefit from the activities of its members in pursuit of their non-Federation careers. In this respect the spring of 1975 was a special moment. Two of Lin's UBC colleagues, whom he had appointed to the WFMH Administrative Committee, completed two-month tours in Thailand as WHO mental health consultants. They were Milton Miller, M.D., head of the UBC Department of Psychiatry, of which Lin was a member, and Edward Margetts, M.D., a professor in the Department. Both were experienced and well-known academic psychiatrists, well-suited to the WHO aim of training mental health specialists, other professionals and paraprofessional workers to serve in public health programs. One goal was to train a large number of people without a professional education, called Health Volunteers and Health Communicators, to supply care for the predominantly rural Thai population. On the basis of Miller's and Margetts' visits the

WFMH Secretariat attempted to prepare a manual,"Mental Health Education for All Health Workers." The project did not come to completion, but the line of thought which it represented remained as an inspiration for what became a WFMH advocacy interest closely linked to that of the WHO. That was the delivery of mental health services in the context of primary health care.

In the same year, 1975, Halfdan Mahler, M.D., Director General of the WHO, designated UBC as a WHO Center for Research and Training in Mental Health. Among the several factors contributing to this decision were Lin's former close association with the WHO, his friendship with Norman Sartorius, now Director of the WHO's Mental Health Division, and the fact that both he and Miller had had extensive research experience in the countries of the Pacific Rim. The Center's formal opening, with Miller as Director and Lin as Co-Director came on 26 March 1976. Former WFMH President Carstairs, now Vice Chancellor of York University in England, marked the reviving relationship with the WHO in his keynote address: "The Role of Psychiatry in WHO's Plans for Basic Health Care."

Later in the year, on 27 May 1976, anthropologist Dr. Rhoda Metraux and Mrs. Francis McFadyen were Federation observers at the UN Habitat Conference on Human Settlements. Metraux, with the help of former WFMH President Margaret Mead, assisted in a position paper on "The Prison Environment and Mental Health." This resulted in a Habitat Forum Conference co-sponsored by the WFMH and the Canadian Ministry of the Solicitor General. Among the speakers were WFMH Regional Vice President for the Western Pacific, Estafania Aldaba Lim and for Africa, Tolani Asuni, and two members of the Administrative Committee, Carlos Leon and Milton Miller.

By now the WFMH was once more recognized as ready and willing to send observers qualified to contribute to WHO conferences. They were all psychiatrists. On 12–17 June 1976 Adly Fahmy Abdou, M.D. of Cairo represented it at a WHO meeting on mental health legislation. On 4–9 November 1976 Marianne Cederblad, M.D., the WFMH European Vice President was joined by Lin's UBC colleague, Professor Morton Beiser, M.D., at the WHO Expert Committee on Children's Mental Health Services in Geneva. They were especially active in focusing attention on the preventive aspects of mental health with children and families.

In 1978 President Lin embarked on a series of voyages aimed at revitalizing Federation activities in the various regions, and strengthening its ties to the WHO. In early April he participated in the inauguration of a WHO Collaborative Center for Research and Training in Cali, Colombia under the sponsorship of the University del Valle where I had been a Visiting Lecturer in 1965. It was directed by Carlos Leon, a former member of the WFMH Administrative Committee and Chairman of the Department of Psychiatry. Leon, with a Master's Degree in Epidemiology from Tulane University, was one of a generation of young South American psychiatrists committed to advancing psychiatric care on their continent. Lin used this opportunity to make contact on behalf of the WFMH with a number of national leaders from other countries who had come to Cali for the inauguration, as well as with mental health leaders in Bogota.

A few weeks later, in Geneva, Lin was able to enlist the interest of WHO Director General Halfdan Mahler in co-sponsoring the 1979 Salzburg Congress. This was the first time in its history that the WFMH had the co-sponsorship of the WHO for its World Congress. Norman Sartorius, in his capacity as Director of the WHO Mental Health Division, expressed his interest in participating in the WFMH policy process, and urged WFMH member associations and Vice Presidents to show their interest in contributing to the WHO's regional and national activities. In response to this Lin invited the Mental Health Advisors of all of the WHO Regional Offices to serve as consultants to the Federation (WFMH, 1978c). Taha Baasher, M.D., of Sudan, WHO Mental Health Advisor to its Eastern Mediterranean Region and Rene Gonzalez M.D., of Venezuela, Mental Health Advisor for the Latin American Region (PAHO), accepted the invitation and Baasher ultimately became the WFMH Vice President for his Region. WHO co-sponsorship of Congresses, and the participation of its Mental Health Division Director became regular features of all of the later World Congresses. Lin's hope that WHO sponsorship would encourage the governments of UN member states to encourage their health professionals to participate in the Congresses was realized in the countries in which Congresses were held.

During his 1978 visit to Geneva Lin also met with Audeoud-Naville and Douglas Deane, who had by now joined her as a WFMH Geneva representative. Deane, a longtime Geneva resident, wondered, in view of the increasing complexity of the WHO's operation and the increasing mental health activities of other intergovernmental or nongovernmental organizations, if "the time has come for the role and function of our representatives in Geneva to be reassessed" (WFMH, 1978b). The suggestion was not followed, but Audeoud-Neville retired at the end of the year to be replaced by Deane who single-handedly represented Federation affairs in Geneva.

Lin was also able to refresh the ties between the WFMH and Unicef in preparation for the Salzburg World Congress which was to take place in 1979, the International Year of the Child (IYC). In February 1978 he was visited by Dr. Herman Stein of Stanford, Special Advisor to Unicef's Executive Director, who encouraged his vision of a joint WFMH-Unicef-WHO world program for the integration of childrens' mental health care with primary health care. Plans were made for a post-Congress Study Group in Salzburg of a small group of WFMH, WHO and Unicef personnel. Its mission would be to prepare a proposal for funding to Unicef to support the hoped for mental health-primary care program for children in developing countries. On 11 December 1978 in Manila, Unicef celebrated its 32nd anniversary and honored former WFMH Executive Board member Aldaba-Lim who had been appointed the UN Special Representative for IYC. The tie with the WFMH was emphasized by Tsung-yi and Mei-chen Lin's presence.

Lin was kind enough to invite me to attend the Study Group after the Salzburg Congress. I made a determined effort to inject family planning and perinatal health issues into the discussion of children's mental health in relation to primary health care. However, while perinatal health measures were recognized as essential to the future wellbeing of mothers and children, there was minimal interest in family planning as a relevant issue. A complete report of the meeting by Morton Beiser noted that while no solutions and no funding proposal were forthcoming there was a general sense of the importance of the WFMH and the UN agencies exchanging information on a world basis. The major job of NGOs such as the WFMH, it appeared, was to continue "the great task of advocating the importance of mental health programs in all of the countries of the world" (WFMH, 1979b). Although this was somewhat disappointing as an opportunity to exert direct NGO influence on UN agencies, the very occurrence of the meeting was encouraging as an indication of the possibility of true collaboration. Zaki Hassan, M.D., a onetime member of the WFMH Executive Board and Chairman of the Executive Board of Unicef suggested as much in a later Unicef Newsletter. He wrote that NGOs can identify emerging problems in the field and "promote projects more easily than either Unicef or governments" (WFMH, 1980).

There was no significant interaction at the leadership level between the WFMH and UNESCO, although Armand-Laroche and Gaston Harnois, M.D., of Montreal, were WFMH observers at its 6–7 October 1979 International Congress on Children of the Fourth World.

Tsung-yi Lin retired as WFMH President during the 1979 World Congress for Mental Health in Salzburg. This ended the longest WFMH Presidency in the organization's history and one marked by the President's intense personal involvement with the agencies of the UN, especially the WHO and Unicef. However, a radical change from Lin's personal attention, especially to the UN, was presaged by the first message to the membership from the new President, lawyer-businessman Gowan Guest, also of Vancouver. In it he wrote: "…if things are done in WFMH they will be done by you, not me…it is simply not possible for one [with] other and primary…responsibilities to do more than intersect from time to time with the activities of the working members of WFMH" (WFMH, 1979b). Guest had neither the interest nor the background knowledge which might have moved him to build upon Lin's achievements. The tasks of forming collaborative relations with the UN agencies, especially the WHO, were delegated largely to Harnois, chairman of a revived WFMH Scientific Advisory Committee. In 1980 Harnois did meet with Sartorius to discuss more effective collaboration. Toward the end of his term, noting that the World Psychiatric Association had applied for consultative status with the WHO, Guest proposed a "working alliance" between the three organizations, WFMH, WPA and the WHO, but no move was made to explore or implement the idea. The WHO Executive Board recommended continuation of "official relations" with the WFMH and the WFMH Scientific Advisory Committee, headed by Gaston Harnois reviewed a WHO questionnaire about possible modalities of affiliation and began consultations about possible input into UNESCO's medium term plan for 1984-1989. It also endorsed UNESCO's Declaration against racial prejudice. Elizabeth Cohen in New York reported her active involvement in committees dealing with the International Year of the Disabled (1981) and the forthcoming International Year of the Aged (1982). In Paris Armand-Laroche became a member of a UNESCO Committee dealing with children, and Veil continued to represented the WFMH at the annual meetings of the International Social Science Council.

THE WFMH AND UN GENEVA AFTER 1981

While our primary Geneva relationship was with the WHO, our representatives there were also charged with maintaining a WFMH liaison with UNHCR, the office of the UN High Commissioner for Refugees, the Commission on Human Rights, and other centers. These will be discussed in Part III of this volume concerned with the WFMH international mental health agenda. The UNHCR relationship will be discussed as an aspect of our work with refugees, which after 1981 was carried out primarily through our Collaborating Center, the Harvard Program in Refugee Trauma, led by Richard Mollica, M.D. The Human Rights Commission relationship will be discussed as part of our work regarding patients' rights led in Geneva by our representative Stanislas Flache, M.D.

Continuing and Strengthening our Relationship with the WHO

Historically, WHO has been the UN agency with the closest and most consistent relationship with WFMH. While the intimacy of the Rees years was never completely restored after 1962, President Lin did much to regain the capacities of the two organizations to work together. Unfortunately, this lapsed during 1979–1981 so it was now up to me as incoming President to renew our collaboration. I did not have the benefit of Lin's background as a WHO staff member, but had, as noted above, considerable contact both with PAHO and WHO Geneva. As late as June 1981, as WFMH President Elect, I joined Henry David and other WFMH colleagues at a Federation-PAHO co-sponsored half-day workshop on "Personal Fertility Regulation: Co-operative Research in the Americas" which he had organized at the annual meeting of the Interamerican Society of Psychology in Santo Domingo. This occasion powerfully underlined the value of Federation sponsorship of socially useful, mental health-relevant research and the power of co-sponsorship with agencies of the UN.

With this background the transition into a smooth WHO-WFMH relationship with the transition of Federation officers in 1981 was seamless. It was also facilitated by the incremental evolution in our agenda. In the WFMH agenda for the 1980s presented in my inaugural talk at the Manila Congress I referred to the WHO's newly expressed interest in "psychosocial" functioning. The WHO was beginning to recognize poor communication between health and educational institutions along with socioeconomic stress, and resultant family instability as a matrix in which illness and inability to function are frequently encountered. This recognition contributed to the new WHO emphasis on primary care carried out by people who while not trained to the most sophisticated medical levels are very familiar with the communities in which they work. With this emphasis in mind I appointed a psychiatrist, Professor Lourdes Ladrigo-Ignacio of Manila, with a strong record in community work, as the WFMH member of a WHO study group on mental health in developing countries. In many of these countries NGOs carry major responsibility for the delivery of mental health services.

An historically significant event, building on the relationships begun with President Lin, was an invitation from the WHO's Mental Health Director Sartorius for the WFMH to be represented, for the first time, at its medium-term mental health planning meeting, this time scheduled for New Delhi from 22–28 October. I asked our Honorary Secretary, New Zealand Professor of Psychiatry Basil James, who was contemplating a move from his professorship to public health administration to attend for us. He skillfully represented the psychosocial perspective which linked the intergovernmental and the nongovernmental organization.

The WFMH at WHO Headquarters, Geneva

One of my first tasks was to find an observer who could keep us informed about developments at the WHO in Geneva and also represent our views there. Douglas Deane, already on the scene, had expressed a wish to retire. A WFMH member since the 1960s, Australian by birth, and an experienced international worker since 1933, he had served in International Schools, four UN agencies, the World Council of Churches and the World Alliance of YMCAs. Since 1965 he had maintained the Geneva office of the Pathfinder Fund, headquartered in Boston, which was concerned with family planning, population problems and women's health. In early 1968, after the late autumn 1967 closure of the WFMH Geneva secretariat, he had accepted the invitation of his friend and fellow Geneva resident, assistant WFMH Treasurer Russell Cook, to assist Audoud-Naville at the WHO. After she retired at the time of the 1979 Salzburg World Congress he had become our sole representative.

Deane was an excellent person for us. We already knew each other since the Pathfinder Fund had supported my 1979 Salzburg World Congress symposium on mental health aspects of unwanted pregnancy. After talking with Henry David who also knew him, I immediately telephoned him in Geneva. He was willing to continue representing the WFMH, but felt that because of advancing age he no longer wished to do the job alone. Luckily he was coming to Boston in the near future so we made an appointment to talk during his visit. We met in the bar of the Copley Plaza hotel where, before too long I was also informed that, despite being 70 years old he could still, while lying supine, press the soles of his feet flat against the headboard of his bed!

With this auspicious beginning, plus our mutual friends and earlier contacts about the Salzburg symposium, we quickly realized that our perspectives on the WFMH and its goals were compatible. He agreed to continue to represent us in Geneva until we could find at least one other person to work with him, preferably as our primary representative. When "Doug," as he asked me to call him, departed I felt much more secure about our Geneva operation.

We didn't have to wait long for an addition to the Geneva team. In 1983, incoming WFMH President Aldaba-Lim found a long-time friend, also known to Deane since 1946, who was willing to serve as our senior representative to UN and WHO, Geneva. Later designated "permanent" representative, he was Stanislas Flache, M.D., who, from 1977 until his retirement four years later, had been assistant director general of the WHO, responsible for several divisions concerned with biomedical information, as well as for the WHO offices outside of Geneva.

Flache, like Deane, had had an international career, but unlike him had shared the experience of the victims of oppression he set out to help. Escaping as an adolescent from Nazi occupied Poland, losing a family whose precise fate he never discovered, he had become a French citizen, graduated in medicine from Montpelier, and in late career under WHO auspices, took postgraduate training at Harvard. He had been a medical officer with the UN Relief and Rehabilitation Agency after World War II in France and Germany; Director of Health for the UN Relief and Works Agency in the Middle East concerned with Arab refugees in Jordan, Syria, Lebanon and Gaza; WHO Chief Medical Advisor to Unicef headquarters, New York; and prior to returning to Geneva, Director of Health, WHO-Western Pacific Region (WPR), Manila, where Fannie Lim had come to know him. Now, having retired from the WHO he was glad to join us in our volunteer operation.

Stan Flache, as I soon came to know him, had the knowledge, status and personal relationships to enhance the WFMH perspective in the councils of the WHO as well as other UN offices in Geneva. After 1983, he rapidly became the chief conduit for informal exchanges of information and opinion between the WFMH and the WHO. An increasing volume of formal requests also began to appear. One such came because the WHO Mental Health Division began to devote increasing attention to the work of the UN Human Rights Commission as it bore on the welfare of people hospitalized because of mental illness. In June 1984 following controversy about an initial Draft Report to the Human Rights Subcommission on the Prevention of Discrimination and the Protection of Minorities, WHO appointed WFMH Board Member-at-Large, and National Director of MIND, Chris Heginbotham, as a consultant for a paper on the rights of persons detained on grounds of mental illness. This was a way station en route to a final Declaration on the rights of such patients and the care of mentally distressed people in general which was passed without a vote by the UN General Assembly in December 1991. That development will be described in Chapter 13.

With Flache on the scene we were able to reinstate a regular WFMH presence at WHO Executive Board and World Health Assembly meetings. Of particular importance was his willingness to keep in touch about WFMH policy in relation to events at the WHO. In order to facilitate this, he was encouraged to telephone at any time and we also supplied him with a fax machine. His presence also stimulated members of the WFMH Board to occasionally visit WHO meetings as observers. The May 1985 World Health Assembly dealing with NGO-WHO collaboration was attended by President Elect Edith Morgan and Heginbotham. She surveyed a range of NGOs in regard to training for delivering mental health services in primary care settings as a contribution to the "WHO Pilot Study on Mental Illness in Primary Care Settings." Among the issues for which WHO wanted WFMH input were alcohol abuse and primary health care.

Within a few months of his return to the WHO as the WFMH representative, Flache was pressed into service by the agency in capacities combining his UN experience with his new WFMH position. In May 1984 in Geneva he chaired an unusual meeting of WHO mental health staff and concerned NGOs on cooperation regarding the problem of alcoholism. This led to a series of meetings over several years on topics including cooperation with NGOs .

The WHO Executive Board meeting of January 1986 was another which, with its emphasis on prevention, was significant for the WFMH agenda. There, Flache spoke in favor of a Resolution to the May 1986 World Health Assembly that it call on all member states to apply preventive measures identified in the WHO Director General's report on the prevention of mental, neurological and psychosocial disorders. At the same Board meeting he supported a WHO resolution that the use of tobacco in all its forms is incompatible with the attainment of the strategy of "Health for All by the Year 2000." In that year it became possible for me to visit him in Geneva on 15-16 December 1986 after the biennial meeting of the International Social Science Council in Paris. There, he arranged for me to talk with several agency heads including WHO Director General Halfdan Mahler, M.D. During our discussion of the role of the WFMH in relation to the WHO and other UN agencies, the fact that Mahler's wife was a psychiatrist with a special interest in aging obviously contributed not only to his knowledge of the field, but to his enjoyment of the discussion.

Only four years after becoming our senior person in Geneva, Flache's contributions were recognized by his being named WFMH President Elect during the Cairo World Congress in 1987. There was some controversy between the Europeans, headed by Edith Morgan his nominator, and members from the African and Eastern Mediterranean Regions who backed Isaac Mwendapole from Zambia for President Elect (to become President in 1989). The Africans felt, perhaps with some justice, that the 1987 Congress' Egyptian location had encouraged more African attendance than might be expected in forthcoming Congresses. The main argument of the Flache supporters was that his election would strengthen our much needed ties with the WHO and Geneva. Finally, they carried the day and he was our official representative, as

WFMH President Elect, when the WHO observed its 40th anniversary, during the 1988 meetings of the World Health Assembly. The WHO Director General also designated him as the leader for the organization and coordination of World AIDS Day on 1 December 1988 with observances in 160 countries. A number of WHO statements on the topic came through my office with requests for written comment which I was usually able to supply, but for which feedback was never forthcoming.

On 3–4 December 1988, at the request of its European members, the WFMH Board meeting in London appointed European Region Vice President Knud Jensen, who had been representing us to most of the European WHO meetings, as "WFMH Liaison to the WHO Regional Office for Mental Health" in Copenhagen. This was intended to give us a continuing relationship with WHO Europe with special reference to issues of prevention of psychiatric illness and mental ill-health. However, this special designation found no WHO group with which to reciprocate. Its consequences were unclear and the position of Liaison was gradually forgotten.

In the following year Flache's role as a WHO-NGO intermediary was expanded as he was appointed coordinator of the several WHO observers at the meeting of the UN Human Rights Commission, 30 January–10 March 1989. There discussion was significantly centered on the human rights of patients with AIDS and mental illness, and of children, as embodied in the Convention on the Rights of the Child. A significant resolution (Draft Resolution 1989–40) was adopted calling for the establishment of a working group to revise an existing draft on the rights of mental patients. These issues with the addition of others recurred at later meetings concerned with human rights where Flache, sometimes accompanied by Deane and/or a new representative, June Spaulding, represented the WFMH. For example, a 5 June 1989 meeting of the Sub-Committee on the Status of Women of the Special Committee of International NGOs on Human Rights also considered the question of female circumcision. Another issue of special WFMH interest at the 8–19 May 1989 World Health Assembly was the WHO document on the prevention of mental, neurological and psychosocial disorders. Spaulding, an American expatriate living in Geneva, took a special interest as the mother of a sometimes hospitalized schizophrenic son in patients' rights and assurances of competent treatment. In 1990 another volunteer, Myrna Merritt-Lachenal with a Master's Degree in Nursing from the Philippines was recruited to the group.

The WHO Mental Health Division's interest in NGO collaboration led its Senior Medical Officer, Dr. J. Bertolote, in 1991, to plan a book on voluntary NGOs. WFMH Board Member-at-Large Hilda Robbins contributed a manuscript entitled,"The Voluntary Sector: Passage to Empowerment for Volunteers, Consumers and Advocates."

Special events in 1991 included a 9–13 September meeting of the Preparatory Committee for the 1993 Berlin World Conference on Human Rights where we were represented by Flache who urged inclusion of mental health in its agenda. The Preparatory Committee for the UN Conference on Environment and Development met on 12 August–4 September 1991 with Douglas Deane as our representative.

By February 1992, his WFMH presidency completed, Flache's reintegration into the WHO had reached the point of his chairing the bi-annual meeting of the Global Coordinating Group for the WHO Mental Health Programme. In 1993 he was appointed chairman of the WHO Working Group on Human Rights, an interdepartmental body established in 1992.

At approximately the same time, in 1992, a new grouping of NGOs in official relations with the WHO, the "Standing Committee of Presidents of International Non-Governmental Organizations Concerned with Mental Health Issues" (SCP), was put together by Sartorius with the collaboration of Harnois (now President of a newly invigorated World Association for Psychiatric Rehabilitation, WAPR) with the initial aim of becoming a funnel through which moneys initially destined for NGOs might flow to WHO mental health projects. Flache was our first representative to this group which evoked significant misgivings in our Board. When, as a Geneva resident involved with but not employed by the WHO, Flache was named as the SCP Secretary General, the group began to occupy more of his energy.

The organizations which composed the SCP, in addition to the World Psychiatric Association which had the dominant role, were fundamentally professional in nature despite some gestures toward general citizen and user representation by WAPR. They included bodies concerned with nursing, psychology,"social psychiatry," "biological psychiatry," and epilepsy. However, its functions, aside from the accumulation of influence and resources, remained ambiguous. Some critics within the WFMH, especially Dick Hunter, pointing to an unusual feature of its structure, i.e., a "permanent" executive group composed of its initial founders, did not hesitate to label its major goal as the accumulation of power. Successive WFMH Boards debated withdrawal from the group, but in each instance concluded that it was important to stay close enough to know and perhaps influence its acts. In 1997 the WFMH Board member most interested in developing the relationship was President Elect Marten de Vries who also saw it as ultimately important for the well-being of his own institute in Maastricht. Other Board members reassured themselves that WFMH remained the only NGO in official consulting status to all of the major agencies of the UN, and the major source of international advocacy for psychologically vulnerable (at risk) persons, as well as those who felt themselves to be or had been diagnosed as mentally ill. Most importantly, it was clear that the Federation's advocacy and public education message differed significantly from that of the professional groups which, by their inherent nature, were concerned with their own survival and welfare.

Because of these considerations the WFMH Board became increasingly uncomfortable, as the 1990s progressed, with Flache as, with increasing frequency, he represented the WFMH as only one of the SCP's several members. This led to their feeling that the WFMH interests were no longer paramount in his mind. This marked the onset of a gradual diminution of his personal influence within the Federation. As indicated at the end of this chapter it indirectly led to the WFMH embarking on a new course of collaboration with the WHO without his involvement.

The WFMH and WHO Regions

As an NGO in "official relations" with the WHO, we were regularly invited to send observers to the WHO's regional meetings some of which dealt with issues of direct mental health relevance. The announcements of Regional Meetings came to my office, and my usual effort, not always successful, was to find appropriate WFMH people in the city or region in which the meeting was to take place.

In 1990, perhaps stimulated by the fact that our senior Geneva representative, Flache, was also our President, the WHO Director General addressed himself for the first time to WFMH regional Vice Presidents as well as regional WHO offices. His emphasis on the importance of regional NGO collaboration with regional WHO offices was sympathetically received. However, his request that regional WFMH Vice Presidents draw up three year plans as the basis for interaction with WHO regional offices elicited no response at all. As noted in Chapter 11, however, close relationships were maintained between the WFMH's European Regional Council and its Vice President and the WHO's European Regional Office.

Africa

We were rarely able to find WFMH observers for the meetings in Africa outside of the Southern tier of states, notably Zambia and Zimbabwe, and it was never possible to identify observers for meetings in Francophone Africa, notably Burundi and Brazzaville. However, some meetings dealing with Africa took place in Geneva. At the 1990 World Health Assembly Flache intervened as an advocate for continued WHO attention to alcohol abuse in Africa. On 11 May 1993 Douglas Deane represented us at a meeting of the WHO's African Mental Health Action Group (AMHAG), a body established in 1977 to foster technical cooperation between African countries in the field of mental health.

The Pan-American Health Organization (PAHO)

The Washington DC site of the headquarters of this hemispheric branch of the WHO facilitated attendance at its meetings by our members on the U.S. east coast. Board member Gaston Harnois, whose Douglas Hospital in Montreal later became a WHO Collaborating Center, was our representative to the Global Coordinating Meeting of the WHO held at PAHO in 1983.

The PAHO/WHO offered many opportunities for NGO involvement. Notable was a March 1986 workshop on psychology training for health personnel in Havana developed by Henry David on behalf of the WFMH with the collaboration of colleagues at the American Psychological Association, Lic. Lourdes Garcia A., of the Cuban Ministry of Public Health, and PAHO/WHO mental health officers.

The long agendas of the PAHO Regional Committee's week long annual meetings usually contained little of direct interest to the WFMH. However we remained in close touch through frequent direct contacts with the Mental Health Advisors, first Rene Gonzalez, M.D. of Venezuela, whom I had known through my earlier work in Latin America, and after 1987, Itzhak Levav, M.D. of Buenos Aires and Jerusalem. Both were friends and colleagues with whom I had worked on many occasions prior to WFMH involvement. In September 1986, 1987 and 1988 we were fortunate to have the late Prof. Bruno Lima of Johns Hopkins represent us. Two PAHO emphases concerned programs for maternal and child care including accident prevention, and a developing program on "Women, Health and Development." Special attention was paid to the status and opportunities of women, and the social and health problems arising from their being stereotyped, discriminated against, and excluded from decision-making roles. This last presaged the later WFMH focus on women's health and mental health as a key to family and community health.

Several months of discussion with Levav resulted in our signing, in early 1990, a contract for the WFMH to administer the funds and participate in the planning of a PAHO Regional Conference on the Restructuring of Psychiatric Care in Latin America. Our talks had begun with a focus on human rights which proved to be too politically sensitive for the WHO; the title had then moved to standards of psychiatric care; and, finally, after much intramural discussion, to "restructuring." However, from my WFMH viewpoint, the issue could still be defined in terms of the rights of distressed people for equitable access to a humane, dignified and competent standard of care. The conference, held on 12–14 November 1990 in Caracas, Venezuela was co-sponsored by the WFMH along with other NGOs. Our representative was Board Member-at-Large, Federico Puente S., M.D., of Mexico, who was to chair our forthcoming 1991 World Congress in Mexico. He was also named by Mexican Health Secretary Jesus Kumate, M.D., to lead the Mexican delegation to Caracas. The Congress ended by the acclamatory adoption of a "Declaration of Caracas," which emphasized community based services as a route to protecting the rights and treatment possibilities of patients.

A major activity at PAHO headquarters, as noted below, was the September 1996 meeting of Rosalynn Carter's WFMH Committee of Women Leaders in Mental Health as the initial collaborative activity of the WHO's new program, Nations for Mental Health. Its stated goal was advocacy for increased attention by Latin American health departments to national mental health programs.

The Eastern Mediterranean

Our re-invigorated presence in the Eastern Mediterranean, following Gamal El Azayem's Mary Hemingway Rees Lecture at the 1983 Washington DC World Congress, and the newly formed World Islamic Association for Mental Health (WIAMH), (see Chapter 10), also enhanced our capacity to maintain a presence at regional WHO meetings. At that in Jordan, in October 1983, attended by all of the health ministers from the region, WFMH member Osama Al Radi,

M.D., from Taif, Saudi Arabia, spoke about the role of the Federation in the region with special emphasis on WIAMH. In October 1986 the WFMH observer to the Regional Committee's meeting in Kuwait was Professor M. Fakhr El-Islam, M.D., of the Kuwait Faculty of Medicine.

Europe

An important set of recommendations came from the WFMH at the WHO Regional Meeting for Europe in Copenhagen, 26 September 1984. There, Knud Jensen reported on the WFMH Regional Conference held the preceding month which had focused on preserving the civil rights of mentally ill people. He urged that this become a WHO priority, recommended that mental health in primary health care be given greater prominence in WHO programs, and noted that the current enthusiasm among psychiatrists for psychopharmacology put patients at risk for "chemical isolation" in place of the geographic isolation which they formerly suffered. In addition he recommended greater WHO attention to the risk of irreversible neurological side effects from the longterm use of neuroleptic drugs. The WHO Regional Committee's recommendations against smoking were also taken up later by the WFMH.

President Edith Morgan was our observer at the WHO Department of Health and Social Security's London, 18–20 March 1986, Conference of Ministers of Health on Narcotic and Psychotic Drug Misuse. WHO Director General Halfdan Mahler made the point, endorsed by the WFMH, that health authorities should invest their efforts in the demand rather than the supply side of the drug abuse problem.

An important addition to the European Region in 1987 was the appointment of J.G. Sampaio Faria, M.D., as WHO Regional Officer for Mental Health. Flache met with him, as well as Drs. Sartorius and Orley from the Geneva office to discuss matters of mutual concern. This was also the occasion when Flache introduced the possibility that the WHO with WFMH help might organize an NGO Group for Mental Health—an idea which required several years before its implementation as an "NGO Committee" in both New York and Geneva. A proposed joint WFMH/WHO effort on AIDS programs did not come to fruition.

On 12–16 1994 for the first time the WFMH European Council sent a representative to the WHO's Regional Committee for Europe. He was Regional Vice President John Henderson, a former Mental Health Advisor for WHO Europe, who presented written and verbal statements on the work of ERC/WFMH.

The Western Pacific

The active WHO-WPR (Western Pacific Region) office in Manila received particular attention from the Federation, both because of Flache's earlier involvement and the availability of Past President Aldaba Lim. Lim, who resided in Manila, was an observer at its September 1985 meeting which emphasized the promotion of childrens' health and the prevention of mental retardation and dementia in old age. At the September 1986 meeting she presented a formal statement on mental health, urging governments to work more closely with NGOs in support of primary health care programs. She also emphasized the importance of manpower training for child health at the primary care level, and the impact of extreme poverty on the rights of children to such care. On 16–20 February 1987 a Mental Health Programmes coordinating group for the Region met in an effort to up-date and expand WHO mental health work in the Region. Division Director Sartorius and other Geneva officers attended along with WFMH representatives Aldaba Lim of Manila and Basil James of New Zealand. WFMH observers at later meetings included a number of Manila members including Regina de Jesus, Executive Director of the Philippine Mental Health Association.

The WFMH in WHO Scientific Meetings

The bulk of WHO-WFMH activity over the half-century has involved organizational planning and the selection of priorities. When they have had the opportunity, WFMH representatives have tried to keep the Federation perspective in view when WHO decisions were being made. At least as often, they have been listeners at meetings and transmitted their impressions to the Board and via Newsletters to the membership.

Only a few meetings have been directly concerned with scientific issues. The 1970 joint consultation of the WHO Mental Health and Human Reproduction Sections with WFMH participation, noted above, was one. Another was a 29 August–2 September 1983 meeting of a joint WHO-NGO Task Force on "Biobehavioral and Mental Health Aspects of Primary Health Care with Particular Emphasis on Maternal and Child Health: Research Possibilities," held at PAHO headquarters in Washington DC. I was able to participate for the WFMH, along with Henry David as an observer. The interdisciplinary nature of the meeting including social and behavioral scientists as well as medical specialists from 18 countries made this an unusual event for the WHO which often tended to be purely medical in its outlook. Its recommendations, compatible with the WFMH agenda, included reducing the hazards of pregnancy and childbirth and enhancing psychosocial development through intervention in the perinatal period; psychosocial stimulation in early childhood; and attention to the consequences of developmental deprivation, including mental retardation, accidents and injuries. An innovative recommendation was for informal study groups on health promotion in adolescence with special reference to the frequency of pregnancy, drug and alcohol abuse and accidents.

On 3–5 November 1986, Professor Sheppard Kellam, Director of our first WFMH Collaborating Center on Prevention at Johns Hopkins, participated in the WHO meeting on Early Brain Development, Environment and Mental Health in Moscow. This focused on the scientific basis for primary prevention of neurodevelopmental, behavioral and mental disorders through early interventions directed to child, mother, family and the social environment at large.

The Johns Hopkins unit's inauguration as a WHO Division of Mental Health Collaborating Center was celebrated with a symposium in Baltimore on 16–17 February 1988. The importance attached to this occasion was reflected in the attendance of several WFMH representatives. In addition to myself they included North American Region Vice President Beverly Long, Board Member at Large Hilda Robbins, and Deputy Secretary General Dick Hunter.

On this occasion it was recognized that Paul Lemkau, M.D., the first Chairman of the Department of Mental Hygiene of which the Center was a unit, was a former WFMH Vice President for North America. Following the inaugural symposium WHO Mental Health Director Sartorius led a consultation of WHO Collaborating Center leaders in North America including Gaston Harnois.

UNESCO AND THE WFMH AFTER 1981

The Revival of the UNESCO Connection

As noted above the WFMH-UNESCO link was interrupted in 1970 when the agency's failure to invite a Federation representative to a meeting precipitated the resignation of Claude Veil as our representative. In the late 1970s psychiatrist Jean Louis Armand-Laroche, M.D., of Paris, already active in the French League for Mental Hygiene, volunteered to become our new representative. As incoming President in August 1981 I had no personal contact with him or with UNESCO., but appreciated the materials which he sent to the Secretariat. The December 1981 Newsletter, still published in Vancouver, carried a full page report on the 1980-1981 activities of UNESCO culminating in its 15–19 June 1981 general conference of NGOs in official relations with it. Here, the organization's Director General publicly thanked the Federation, represented by Laroche, for its participation in the International Year of the Child, especially during the 1979 World Congress in Salzburg. Laroche also did his best to create a working group of NGOs within UNESCO which would focus its attention on mental health. This unsuccessful effort was one of many such tries made over several years in the context of the UN specialized agencies. The effort finally succeeded in 1996, as described below, when a Mental Health Committee was created within the group of NGOs associated with ECOSOC at UN Headquarters in New York. However, it was not a scientific body as originally envisioned, but one combining advocacy and education for the UN Community, including country representatives. Meanwhile, I was impressed by Laroche's attitude and effort and took the first opportunity of a later trip to Paris supported by the International Social Science Council to meet him.

Another renewal of our connections with UNESCO came through President Dr. Estafania Aldaba Lim of Manila who succeeded me during the 1983 World Congress in Washington, DC. Her ties with UNESCO were mainly by virtue of her personal status as a former government official and UN leader. Thus, she served on UNESCO's International Commission for Peace in the Minds of Men. As part of the Philippine delegation she attended the 29 November-4 December 1983 regional meeting of all UNESCO national commissions in Asia and the Pacific and chaired the biennial conference of the Philippine National Commission on UNESCO on 5–6 December 1984. Shortly thereafter, on 9–14 December, she was in Dubrovnik, Yugoslavia at an Expert's Meeting on "Factors Influencing Women's Access to Scientific Life." This focused on measures to increase women's access to and responsibilities in scientific fields. The group concluded that despite the UN decade of women ending in 1985 there had been almost no progress in women's political, economic and scientific status during this period. Their finding helped provide the background for a later concern, both by UNESCO and WFMH with women's issues. On 14–18 November 1986 Aldaba Lim contributed a paper on the "Plight and Rights of Women and Children in the Context of Poverty and Development" to a UNESCO "Expert's Meeting."

During this period Laroche was quietly available if we needed him, and continued as our official representative to UNESCO. But his developing role for us was interrupted when Edith Morgan, who became WFMH President during the Brighton, England World Congress in 1985, appointed Dr. Elena Millan Game as our representative to both UNESCO and its closely related organization, the International Social Science Council (ISSC). Laroche had received no advance warning, but offered no objection and indicated his continuing willingness to help if called upon. I met Game in London before the Congress, and we stayed in touch by mail afterwards. However, although she was conscientious her personal investment in the position of being our liaison person was not high. Eventually, it became necessary for her to move out of Paris and for a time Laroche, again, faithfully filled the breach. Then, in the summer of 1993 after the Tokyo World Congress, at his first Board meeting as President, Federico Puente announced that he was appointing psychiatrist and psychoanalyst Madeleine Riviere, M.D. of Paris as our representative to UNESCO and ISSC. Neither Laroche nor I had had prior notice of this latest presidential move, and we were unsure about what to expect. However, Riviere turned out to be a highly interested, competent and conscientious representative for us.

The WFMH and the International Social Science Council (ISSC): After 1981

Not long after becoming WFMH President in August 1981 I began to receive communications from this body, ISSC. Although it identified itself as an NGO, and received project funds from a variety of sources, it was in fact a financial dependency of UNESCO in whose Paris headquarters it had its offices and held its meetings, functioning very much as an arm of the parent body. It was founded in October 1952, following a Resolution adopted at the VIth UNESCO General Conference in 1951. The sponsors of the Resolution "wished to add to the network of international interdisciplinary Associations (established under UNESCO auspices between 1945 and

1950) a new interdisciplinary body to facilitate the drawing together of the different branches of knowledge and to accelerate the resumption of intellectual communication between the nations of the world" (ISSC, 1992–1993 p.16). These Associations were scientific and scholarly dealing mainly with established branches of academic study such as anthropology, economics, geography, political science, psychology and sociology. In that era the WFMH was conceived by many of its leaders, beginning with Rees, as an organization which would bring social science together with applied mental health fields such as the medical specialty of psychiatry. Although the WFMH was not one of the original members it maintained a presence and gradually became a participant in ISSC's occasional meetings through several of its founders, most prominently Otto Klineberg and Margaret Mead. By 1972 when ISSC was transformed into a formal federation of eleven interdisciplinary associations, the WFMH was one. In time additional associations were admitted, some with "associate status." Some, such as the Russian Academy of Science, the Mexican Council of Social Sciences, and the U.S. Social Science Research Council (all admitted in 1992), had national rather than international purviews. Its aims were defined as the advancement of "social sciences and their application to major contemporary problems by means of cooperation...at the international and regional level" (ISSC, 1992–1993 p.18). While it was apparent that the WFMH did not fit easily into this group of organizations, I hoped that it might become possible to introduce mental health issues into their agenda.

The main ISSC governing body was and continues to be its biennial General Assembly to which the WFMH had not sent representatives to it for some years. I was happy to receive an invitation to attend its December 1981 meeting, the first after I became WFMH President. However, at that point I was still coping with the Federation's administrative problems, and, with Dick Hunter, faced the daunting task of staging a 1983 World Congress for Mental Health with minimal resources. The Council's next meeting, the fifteenth since its founding, was scheduled for December 1983 at UNESCO headquarters in Paris. This was shortly after Dick and I had assumed our new posts as Deputy Secretary General and Secretary General, respectively. We had just moved the existing WFMH records from Vancouver and opened a new business and membership operation in Alexandria, Virginia so, again, I was in no condition to make a trip to Paris for a meeting which promised little immediate reward for the Federation. However, the ISSC office expressed interest in our status, requesting a copy of my curriculum vitae and bibliography, and I decided that we should re-establish our dormant ties with it. After considerable consultation I managed to identify a Parisian to represent us at the meeting. He was Marcel Henri Boisot, a much decorated veteran and officer of Frances Legion of Honor, a physicist, educator, and author in the fields of political and social theory. He attended and reported back, but mental health was not his field and we did not maintain our connection.

Then the ISSC office, itself, got in touch to inform me that the 1983 Assembly had established a Scientific Activities Committee to study and make recommendations on research priorities in areas of general international and multidisciplinary significance. I was pleased to be appointed a member of this Committee which scheduled its next meeting in June 12–15, 1984 to consider such general and familiar subjects as the peaceful resolution of international conflict and consequences of technological change with emphasis on "problems of youth and unemployment." By this time our new offices were functioning, and, since ISSC supported the travel, I attended that meeting and by invitation the ISSC's Executive Committee. There I became acquainted with the ISSC President, Dr. Candido Mendes de Almeira, a major financial benefactor who had the unusual distinction of owning a private university in Rio de Janeiro. I also met its Secretary General, Dr. Luis Ramallo, Professor of Social Psychology in a Barcelona business and technical college. Perhaps of greatest significance for the WFMH was meeting Ramallo's recently appointed Deputy, Dr. Stephen Mills, an industrial psychologist from Birmingham, England, who was familiar with Western academic life and in time developed a good understanding of the WFMH's potential value for ISSC. These contacts allowed me for the first time to arrange an annual financial contribution from ISSC to the WFMH earmarked for the support of our

Newsletter which I had revived in March 1984 after an approximately 18 month hiatus associated with the Secretariat's move from Vancouver to Baltimore-Washington. It was less than $US7000 yearly, but paid our newly assessed ISSC dues as well as providing a welcome addition to our slender budget.

Perhaps the most gratifying consequence of that first ISSC activity was the opportunity to spend some time with Otto and Selma Klineberg. My wife and I were invited to a dinner at the Hotel Crillon given by Mendes in honor of Director General M'Bow of UNESCO, and upon arrival discovered that we were seated at the table for which the Klinebergs were hosts. This afforded an opportunity for much story telling about the early days of the Federation. It was a long evening because the guest of honor was very late. Dinner had been scheduled for sundown in respect for Ramadan, as M'Bow was a Muslim. However, he did not appear until an hour afterwards when it was sundown in Mecca. After dinner Mendes presented him with an abstract expressionist white-on-white painting, and he responded with a speech of more than an hour's duration.

Another pleasant and important opportunity was that to meet Dr. and Mrs. Laroche. My wife and I visited them in their charming antique apartment in an enclave off the Champs Elysee near the French President's home. I was very glad to know our long-time representative to UN Paris, and this meeting made it much easier for us to keep in touch during the years which followed.

The ISSC in that era had a special interest in peace research and one of its member organizations, the International Peace Research Association (IPRA) was planning a Paris "issues group on peace" meeting on 19–20 September 1984. I was asked to appoint a recognized scholar in the area to represent us there and was able to persuade an old friend, Jerome D. Frank, M.D., Ph.D., Professor Emeritus of Psychiatry at Johns Hopkins University to be our representative. He was one of the few world leaders on the subject having attended the early Pugwash Conferences on Science and World Affairs, and served on a broad range of Boards and advisory groups, as well as published widely on the prevention of nuclear war. While in Paris he also attended the "Informal Consultation on Links Between Peace, Disarmament and Development" sponsored by UNESCO on 17–18 September.

Another "issues group," this one on "the impact of unemployment on youth" was to be convened in Paris on 8–9 November 1984 by another ISSC member organization, the International Sociological Association. Again I was able to persuade a colleague to represent us. He was Dr. Harvey Brenner, Professor of Health Policy and Management and of Behavioral Sciences at the Johns Hopkins School of Hygiene and Public Health, and author of the definitive work relating unemployment to mental illness. These appointments seemed to me to bear on the WFMH's developing concern with prevention, as well as to some of the earlier concerns with international harmony and the social context of behavior which had marked the Rees era

We received stimulating reports of the ISSC discussions from both Frank and Brenner, along with recommendations for WFMH research. However, the WFMH was not equipped to follow them up and they emphasized our difference from the other participating associations all of which were composed of academic investigators and had regular meetings where they reported their research findings. It was this experience which led me to think seriously about how the WFMH's historic interest in a scientific base for its advocacy might be renewed. That was realized with the identification of our first Collaborating Center, that on Prevention at Johns Hopkins University, in 1986. In 1988 when the Issue Group on Peace met in Washington DC to discuss "Conflict Resolution and Conflict Transformation" I was able to persuade Jerrold Post, M.D.,Professor of Psychiatry and Public Policy at George Washington University to represent us. He agreed and gave us a full report, published in our Newsletter, of the relevance of the WFMH perspective to the problem.

The ISSC was also interested in developing new "issue groups" on Women and Development in a World in Crisis. This was the topic of a special General Assembly in Paris on 16–18 December 1985 attended on our behalf by WFMH President Edith Morgan. She was one of 11 invited delegates to a follow-up meeting in Paris, 8–9 April 1986 to consider establishing an interdisciplinary issue group on women. This provided added impetus to Morgan for her work with women's status in Europe, but there was no significant follow-up from ISSC.

In that year, 1986, our immediate Past President Aldaba Lim expressed an interest in becoming personally active with ISSC. With the agreement of our Board, I attended the ISSC General Assembly in Paris on 9–11 December 1986, spoke for her nomination to the ISSC Board and had the pleasure of seeing her elected. With adequate travel support from Philippine sources she was able to attend its meetings as our representative. I had not expected to attend for the time being, but in consequence of the discussions on biomedicine and human rights (see below) was specifically requested to give a report to the 7–9 December 1988 General Assembly which convened in Barcelona. There I was elected to the ISSC Executive Committee succeeding Aldaba Lim. Among the other members who formed a congenial group were representatives of the International Unions of Psychological Science (from West Germany), Anthropological and Ethnological Sciences (from the Netherlands) and Sociology (from Norway). A major project was the continuation and elaboration of the Council's program,"Human Dimensions of Global Change," initiated just a few months before. A Committee headed by Canadian Professor L. Kosinski of the International Geographical Union undertook the task of identifying primary areas of concern for the social sciences and the role of ISSC and its member unions in the project. Although I made a case for including the psychosocial elements of "human dimensions," this was obviously a low priority item.

The ISSC, UNESCO, and the Biomedicine and Human Rights Project

This project marked the most significant chapter in the contemporary ISSC-UNESCO-WFMH relationship, i.e. that existing after 1981. 1t began when I was invited to participate in an ISSC-UNESCO Division of Human Rights and Peace conference on the "Effects of Recent Technological Advances on Human Rights" in Barcelona, 25–28 March 1985. On behalf of the WFMH I discussed human rights issues inherent in the neuroleptic drug treatment of persons involuntarily committed to mental hospitals. Other papers dealt with genetics, neuroscience, and behavioral manipulation. The conference was attended by ISSC's Luis Ramallo and Stephen Mills and the UNESCO Division's Senior Programme Specialist, Georges Kutukdjian, Ph.D., an anthropologist, who, along with Mills, became my major liaison to UNESCO.

I reported the outcome of this conference not only to our Board and, via the Newsletter, our membership, but to Dr. Henry David and Professor Lucile Newman Ph.D., co-chairs of new WFMH Committee on Responsible Parenthood established during the 1983 Washington DC World Congress for Mental Health. Newman, an anthropologist in Brown University's Department of Community Health and an early contributor to the study of women's contraceptive behavior, responded with particular enthusiasm, suggesting that the next step should be a focus on reproductive technologies and women's rights. I transmitted her ideas to Kutukdjian, with an almost immediate result. He developed a contract with the WFMH to set up an international, multidisciplinary working group of medical and social science specialists "to consider the impact of new reproductive technologies on the human rights of women including the ethical issues involved" as well as the changing roles of women in public and private life. The technologies would include those involved in contraception, pregnancy termination, genetic counselling, the prediction of fetal gender and other socially or biologically significant characteristics, and social attitudes toward the treatment of infertility including such procedures as in vitro fertilization and various types of artificially induced pregnancy. The contract would require regular progress reports in the WFMH Newsletter and a final report to be submitted to UNESCO no later than 30 June 1987. All of this reflected the importance attributed by UNESCO to clarifying the issues and raising the level of public education and discussion regarding human life in an environment increasingly shaped by science and technology. These last clearly influence our understanding of human rights, personal diversity and personal choice.

This was, in a sense, an historic moment for the WFMH as it was the first such contract since those eventuating in two publications by Margaret Mead in the Rees era. After reflection and consultation I accepted it for the Federation, asking Newman to join me as a Co-Principal Investigator and to be the main contact point for the project work. She agreed and put the resources of her department and considerable personal network of investigators at our disposal. Before long an appropriate moment for a first International Working Group meeting presented itself with the WFMH co-sponsored Conference of the International Association for Child and Adolescent Psychiatry scheduled for Paris on 21–25 July 1986. We identified members of the new Working Group and, as our first activity, organized a symposium for the Paris meeting on "The New Reproductive Technologies: Framing the Ethical Issues." Our members in addition to Newman, Kutukdjian and myself included psychologist Professor Nila Kapor-Stanulovic, Ph.D., of the University of Novi Sad, Yugoslavia; anthropologist and demographer Maria MacDonald, Ph.D., of International Planned Parenthood, London who had reviewed my book on personal fertility regulation in Jamaica (Brody, 1981); Professor Eylard van Hall, M.D., Chair of the Department of Obstetrics and Gynecology of the University Hospital in Leiden, the Netherlands, a colleague from the International Society for Psychosomatic Obstetrics and Gynecology (ISPOG); and anthropologist, Professor Phyllis Palgi, Chair of the Department of Behavioral Science at Tel Aviv University, Israel whom I had known since an ISPOG meeting in Rome which I had attended at the invitation of Paris psychiatrist Leon Chertok. We, thus, had a congenial as well as accomplished and knowledgeable group ready to begin the required dialogue. Newman's friend and one time colleague, sociologist and demographer, Professor T. Pearce of the University of Ife, Nigeria was unable to be present. Dr. C. Ambroselli, Director of the Center for Ethics Documentation and Information of the French National Institute for Health and Medical Research was present as an observer.

We soon agreed that "new" technologies could not be effectively separated from "old" ones, and that the work of the Group would be more usefully conducted in the language of rights and roles rather than the professional language of ethics. Three categories of issues were identified as salient. First were those at the interface of science/technology and human rights; second were those related more immediately to the rights and roles of women; third were issues of a collective, social and institutional nature. Examples of these last were cultural rights as an aspect of a community's perception of the continuity of its lineage, affiliative rights and knowledge of parenthood as an aspect of identity, and the development of institutional forms, such as ethics committees, to consider these issues.

At this meeting the Group adopted Newman's suggestion to develop regional meetings in their own areas of the world. She obtained a grant from the New World Foundation of New York City of which she was a Board member to support meetings in the U.S. They were held with groups of female undergraduate and medical students, disadvantaged refugee and minority status women. Within all of the groups there was general agreement that birth limiting and spacing technologies had greater personal and public health significance than the more advanced techniques of noncoital ("artificial") reproduction. At the same time there was general recognition of the importance of raising the level of public debate about ethical aspects of the newer technologies as they have a potential impact upon human rights and mental health. Areas of special concern included: prediction and manipulation of gender; the use of surrogate mothers with special reference to their commercial exploitation; the medical compulsion to use all available, although not fully assessed, technologies; and the social control roles of physicians and ethics committees.

Newman also established a lecture series at Brown University with that institution's financial support, on the ethical and human rights significance of reproductive technologies for which I served as an occasional discussant. On 28 November 1986 she met in Melbourne, Australia with a group convened by psychiatrist Lorraine Dennerstein, M.D., President of ISPOG. Discussions there reflected the current Australian concern about the "new eugenics" made possible by eliminating the genetic expression of trait faults as well as the high level of interest in treatments of infertility including in vitro fertilization. Among the rights discussed were those to do research essential to human well-being; for practitioners not to treat if they felt that was the correct course; the rights of children ensuing from artificial reproduction; and the right of access to treatment if desired.

In January 1987, with the help of its President Dr. Wayne Holtzman, I was able to organize a regional meeting in Texas supported by the Hogg Foundation for Mental Health of which I was a National Council member at the time. In addition to members of our Working Group we were joined by Drs. Toni Falbo of the University of Texas, Susan Pick de Weiss and Annemarie Monroy of Mexico City.

The final meeting of the Working Group arranged by Newman was held at the Alton Jones Conference Center of the University of Rhode Island, U.S.A., from 3–5 March 1987. All members were present except for Dr. Pearce who submitted a paper. Attending as consultants were Professors Lina Fruzetti of the Sudan and J. Waage, both affiliated with Brown University. By June the final report had been submitted to UNESCO (Newman, Brody, 1987).

This report was one of two discussed at a second "International Consultation on Biomedical Science and Technology and Human Rights" sponsored just six months later by ISSC and UNESCO in Barcelona, 30 November–5 December 1987. The second paper was one which I had prepared, commissioned by UNESCO at the request of Mills and Kutukdjian on "An Inventory of Biomedical and Clinical Research Domains Relevant to the Expansion or Limitation of Human Rights." This gathering proceeded with some ceremony as it was opened by Ramallo with greetings from the new UNESCO Director General Dr. Federico Mayor Zaragosa, a Catalan native, who had participated in the 1985 Barcelona meeting. In addition to Mills, Palgi, Newman, and Kapor-Stanulovic, the group included a UNESCO nominee, Dr. W. Muller Freinfels, Professor of Comparative and Family Law at the University of Freiburg in Breisgau, West Germany. Observers were Dr. Felix Marti, Director of the Centro Unesco de Catalunya and Professor of Theology at the University of Barcelona. The discussions were more focused. In addition to presenting one of the two working reports I served as Rapporteur for the discussions. The aim of the final Report as enunciated by ISSC/UNESCO was to "(1) arrive at cross-culturally acceptable value formulations useful for the construction of an international human rights instrument regarding the impact of advancing science and technology with special reference to biomedicine; (2) make programmatic recommendations for UNESCO's medium-term, i.e. 6 years, program; (3) make short-term project recommendations to be included within the medium-term program."

There were several consequences to the Report. An immediate one was that ISSC supported my travel to organize and moderate a symposium on "The New Reproductive Technologies and Women's Rights" at the International Congress of Anthropological and Ethnological Sciences held 24–31 July 1988 in Zagreb, Yugoslavia. Several members of our original Working Group were able to participate in this. A number of published papers, all listing WFMH sponsorship of the project, also ensued (Brody, 1987b, 1988a, 1989a and b; Newman, 1989).

A more important consequence signalling a new role for the WFMH as an NGO concerned with human rights and biomedical ethics, and an active contributor to the development of international human rights instruments, was a request by UNESCO-ISSC to produce a "Draft Report on Human Rights Aspects of Traffic in Body Parts and Human Fetuses for Research and/or Therapeutic Purposes." I hesitated to accept this assignment, wondering if it would fit the mission of the WFMH, and might even diffuse it away from its mental health goals. Consultation and reflection, however, suggested that it did fit our perspective on prevention of mental illness and emotional distress, broadly conceived, and that its international ramifications certain fitted the implicit intentions of our founders to promote international harmony. The preparation of this Report involved consultations with a multi-disciplinary group of experts whom I visited between 1988 and the spring of 1989. They included Professors H. Tristram Engelhardt, Jr., M.D.,

Ph.D. of Baylor University, in philosophy and medicine; Robert C. Cefalo, M.D., Ph.D.,of the University of North Carolina in Obstetrics, Gynecology and Maternal-Fetal Medicine; George J. Annas, JD.., M.P.H.,of Boston University in Health Law; Margaret Somerville, LL.B., of McGill University in Law and Medicine; Larry O. Gostin, J.D., of Harvard in Health Law and Public Health Policy; Anthony E. Reading, Ph.D., Director of Psychological Studies for UCLA's Center for Reproductive Medicine; Dr. James Childress, Professor of Religious Studies and Medical Education at the Universit of Virginia and a member of the US Commissions on Organ Transplantation and Fetal Research; and from our initial group, Professors Dennerstein, Newman and van Hall. By April 1989 I had completed an initial draft of the requested document and sent it to UNESCO as well as a number of consultants for preliminary review. It emphasized psychosocial, cultural and mental health issues with particular reference to the needs of populations which might need transplants, and mental health and ethical issues in the processes of obtaining, distributing and transplanting the materials. After the 28–31 May Congress of ISPOG in Amsterdam I convened a workshop of consultants to discuss the most sensitive ethical issues involved. The 21–25 August 1989 World Congress for Mental Health in Auckland, New Zealand made it possible for me to visit Dennerstein and her group at the Key Center for Women's Health in Society at the University of Melbourne in Australia for further examination of my findings and conclusions. She invited me to speak at the Mercy Hospital in Melbourne on 17 August under the auspices of the Center which she headed. I felt a little uncertain about speaking on artificial reproduction at a Catholic hospital, but the Sister who directed the hospital was not only welcoming, but impressively well-informed in her comments and questions. Afterwards I conducted a workshop for 20 participants, chaired by Dennerstein, on human rights aspects of transactions in human fetal tissue. Among the participants were Professor Louis Waller of the University of Monash School of Law, author of the influential "Waller Commission" Report on In Vitro Fertilization, Professor Peter Singer, a well-known ethicist from the Melbourne Department of Philosophy., Dr. Graham Schofield, former Dean of the Medical School and Professor of Anatomy, and visiting Professor Franca Bimbi of the University of Padua, Italy.

By 19 September 1989, I was able to submit the completed document (Brody 1990a). Although it was for UN interagency use only, the subject elicited many invitations to speak, especially in Mexico where it turned out to be a particular interest of Manuel Velasco Suarez, M.D. Honorary Chairman of the 1991 World Congress. Later, it became the topic of one paper in a medical journal (Brody 1990b).

UNESCO and ISSC required my presence again in Paris in 1989. There, on 17 November, I had the privilege of a personal conference with UNESCO Director General Federico Mayor who, prior to his appointment, had been part of the March 1985 Barcelona Symposium. He affirmed UNESCO's co-sponsorship for the 1991 World Congress for Mental Health in Mexico; his support for my request to advance the WFMH from a Class B to a Class A (with the opportunity for a direct voice influencing UNESCO policy) relationship with UNESCO; and invited me to be an advisor and participant on behalf of the WFMH in a planned UNESCO workshop on biomedical ethics tentatively scheduled for mid-1990 for which my interagency document would be distributed as a background paper.

I also conferred with Georges Kutukdjian regarding the uses of the not yet published interagency document (Brody 1990a) for UNESCO, and the possibility, since it was becoming a more central concern for UNESCO, of continuing WFMH sponsored contributions to the field now widely known as "bioethics." Stephen Mills also wondered about a possible ISSC workshop on "Human Response to Global Change" at the Mexico Congress, and the ways in which the WFMH could contribute to the "Human Response" program. I felt that this was a worth-while move and encouraged it. Later discussions, however, made it clear that our particular concerns with mental health and human behavior in general were not part of the project leaders' perspective.

I was not eager to undertake more at that time, but did feel an obligation to respond posi-
tively to Mills' request that I produce a book for ISSC, based on our working group meetings,
with the working title,"Biomedical Science and Human Rights." These and other projects were
on the agenda for the 26–27 April 1990 meeting of the ISSC Executive Committee in Madrid.
There it became apparent that the WFMH was one of the few ISSC member organizations with
no working group on the "Human Response" project. Through the Newsletter and other channels I looked for individual or organizational WFMH members who might be interested in
developing such a group for which there was a possibility of ISSC funding. President Elect Max
Abbott identified a colleague, Professor Manfred Cramer of the University of Munich, with a
long involvement in the environmental-mental health interface. He was interested and agreed
to become our liaison person to the ISSC project, to go in my place to the ISSC General
Assembly, 28–30 November 1990, and to its Symposium on "Human Dimensions of Global
Environmental Change" in Palma de Mallorca. He did attend and we received a report on the
happenings in Mallorca, but that was the extent of the Federation's involvement in the Human
Dimensions project.

The biomedical ethics meeting planned for 1990 eventually took place in Moscow, organized
by the USSR National Center for Human Sciences with UNESCO cooperation, on 13–15 May
1991. The working title was "Bioethics and the Social Consequences of Biomedical Research"
and I was invited to keynote the discussions on informed consent. Unfortunately, previously
scheduled activities made it impossible for me to attend. I had also become very ill after a 1990
visit to the USSR (see Chapter 11) and was not eager to return. Therefore, I suggested an alternate WFMH representative.

By 1991 it had also become apparent to me that the working papers for our several group meetings stimulated by the 1985 Barcelona conference would not be an adequate basis for the edited book
proposed by Mills. The papers were not sufficiently deep for scholarly purposes, the literature cited
was mainly out of date, and the coverage was too narrow. I told this to Mills who suggested that I
scrap the idea of an edited volume and start from the beginning to write a completely new book with
the meetings as background for my thinking. At first I refused, but upon reflection realized that this
was an unusual opportunity, especially as the publication would be financed by UNESCO and the
volume would be issued under the joint imprimatur of UNESCO/ISSC/WFMH. Writing this volume occupied the better part of my spare time during 1991 and 1992. It was finally published in the
spring of 1993 (Brody, 1993) and distributed to relevant UN offices and elsewhere throughout the
world. Since UNESCO held the copyright I could not benefit materially, but took great pleasure in
the several good reviews which the book received, and, especially, in putting the WFMH firmly on
the map in this very important area of mental health.

In 1993, following the book's publication, UNESCO established an International Bioethics
Committee led by Kutukdjian. It was created by Director General Mayor to examine ethical
questions raised by advances in genetics and biology, and brought together scientists, philosophers, lawyers and sociologists. Its first meeting was in UNESCO House on 15–16 September
1993 to discuss a possible international instrument for protection of the human genome. Among
those present was Lord Kennett who some time later on 27 June 1994 wrote me a letter about it.
He said,"Like everyone else I used your book as the general mine of information about the ter-
ribly dispersed field of bioethics." I was appointed ISSC's "Permanent Representative" to the
Unit, but in the absence of travel support did not attend its regular meetings which took place
largely in Paris, but occasionally in other parts of the world.

The WFMH and ISSC after 1992

In early 1992 ISSC President Candido Mendes circulated suggested changes in its
Constitution and By Laws to the Executive Committee. In my response of 10 February I tried

once more to stimulate interest in bringing health-related research into the ISSC program. This effort was not successful. My last attendance at an ISSC Assembly was in Paris in December 1992 after I had had a final consultation with Kutukdjian about my book and his and UNESCO's plans in the bioethics area. At ISSC I encountered a great deal of intra-Council turmoil over the succession of its staff officers. Approximately a year earlier Candido Mendes had retired as President to move up to a position, which he had helped create, as Chairman of a new "Senior Council." Luis Ramallo had taken his place, and in turn was replaced as Secretary General by Stephen Mills for the year 1993–1994. Mills was, for reasons which never became completely clear, not popular with the most politically energetic ISSC members and he, rightly, surmised that they wanted him out. Perhaps this was a reason why he urged me to attend the 11–12 December 1993 meeting of the Executive Committee in Paris although he was unable to support my travel. I couldn't make it and not long thereafter received a letter dated 16 December 1994 from the Chairman of the Nominating Committee who also chaired the Search Committee for the Secretary General's post. It indicated general distress with what constituted a "financial and administrative crisis" in the Council. He asked if I wished to stand for re-election to the Executive Committee and later telephoned to press his inquiry. I demurred, uncertain about whether I would be able to attend the meetings without support. Nor was it possible for me to attend the next Executive Committee which took place on 23 February 1994 but its minutes again revealed significant dissatisfaction with Mills, especially regarding his capacity for "leadership." During 1994 the pressure not to re-elect Mills was building. A 7 June 1994 letter from the Nominating Committee Chairman reminding me that the position of Secretary General was to be voted on, asked me once more if I intended to stand for re-election. This time I was certain, and by fax let him know that I did not intend to become a candidate for any ISSC office.

Meanwhile, Madeleine Riviere, our new liason to UNESCO, was becoming known. She represented us at the first meeting of UNESCO's Management of Social Transformations (MOST) Programme in Paris, 7–10 March 1994 and also established good working relations with Kutukdjian. Thus, she was able, at his invitation, to attend the third session of the Bioethics Committee on our behalf on 27–29 September. On 3 December 1994 she was invited at my request to attend the ISSC Executive Committee in my place. However, she was not admitted to discussion about the choice of a new Secretary General. By this time she had gotten to know and appreciate Mills, and agreed to cast the WFMH vote for him, or if his name was not on the ballot, to abstain from voting. The vote took place on the next day, and terminated Mills' period of ISSC stewardship. Riviere in her report to me noted that he had been informed ahead of time by Ramallo and Mendes that he would not be re-elected. He did not seem too upset and had already made new plans for his future.

1994 in Paris was significant for the WFMH for other reasons. I had asked Riviere to get in touch with Laroche. She passed the request on to her colleague, psychiatrist Roland Broca, M.D., who invited him to a meeting on 10 December 1994 to discuss the founding of a French Federation for Mental Health. Ultimately, this led to what was, perhaps, the major event organized by French colleagues in relation to UNESCO: a 10–11 October 1996 conference on "Ethics and Psyche." Sponsored by the now viable French Federation for Mental Health (FFMH) with the collaboration of the WFMH and UNESCO's Bioethics Unit it was held at UNESCO House. The primary conference organizers were Roland Broca, President of FFMH, and Riviere who, in addition to being our representative, was the FFMH Vice President. Kutukdjian, also a speaker, was a consultant for the conference organizers. This was an important, multi-disciplinary, intellectual and professional event in the best UNESCO tradition under the patronage of Mme Chirac, wife of the French President, with the participation of leading psychoanalytic, psychiatric, psychological, historical, social science and juridical scholars, including representatives of the French National Committee on Ethics and an advisor on human rights to the European Community. I was much pleased to sit with UNESCO Director General Mayor at the opening, and present my views on patient autonomy to this gathering, as part of the same program with Broca, Riviere and Kutukdjian (Brody, 1996).

By 1996 ISSC's reorganization by Mill's successor was well under way. He was French, Polish and English speaking Canadian Professor of Geography, Leszcek Kosinski, Ph.D., who had been a leading figure in the "Human Response" project. Kosinski, clearly an able administrator and an accomplished scholar, was faced with significant financial problems because UNESCO, itself, was in the process of decentralizing its system of dispensing subsidies. In mid-1996 we lost the small but regular grant earmarked for the Newsletter. We were already in frequent touch with Kosinski through the mails, telephone and fax, and had learned that we might have a chance for two small grants through the ISSC Tunis office dominated by Palestinians I submitted one proposal from Dr. Leila Dane, Director of our member organization the Institute for Victims of Trauma and one from Dr. Nancy Dubrow. Dane's proposal was for funds to edit the proceedings of the 1994 Cairo conference on building tolerance for diversity. Dubrow's was for planning toward a children's "Peace Museum" in East Jerusalem. Before long we were notified by ISSC that both had been rejected by the Tunis office.

When Kosinski visited the U.S. in autumn 1996 we took advantage of the opportunity to know him better and I invited him for dinner at the Cosmos Club in Washington. I especially wanted to solidify the working relationship between his office and Dr. Elena Berger to whom I was giving increasing responsibilities for the Secretary General's Baltimore operation. He also came to our PAHO conference with the Committee on Women Leaders two days later where he met President Beverly Long and President Elect Marten de Vries.

Before the end of the year a new project possibility opened up. It was presented initially as a request from Palestinians in Gaza to help develop a center for Youth activities. Clearly, this did not fit our capabilities. However, I called Nancy Dubrow, already working in the area and asked her to look into the matter and to consult both with Fathi Arafat, M.D., Director of the Palestine Red Crescent Hospital in Cairo where I had visited some years earlier, with Elia Awaad, Ph.D., of Birzeit University on the West Bank, as well as with our Regional Vice President Ahmed El Azayem. Finally, there emerged a fundable project centered on a survey of Palestinian youth attitudes bearing on their ability to participate in main stream community building activities, rather than simply to focus on continuing hostile interaction with the Israelis. The amount of money was small, the equivalent of two years support for the Newsletter, but we were permitted to take our ISSC dues from it.

UN NEW YORK: ECOSOC, Unicef, AND OTHER AGENCIES

The Agencies

WFMH representatives to UN New York have acted as liaisons primarily to units of ECOSOC, the Economic and Social Council. This is not properly an agency but a forum for discussion with its own Office of Secretariat Services for Economic and Social Matters. Its subsidiary bodies of most immediate interest to the WFMH have included the Population Commission, the Commission for Social Development, the Commission on the Status of Women, the Commission on Narcotic Drugs, and the Commission on Human Rights which includes among its Subcommissions one on the Prevention of Discrimination and Protection of Minorities. Much of the WFMH work in relation to ECOSOC has been in the context of NGO Committees for such issues as Aging, Human Rights and Women.

The various NGOs in consultative status to ECOSOC come together in the Conference of Non-Governmental Organizations known as CONGO. CONGO has meetings in both Geneva and New York and is the forum in which different NGOs are able to establish their differences and commonalities in relation to UN initiatives.

In addition to ECOSOC we tried to maintain the WFMH connection with Unicef. One of 136 NGOs in consultative status to Unicef we are the only one with an explicit interest in mental health. We have related to Unicef in an irregular basis, usually in regard to such broadly defined issues as "street children" or "children in extremely difficult circumstances." In these respects we have often been informally allied with other NGOs concerned with parenthood, reproductive behavior and children's rights. As noted above President Tsung-yi Lin arranged a consultation with Unicef after the 1979 Salzburg World Congress as part of the International Year of Youth program.

Through my earlier collaborations with Henry David I became familiar with UNFPA, the United Nations Fund for Population Activities. We had no formal relationship with it, but were successful in persuading Pakistani obstetrician and gynecologist Nafis Sadik, M.D., its Deputy Director (and later Director), to address a plenary session on family planning, responsible parenthood and mental health at our 1983 World Congress in Washington DC. In 1987, as part of the research for the UNESCO-ISSC project on reproductive behavior and women's mental health, Lucile Newman and I visited the UNFPA office to discuss the cultural problems which it encountered in its work.

UN New York (ECOSOC, Unicef): 1981–1990

Since New York was the UN office closest to Baltimore, that became my first destination in the role of President. By late October 1981 I had met on several occasions with our long-term representative, Elizabeth Cohen. She was a living connection with the Federation's founding era, and an ardent advocate of mental health as it was broadly defined by the founders. While her interest in mental health encompassed the welfare of mentally ill people, it was more oriented to the maintenance of intergroup harmony, and the prevention of mental ill-health. It had become important to her in 1947 when, following the appointment of her husband, Dr. Myer Cohen, as Assistant Director General of the International Refugee Organization (predecessor of UNHCR) she moved her family to Geneva. There she met Brock Chisholm who had just become WHO Director General and had already made the initial moves toward founding the WFMH. The other WFMH prime mover, often at the WHO, was Jack Rees. Cohen became a WFMH member at its 1948 London founding Congress when Rees was elected its first president and remained in close touch with him when he served as its first Director. She recalled taking part with him "in an early seminar on the mental health problems of displaced persons and refugees" (letter to the author, 4 September 1995). From 1952 to 1956, she lived in Yugoslavia where her husband directed the UN social and economic programs. After their return to New York in 1956 she began working with Helen Ascher, the first WFMH representative to the UN and Unicef in New York City (see above). In 1960, after Ascher's death, she was the WFMH's senior person at UN New York.

When we met in 1981, Elizabeth Cohen was 77 years old. She impressed me as the best Federation representative for whom we could hope: knowledgeable and effective with the charisma of someone who had been present "at the creation." When my wife and I first had dinner with her and Myer in New York, I realized that she was a fount of information about this organization of which I had become President with broad, but shallow, knowledge. Looking backwards she identified her most significant contribution to the WFMH. It was "rectifying the omission of any reference to mental health" in the Declaration of Alma Ata emerging from the 1978 primary health care conference sponsored there by the WHO and Unicef. In retrospect (her letter of 4 September 1995), she identified as "most satisfactory" her success in achieving "the proper status for WFMH as an NGO." She also regarded as significant her participation in dealing with a request from Unicef in the early 1970s for studies regarding its activities in several of the less developed countries of Asia and Africa. I resonated especially to her recalling that Margaret Mead, my predecessor as a U.S. WFMH President, was particularly helpful, in enlisting her fellow anthropologists to advise and consult on such issues. Cohen was most sympathetic to my feeling, similar to that of Rees and the other founders, that the WFMH should pay more attention than it had to the cultural variability of the peoples with whose mental health we were concerned. As she put it,"WFMH is strategically placed to have an important interdisciplinary role in the work of the NGOs." I felt her compatibility and very much wanted her to stay in her volunteer post with us. However, she felt that advancing age was beginning to reduce her available energy, and had already initiated plans to move to a retirement community in Pennsylvania.

That made it clear that we needed to find another person or persons to represent us. At a later visit, she introduced me to Mrs. Dorothy Miller, a friend whom she had recruited to work with her. I had also heard from Andrea Delgado, M.D., President of the Black Psychiatrists of America who attended the Manila Congress and talked with her about possibly joining the UN team. On another occasion, now in 1982, I was able to meet with Executive Director Bertie Beiser, in town with her husband Professor Morton Beiser to attend a regional meeting of the World Psychiatric Association. We conferred together with Varinda Vittachi, Sri Lankan Assistant Deputy for External Affairs and Dr. Herman Stein, Senior Advisor to Unicef's Executive Director about how the WFMH might best function in relation to Unicef programs. Later Dr. Stein sent me records of the WFMH-Unicef meeting arranged by President Lin in Salzburg and copies of Unicef discussions after that meeting. I studied them and found them very supportive of the roles of NGOs in relation to their work, but realized that the WFMH as an advocacy and educational organization did not have the capacity to engage in the direct service operations of most NGOs which assisted Unicef in its essentially relief-oriented work.

In January 1982 the Cohens moved to a retirement village in Pennsylvania. Dorothy Miller then took Elizabeth's place as our Main WFMH Representative to UN New York. Her career had been in public relations, and she was knowledgeable and sensitive to important aspects of advocacy. After retirement, in addition to travels to remote areas of the world, she had pursued a new career as a volunteer working with various social service agencies and brought this perspective to the UN. My wife and I met her in New York on several occasions. We became friends, and I acquired great respect for her capacities as our representative. As the WFMH liaison she attended briefings on general UN concerns such as disarmament and arms limitation, prevention of nuclear war, the peaceful uses of outer space, and apartheid. She was especially active as a member of the NGO Committees on Youth, Aging and Population and contributed a note to the March 1982 WFMH Newsletter on the importance for child development of a stable family structure supporting the use of foster care rather than institutionalization whenever possible.

She later joined the NGO subcommittee to address the world wide problem of unwanted children formed in consequence of the December 1983 conference on street children sponsored by Covenant House, New York with WFMH President Aldaba-Lim as a leading participant. She also represented us at meetings of a special committee established by CONGO to prepare for the International Population Conference in Mexico in August 1984.

A WFMH Regional Meeting that fall, 30 September–4 October 1984, was held at Ben Gurion University in Beersheba, Israel. It brought me in contact with Yael Danieli, Ph.D., an Israeli psychologist living in New York who had founded and directed the Group Project for Holocaust Survivors and their Children. Especially impressive was her conduct of a group discussion of survivors which elicited for the first time from one of our hitherto restrained colleagues a public account of her traumatic childhood memories in Nazi Germany. Danieli's unusual mixture of intelligence and high emotional intensity led me to ask if she might be interested in working with the WFMH in New York. Upon her return she lost no time in getting in touch with Dorothy Miller who immediately involved her in our UN work. When, within the year, Miller decided to devote more time to other causes, Danieli accepted my invitation to become our new Senior Representative. Although Miller, Cohen and Hilda Robbins our Regional Vice President for North America all participated to some degree in the UN activities, Danieli's energy, commitment and self-confidence rapidly made her the dominant force and a known quantity among both UN NGO and country representatives. Her particular interests led her to represent us at the Seventh UN Congress on Prevention of Crime and Treatment of Offenders in Milan, 26 August–6 September 1985, along with Dr. Micheline Basil and Professor Irwin Waller of the University of Ottowa School of Law who had been members of a WFMH Committee on Victims of Violence established in 1980. This WFMH group, led by Waller, was active in circulating background materials to Congress delegates, talking with them and drafting what became the United Nations Declaration of Basic Principles of Justice for Victims of Crime and Abuse of Power, ultimately passed by the General Assembly in November 1985. Although it has not been enforced this was a landmark statement, eroding the principle of national sovereignty by specifying the right of international organizations to enter countries to help care for victims of government abuse of their own citizens. It also made explicit that emotional and mental injuries following such abuse were grounds for assistance and compensation.

From 4–6 September 1985 Miller joined Hilda Robbins at the NGO Conference staged by the UN in San Francisco which focused on how NGOs might mobilize support for issues before it. However, just a few months later, in mid-1986, Miller, having been elected to the presidency of a major organization requiring most of her time, and then suffering an injury in an automobile accident, felt it necessary to withdraw completely from UN work. I was most grateful when she agreed to remain until we could find another person to deal with some of the issues which Danieli did not have time to cover. In the fall Danieli recruited Leonard Feinberg, Ph.D., a Rochester and William Alanson White trained psychologist and psychoanalyst to be our liaison with ECOSOC and Unicef. When Danieli organized WFMH participation in the 23 January 1987 UN Department of Public Information Conference he was a competent participant. The Conference theme was "Bettering the Human Condition" and Danieli had been appointed chair of one its four subthemes,"Narcotics and Substance Abuse Control." This also gave me an opportunity to present the WFMH perspective to a broad UN audience, as well as to talk at length with our 2 representatives.

Perhaps Danieli's most effective contribution, and her NGO event with the greatest impact at the UN, was a half day consultation on the 1985 "Declaration" aimed at bringing its significance before a mixed UN and public audience. She moderated it at UN New York on 23 April 1987, tracing the Declaration's development and the WFMH's role in it, noting its significance and drawing implications for further action. This was a major event co-sponsored by most of the New York UN offices. It drew an audience of approximately 150 including UN delegates from many countries, NGO representatives and UN officials. In addition to a number of public figures, WFMH participants included Richard Mollica, M.D., of Harvard, who chaired our Committee on the Mental Health of Refugees and other Migrants; Dr. Robert Rich of Princeton, chair of our Committee on Victims who was Director of the Institute of Government and Public Affairs at the University of Illinois; Dr. Susan Salasin of NIMH the founding chairperson of our Committee on Victims; and myself.

Danieli's personal impact and understanding of the importance of public relations for advocacy began, before too long, to increase our general visibility in the New York NGO world. On 7 April 1988 she was elected to the Executive Committee of the NGOs Associated with the UN Department of Public Information (DPI) and subsequently became its Vice President. This led to her appointment for a term as Chair of the DPI's NGO Publications Committee.

She also renewed our dormant connection with Unicef, representing us later in the month at a 15–19 April conference organized by the NGO Committee on Unicef dealing with "Children's Rights—an Agenda for Action: A Forum to Promote the Convention on the Rights of the Child and Meet the Global Challenge of AIDS." She became a resource person for the conference's working group on "Street Children in Especially Difficult Circumstances." At this meeting she met Nancy Dubrow, a child care worker and consultant enrolled in the PhD program in child development at the Erikson Institute in Chicago. After talking with Dubrow in New York I appointed her as our representative to the NGO Committee for Unicef and related child and youth activities. This was possible because the Erikson Institute was willing to pay for her travel to NY from Chicago in order to participate in Unicef work. Dubrow was our liaison to the 29 November 1988 meeting of the NGO Committee on Unicef on the use of children in situations of armed conflict. This introduced us to what would later become one of our human rights concerns. By spring 1989 she was elected in her WFMH role to the Executive Committee of the NGO Committee. In this capacity supported by a letter from my office representing our Board she added the Federation's weight to the NGO advocacy effort for the Convention on the Rights of the Child scheduled for debate and adoption by the UN General Assembly in New York on 20 November 1989. On the day after this debate, on 21 November, I came to New York for a briefing of NGO officers at Unicef House. The agenda included the NGO Committee, the Convention, a forthcoming Summit on Children by government leaders, and Unicef's strategies for improving the lot of children worldwide in the 1990s. The General Assembly had adopted the Convention which was scheduled for ratification by individual nations in January 1990.

During that visit I was also able to participate in the Unicef Working Group on Street Children and Children in Especially Difficult Circumstances co-chaired by Dubrow who had suggested its formation. This group met again on 29 January 1990 with special reference to children in armed conflict, street and family violence and parental loss. I came to New York again on 19–20 April for the 6th Annual Forum of the NGO Committee on Unicef, during which the Working Group heard from Dubrow about her recent experiences surveying trauma to children in Mozambique and Central America under the auspices of the Erikson Foundation. This foreshadowed a decade during which, sometimes carrying the flag of the WFMH but supported by other sources, Dubrow spent many months in war torn areas gathering data and collaborating with others in the effort to improve the emotional state of the traumatized children there.

Danieli's activities were further recognized in February 1990 by her election to the position of Treasurer of the Alliance of NGOs on Crime Prevention and Criminal Justice. Early in that month, 5–16 February, along with Dr. Maria Simon she represented us at the meeting of the UN Committee on Crime Prevention and Control in Vienna. There, with my approval, she also represented the Society for Traumatic Stress Studies, submitting on its behalf a Report on Curriculum, Education and Training for people engaged in treating survivors of traumatic events. There was some concern by our Board members about her representing more than one organization, but I felt that useful coalitions of this sort should be encouraged. At the 27 August–7 September 1990 8th UN Congress on the Prevention of Crime and the Treatment of Offenders she represented both organizations. She returned in time to serve on an NGO Committee preparing for the World Summit for Children held 29-30 September at UN New York. This was the "World Safe for Children Conference Committee" which facilitated the passage of a resolution,"Family—Zone for Safety," as part of the Summit proceedings. Dubrow was part of the NGO Working Group Response to the Draft Declaration and Plan of Action for the Summit.

UN New York: 1991–1997

As I became more familiar with the nature of NGO work at UN headquarters it was increasingly apparent that, in addition to the stellar performance of our senior representative we needed a group of people who could work together as a team. I hoped that we would eventually be able to have a WFMH representative in each of the NGO committees. With this in mind I urged Danieli to pay particular attention to friends and colleagues in the New York area who might be interested in joining our UN group of representatives. However, the beginning of a new era in our representation at UN New York did not take place until August 1990.

In that month, the late summer of 1990, I escorted a small group of WFMH members and their friends under the auspices of the American Ambassadors Program, begun by President

Eisenhower in 1952, to visit mental health institutions and personnel in the Soviet Union. One of our group was Kay C. Greene, Ph.D., a clinical psychologist with broad social interests. Prior to becoming a psychologist she had been a concert artist and stage and television actress, and later a management consultant. In addition to her private practice she was a lecturer and writer and served as a workshop leader and consultant for a number of agencies in New York City. We talked at length about the WFMH and especially opportunities at the UN in New York where I told her we needed the help of knowledgeable colleagues. She expressed interest and upon our return to America I introduced her to Danieli who greeted her warmly and briefed her on the situation. I had already identified aging as an area in which there was little WFMH activity and was pleased when she chose the NGO Committee on Aging as her special area of interest, expecting to devote approximately an hour monthly to it. Her first meeting with the Committee was on 7 February 1991. She identified a number of the WFMH concerns and was quickly recognized as a contributor, accepting a place on its Questionnaire Design Subcommittee and on the Planning Committee for the 1992 Celebration of the tenth Anniversary of the World Plan for Action on Aging. At that meeting she suggested broadening its perception of good mental health beyond the absence of neuropsychiatric impairment to include the entire aging population and approaches to preventing the occurrence of psychiatric difficulties. By her third meeting she was involved on several fronts, including writing press releases for the DPI. At its 2 May 1991 meeting she was elected Secretary of the Committee, devoting much more time to the work than the originally contemplated one hour per month. Her awareness of "so many opportunities for changing people's perceptions about mental illness and mental health at the UN" fired her enthusiasm for the work, and especially her interest in recruiting other representatives to build our much desired WFMH team (Greene, 1997). With little delay she began to recommend new representatives and increased the pace of her involvement. Danieli for her part increasingly focused her attention on her own special areas of interest. By year's end when I was required to renew our representative appointments with the UN NGO office Danieli decided to withdraw as our Senior (in UN parlance,"Main") Representative to UN New York, understanding that Greene, by now a proven organization builder, was ready to take her place. Thus it happened that less than a year after starting to work with us Greene became our Senior, i.e,. Main, Representative to UN Headquarters in New York. The new team which she headed included at one time or another, between 1990 and 1995, fifteen people who served for shorter or longer periods with her as their leader. As she suggested in a summary written at my request, it is impossible in retrospect to do justice to their many contributions. Looking back, though, her five years of work could be understood in terms of two perspectives: "building the WFMH UN NY team, and creating an environment in which comprehensive mental health issues would merit recognition as priorities and deserve the focus of an official NGO Committee." She went about the task of team building through attending meetings of many NGO groups, consulting with UN officials especially those who handled the accreditation of representatives, and scheduling "mentoring" sessions with seasoned representatives in responsible positions. In this way she derived her criteria for effective NGO volunteers: "a strong interest in mental illness and mental health, an aptitude for advocacy, a dedication to volunteerism" and "an understanding that at the UN they would represent WFMH issues and policies and not their personal agendas" (Greene, 1997). The aim was to find a WFMH representative for each committee in order to deepen the Federations' impact on the work of other NGOs and at the same time broaden its influence across all areas of the UN s system. As new people became available and chose committees for themselves, Greene accompanied each to their first meeting.

   The following account is informed by Greene's summary and by items in the WFMH Newsletters of the period, written mainly on the basis of materials periodically sent by her or by others in our New York group. It affords a picture of the intense Federation activity within the NGO community at UN New York which did a great deal to make mental health issues visible and a matter of concern to UN officials and country representatives after 1991.

In the beginning, despite the years of work by earlier WFMH representatives in New York, and the significant ongoing activity of the WHO's Division of Mental Health in Geneva, Greene encountered "widespread reluctance to discuss mental health issues. The consensus both in the NGO community and the UN system was that mental health was a low or non-priority." In June 1991 Drs. Hedwin Naimark and Selma Sapir, representing the Society for the Psychological Study of Social Issues and the International Council of Psychologists, respectively, asked her if the WFMH would work with them and other organizations over the next few years "to convince the NGO community that mental health issues were of prime importance to everyone" (Greene, 1997). We discussed this, I agreed that an NGO Committee on Mental Health would be an appropriate goal, and arranged a luncheon meeting for her with some of our representatives and relevant UN officers. One of the DPI officers revealed a profound personal interest in mental health, saying that it was necessary to create "a groundswell" by applying mental health issues broadly across many areas of UN work and to link them to a current UN focus. It was to him that she later took her plan for a full-day mental health conference dedicated to UN Secretary General Boutros Boutros-Ghali's "Agenda for Peace." It was to open with a briefing on the 1991 UN Mental Health Resolution,"The Protection of Persons with Mental Illness and the Improvement of Mental Health Care," for which our Geneva representative Stanislas Flache, M.D., had been so active. It was finally realized as a 13 May 1993 conference called "No Peace Without Peace of Mind: Better Mental Health for All" which focused on refugees, victims of natural disasters, the AIDS crisis, and a variety of interrelated issues. Organized by Greene and Linda Pelerin (see below) it was co-sponsored by DPI, WHO and UNESCO. Organizational credit was given to the WFMH for the first such NGO program ever to be printed on UN stationery. Flache identified Lic. Hernan Fuenzalida, chief of the PAHO Legal Office who had already worked with us at the WFMH, as a resource, and, at Greene's invitation, he came to New York to be the UN briefer. Other speakers, besides Greene who served as moderator, included Hilda Robbins, Chair of our WFMH Committee on Mental Health Associations, Paolo del Vecchio, Vice Chair of the World Federation of Psychiatric Users which we had helped form at the Auckland World Congress in 1989, WFMH UN representatives Anie Kalayjian and Alexander Nader (see below), and myself. The event, filling one of the auditoriums at the UN, was an impressive testimony to Greene's organizing ability, and her sense of the WFMH mission.

During 1990, Danieli and Dubrow (who had not yet obtained her doctorate) continued to pursue their particular interests independently of the team which Greene, not yet our senior person, was organizing. For both—as for the new people being recruited—their professional knowledge was essential to their volunteer work. Dubrow was becoming increasingly focused on children in war. She represented us at the 19 February 1991 special session of the NGO Committee on Unicef and participated in planning for their April general and strategic planning meetings, helping to organize a special consultation on 20 April on adult responses to children in time of war. In September 1991 Danieli, as Treasurer of the Alliance of NGOs on Crime Prevention and Criminal Justice, represented the WFMH at the meeting of its International Advisory, Scientific and Professional Council in Milan. At about the same time, although I expressed doubts about her ability to be an effective WFMH liaison to so many groups at the same time, I acceded to her request and appointed her to the newly formed NGO Committee on Indigenous Populations. She also continued to attend the NGO Committee on the Family.

Greene's first team-building recommendation (to me and to still Senior Representative, Danieli) came in April 1991. It was for the recruitment of Nancy E. Wallace, C.S.W., a social worker, active in the field of Employee Assistance and a long time advocate for womens' rights. Wallace chose the NGO Committee on the Status of Women as her special assignment, and by 1992 became its Secretary. Along with Danieli and Greene she attended the Annual Conference of NGOs in September 1991 sponsored by the DPI in which Danieli had remained active. The topic was "Peace, Justice and Development—Ingredients." Among other activities she was the Facilitator of Working Groups on Entrepreneurship and Unemployment, and a member of

Working Groups on Health and Mental Health which Dr. Ricki Kantrowitz (see below) helped organize. As a WFMH representative Wallace attended the 37th Session of the UN Commission on the Status of Women in Vienna in 1993, and its 38th Session in New York in 1994. During its 39th Session she, along with Kantrowitz, took part in a panel on violence against women, where Kalayjian presented a talk on post-traumatic stress disorders. In autumn 1995 she played a leading role in preparations for the NGO Forum and the Fourth World Conference on Women in Beijing, China which she attended as a key member of the WFMH delegation headed by our 1995–1997 President Beverly Long.

In June 1991 Greene recommended Benjamin D. Reese, Jr., Psy. D., Director of Psychology and Clinical Supervisor at the Fifth Avenue Center for Counseling and Psychotherapy who chose to become a member of the NGO Committee on Human Rights. Reese' s background as a consultant in such diverse areas as cultural sensitivity and conflict resolution had taken him to a range of countries. He hosted his own weekly mental health education program and was adept at public communication. However, he stayed with us for less than two years, resigning in 1993 to accept an appointment as Ombudsman for the Rockefeller Foundation which left insufficient time for the demanding volunteer work at the UN.

In July 1991, Greene persuaded Ruth Warrick, a well-known film and television actress, author and consultant for job training programs for school drop-outs during the Kennedy, Johnson and Carter administrations, to take a limited assignment for the 1992 Tenth Anniversary Celebration of the International Plan of Action on Aging. Warrick also became a member of the NGO Committee on Shelter and Community.

In September 1991 Dr. Janice E. Williams, with an M.A. in Psychiatric Nursing and a Ph.D. in Clinical Psychology was recruited by Greene to become the seventh team member. An Adjunct Assistant Professor at the Columbia University School of Social Work and consultant to several programs serving children, she chose to work with the NGO Committee on the Family for which she was elected Vice Chair in 1993. Among other projects she organized three joint programs between the NGO Family, Narcotics and Substance Abuse, and Status of Women Committees, and Unicef. Her service as Chair of the Planning Task Force and NGO-UN Liaison for the 1994 International Year of the Family (IYF) won her an award from Henryk J. Sokalski, the UN-IYF Coordinator in Vienna "in recognition of [her] important contributions towards the cause of families and the promotion of the United Nations Programme on the International Year of the Family." She made an effort to learn about the Federation's activities outside of the UN context, attendeding several meetings, the last the 1993 World Congress in Tokyo. In 1995 serious injuries from an automobile accident ended the UN work of this "gifted and sensitive" person (Greene, 1997).

Meanwhile, Greene, herself, as a member of the Committee organizing the Ten Year Anniversary Conference scheduled for 3 October 1992, was working with the Chief of the NGO section in the DPI. She also extended her reach to build bridges to other organizations. On 14 October 1991 she met in Washington DC with members of the Minority Affairs Division of the American Association for Retired Persons to assist in planning their national research agenda. She also chaired an NGO Committee on Aging Subcommittee on "Mental, Emotional and Spiritual Well-being of the Elderly." This led to her presentation of a workshop entitled "Productive Aging: Conscious Living, Conscious Dying" as part of the Tenth Anniversary Conference.

By December 1991 a new WFMH- UN team had come together largely because of Greene's recruiting, organizing and nurturing skills. It was increasingly evident that we would want to formalize new leadership for the group which was becoming a cohesive unit under her leadership. In this month she also brought aboard Linda N. Freeman, M.D., a child psychiatrist who was the Marion E. Kenworthy Assistant Professor of Psychiatry at the Columbia University School of Social Work. Recipient of several national awards, including an NIMH Minority Fellowship, she had co-authored a book and produced an award winning television series. She accepted many WFMH assignments including the NGO Committee on Youth and those involving the UN Conference on Environment and Development in Brazil, the NGO Committee on Sustainable Development and the NGO Committee for the International Year of the World's Indigenous Peoples for which she helped organize an NGO briefing on 8 October 1992. In the summer of that year she also visited Brazil for the NGO Committee on Unicef's Sub-working Group on Exploited Children. However, with the birth of her first child, she left both her professional and volunteer careers for full-time motherhood.

Each year's start was reappointment time for NGO representatives to the UN. Danieli indicated that she did not expect to stay on as our Senior Representative. In 1992, after several consultations with her and with the agreement of the WFMH Executive Committee, I appointed Greene as our Main Representative to ECOSOC and Wallace as Main Representative to DPI. Danieli remained a member of the team, immersing herself more deeply in the Alliance, participating in a 10–14 March 1992 consultation at the University of Limburg in the Netherlands on the right to restitution and rehabilitation for victims of human rights violations, and representing us at the first session of the Commission on Crime Prevention and Control at the Vienna International Center on 21–30 April. She also served on the Advisory Committee of the UN Environmental Programme's 1992 Global Youth Forum held in the UN General Assembly Hall on 14–15 May. As time went on, though, she began to shift her identification away from the WFMH reflecting her greater personal and professional involvement with the Society for Traumatic Stress Studies, and its new overarching International Association which was initiating moves towards its own UN associate status.

A major NGO project was preparation for the 1994 UN international Conference on Population and Development in which our WFMH Committee on Responsible Parenthood chaired by Henry David and co-chaired by Lucile Newman had a special interest. David had attended the first UN conference in Bucharest in 1974 and, for the first time as our official representative, in Mexico City in 1984. He would attend this one scheduled for 5–13 September 1994 in Cairo in the same capacity. The first NGO planning meeting at UN New York was held on 12 March 1992 with Newman and Greene in attendance for the WFMH. I was not able to attend follow-up conferences and Greene, sometimes with Newman or David, maintained the WFMH connection. Formal consultations by the Conference planners did take place with the WFMH through David in 1993. WFMH contributions included attention to the importance of mental health, issues of wantedness, care and support at the beginnings of life, family wellbeing, the position of women in society, and problems of migration and refugees.

In April 1992 Greene, now our officially designated Main representative to ECOSOC (and informally, along with Wallace, to DPI as well as the rest of UN New York) asked Alexander Nader, former Orientation Officer for Displaced Persons at the U.S. State Department in Germany, to assist her with her work with DPI and the NGO Committee on Aging. He agreed and chaired a Sub-Committee on Media, Promotions, and Public Relations of the aging group. A graduate of the Georgetown University School of Foreign Service with an M.A. from the American University in Beirut in Middle Eastern and Islamic Studies, he was a devoted worker for WFMH causes until his premature death in 1994.

In September 1992, Linda P. Pelerin, a lawyer currently on leave from studies in anthropology and psychology at the University of Michigan, came on special assignment to DPI to produce videos on UN/NGO collaboration, now part of the UN Film Library. At Greene's suggestion she was appointed WFMH representative to the NGO Committee on Disarmament. Her most important contribution to us was making her UN contacts available to our WFMH team. She returned to Michigan in 1993.

In November 1992 Dr. Anie Sanentz Kalayjian with degrees in nursing, psychosocial gerontology and mental health education became the 12th member of the WFMH team. Founder and President of the Armenian American Society for Studies on Stress and Genocide her collaborative research covered Armenia, the Netherlands and Russia. She joined the NGO Committee on

Human Rights and was elected its Secretary in 1994. She also served as Corresponding Secretary for the NGO Committee on the UN University for Peace and the Unicef Working Group on Children in Especially Difficult Circumstances for which she compiled international NGO position statements on child labor. One of the most vocal and committed workers on the WFMH team, Kalayjian continued throughout her work with us to be a passionately committed advocate for the Armenian cause.

In the fall of 1992, again under the auspices of the American Ambassadors Program, I had escorted a group of WFMH members on visits to psychiatric personnel and institutions in Poland, Hungary and Czechoslovakia. One was Haydee Montenegro-Gonzalez, Psy. D., who identified herself as a forensic psychologist. We talked about the Federation and I suggested that she get in touch with Greene. This she did and in March 1993 she became our representative to the Alliance, where Danieli, still our representative, served as Vice Chair. By 1994 Montenegro's energy and intelligence led to her election as Secretary in 1994. In 1995 she participated in preparations for the Ninth UN Congress on the Prevention of Crime and Treatment of Offenders held in Egypt.

With increasing exposure to the UN system, Greene became interested in the overall issue of effective NGO-UN relationships, a topic which emerged regularly in UN conferences. On 5 August 1992 she joined Danieli at a meeting of CONGO, the Conference of NGOs in Consultative Status to the Economic and Social Council, which addressed this issue. Danieli volunteered to serve on a committee to review situations where NGOs, singly or in groups, had interacted successfully with UN delegations. One opportunity for direct influence came at the 15–16 October 1992 General Assembly discussion on aging when members of the Committee, including Greene, addressed representatives of member states immediately following adjournment of the formal opening ceremonies. Another was the 13 May 1993 mental health conference organized by Greene with DPI cooperation. Yet an additional opportunity came with her appointment in early 1993 as Chairperson for the UN International Day of the Elderly scheduled for the autumn.

A new team member recruited by Greene in May 1993 was Dianne Davis, Ph.D., board member of several organizations, co-author of "Hospitable Design for Healthcare and Senior Communities" and designer of a program using NGO volunteers to support the work of DPI. We appointed her as our representative to the NGO Committees on Shelter and Community and on Aging where she became Chair of the Communications Subcommittee. In that capacity she organized a conference at UN Headquarters on 10–11 January 1995 on "Better Living—Adding Life to Years" where Greene moderated a session promoting intergenerational links. This was the first in a series of international meetings focused on city planning initiatives to create integrated neighborhoods supportive of older persons who, ideally, would participate in a full range of community activities. Her primary affiliation was with the International Council of Caring Communities, and through it, in cooperation with various UN agencies, she organized conferences at the UN, in Costa Rica and Chile, and was preparing for the 1996 Habitat II Conference in Turkey. While the WFMH was not primarily involved in these activities we determined that they did further our broadly conceived mission, and gave them whatever publicity and support we could.

The last UN representative brought in by Greene was psychologist Ricki Kantrowitz, Ph.D., of Boston. In May 1993 she asked Greene if she could work on women's issues for the WFMH at the UN. Wallace brought her on to the NGO Committee on the Status of Women, where she became a member of the WFMH team.

In the April/May 1993 number of our Newsletter Greene reported that "mental health concerns are mentioned more frequently at UN meetings." Williams arranged a program on family involvement in rehabilitation of their mentally ill relatives which elicited favorable comment. Wallace, at a March 1993 consultation at UN Vienna preparing for the 1995 NGO Forum on Women, was co-facilitator of a workshop addressing psychological trauma in female victims of violence. Greene spoke to the New York NGO Committee on the Status of Women on "Women's Attitudes Towards Themselves: A Key to World Mental Health."

On 8–10 September 1993 Greene was Vice President of the DPI's NGO Conference which dealt with poverty, unemployment and social integration. It included representatives from all of the UN regions and marginalized and activist groups from the United States. In his keynote address to the Conference's opening session UN Secretary General Boutros Boutros-Ghali mentioned "mental health rights," noted that the WHO and UNESCO "work in close consultation with the World Federation for Mental Health" and referred to the recent contractual arrangement between the UN High Commissioner for Refugees (UNHCR) and the WFMH (see below). In preparing his remarks he utilized the references to the WFMH and its UN affiliations in an outline submitted by Greene. This working relationship, reminiscent of that between WFMH and the UN agencies in the Rees era, was referred to by DPI staff as "unprecedented" (Greene, 1997).

In early 1994 there was an unanticipated challenge to NGO team building when, in response to a series of security threats, the UN declared that ECOSOC organizations would be limited to a Main Representative and four Alternates. Elena Berger in my office spent a great deal of time on the telephone with Greene and the UN NGO office, and eventually secured continuing accreditation for our then six representatives for the current year. Later Greene learned how to obtain official approval for seven entry badges and how to bring in additional uncredentialed representatives. By this time Berger had established good telephone relations with her and members of her group as well as with the relevant UN staff, and was able to deal independently with most of the administrative issues arising there. WFMH President Elect Beverly Long (to become President in 1995) was also establishing her own relationships with our UN group. Her work and that of Berger freed me to a considerable degree from liaison responsibility for the UN group, but I did my best to remain informed and offer programmatic suggestions when possible.

Greene, now widely identified as an effective, conscientious contributor to the NGO community continued to accept added responsibilities which consumed her already limited time. She was elected Vice President of the NGO/DPI Executive Committee and Editor of the NGO/DPI Reporter the Committee's quarterly Newsletter for the NGO community. In addition she accepted an appointment as President and Chair of the Planning Committee for the 47th Annual DPI/NGO Conference scheduled for 20–22 September 1994 at UN Headquarters to coincide with the opening of the General Assembly. Davis and Kalayjian assisted her, but the basic responsibilities for these enterprises could not be delegated. The conference theme, following a recurrent concern, focused on collaboration between NGOs and the UN, this time in pursuit of global human security, broadly defined. Entitled,"We the Peoples: Building Peace," it offered an unusual opportunity for an exchange of ideas between NGOs and UN officers. Among the speakers were UN Secretary General Boutros Boutros-Ghali; President of the Republic of Ireland, Mary Robinson; Astronaut Valentina Tereshkova, the first woman in space; and Bianca Jagger who was working as a human rights advocate on behalf of women and children in former Yugoslavia. Greene addressed the opening session and gave the official summary speech on the last day, relying on notes provided by a team of 35 rapporteurs who had attended all of the sessions. She concluded: "Institutions…must function under an agenda for peace that has, at its center, the protection of human rights." Following this success Greene was appointed as an Advisor to the Planning Committee for the 1995 DPI/NGO Conference and its ex-officio President.

The most encouraging harbinger of future collaboration between NGOs in the cause of mental health came in early 1995 with the establishment of a Mental Health Consortium (also known as a Caucus on Psychosocial Issues) made up of groups including the International Council of Psychologists, a WFMH voting member organization. The intent was to provide support and signatures for UN-initiated advocacy moves with mental health significance. Greene and Kalayjian, now Secretary Treasurer of the NGO Committee on Human Rights, also tried to create a CONGO or Task Force Subcommittee of organizations devoted to mental health-related human rights issues which could collaborate with a counterpart subcommittee at UN Geneva which our Representative Stanislas Flache was trying to organize. A primary goal would be to promote the implementation of UN Resolution 46/119,"The Protection of Persons with Mental Illness and the Improvement of Mental Health Care." This effort fit Kalayjian's work at the NGO Committee on Human Rights where she had recently helped to organize panels on the prevention of discrimination against minorities and on women's rights. In mid-1995 Flache did establish a Special CONGO Committee of International NGOs on Human Rights of the Mentally Ill in Geneva (Greene, 1997).

In this spring of 1995 our UN New York representatives were active on many fronts. The 9th UN Congress on the Prevention of Crime and Treatment of Offenders took place in Cairo, Egypt from 29 April to 8 May. Our NGO Crime Prevention Committee representative, Montenegro, was involved in planning some of its auxiliary meetings with former President Gamal El Azayem, M.D. Our Unicef Representative Nancy Dubrow, who had by now received her Ph.D., participated in a panel on "Reintegration of Children Following Wars and Other Situations of Community Violence" presenting her recently completed Unicef supported study, "Child Soldiers in Liberia: An Exploratory Study of the Psychological Effects of Participating in War." The panel was chaired by Yael Danieli, who had finally severed her ties with us to represent the International Society for Traumatic Stress Studies.

On 15 May 1995 a Harvard produced volume on mental health in low-income countries, for which both Beverly Long and I (among a great many others) had been consultants, was officially released at a special briefing at UN Headquarters addressed by Secretary General Boutros Boutros Ghali. He stated that the report "puts the issue of mental health and well-being firmly on the international agenda…Psycho-social disorders affect the development and the peace and security of many societies. The international community must mobilize to address them." Elaborating on this theme in his closing remarks, he stated that "when the United Nations promotes sustainable human development, it is working to remove some of the root causes of mental distress." The WFMH delegation to this briefing led by President Elect Beverly Long included Greene and Deputy Secretary General Richard Hunter. In order to underscore WFMH participation in this event Long decided that we should give Professor Arthur Kleinman, the moving force behind the Harvard volume, the first WFMH Good Citizenship Award. This was done with modest fanfare at our May 1996 spring Reception at the Finnish Embassy in Washington, DC.

The book launching at the UN was the last major event which Greene attended as our Senior and Main Representative to UN Headquarters, New York. Not long thereafter, in August 1995 just before the Dublin World Congress, she submitted her resignation in order to have more time to devote to other activities including family matters. But she departed with a sense of achievement. As she put it, the Secretary General's words told us that "the long battle to establish an official NGO Committee on Mental Health at UN New York would soon be won" (Greene, 1997).

With Greene's decision to relinquish her post, we were faced once more with the problem of UN New York leadership. After much discussion Long and I agreed that Greene's first nominee to the WFMH UN team, Nancy Wallace, should be designated as its new Main Representative. Her nomination was unanimously confirmed by the Board which met prior to the World Congress. Wallace, herself, was eager for the new responsibilities, although they did not significantly change her activities. She was already deeply and extensively involved in a variety of UN projects and her life within the NGO community was already integrated with that outside it.

Many of her UN projects anticipated the NGO Forum (30 August–8 September) and the World Conference on Women (4–15 September) scheduled for Beijing, China. In the late spring I had reminded then President Elect Long of this event, suggesting that she should lead the WFMH delegation for which much of the preparatory work had already been undertaken by Wallace with the important collaboration of Kantrowitz. After assuming the WFMH presidency in Dublin, Long began her involvement in the Beijing events by joining the thousands who sent messages to the UN Secretary General and the China Organizing Committee protesting the banishment of NGOs to a remote site with inadequate facilities and accommodations. She also participated with Wallace and colleagues in the preparation of a WFMH Resolution urging governments to include mental health needs, services and rights of women in the forthcoming Platform for Action. The Resolution was adopted by the WFMH Board meeting in Dublin, on 19 August 1995.

The final WFMH delegation to Beijing included five official volunteer observers: Long; Wallace, Kalayjian and Kantrowitz of our UN New York team; and Susan Feldman, M.A. of Melbourne, affiliated with our Collaborating Center on Women's Health there. Six others in the delegation were interested WFMH members who had asked to be included. With the addition of former WFMH President Estefania Aldaba-Lim, as a government delegate representing the Philippines, they were able to engage in effective advocacy with government delegates and UN agencies. The advocacy focus was two-fold: first, to educate and raise awareness by introducing in the Platform document the words "physical and mental health" to replace "health" wherever it appeared; and second, to include the provision of counseling services in relevant sections such as violence against women, and migrant and refugee women. The WFMH conducted a standing-room only workshop on "Mental Health and Women in a Global Context," moderated by Long and led by Wallace and Kantrowitz. It also led a mental health caucus attended by approximately 100 women from diverse cultural, religious, social and professional backgrounds. The September 1995 WFMH Newsletter carried a report of the Beijing activities and a copy of the WFMH Resolution. The impact of the meeting continued in New York as our representatives who had been there were all featured speakers at community and college programs and several wrote articles for newspapers and magazines. Wallace, Montenegro and Kalayjian were all elected to leadership positions in their NGO Committees.

Post Beijing activities continued through the end of the year and into 1996. In January, Long and Wallace met with members of the U.S. President's Interagency Council on Women which was charged with coordinating the federal implementation of the Beijing Platform for Action. The WFMH recommended that the Council give mental health programs priority in regard to health, economic security and violence against women. Following Diane Davis' lead other members of the team also became involved in planning for Habitat II, the second UN Conference on Human Settlements scheduled for Istanbul, Turkey from 3–14 June 1996. At the request of CONGO and DPI, Wallace as a representative of the NGO Committee on the Status of Women discussed linkages between the Beijing Conference and Habitat II.

Meanwhile, the NGO-UN relationship, particularly with ECOSOC, was an increasingly intense focus for discussion, both at the NGO and the UN level. The concern, occasionally arising in earlier years, about how if at all the activities within the NGO community actually influenced the UN, faded into the background. Our team's preparation for closer collaborative work with the UN itself was facilitated by Long's decision to make it one of the major concerns of her WFMH presidency. On 19 November 1995, after taking office during the Dublin World Congress in July, she met with the UN New York group to discuss policy and procedures and the future role of WFMH representation at the UN. On the next day they attended a special session of ECOSOC honoring the UN's 50th anniversary. Addressed by the Secretary General and sponsored by CONGO, a coalition of NGO Committees, and the DPI/NGO Executive Committee, it was entitled "The NGO/UN Partnership—the Way Forward." An audio-visual link to a parallel meeting in Geneva enlarged the meeting.

A major triumph for the WFMH and the other mental health NGOs, with the WFMH contributions building on the work of Kay Greene followed by Nancy Wallace, was the establishment of a new UN NGO Committee on Mental Health in New York. CONGO voted in its favor at its meeting of 28 May 1996. The work of the Committee was expected to be primarily education and advocacy in the prevention of mental illness, the promotion of psychological well-being and the improvement of mental health care services. In this sense its proposed agenda overlapped significantly with that of the contemporary WFMH. It would also cooperate with other CONGO

Committees, and the UN, to ensure the inclusion of mental health issues within a broad context of concerns such as human rights, poverty, violence, children, refugees and substance abuse. Wallace was asked to serve as Convenor for an Interim Bureau to develop the Committee's structure, mission and By Laws, and prepare for the future election of permanent officers. At the same time she and all of the members of the WFMH team continued their involvement in other areas: human rights, children in difficult circumstances, the interface of mental health and housing, and the status of women. Kalayjian as workshop coordinator of the annual DPI conference in September was the facilitator for a discussion on "Conflict Resolution." Davis spoke at an October Conference on Gerotechnology in Finland. Another WFMH member, Tom Dessereau began, with Wallace's encouragement, to attend meetings of the revitalized NGO Committee on Narcotics and Substance Abuse, as well as ECOSOC's sessions on the matter in an unofficial capacity.

By autumn 1996 the Interim Bureau of the Mental Health Committee included representatives of nine associations including the WFMH. One of its first program activities was preparation for a 10 October, World Mental Health Day NGO Briefing in collaboration with DPI on "Women and Mental Health." Wallace's 1996 activities report to my office notes the very high level of interest in the new Committee's future course and significance. Of greatest significance for the future power of NGOs was a new resolution by ECOSOC governing the arrangements for consultation with NGOs. In the fall of 1996 WFMH representatives had been engaged in active dialogue with representatives of other NGOs, governments and members of the UN secretariat during ongoing meetings of at least three groups. These were,"The Future Role of the ECOSOC Committee on NGOs," the "Open-Ended Working Group on the Review of Arrangements for Consultation with NGOs" and "Meetings on the Future of CONGO." All dealt with how NGOs could gain greater access and strengthen their influence ("cooperation and collaboration") within the UN process. A nodal point was an October meeting of the chairs of CONGO with the President of the UN General Assembly and the chairs of its main committees to discuss how NGOs might more effectively participate in the work of the General Assembly.

By spring 1997 Wallace had been elected the first chairperson of the new NGO Committee on Mental Health at UN Headquarters, New York and a new chapter in NGO-UN relations seemed to be at hand.

THE WFMH AND UN VIENNA, 1981–1997

Among the many posts which needed filling in 1981 was that of liaison person between the WFMH and the UN's Center for Social Development and Humanitarian Affairs (CSDHA) which remained in Vienna until 1993–1994 when the bulk of its operations were moved to UN Headquarters in New York.

The Center's title suggested that its aims might overlap with ours and its component units heightened that impression. They dealt with Aging, Youth, Disabled Persons and "Developmental Social Welfare." However, repeated inquiries from my office yielded little to illuminate their goals and activities and no indication about the role of NGOs in relation to CSDHA. Further, unlike UN New York, I could not take the train from Baltimore and evaluate the situation for myself. Under the circumstances we were fortunate to have two colleagues, Drs. Springer-Kremser and Jandl-Jager to represent us. But our communication was only occasional and, seemed to confirm that there was no well defined role for NGOs in Vienna. This, coupled with the fact that my energies were almost totally consumed with the effort to sustain the Federation's operating capacity and with preparations for the 1983 World Congress in Washington, DC, contributed to a tendency to treat the undemanding Vienna office with "benign neglect."

By the end of 1983, with the Congress over, the new Baltimore-Washington Secretariat established, and my move to the post of WFMH Secretary General completed, the problem of Vienna UN representation again emerged. But again, it was a low priority. Perhaps in part because of this, Springer-Kremser and Jandl-Jager concluded by 1985 that they could not give the necessary time to develop a relationship on behalf of the distant WFMH with the relatively disinterested Vienna Center. However, they were good enough to recruit two volunteers with more time and greater motivation to replace them. These were the Chairman of the Austrian Association of Families of the Mentally Ill, Mr. Kurt Kirszen and his Deputy, Dr. Maria Dorothea Simon, a clinical psychologist and retired Dean of the University of Vienna School of Social Work. In time. Kirszen dropped out, but Simon remained, despite many competing demands for her time. These included her work, beginning in 1991, as Director of the Austrian Association of Relatives and Friends of the mentally ill. But this, and the fact that her own adult son suffered from schizophrenia, served to strengthen rather than weaken her ties to us. Her personal interest in addition to her professional accomplishments which commanded significant local respect were important in her capacity to act as our liaison person. In response to my request she wrote a summary of her years as our representative, and much of what follows is adapted from her account (Simon, 1997). Additional material comes from my own records and the WFMH Newsletters produced by my office.

Discovering at the outset that the Director of the Vienna Center was opposed to the idea of an NGO Committee for Mental Health, Simon decided to organize an informal group of motivated persons to participate in the activities of the several NGO Committees concerned with social and health issues. It s objectives were monitoring the activities and discussions of already established NGO Committees; providing appropriate input about mental health aspects; joining forces when possible in regard to particular resolutions and actions; and participating actively in meetings and conferences of the various UN bodies taking place in Vienna.

It was difficult to recruit a team because many interested people lacked the requisite facility in English or were too busy at their jobs. Some who did join left because they found the tasks unrewarding. This, as Simon saw it, was due to the difficulty in establishing a working relationship with UN personnel. "It was difficult even to understand the workings of the organization (e.g. who is who, who does what, what are the rules?)" (Simon, 1997). In her first year of representing us Simon made a point of attending the 1985 Brighton World Congress where we had a chance to meet and talk briefly about the Vienna situation. I was impressed with her overall grasp of mental health issues, with, understandably, a special focus on psychiatric research and the problems of familial caregivers for young adults with severe, chronic mental illness. But the CSDHA, itself, was not very helpful, providing only a single briefing for NGO volunteers in 1985–1986. On 12 December 1986 her interest was stimulated by a meeting on "Violence in the Family" with special emphasis on its effects on women. Her report on this event for our Newsletter served to alert our membership both to the topic and the existence of UN Vienna. This was the first of a valuable series of reports which she contributed.

Despite frustrations Simon was successful in finding interested and highly qualified people. This made it possible for the WFMH to be regularly represented at several key NGO Committees during the Center's stay in Vienna. These were the Committees on Aging (Dr. Vijaya Rao and Marion Kalousek, M.D.), Disabled Persons (Simon and Ernst Berger, M.D.), and the Family (Dr. Monika Vysloucil who also represented Help Age International). There was also intermittent liaison with the Committees on the Status of Women (Drs. Vysloucil, Beate Wimmer-Puchinger, Hilde Rosenmayer and Ms. Rosa Loger), Narcotic Drugs and Psychotropic Substances (Peter Herrman, M.D., Simon and Mrs. Marlene Prenzan), and Youth (Gertraud Czerwenka-Wenkstetten, M.D.). Kalousek, a senior psychiatrist and geriatric specialist was intermittently active throughout the whole period. In early 1993 at the suggestion of WHO's Regional Office for Europe she prepared a brochure on the symptoms of depression with special attention to the needs of care-givers for advice. Wimmer-Puchinger, a colleague from the International Society for Psychosomatic Obstetrics and

Gynecology joined the group in June 1988 and was active for a time. Hermann, a psychiatrist and director of a substance abuse clinic, joined the group in mid-1992. Berger, a child psychiatrist came aboard later in the same year. Czerwenka-Wenkstetten, with advanced training in psychotherapy and family therapy, was particularly interested in the political aspects of promoting mental health prevention. Most representatives communicated directly with me, at Simon's request, as well as with her, and my office also heard from time to time from UN officials in Vienna. Eduardo Vetere of the Crime Prevention and Criminal Justice Branch of the UN Center had been especially interested in the Federation's earlier efforts, headed by Yael Danieli to promote the Declaration of Basic Principles of Justice for Victims of Crime and Abuse of Power. This meant that the WFMH Newsletter regularly carried stories about happenings at UN Vienna. Rao, a major Newsletter contributor left Vienna in August 1990 to accept a teaching position at Weslyan University in West Virginia, USA.

The group of representatives convened by Simon met monthly until 1993–1994 when CSDHA was moved to New York. They exchanged information about the work of their NGO Committees, discussed relevant policy issues (e.g. in regard to family planning or bioethics), and considered how they might raise the visibility of mental health. The meetings also afforded opportunities for Simon to distribute WFMH materials which my office sent regularly to her. She secured a wide dissemination among Vienna based NGOs of the WFMH Luxor Declaration of Human Rights and Mental Health and the UN Resolution on the Protection of Persons with Mental Illness and the Improvement of Mental Health Care. After the Luxor Declaration was revised and officially adopted by the Federation at its New Zealand World Congress in 1989, Simon distributed copies of it during the 11 December 1989 celebration of Human Rights Day at UN Vienna and discussed the Federation's efforts in this field with Austrian Justice Minister Egmont Foregger, and Mr. H. Sokalski, Director of the UN Division of Social Development.

She identified several of her group's activities as worthy of note (Simon, 1997). Between 1988 and 1992 Rao and Vysloucil were especially active in the NGO Committees on Aging and the Family respectively. Vysloucil became the editor of a newsletter, *Families International*, in which she accorded a prominent place to mental health issues. Both took part in the NGO Consultations on the Status of Women and the Commission on the Status of Women. In October 1989 Rao became chairperson of the Vienna NGO Committee on Aging. In this capacity, and before, she contributed to many discussions regarding the International Plan of Action on Aging, also a major concern of our representatives to the NGO Committee on Aging at UN New York.

Simon's own activities centered on the NGO Committee on Disabled Persons and she was involved in meetings, conferences and consultations in connection with both the Year and the Decade of the Disabled. She represented us at the 1989 and 1993 sessions of the Commission on Social Development and in 1992 participated in the NGO Consultative Meeting on Disability preceding the Tenth International Meeting on the UN Decade of Disabled Persons where she delivered written and oral reports about relevant WFMH activities.

The 1992–1993 meetings led to a plan for closer cooperation between members of the WFMH group and representatives of the Richmond Fellowship International, and the recently reactivated World Association for Psychosocial Rehabilitation (WAPR). In May 1992 the group assisted with arrangements for a symposium on Children and Youth with Disabilities, at which team member Ernst Berger was a featured speaker.

After CSDHA's relocation to New York, the WFMH team at UN Vienna effectively dissolved. However, during 1996–1997, without formally joining it, Simon attended meetings of the remaining NGO Committee on Narcotic Drugs, acquainting it with the WFMH objectives and activities. She has continued to be a voice and a listening post for the WFMH with the remaining UN Vienna offices.

TOWARD A NEW PHASE IN WFMH—WHO RELATIONS: NATIONS FOR MENTAL HEALTH

At the 1995 World Health Assembly, Norman Sartorius, M.D. (who had resigned as WHO Mental Health and Substance Abuse Director to become a Professor of Psychiatry at the University of Geneva) was replaced by Jorge Alberto Costa e Silva, M.D., of Brazil. This coincided with the development of a new program, Nations for Mental Health (NMH), financed by a two million dollar grant from Eli Lilly and Company. It was intended to initiate programs suggested by the Harvard Report on world mental health. In remarks, which I published in the WFMH Newsletter, Stanislas Flache asked that the WHO be given "executive responsibility" for administering the new program. This request moved incoming WFMH President Long to note that it had not been discussed with the Board and did not represent WFMH policy.

She began to deal directly with new WHO Mental Health Director, Costa e Silva and his head of the NMH program, Benedetto Saraceno, M.D., by-passing Flache. With new WFMH Board member, psychologist Dr. John Gates, Director of the Carter Center's mental health program, she discussed the possibility of the WFMH Committee on Women Leaders led by former First Lady Rosalynn Carter appearing at a meeting of PAHO Health Ministers in order to raise their awareness of the need for mental health programs. We had a meeting, organized by John Gates, with the Carter Center group and several WFMH representatives on 15 January 1996 and agreed that the idea was a good one, and that an appropriate focus, compatible with one of the Harvard Report's themes, would be womens' status and mental health. The new WHO-Geneva team embraced the proposition, the details were organized by the PAHO staff and a coordinator, Marilou McPhedran, LLD of Toronto (reflecting a corporate Toronto source of funding for the meeting), and the event was held at PAHO headquarters on 26 September 1996 immediately after the annual PAHO meeting of regional health ministers—several of whom were able to be present. Twenty-five countries sent representatives, including eight First Ladies who spoke or were discussion leaders. The main plenary was addressed, among others, by WHO Director General, Hiroshi Nakajima, M.D., WFMH President Long, and PAHO Director, Sir George Alleyne, M.D. who suggested a relationship between this meeting, the Declaration of Caracas six years earlier, and its PAHO followup in Panama earlier in 1996. The official convenors of the meeting were the WFMH and the Carter Center, in co-sponsorship with the WHO, PAHO and the Harvard University Department of Social Medicine. It was the regional launching of the new NMH program of the WHO intended to bring UN agencies together with NGOs to work on designated projects with special reference to mental health in national public health policies and the improvement of mental health care.

This was the beginning of a new phase in the WFMH-WHO relationship based on Costa e Silva's and Saraceno's recognition of the WFMH as the most reliable, genuinely global, and representative mental health NGO. It also recognized the social and political potency of the WFMH Committee of Women Leaders in Mental Health headed by Rosalynn Carter. Within the WFMH it underscored the importance of John Gates as the Carter Center's mental health leader. The next step in this new era was to be the WHO's invitation of Long and Gates to its Regional Meeting in Hong Kong to explore the possibility of a similar activity there. This was deferred, but another event was arranged for the last day of the 1997 World Congress for Mental Health in Finland. The Congress was to be held in Lahti, an hour away from Helsinki, but a WFMH-WHO meeting with the First Lady's Committee was to be held with a limited attendance in Helsinki on 12 July 1997. During preliminary planning for this event at the time of the Airlie House retreat in May (see Chapter 5), there was a generally good feeling about the WFMH's relationship with WHO Mental Health—that it was, indeed, unique among the mental health advocacy NGOs in its relation to WHO as it had been in its founding years. It was the organization chosen to achieve the heightened awareness by governmental health ministries which was a major aim of NMH. At the same time we realized that this conclusion was uncertain and were prepared to cooperate with the UN health agencies during the inevitable shifts in outlook and context which would occur as the century ended.

Part II

REGIONS AND REGIONALIZATION

Regionalization: The Concept and Its Elaborations in the Caribbean and Latin America

GEOGRAPHICAL CONSIDERATIONS

In 1948–1949, the World Health Organization (WHO) began creating its regional structure. As indicated in Appendix III, this began with agreements for the integration of WHO into the Alexandria, Egypt Sanitary Bureau; it became the WHO Eastern Mediterranean Region in July 1948. The PanAmerican Sanitary Organization became the PanAmerican Health Organization (PAHO/WHO) on 24 May 1949. Asia was divided into Western Pacific and Southeast Asian Regions. A last agreement was for the regional office for Europe in May 1954.

The World Federation for Mental Health (WFMH) did not follow the model exactly, dividing itself into six regions: Africa, Asia, Australia, Europe, North/Central America, and South America. This division was intended to facilitate more effective two-way communication between the Board, the Secretariat, and member associations in the various regions; to encourage participation in local/regional mental health relevant activities; to empower local groups; and to decentralize administratively for efficient action. Although there was no formal position of regional vice president, an effort was made to approach equable geographic representation within the membership of the Executive Board. The focus was not on regions as entities in themselves but on the member organizations, encouraging them to establish and maintain a working relationship with the Secretariat, the Executive Board, and the Interprofessional Advisory Committee. One way of encouraging such relationships was suggested by H.C. Rumke, M.D., Professor and Chairman of Psychiatry at the University of Utrecht and first chairman of the Federation's Executive Board. He suggested that when the Executive Board was convened, it should hold public meetings with the national mental health association(s) of the country in which it met. There was also an early concern with the potentially split allegiance of Board members. Would some function primarily as regional representatives or advocates to the Board rather than as members of the global WFMH? In an 11 May 1949 letter to Interprofessional Advisory Committee members, Executive Board member George S. Stevenson, M.D., commented on the effort to have it include representatives from the six continents: "Obviously a member of the Executive Board cannot represent a country [or a Region or a continent] but must represent the interests of the world." Similarly, the 18 February 1954 minutes of the British National Association for Mental Health expressed "concern with the relationship of WFMH to various regional bodies" noting that "regionalization might be undesirable" from the point of view of maintaining the Federation's global status and outlook.

It appears that the original forerunner of the system of regional representatives was established at the 27–28 August 1950 Executive Board meeting in Paris. This was the newly established Credentials Committee chaired by E. E. Krapf, M.D., of Argentina. It had six members representing each of the WHO/WFMH continental regions. The rest of the Board constituted the Finance and General Purposes Committee. The Credentials Committee (as well as that on General Purposes) did not survive for long, however, and 21 years elapsed before formal regional representation on the Board was initiated in 1971.

Meanwhile, WHO was uncertain about the optimal dimensions of its regional divisions. In 1950, it combined the Americas into a single region under the PAHO, which had existed earlier as the PanAmerican Sanitary Bureau.

But the WFMH Board was not satisfied that the new WHO megaregion of the Americas accurately reflected the situation on the ground. Instead of combining the Americas into a single unit, the WFMH Board chose the opposite solution: dividing it, first, into two (retaining the North America/Central America unit) and, then, into three Regions, based on differences in socioeconomic development, culture, and geography. These were continental South America; North America, including the United States, Canada, and Bermuda; and a new Caribbean region, including Meso (or Central) America where Mexico was the dominant country.

By 1954, having gained some experience with Board meetings, the first Federation Treasurer and 1954–1955 President, Frank Fremont-Smith, M.D., recognized additional complexities in regional development. He tied its significance to the Federation's overall financing problem, noting that representatives of member associations who attend annual meetings are usually those in a position to travel without financial assistance and may not even be knowledgeable about the interests and needs of their own organization. Nor, upon their return, are they necessarily in a position to communicate an authentic picture of the Federation to their associations. Improving the liaison between member associations, the Executive Board, and the Secretariat, he felt, would require the systematic development of meetings of member associations within regions.

The first part of the world to receive systematic WFMH attention as a region was the Caribbean. Jack Rees had already attended several meetings of the Caribbean Federation for Mental Health (CFMH) and saw work in the region as an opportunity for WFMH to get away from European and North American dominance and extend its influence into a not fully industrialized part of the world. With this in mind, he urged the WFMH Executive Board to hold its 1951 World Congress in the new region and use it as a means of promoting the election of a first Caribbean WFMH President. The only country with resources adequate to hold the desired World Congress and the only one with a prominent mental health leader already involved with the Board was Mexico. The 1951 Congress was held in that country, and its Assembly of voting delegates elected the leading Mexican Professor of Psychiatry, Alfonso Millan, M.D. (see below), as the first "Caribbean" WFMH President (1951–1952). The designation "Caribbean" for the Mexican nation with its Hispanic and Meso-American identity did not seem totally appropriate, but the name and composition of the region remained through Michael Beaubrun's Jamaica-based presidency extending through 1974 (see Chapter 5 and below).

By this time, at the WFMH Annual Meeting in Hong Kong in 1971, revised bylaws had been approved introducing a new office, formally designated as Regional Vice President, one for each region. This was a first step toward a concept of regions understood as geographical areas containing a cluster of national mental health associations with common problems and aspirations.

At the Copenhagen World Congress in 1975, Beaubrun's successor, President Tsung-yi Lin (see Chapter 5) introduced a new "emphasis on regionalization through the promotion of regional programs and the strengthening of the Vice Presidents' offices" (WFMH, 1975a). In 1978, anticipating the Salzburg Congress of 1979, he said that "the dawn of an active regionalized movement in mental health seems to be at hand" (WFMH, 1978c). During this period, the former Caribbean Region was absorbed into a newly designated Latin American Region, while the United States, Canada, and Bermuda were combined to constitute a North American Region. It was not until the April 1980 Board meeting that a new Oceania Region, encompassing Australia and New Zealand and accepting the possibility of Pacific Island membership, was approved.

However, after I became President in 1981, I was faced with continued questions regarding nomenclature and boundaries within the Americas. In 1982, therefore, I asked Alvaro Gallegos-Chacon, M.D., of Costa Rica, a long-time PAHO consultant and friend from Interamerican Council days, who was broadly knowledgeable about the Americas, to chair an Ad Hoc Committee on Possible Redefinition of the Latin American Region. The Board, meeting on 24–25 April 1984 at Sheppard Pratt Hospital in Baltimore, voted to adopt his suggestion that the Latin American Region be subdivided into a South American and a Central American/Caribbean Region. This, however, was not satisfactory to Mexican colleagues who desired more explicit recognition. Therefore, on 12-13 July 1985, at its meeting in Brighton just before the World Congress, the Board, chaired by outgoing President Estafania Aldaba-Lim, revised the proposal and voted, "in recognition of continuing debate about Mexico's proper geographical designation" to rename the area as the Mexico/Central America/Caribbean Region.

A never fully resolved issue, despite intermittent debate, has concerned the inclusion of island communities, or those socioculturally or politically at odds with most others, in particular WFMH regions. The matter has been treated flexibly in accordance with the requirements of current Federation activities or regional politics. Puerto Rico, for example, although it could be considered part of the North American Region because of its political association with the United States, functioned as part of the Mexico/Central America/Caribbean Region. Questions persist as to whether some of the islands of the Pacific should be considered part of Oceania or of Southeast Asia. Israel, not welcomed by the Arab states of the Federation's Eastern Mediterranean Region, was considered (following the WHO designation) as part of the WFMH European Region. As additional mental health associations are added to WFMH membership, the possibility of further subdividing existing regions also arises. Examples are Europe, where the creation of an Eastern European Region has been considered, and Africa, where new associations are coming from discrete ethnic-linguistic groupings, which may, in time, require new regional designations.

VALUE CONSIDERATIONS: UNIVERSAL AND PARTICULAR, GLOBAL AND LOCAL

Aside from geography, the matter of local values and resources has been important. The WFMH membership includes people with uneven access to resources, linkages to other groups, historical traditions and beliefs, and moral standards. The much-used phrase, "think globally, act locally," requires sufficient knowledge of regional cultures and socioeconomic organization to ensure that programmatic prescriptions are acceptable and can be carried out within the limits of existing resources. However, difficulties persist in reconciling a universal standard with local values to carry out a global program in a locally appropriate and feasible manner.

For example, a value position is inherent in WFMH's advocacy for a universal standard of competent, humane, and dignified health care based on respect for the autonomy and rights of all individuals. It recognizes the rights of minorities, including women. However, some societies, cultures, and governments, despite their subscription to the 1948 UN Universal Declaration of Human Rights and the 1989 WFMH Declaration of Mental Health and Human Rights, constrain the freedoms of their citizens on grounds of gender, sexual orientation, race, ethnicity, nationality, or religion. Lack of resources has been a frequent justification by some regimes for their failure to observe internationally accepted standards of human rights. These issues will be addressed again in the chapters on the international mental health agenda.

ADMINISTRATIVE CONSIDERATIONS AND THE IDEA OF REGIONAL COUNCILS

These aspects of regionalization have been issues in the evolving internal organization of WFMH and its recurrent financial difficulties (reviewed in Chapters 5 and 6). They pose questions of central versus decentralized administration, regional representation, and the functions of Regional Vice Presidents. Recurring questions have included the designation of substitutes. The poor attendance of some Executive Board members, including Vice Presidents, was noted as early as the Rees era, beginning in 1948 and continuing through the end of the Geneva Secretariat in 1967. It was understood that financial requirements and conflicting obligations might make it impossible for Board members to attend every meeting. The problem was met by the election of substitute members, each serving a one-year term. This practice was abandoned with the demise of the Geneva Secretariat and the onset of the era of working presidents.

After the Washington-Baltimore Secretariat was established in 1983, the idea of Board substitutes reemerged on several occasions but was rejected. This despite the complaints of Regional Vice Presidents who sometimes felt themselves perceived as less central than the others in the work of the global governing body and wanted the regions to be represented even when they, personally, could not be present. Lack of personal interest, as in Latin America between 1979 and 1983, and Southeast Asia between 1995 and 1997, did lead the incumbents to send substitutes who were accepted by the Board as observers but were not granted official voting status.

As noted in Chapter 5 and described especially in Chapter 11, the development of WFMH interests in Europe, and the decision of the European League for Mental Hygiene (ELMH) not to join with WFMH, accelerated the movement toward forming a European mental health alliance under WFMH auspices. This fanned the enthusiasm of Board members for regional development in general. As President, I placed the issue on the agenda for the 1983 Board meeting at the time of the Washington DC World Congress for Mental Health. I was very much in favor of it and backed it strongly. The vote was favorable and regionalization became an organizational priority for the Federation. This did not explicitly direct the formation of Regional Councils but was intended to facilitate the work of Regional Vice Presidents, especially to encourage the collaboration of member organizations in Regions. The discussion, thus, included the idea that some kind of Regional office, tentatively called a "Regional Desk," would be essential for the Regional Vice President to operate effectively. As the concept grew from Regional Desk to Regional Council, each Vice President, with the new potential status of the Council's President or Chairperson, acquired what could become a powerful leadership post with a regional constituency. In that context, the Vice Presidents interested in developing such Councils (notably Europe but also Latin America—including South and Central America/Caribbean—Africa and the Eastern Mediterranean) became more active. Oceania, North America (despite having declared a Council), the Western Pacific, and Southeast Asian regions lagged behind. At the 1986 Board meeting in Cumberland Park, England, President Edith Morgan (1985-1987) convened a meeting of Regional Vice Presidents chaired by Vice President for Oceania, Max Abbott, Ph.D., of New Zealand. The group produced a job description for the vice-presidential position, which was published in the WHMH Newsletter, but its requirements were difficult for individuals without office support and have been only variably followed.

Since the early 1990s, the Vice President for Europe has been increasingly occupied with the activities of that Region. A Latin American Council, embracing both the South American and

Mexico/Caribbean/Central American Regions, was formed after the 1991 World Congress in Mexico. Its leaders, exclusively in Mexico, were inevitably more concerned with events in their own country. Despite communication difficulties, contact with mental health (including professional) associations in other Caribbean and Central American nations has been established, mainly by telephone and telegraph, and plans for a General Assembly formulated. With the first South American Regional meeting since 1967 convened in Chile in December 1996 (see below), the Latin American Council began the process of dissolution, changing its name in January 1997 to the Mexico, Central American and Caribbean Regional Council.

At the same time that the Latin American organizing activities began, mainly after the 1991 World Congress in Mexico, hard work against significant odds, and with grossly insufficient financing, resulted in the establishment of the African and Eastern Mediterranean Councils as significant entities (see Chapter 10).

Also in the 1990s, the strength and increasing independence of the European Council (see Chapter 11) led to increasing concern about the future of strong Regional Councils as arms of the global organization embodied in its Board of Directors and Secretariat. The question was raised as to whether WFMH might become, in effect, a federation of Regional Councils, with their member associations belonging to the Councils rather than to the Federation. Some of the uncertainty associated with these general questions became focused in the course of Dick Hunter's attempts to have the European Council submit its financial records to his office and that of the Treasurer. These attempts gave rise to long and intense discussions, by both the 1991 Pre- and Post-Congress Boards in Mexico focusing on the relationship of developing regional councils to the parent body. Incoming President Max Abbott, reviewed the Regional Vice Presidents responsibilities as adopted at the 1986 Board meeting. This review prompted the Board's adoption of several points in principle. Background was the sometimes forgotten fact that the Federation is a legally constituted corporation accountable to the public for all activities and management taking place in its name and that its Board of Directors, including the Regional Vice Presidents, is the body responsible for such accounting. With this background, the Board agreed on several points.

The first point of agreement was that although voting member organizations are independent and not accountable to the corporation, Regional Councils that act in the name of the Federation in raising funds and conducting their business may not consider any of their activities to be private or free from inquiry from the Board, which is ultimately responsible for all actions of a Region taken in the name of WFMH.

Second, it was agreed that the Board in its own public accountability must be able to expect accountability regarding the action of its Councils.

Third, all member associations of Regional Councils must be members of WFMH.

Fourth, all proposals for Regional Council sponsored meetings should be submitted to the Secretary General's office for circulation to the Executive Committee. An earlier decision, already put into practice, required that a WFMH sponsored or cosponsored meeting, which was not sponsored by a Regional Council, be submitted for information and discussion to the Vice President of the Region in which the meeting is to be held. Implicit was the idea that the Council might, if it were appropriate, become a cosponsor of the event.

As noted in Chapters 5 and 11, the European Council, once formed, became especially vigilant in monitoring new European-based WFMH member associations to make sure that they belonged to the Council. In 1995–1996, for example, a new WFMH member, the French Federation for Mental Health, felt itself discouraged by the European Council from relating independently to the WFMH Board and Secretariat. In 1996, similar uncertainties were reported by the Austrian Federation of Mental Health Associations. A problem lay in the organization of the ERC/WFMH's deliberative Assembly with representation allotted by countries so that the delegates, in effect, represented national rather than organizational entities. To avoid such difficulties, WFMH from the beginning had defined itself as a federation not of national/political entities but of associations. As noted elsewhere, this issue, the basis of representation at the general Federation Assemblies, has not been totally resolved.

These organizational concerns, however, have had little impact on the Federation's actual functioning. In its fiftieth year, the evolution of regional groupings has followed a practically feasible, and, except for Europe, relatively informal path. The Councils operate within the framework of WFMH, and member associations are expected to belong to both the regional and the global organization. Reciprocal communication between member associations and the global headquarters, including the Board, may bypass the Regional Council if necessary, although information about the transaction is expected and desired. If the Federation Board cosponsors activities within a Region, the concerned Regional Vice President is notified as a matter of courtesy and information, and the Regional Council, where one exists, is welcome to become a cosponsor if appropriate. United Nations organizations, except for their regional offices, are not regarded as regional but as global entities that interact with the Board and Secretariat rather than the Regional Council.

As described more fully in Chapter 11, the only Council to have achieved a mature, independent status as of the Federation's fiftieth year was that in Europe. This is a consequence in part of the years of preliminary work on a European mental health alliance, with the European League for Mental Hygiene beginning in 1926. However, its accelerated development since 1985 could not have occurred outside the context of the increasing post-World War II movement toward European political unity and without the support of the European Union. No other Council can depend on that kind of context. At the 6–8 May 1996 meeting of the WFMH Executive Committee in Alexandria, Virginia, doubt was expressed as to whether it could be a realistic model for the other regions. The main reason given was that most regions do not have the political infrastructure—the formal relationships between the states within them—that would permit such development. Additionally, the North American Region was not considered comparable to Europe with its many national mental health associations, because it is dominated by two powerful national organizations, one in the United States and one in Canada, that already span the continent. Although the universal applicability of the ERC model was in doubt, there was general agreement that the future effectiveness of WFMH would require strengthening the relationships between the Board and Secretariat on one hand and, on the other, the network of mental health associations that constitute the Federation's heart.

WFMH AND THE CARIBBEAN FEDERATION FOR MENTAL HEALTH: 1948–1968

An Opportunity in the Less Developed World

It was in the Caribbean that WFMH with its historically European base first attempted a systematic expansion of its influence into a new Region. This was initially the work of Jack Rees. He was motivated by several factors. One was his concern that a perception of the new Federation as Eurocentric, and dominated largely by former colonial powers, could detract from the original concept of an egalitarian global mental health organization. The global identity was essential to the ideal of "world citizenship" enshrined in the Federation's founding document, which he regarded as its "bible" (Rees, 1966). Besides, according to Bill Beaty (1995), "Jack always had trouble with the Europeans—they always wanted to do things in their own way." However, the North Americans were also factors as they threatened the pride of the Europeans whose continent they had so recently rescued from the Nazis. There was also the traditional European stereotype of American insensitivity to issues outside of North America. Whatever the reason, there was a general feeling that it would be as detrimental to the Federation goals if it were perceived as "too American" (Beaty, 1995) as if it were regarded as "too European."

Beyond these factors, Rees, following WHO, had a particular interest in mental health in the less industrialized world. Much of that world had neither an infrastructure nor a cultural history conducive to collaboration with an international, voluntary mental health organization. Voluntarism as a concept was unfamiliar. So most of them were effectively out of reach. An exception was the Caribbean basin with its nearby island nations, potential partners in America's backyard. Here the Federation might be able to follow its preferred working style: using others to put into action the ideas for which it was an advocate. Rees, in fact, made a special point of noting that the Caribbean work illustrated "the way in which local activities are developed" (Rees, 1966, p. 120).

The region was also ripe for overall organization, whether in the name of science, mental health, or political self-determination. One factor encouraging a receptive climate for inter-island organization was the high prevalence of family connections between islands, especially among the leaders, political, professional, and artistic, of the various small nations. A salient feature of the late 1940s and early 1950s context was the ideal of political federation, particularly of those islands sharing a connection with the British Commonwealth. The idea of inter-island federation was illustrated in a fictionalized history, *The Black Jacobins* (James, 1938), brought to my attention by Matthew Beaubrun, M.D., of St. Lucie in Paramaribo at the 1971 CFMH meeting, where, at Carstairs' request, I represented WFMH. CFMH President Matthew Beaubrun, a general practitioner, was the cousin of Michael Beaubrun, Professor of Psychiatry at the University of the West Indies (UWI) in Jamaica and an earlier CFMH President. Matthew was also a significant political figure who later became Jamaica's Ambassador to Venezuela. The author of *The Black Jacobins*, C. L. R. James, was a native of Trinidad, Michael's home for many years. He lived in Britain and the United States as well as his home country, developing a reputation as a Marxist author and thinker and a romantic revolutionary. His book, devoted to the Haitian revolution of Toussaint L'Ouverture, was recommended by both Beaubruns as a route to understanding the political ethos of the region. Michael's enthusiasm for the volume during his periods as a CFMH and Federation leader (President 1972–1974) made it seem plausible that WFMH could also be a vehicle for regional political organization.

The Emergence of Mental Health Activities and of Michael Beaubrun

The early awareness of psychological issues in the Caribbean included, as it often has in the less developed world, the study of its culture by outsiders from a more powerful culture. Perhaps the pioneer was anthropologist, Dr. Vera Rubin, head of the Research Institute for the Study of Man based at Columbia University in New York City. However, Western biomedical psychiatry had been a presence in the islands for some years before. An address by Beaubrun to CFMH (Beaubrun, 1994a) and a long letter from him (Beaubrun, 1995) gave many details of the period. His own professional history indicates the strong British influence on the practice of medicine and psychiatry in the Caribbean. After premedical studies at McGill University in Montreal, and graduating in Medicine at Edinburgh University in 1949, he had an assignment for six months with the Professor of Psychiatry, Sir David Henderson, and then returned to the West Indies where he worked in St. Lucie as a District Medical Officer beginning in April 1950. In mid-1951 he spent some time in medicine and surgery at the General Hospital in Trinidad before returning to London to complete his graduate training in psychiatry at the Maudsley Hospital in 1955. Considerable interest in psychiatry and mental health had already surfaced on the island. Psychiatrist Roger de Verteuil, M.D., a Trinidad native, had attended the 1951 WFMH Congress in Mexico City and returned "full of enthusiasm for founding a Mental Health Association." In the following year, 1952, Beaubrun was invited to give radio lectures on mental health and on alcoholism (Beaubrun, 1952, 1957). One of his lectures, printed in the Trinidad Guardian, gave him some notoriety. He had interpreted Carnival as a cathartic strategy for dealing with the frustrations of Caribbean life. The headline alleged that he had described it as "a symptom of our frustration and that our reckless pursuit of hedonism at Carnival symbolized this" (Beaubrun, 1995). This may have had a consciousness-raising effect because at the next Carnival, there appeared a Calypso band called "Dr. Beaubrun's Frustrated Men." Its characters portrayed "artistic poverty," "economic frustration," "racial prejudice," and other factors that he had listed as causes of impaired mental health.

Rees and WFMH, Beaubrun and CFMH

The possibility of WFMH work in the Caribbean arose concretely when Jack Rees was invited, as a specialist in "international psychiatry," to attend the 1956 meeting of the U.S. Group for the Advancement of Psychiatry (GAP). This was a group of so-called "young Turks" founded by William Menninger and others who had been associated with him in the American army. There, as senior officers, they had known their counterparts, Rees from the United Kingdom and Chisholm from Canada. At the time of Rees' visit to GAP, I was one of its younger members, having been recruited in 1952 by Fritz Redlich, M.D., Professor and Chairman of Psychiatry at Yale, where I was an Assistant Professor. Because I had spent some time in school in France as a child and had served as a medical officer in Germany from 1946 until early 1948, I listened with interest to Rees' account of his international work. He impressed me as a superb organizer, a witty and literate person able to inspire colleagues to effort on behalf of an idealistic goal. By that time, also, the Federation was "well advertised" as a source of consultation for international work (Beaubrun, 1992). His presence, therefore, attracted the attention of another guest, Dr. Robert Turfboer, a Dutch physician attached to the Esso Refinery on Aruba.

As Rees recalled the encounter, it led to a meeting at which he, representing WFMH, was one of the ultimate initiators of CFMH. He also mentions the future role of Bertram Schaffner, M.D., in stimulating the development of mental health services under WFMH auspices (Rees, 1966, pp. 120–121): "Dr. Turfboer was largely concerned with the psychosomatic problems of the workers on that multiracial island [Aruba]. We discussed the possibilities of a conference on mental health for the whole Caribbean area to be held at Aruba. Under his leadership, this conference came off in 1957. I presided at an extremely useful meeting out of which grew the idea, then the formation, of the Caribbean Federation for Mental Health (CFMH), now a member of WFMH. The Caribbean Federation has held three further conferences at two-year intervals. With the encouragement and leadership of Dr. Bertram Schaffner of New York, who has dedicated an immense amount of his time as a voluntary consultant to the area, great developments have taken place."

This first, 1957, Caribbean Conference on Mental Health was held with the cooperation of the Virgin Islands and Puerto Rico "under the auspices of WFMH." Its main theme was alcoholism, perhaps reflecting the interests of the U.S. Department of Health Education and Welfare's Caribbean consultant, John Lewis, M.D. Rees was invited in his capacity as WFMH Director, and Otto Klineberg also attended as a WFMH representative.

Beaubrun recalls (1995) that, perhaps because of the notoriety associated with the Trinidad Carnival events, Turfboer had invited him to the 1957 Aruba meeting. However, Earl Lewis, M.D., Senior Psychiatrist at St. Ann's Hospital was chosen as the government representative. Beaubrun became involved afterwards as he spoke at public meetings in Trinidad arranged by the Mental Health Conference steering committee. These helped spur the development of mental health associations throughout the Caribbean. One of the first was the Trinidad and Tobago Association for Mental Health founded by Lewis in 1958. Lewis, who died in 1994 at the age of 86, helped revise his country's mental health laws and chaired its first committee to produce a comprehensive plan for mental health services (Beaubrun, 1994b).

By 1959, a second biennial meeting of the group formed in Aruba was held in St. Thomas. At this time the CFMH was formally launched. Its founding members represented associations in Aruba, Barbados, Haiti, Martinique, Puerto Rico, St. Croix, St. Thomas, and Trinidad and Tobago (Beaubrun, 1995). Rees also attended the 1959 meeting, which featured "a glittering array of internationally famous people" (Beaubrun, 1992, p. 375) including such psychoanalytic notables as Bruno Bettelheim and Eric Erickson. Lewis was elected its first President, and Beaubrun was on the Executive, first as Deputy Chairman and then as Chairman of the Executive Board. Robert Turfboer has been called the father of CFMH, and Eldra Shulterbrandt, Director of Mental Health in the Virgin Islands, its mother (Beaubrun, 1994a).

A third CFMH meeting was held in Jamaica in 1961 with the theme, "The Adolescent in a Changing Caribbean." Aside from its scientific value, it moved Beaubrun along the path that would ultimately bring him to the WFMH Presidency. Although Sir Philip Boyd was elected CFMH President, he was unable to take up the post, and Beaubrun as Executive Board Chairman often acted for him. He was actually elected President in 1963 in Curacao at the fourth Caribbean Conference on the topic, "Family Relationships and Mental Health."

Jack Rees' recollections recognize, but do not pay significant attention to, the intense activity by local professionals in such major Caribbean centers as Trinidad, Jamaica, and a few of the other islands. Instead they emphasize the role of American volunteers: "A plan, begun in 1962, was developed for assuring a psychiatric service throughout the scattered islands of the Caribbean, linked with a voluntary professional service programme for U.S. psychiatric personnel. The amount of psychiatric help available has been limited to the islands of St. Thomas, Jamaica, Barbados, Trinidad and Martinique. Donations of the drugs used in mental hospitals were obtained from January, 1964, onwards, and intensive courses for general physicians and nurses in the treatment of acute mental illness were started in Barbados in the spring of 1964" (Rees, 1966, p. 121). It is true, of course, that the local professionals became involved as partners with and advisors to their colleagues from the easily accessible U.S. mainland. Much mutual learning took place. The Americans were glad to spend time in the exotic, tropical Caribbean, but they were also interested in learning about its new cultures and in the challenge of building mental health services where few had previously existed.

All of these elements and more favored the ultimate establishment, in 1965, of a pan-Caribbean Department of Psychiatry headed by Michael Beaubrun at the University of the West Indies (UWI) in Jamaica. It was conceived as a unifying professional force between the peoples of the 14 nations it would serve. Educated islanders felt that their people would be better cared for by professionals trained within the Caribbean environment, rather than the émigrés from Eastern Europe or visitors from the United Kingdom who were often in leadership roles. They wanted psychiatrists capable of work compatible with the island cultures. This would be preferable, they felt, to the transplantation of Northern viewpoints and techniques alien to the tropical, agrarian Caribbean with its infusion of African-based religions and beliefs. This view was officially embraced. However, despite efforts to produce culturally sensitive students for work in the islands, the hope was only partially fulfilled. By the time that, at Michael Beaubrun's invitation, I became an intermittent visiting Professor of Psychiatry at UWI from 1972 to 1975 (see Chapter 5 and Brody, 1981), the exports from Jamaica to the rest of the world included a large percentage of the physician graduates of UWI.

The Contributions of Bertram Schaffner and Some Early Friendship Networks Linking WFMH and the United Nations

The person behind the "plan," and the "Caribbean developments" to which Jack Rees referred, was Bertram Schaffner, M.D., a New York psychiatrist and psychoanalyst. Michael Beaubrun believes that he first encountered him at one of the post-Aruba meetings in the

Trinidad Public Library in 1957. At that time, he was already known for his well-received book on authoritarianism in the German family, *Fatherland* (Schaffner, 1948). I first heard of Schaffner's work in the Caribbean in 1962 when I became a consultant for the PAHO of WHO. Thirty-three years later, in November of 1995, I visited him in New York to obtain his personal perspective on the period. At that time, he was 83 years old and long removed from his Caribbean era, but his memories were fresh. He was also widely known for another reason: having been President of the Gay and Lesbian Psychiatrists of New York and Chairman of the Committee on Human Sexuality of GAP, he had been in the forefront of those psychiatrists dealing constructively with gay and lesbian issues.

Bert Schaffner's reminiscences offer a perspective on Caribbean mental health developments, which is different from, but not totally incompatible with, that of the professionals who lived there—the insiders who would acknowledge that his "Mental Health Peace Corps" was tremendously important, but regarded it more as "aided self-help" (Beaubrun, 1995a). Shaffner also afforded a view of the early days of the Federation through the eyes of a cross-cultural scholar and clinician. This view recognizes the role of social and friendship networks as a route to involvement in the kind of work to which the Federation has been happy to lend its name. He even knew John Lewis. In 1952, concerned with alcoholism in the Virgin Islands, Lewis had encountered Schaffner's book on Germany and found it illuminating as the Danes had left the islands with a culture, perhaps as strongly influenced by authoritative Lutheran teaching as Germany.

Schaffner's interest in the multicultural Caribbean stemmed ultimately from his own divided cultural background. Although he was born in the United States, his mother was German, and with a mixed European and American education, he became fluent in German as well as French and English. Because of having grown up half in Europe and half in the United States, and perhaps because of his minority sexual orientation, he "never felt totally at home in the U.S." but was "very comfortable in the Caribbean." As he said, referring to his work with local leaders of African and to a lesser degree East Indian background, "this was the period before civil rights, and I felt like something of a revolutionary." He emphasized that this personal sense of participating in a "revolutionary" activity was only in reference to his identification with the dark-skinned natives of the islands. His sensitivity to other cultures, and his concern with minority rights, had already been honed by close contact, much earlier, with an outstanding student of culture. This was the world famous anthropologist and Africanist, Melville Herskovits, who, after Bert's mother's death, lived in the Schaffner household. Bert's experience with his own austere father sensitized him during his service as a U.S. medical officer in Germany to the hierarchical nature of the German family. Back in the Unites States, he conducted a study of German prisoners in search of the roots of authoritarianism in German culture. This interested many U.S. and UN thinkers concerned with how to train a democratic leadership in the new Germany. It led to his book and enhanced his friendship with persons important in the Federation's early years. Among them was Margaret Mead whom he had consulted about the different clusters of physical symptoms he was finding in people from different European cultures. Mead was so impressed with his work that she wrote the foreword to his book. When he happened to be in London in 1948, knowing nothing about WFMH, she invited him to join her at a Federation party. He had already known Henry Dicks, M.D., one of the Roffey Park group and an early Federation Board member, through military connections and knew that Mead and Harry Stack Sullivan, also involved in the Federation's founding, were good friends.

Outside of the Federation, other links developed, illustrating the interconnectedness of the internationally sensitive psychiatrists of the era. One was Mottram Torre, M.D., a U.S. State Department psychiatrist, stationed in Paris, who traveled to U.S. embassies where diplomats were having psychiatric difficulties, many of which were alcohol related. When a State Department officer committed suicide shortly after his return to the United States from abroad,

UN Secretary General, Trygve Lie, became concerned with possible difficulties among his own personnel. Lie organized a 10-person UN Expert Committee to deal with mental health problems in his domain. Torre, known to Lie through his State Department post, was appointed by him as an initial member of the UN Committee. Through the friendship network, Schaffner also became part of this Committee, and it, indirectly, helped lead to his work in the Caribbean. Torre was also a friend of Frank Fremont-Smith, who as the influential Medical Director of the Josiah Macy Jr. Foundation was among the informal advisors to the early UN leaders in New York. At Torre's suggestion, Fremont-Smith spoke with Schaffner about the Committee; Schaffner recommended him to Lie who appointed all three to the Committee. They remained mental health advisors to the UN for 10 years until the group was dissolved by then Secretary General Dag Hammerschold. During his 10-year service on the Expert Committee, until the late 1950s, Schaffner was often involved in Fremont-Smith's Macy Foundation conferences and through them became more familiar with WFMH, because Jack Rees was frequently in attendance. According to Schaffner, when Rees attended the 1957 Aruba meeting "he saw the Caribbean as an opportunity for a mental health organization which would approximate a miniature World Federation" (Schaffner, 1995). However, as he put it, "Jack, of course, had no money." So he, Schaffner, offered to help start mental health associations in the area if he could combine it with his vacations. Rees responded favorably, giving him official status in the venture as a representative of WFMH. Because he was already on Trygve Lie's Committee, he was able to enhance his organizing power by presenting himself as an agent of the United Nations as well as WFMH (Schaffner, 1995). His work in the islands, beginning in 1958, must have contributed to a favorable context for the development of CFMH in 1959. By that year, stimulated by the CFMH conference, several island governments (including Trinidad and Tobago as noted above) beginning with St. Kitts and Nevis, became interested in helping to form associations and, particularly, in developing mental health services. However, as recalled by Schaffner, "they said, we don't have a penny." The message was clear. If he were to carry out any service or organizational projects in the area, he would have to finance them himself. He continued to familiarize himself with the area, and in 1960 went to Trinidad "and there found Michael Beaubrun," an obvious candidate for a professorial post. Schaffner was among those involved with the CFMH in persuading the Foundations Fund for Research in Psychiatry, headquartered at Yale, to give money for a new Department of Psychiatry at UWI in Jamaica. The Department, serving 14 Caribbean governments, was founded in 1965 with Michael Beaubrun as its first Professor and Chairman. It seems safe to say that, however remotely, WFMH was a contributor to this important development.

Between 1960 and 1965 Schaffner went to every island at least once a year. In 1962, almost single-handedly, he began to raise funds and recruit volunteer psychiatrists, social workers, psychologists, nurses, and occupational therapists from the United States to work in the islands for periods of about a month during their summer vacations. He remembers Francois Cloutier's being present in his living room during some of the planning meetings but does not believe that he (Cloutier) contributed significantly.

The island governments provided no money, but they did supply a house and car for an American mental health professional with his or her family. They participated in short-term projects, public education, and clinical work coordinated by CFMH. This work stimulated CFMH to conduct the first intensive courses in the area for general practitioners and nurses in the care of the mentally ill.

Schaffner's main local advisor was Kenneth Royes, M.D., Director of the Bellevue Hospital in Kingston, Jamaica, and he always stayed with the Royes family. Royes emphasized the importance of local treatment. He initiated the training of public health service personnel for mental health work, training for the police in mental health; and established mobile teams to take patients from one island with no services, such as St. Lucie, to another where they were available, such as Guadeloupe. Most islands had no services and no medications. Because of that, people were sometimes sent from St. Thomas to St. Elizabeth's Hospital in Washington, DC where they might die without ever seeing their families again.

Royes also advised that medications were a primary need, so Schaffner organized a campaign to get psychiatrists from all over the United States to send him sample drugs. They would come to his New York apartment in boxes. West Indian women in New York would pack them and they would be sent directly to hospitals. Finally it became more than he, Schaffner, could handle. Royes suggested getting in touch with the island benevolent associations. Each island had its own association that lent money to natives who were in trouble. Schaffner spent months phoning them and overcoming their suspicions by inviting them to New York where, for years, they participated in meetings in his home. Their discussions provided the basis of a new, but temporary, organization, the U.S.-Caribbean Federation for Mental Health. They gave West Indian dances with a $5.00- to $8.00-admission charge to which people brought their own food and liquor. In this way, they were able to raise about $12,000 yearly, a significant figure in that era. Each fund raiser was advertised as "under the auspices of WFMH," and Jack Rees always had a copy of what went on.

These activities supported the "great developments" to which Rees alluded in *Reflections*. By 1964, they included the formation of 22 mental health associations and 9 mental health committees in the area, the first census of patients in Caribbean mental hospitals in 1960, and the procurement of funds for a Department of Psychiatry in the Medical School of UWI. Schaffner was a significant actor in this long process of achievement. He reported, however, that as time passed, his conviction about the importance of local leadership became an issue between him and the American organizers of the fourth Caribbean Conference on Mental Health scheduled for 1965 in Martinique: "The time had come," he felt, for the Americans to step back and for the people native to the Caribbean "to take over." Looking back, he felt that the American organizers' failure to invite him to participate in that fourth Conference was due to his "unacceptable political stance," which was a threat to their own domination of the process. Their rejection, he said, led to his temporary disillusionment not only with his erstwhile colleagues but with WFMH in general, which he now perceived as a racist organization.

Whether or not Bert Schaffner's rejection was due solely to the conflict described above is uncertain. Caribbeans rather than Americans were, in fact, in the senior positions of CFMH. His rift with the leadership widened after the Martinique Conference when Michael Beaubrun was succeeded as CFMH President by his cousin Matthew. At the end of Matthew Beaubrun's four years as CFMH President, encompassing two more biennial CFMH conferences, Schaffner was removed from the list of Consultants to the organization. It is possible that the issue may have been complicated by a public perception of his sexual orientation. My own research on sexual behavior and personal fertility control in Jamaica (Brody, 1981) suggested that many Caribbeans, including professionals, were intolerant of homosexuality, and this could have influenced attitudes toward him. Whatever the cause, this termination of his recognized status was a severe blow for the man who, perhaps, had done more than any other single individual to establish mental health services in the area. In consequence, he felt that he was operating alone in the Caribbean and abandoned what had been a significant life activity. His legacy, though, has survived him.

Caribbean Mental Health Organizations in the Beaubrun Era

Schaffner's withdrawal from the Caribbean marked the effective end of active North American involvement and an acceleration of local Caribbean responsibility for the development of psychiatric services in the Region. At the same time Michael Beaubrun, already a prominent contributor, was becoming the dominant mental health figure in the Region. His ascendancy was marked by his 1963–1965 Presidency of the Caribbean Federation for Mental Health, his 1965 appointment as Chairman of Psychiatry at UWI, and his presidency of the Caribbean Association of Psychiatrists, which he founded. We first met, as noted above, at the August 1971 CFMH Conference in Paramaribo, Surinam where I had been sent by President Morris Carstairs as the representative of the global Federation. At the Conference, Beaubrun steered the passage of several resolutions. The first concerned a major Caribbean problem, alluded to above. That was the "brain drain" of its most educated citizens, especially its physicians, to countries in the North offering better job opportunities. The Conference recommended that Caribbean governments make the repayment of student loans "less onerous," that candidates should be selected "who are not already alienated from their culture," and that overseas training "be resorted to only after a significant period of local training" (WFMH, 1971a). Other recommendations referred to the rights of women, children, and psychiatric patients, to drug dependence, and to family planning in relation to mental health. These will be discussed in more detail in Part III of this volume.

The revival of mental health interests in the Caribbean during Beaubrun's nearly two-year (1972–1974) WFMH presidency—with the Federation Secretariat in his office at the UWI—is detailed in Chapter 5. In this period, WFMH became a widely known entity in the Region, and Beaubrun was much evidence at ceremonial occasions in Jamaica and other island nations. He also brought the Caribbean to the attention of the rest of the world through his participation in meetings in Quebec, the United States, Colombia, Africa, Europe, and Latin America. As an occasional consultant for PAHO, I was able to work with him representing WFMH to its consultative meetings. An example was a meeting held in Bogota, Colombia from 26–30 June 1972 on the training of psychiatrists in the developing countries of Latin America. The participants were professors of psychiatry, many of whom I knew from my work in the 1960s as a participant in professional meetings while a Visiting Professor in Rio de Janeiro, and as a PAHO consultant. I also knew most of them from my 1966–1968 work as Director of the Interamerican Mental Health Studies Program, of the American and Latin American Psychiatric Associations. Many had also been present at an earlier PAHO meeting in Lima, Peru in 1967, where we focused on defining the needs for undergraduate education in psychiatry. It was on the plane en route to Lima on that occasion that I sat next to Henry David and continued my education about WFMH begun by Morris Carstairs in 1966. In 1972, I was able to participate with Michael in educating our academic colleagues from Latin America about the work and principles of WFMH and ways in which training programs could collaborate with mental health associations in their regions. We were especially pleased when the final report emphasized not only the clinical role of psychiatrists but their importance as change agents promoting better conditions for mental health in their countries.

This period of Beaubrun's active leadership was stimulating. However, after he announced his resignation from the WFMH presidency at the end of 1973 and resigned in 1974 from the chairmanship of psychiatry at UWI Jamaica to return to Trinidad, mental health activities in the Caribbean began to fade. For a time, CFMH was succeeded as the main regional change agent by organizations it had helped to originate, namely the Caribbean Association of Psychiatrists and the Caribbean Association of Social Workers. In the 1990s, CFMH was revived with the aim of providing "the resuscitation" of which 11 of the Caribbean's 22 former mental health associations were "seriously in need" (Keens-Douglas, 1994). This renewal was outlined in a five-year plan initiated in 1993. Its major goals were preserving good mental health and improving the quality of life of those who had succumbed to illness. To accomplish these aims in the face of "difficulty in communication…and limited finances," CFMH sought interaction with mental health associations outside of its region. As its President Gloria Keens-Douglas wrote: "This potpourri of races, religions, cultures, post-colonization attitudes and effects is still in the process of forging some kind of destiny as 'one people, one destiny.'" Among the specific problems she cited, "inferiority complexes, socioeconomic problems, racial inequities or disharmony" (Keens-Douglas, 1994). These are all themes that I heard frequently from fellow faculty members at UWI between 1972 and 1975.

WFMH IN LATIN AMERICA
During the London and Geneva Secretariats
1948–1954

Although Jack Rees' desire to extend WFMH influence to the less developed world found a ready outlet in the English-speaking Caribbean, there was no comparably receptive or cohesive Latin American mental health community. The new Federation depended for its growth, status, and effectiveness in the Spanish- and Portuguese-speaking Americas upon the recruitment of well-known psychiatrists, typically that handful of university professors repeatedly encountered at international meetings. The first Executive Board included Eduardo E. Krapf, M.D., of Argentina, then an Associate Professor of Psychiatry at the University of Buenos Aires, who was already a consultant for the embryonic WHO. Another South American was Professor H. de B. B. Roxo, M.D., of Brazil, then Professor Emeritus of Psychiatry at the University of Brazil. Each belonged to the psychiatrist-dominated national mental health association in his country, which confined its activities largely to an occasional public lecture.

Participants in the second WFMH annual meeting, in Geneva from 22–27 August, 1949, included another politically powerful Brazilian Professor of Psychiatry, A. C. Pacheco e Silva, M.D., of Sao Paulo. There were also individual physicians from Mexico, Puerto Rico, and Venezuela. National mental hygiene associations from Brazil, Chile, Cuba, Mexico, Peru, Uruguay, and Venezuela were already members with voting privileges.

At the third WFMH annual meeting, in Paris, September 1950, the decision was taken to have the next meeting, along with a World Congress for Mental Health, in Latin America. Mexico was the best known and most convenient venue for the Europeans and North Americans who dominated Federation affairs, and the Professor of Psychiatry at the University of Mexico, having expressed interest in the field of mental hygiene, was already an Executive Board member. He was Alfonso Millan, M.D., who was also President of the *Liga Mexicana de Salud Mental*. Dr. Millan was elected Vice President at the Paris meeting, with the expectation that he would succeed to the WFMH presidency at that Federation's fourth International Congress, now scheduled for December 1951 in his home city. During his presidential term, 1951–1952, Millan helped recruit other Latin American psychiatrists to the leadership group.

The first was Carlos Alberto Seguin, M.D., Professor of Psychiatry at the San Fernando Medical School of the ancient University of San Marcos in Lima, who was elected to the Executive Board for a three-year term. However, his interest did not persist beyond his initial term. Although politically influential and organizationally adept, his first love was scholarship. An unusual combination of clinician and scholar, psychoanalytically trained as well as a knowledgeable ethnographer and student of indigenous Peruvian cultures, present and past, he was reluctant to devote much of his energy to this international organization with somewhat abstract aims. He was also critical of what he considered its anglophilic tendencies. We first met in 1964 when, at the request of Dr. Daniel Blain then President of the American Psychiatric Association, I addressed the *Asociacion Psiciatrica de America Latina* (APAL) as part of an effort to form a joint Interamerican Council of Psychiatric Associations. The meeting, held in Lima's historic city hall, attracted Dr. Seguin, and we became friends. Not long thereafter, I became a Board member of his new Institute of Social Psychiatry, and we maintained a close relationship for several years. During this time, he was an active member of the research-oriented Interamerican Society of Psychology, but WFMH was not one of his concerns.

Two other *Limeno* friends and colleagues interested for a time in the Federation were Professors Humberto Rotundo, M.D., a student of the psychosocial impact of migration from the high Andes to Lima, and Baltazar Caravedo, M.D., head of the Health Ministry's Department of Mental Health. Rotundo like Seguin was primarily a scholar and did not develop a lasting interest in this association of volunteers. Caravedo, on the other hand, a government administrator concerned with international contacts as well as the practical application of knowledge, was deeply interested. As noted below, he eventually became a Board member and Vice President.

The first Chilean named to the WFMH leadership group was another colleague who also became a friend in the decade of the 1960s. He was Professor Ignacio Matte Blanco, M.D., an internationally known psychoanalyst who was Chairman of Psychiatry at the University of Santiago in Chile. Elected a substitute Executive Board member for a one-year term in 1951, during Millan's presidency, he was never an active participant in its deliberations. In 1952, however, at the Federation's fifth Annual Meeting in Brussels, from 24–30 August another Chilean, child psychiatrist Carlos Nassar, M.D., Professor of Mental Health in the University of Santiago's Educational Faculty and President of the *Asociacion Chilena Pro Salud Mental*, was elected to substitute Board membership. He participated actively and his efforts to combine mental health and developmental knowledge were of great interest to the North American and European Board members.

Two new member associations from Latin America were also welcomed into the Federation in 1951, the Mental Health Association in Costa Rica and the Argentinean Psychoanalytic Association, one of the first professional societies to become a member. Other Latin American representation came from Cuba, Guatemala, and Venezuela.

In 1952, Eduardo Krapf became Chairman of the Executive Board. When, at the sixth Annual Meeting in Vienna, August 16–22, 1953, he moved to the still active position of Past Chairman, Pacheco e Silva from Brazil was elected a Board member for the 1953–1956 term. Baltazar Caravedo was also nominated, first to the Executive Board and then as a substitute; perhaps because he was primarily an administrator rather than a university-based scholar, he was not elected to either post. At this 1953 meeting, which was still influenced by Krapf, Seguin gave an opening plenary presentation on recent mental health activities in South America. This offered most Federation members their first knowledge about mental health in Latin America, hitherto an unknown region and appeared to act as a stimulus to Jack Rees' desire to learn more about it. That year also saw the WFMH membership of the first international Latin American association, the *Asociacion Latina-Americana Pro Salud Mental*.

The Director's Visit to Latin America, 9 June – 27 July, 1954

A major breakthrough for WFMH involvement in the countries south of Mexico was Rees' personal visit to the area. Long desired, it had been discussed since the Mexican Congress. He wanted to meet mental health leaders in the region and directors of the ministries of health and education. The preferred aim, as usual, was to exert direct influence on the governments of the region. It was also to "create closer and better links between the Federation and the countries we serve, and at the same time to do whatever seemed possible to stimulate thinking and activity in the mental health field in this vast continent" (WFMH, 1954, p.36). The trip was supported by a special travel fund from the Ittleson Family Foundation, almost all of which was eventually paid back by South American colleagues. It included Havana, Cuba; San Jose, Costa Rica; Caracas, Venezuela; Quito, Ecuador; Lima, Peru; Santiago, Chile; Rio de Janeiro and Sao Paulo, Brazil; and Panama, Republic of Panama.

The details of visits in each country are faithfully recorded in the 1954 Annual Report. Many aspects are familiar: the warm hospitality and easy access to notables in the health field; the dominance of physicians, not all psychiatrists, in most national mental health associations— except for Costa Rica and Venezuela, which had multiprofessional and lay citizen representation; the old, decaying mental hospitals, many lacking basic amenities; the immense need for trained personnel; the eagerness of local professionals to have the distinguished foreigner discuss their problems and possibly offer solutions; and the presence in each country of one, or at most a handful, of psychiatric personalities occupying the few available high status leadership positions, while engaging in individual private practice or owning a private psychiatric hospital or clinic. In every country, Rees also reported meeting a few "promising and useful" young professionals. In 1955, looking back, he felt that his brief visits to each country, as in other parts of the world, had acted in catalytic fashion: "New lecture courses and training projects, more adventurous planning with Ministries of Health and Education, new societies, research projects, sociological inquiries and surveys" undertaken by member societies "are said in part to be stimulated by our activity as a Federation" (WFMH, 1955a, p. 11).

One important step was to foster the development of Regional meetings. This was a truly international bridge building effort. It was done by bringing together knowledgeable officers of member associations with observers from neighboring countries without mental health associations. They would discuss the mental health problems of their countries and how to approach them, exchanging information about methods, successes, and failures. In May 1955, a meeting for officers of WFMH member associations in Latin America was held in San Jose, Costa Rica with the cooperation of that country's Ministry of Health. In addition to representatives of the Costa Rican mental health association, there were observers from El Salvador, Guatemala, Nicaragua, Cuba, and Puerto Rico. Consultants besides Rees included Ms. Desjardins, a Canadian social worker employed by the UN in Panama, and Ernest Gruenberg, M.D., a New York psychiatrist and public health specialist supported by the Milbank Fund who later headed the Department of Mental Hygiene of the Johns Hopkins University School of Public Health.

1955–1967: Toward the Peruvian Annual Meeting

In 1955, Eduardo Krapf was elected Vice President. In 1956, he succeeded to the post of President but had to resign the office prematurely as he was appointed Chief of WHO's Mental Health Section in the same year. In 1956, Mariano Coronado, M.D., Professor of Psychiatry at the University of Costa Rica and President of Costa Rica's National Committee for Mental Health, joined the Executive Board. This was a consequence of his having met Jack Rees during the latter's expedition to Latin America .

It was not until the tenth Annual Meeting, 11–17 August 1957 in Copenhagen, that Baltazar Caravedo, who had been nominated on several previous occasions, was finally elected to the Board. In the ensuing years, there were gradual increments in Latin American individual and organizational membership in WFMH. At the sixteenth Annual Meeting in Amsterdam, 22–26 July 1963, Caravedo was elected for another term on the Board, this time from 1963–1967. The high point of Latin American activity for the Federation was reached in 1967 with his organization of its twentieth annual meeting in Lima, Peru the first to be held in South America. However, this happened almost by default because not only Peru but Canada, the Caribbean Federation, and the United States had issued invitations, and the Executive Board had approved the U.S. location. Caravedo, now the senior mental health officer of his government, very much wanted the annual meeting as a national honor and promptly issued another invitation. This time it was for 1969 because it had already been agreed that the 1968 twentieth anniversary meeting would be in London. However, a combination of factors, partly financial, led the Executive Board in late 1966 to shift the 1967 location from the United States to Lima and to reschedule the 1969 meeting to the United States.

This necessitated intensive last-minute preparations led by Caravedo. The Lima meeting, the last under Cloutier as Director General, finally took place from 26 November to 1 December 1967, attended by 450 participants from 32 countries. With particularly large delegations from South America, as well as other Latin nations of the region including Cuba, it was perceived as the beginning of a significant expansion of WFMH into the region. Many participants took advantage of the occasion to visit other countries of South and Central America, where it was possible to engage in useful local consultations and exchanges of ideas and experiences.

The Assembly of voting member associations held during that meeting on 29 November with representation from 107 voting associations, elected A. Mateo Alonso, M.D., of Venezuela and C. Gonzales-Orellana of Guatemala as two of four members of the Executive Board for the 1968–1972 term. Riding on the crest of popularity engendered by the meeting, heavily sponsored by Peruvian government dignitaries including the President of the Republic, Caravedo was elected Vice President for 1967–1968. It was expected that he would succeed to the WFMH presidency in 1969 during the U.S. Annual Meeting, which had been put off until that year. However, this expectation and that of a productive Federation future in Latin America were not met. This 1967 gathering was the final annual meeting of what might be called the "old" World Federation with its central Secretariat first in London and then in Geneva. As noted in Chapter 5, Morris Carstairs, who had been the 1966–1967 Vice President, took office as President during the Lima meeting, expecting the usual single-year term; i.e., 1967–1968. However, the Federation's financial collapse with the closing of the Geneva Secretariat led the Executive Board to request that he remain in office for four more years to conduct a rescue operation. He reluctantly agreed. This superseded Caravedo's expected ascension to the presidency and ended the Federation's thrust into Latin America. It was not to be revived for more than 20 years until preparations for the 1991 World Congress for Mental Health in Mexico. By that time, Caravedo was old and ill. When he died in 1992, his obituaries noted that he had been a member of the WFMH Executive Board.

WFMH in Latin America during the Era of Working Presidents

1968–1980: The Period of Minimal Activity

WFMH activity in Latin America rapidly receded from its 1967 high point achieved in Lima to a level of obscurity. Carstairs' energies from 1968–1972 were focused on resuscitating the organization, although under the influence of his successor, Michael Beaubrun of Jamaica and Trinidad, he developed an interest in the Caribbean. Beaubrun, himself, during his 1972–1974 Federation presidency, limited his regional activity, with a few notable exceptions, to the British Commonwealth Caribbean.

It fell to Tsung-yi Lin (President 1974–1975), whose global interest and energies were undimmed, to try to revive the Federation's Latin connection. In 1976, with his encouragement, a number of Mexican psychiatrist friends led by Guido Belsasso, M.D., brought one mental health and two psychoanalytic associations into the Federation. A WFMH Committee was formed in Mexico and became active in disseminating information about the forthcoming 1977 Vancouver World Congress. In a burst of activity, it established contacts with many private and governmental groups and individual leaders, among them Manuel Velasco Suarez, M.D., a neurosurgeon who was Governor of the State of Chiapas. A long-time mental health leader in Mexico, he was preparing the opening of a community mental health center in his state. Dr. Velasco Suarez was later to become the senior health officer of his country and Honorary President of the organizing committee for the 1991 World Congress in Mexico City.

My old friend and colleague, Carlos Leon, M.D., Professor and Chairman of the Department of Psychiatry at the Universidad de Valle in Cali, Colombia had also been enlisted to recruit Latin American mental health professionals to participate in the forthcoming Vancouver Congress of 1977. Carlos was an excellent scholar in the field of psychiatry and culture, with special training in epidemiology. I had visited him in Cali in the mid-1960s in my capacity as Director of the Interamerican Mental Health Studies Program of the American Psychiatric Association and the *Asociation Psiciatrica de America Latina*. He was a native of Ecuador, and at his request, I also visited his former teacher and mentor, head of the medical school and teaching hospital in Quito, Julio Endara, M.D. In that era, in the tradition of academic exchanges, he had also spoken in my department at the University of Maryland in Baltimore.

In April 1978, 11 years after the Federation's annual meeting in Lima, to be its first and last in South America until 1996, President Lin traveled to Colombia and Mexico, a trip "intended to be the beginning of revitalization" of WFMH's regional programs in Latin America (WFMH, 1986). On 3 April at the Universidad del Valle Cali, Colombia, he attended the inauguration of a WHO Collaborative Center for Research and Training headed by Leon. In the mid-1970s, Leon became a member of the WFMH Administrative Committee and welcomed WFMH participation in his new Center. The possibilities were outlined in the conference following the inauguration, "Perspectives in Mental Health in Latin America." This was a matter of considerable excitement for Tsung-yi Lin because it marked the apparent beginning of a collaboration between Colombia, Mexico, Costa Rica, Panama, Peru, Argentina, Brazil, Venezuela, and Ecuador and WHO/PAHO with an opportunity for some kind of WFMH involvement. Unfortunately, there was no way in which WFMH, an educational and advocacy organization, could participate actively in the research programs of the new Center in Cali. Nor did any channel open up to encourage WFMH influence on its investigations. Nonetheless, Lin renewed WFMH contacts with this group of Latin American psychiatric leaders and secured a promise from, perhaps the senior Bogota psychiatrist, my friend Humberto Rosselli, M.D., to revive the inactive Colombian League of Mental Hygiene and affiliate it with WFMH. Carlos Climente, M.D., of Leon's department, President of the Colombian Psychiatric Association, also expressed interest in participating in future WFMH programs.

Buoyed on the wave of enthusiasm typically felt by foreign visitors receiving the royal treatment from gracious Latin American hosts, Lin then proceeded to Mexico City. Here, too, he was greeted effusively. Within two days, he met with the leaders of all of the mental health professions as well as educators and government officials. The culmination was a warmly expressed interest in having the Federation's 1981 World Congress in Mexico. Unfortunately, after Lin's departure, there was no further expression of interest from Mexico in hosting a World Congress.

It fell to Lin's successor, Gowan Guest (1979–1981), to attempt another revival of the Latin American connection by scheduling a Board meeting in Mexico in the spring of April 1980. His proposal for the meeting came at the beginning of his presidency, after the Salzburg Congress in early autumn 1979. Although I understood the attraction of opening a new door for WFMH in Mexico, my experience in that country as a lecturer and consultant beginning in December 1961, and later as a member of the Interamerican Council of Psychiatric Associations, made me hesitant. I was particularly concerned because of the long-standing adversarial relations between the two major factions of Mexican psychiatrists. One was led by Professor of Psychiatry and Director of the Mexican Institute of Psychiatry, Ramon de la Fuente, M.D., institutionally, the most powerful psychiatrist in the nation. He was an adherent not only of traditional biological psychiatry but of the psychoanalysis of Eric Fromm, his former analyst, who had been a long-time resident of Mexico City. The most prominent figure on the other side, a member of the multi-disciplinary, Mexican Society for Neurology and Psychiatry, and the Freudian psychoanalytic association, and also the best known in United States psychoanalytic and medical anthropological circles, was the psychoanalyst and cultural psychiatrist, Ramon Parres, M.D. I had known him for years as an impressively scholarly colleague, first through earlier visits to Mexico and later as a fellow member of the American Psychiatric Association's Committee on Transcultural Psychiatry. Another source of disquiet, apparently unknown to either Guest or Lin, was the long-time membership in WFMH of the Society for Neurology and Psychiatry, and the fact that it was the rival organization of the Mexican Psychiatric Association of which de la Fuente was the leading patron.

Because of these concerns, I sent a long letter on 20 November 1979 to Guest and his closest advisors, Mary Chase Pell, North American Vice President for WFMH; George Rohn, the senior executive of the Canadian Mental Health Association; and Roberta Beiser, whom Guest had recently elevated to the post of WFMH Executive Director. In it I wrote that I had "reservations about a full Board meeting [in Mexico] being exploited for local factional gain. It would be better, I think, at this moment, to consider as a first step toward a possible Mexico City Congress a small delegation empowered to meet with a variety of people representing the range of groups there. (It is important to remember, also, that in most of the Latin countries 'mental health' is still pretty much the captive of and a springboard for the activities of psychiatrists who do not have the institutional bases, e.g. in universities, of those in North America and Europe)." Pell, who in any event preferred a meeting at the same time as the International Hospital Federation in Belgium (see Chapters 11 and 13) responded favorably. The others did not react.

1980, The Hope for a New Beginning

One basis for Guest's decision to meet in Mexico was then President Lin's 1979 appointment of de la Fuente as Vice President for what was then the Federation's Latin American Region, the huge expanse encompassing South and Central America, including Mexico. However, Dr. de la Fuente had no vested interest in the Federation as an organization or in its goals. A distinguished figure in his country—the Mexican Institute of Psychiatry was the equivalent of a National Institute of Mental Health—he was a traditional conservative gentleman of his culture and dubious about the soundness of a "mental health" organization, which included not only physicians but nonmedical volunteers with avowed interests in social change. WFMH was clearly not a supporter of traditional, biologically oriented, hospital-based psychiatry and could even be seen as a danger to the long-standing structure of thought and practice that supported the Mexican psychiatric and professional establishment. The WFMH mission also suggested a modification of the paternalistic relationship of doctors and patients, removing a major source of the former's authority by fostering community-based facilities.

For the first year after becoming a Regional Vice President, de la Fuente was silent. However, he graciously acceded to the new President Guest's request that a Federation Executive Committee meeting be held under his auspices in Mexico City in April 1980. That meeting was marked by two developments. First was the failure of Guest's attempt to impose some element of unity on the Mexican mental health (essentially psychiatric) community in support of the WFMH goals. The attempt reflected his lack of knowledge about the entrenched disagreements between the two major factions of Mexican psychiatry. Guest invited the leading members of both groups, who had typically avoided each other for nearly a quarter century, to a WFMH reception. Predictably, attendance was spotty and the WFMH was identified as naive and insufficiently knowledgeable about what was going on in the region to be taken seriously.

The second consequence of the Mexico Committee meeting was the appearance on the WFMH scene of de la Fuente's chief assistant, Federico Puente Silva, M.D. Unlike his chief, Puente was a confident English speaker, having studied in London. With an M.A. in Epidemiology as well as psychiatric training in London, he knew the language of American and British academic psychiatry and was easy to communicate with. He readily assumed the tasks of representing de la Fuente to the Federation, when the latter was routinely reappointed *in absentia* as Latin American Vice President by the 1981 Board meeting in Manila. However, Puente was still not well known and was perceived as a representative of de la Fuente rather than a potential Federation leader in his own right. His immediate access to influence was also impeded by the presence, as noted above, of Alvaro Gallegos Chacon, M.D., of Costa Rica. Alvaro, well known and accomplished, was brought into the Federation in 1982 to reconsider the existing divisions of the Americas. Among other distinctions, he had that of being born in a mental hospital, the one in San Jose where his grandfather had been superintendent. Professor of Psychiatry at the University of Costa Rica and advisor to his country's social security system, he was a frequent consultant to the PAHO in Washington, DC and to WHO's Mental Health Division in Geneva. I had known him as a colleague in the Interamerican Council of Psychiatrists, and, long before I had heard of the Federation, my wife and I had visited him and his family in Costa Rica. Not only did we see the hospital of his birth in San Jose, but he arranged for us to be driven down the bumpy Pan American Highway to the coastal retreat where the family gathered on holidays. It was quite natural, therefore, that at the 1983 Washington DC World Congress, in the same year that he was a Visiting Professor of Psychiatry at Johns Hopkins University in Baltimore, I recommended him to the Board to succeed de la Fuente as Regional Vice President for Latin America.

After 1983 and the Baltimore-Washington Secretariat

The years since 1983 have seen intermittent WFMH participation in the mental health activities of Latin American nations including Cuba. Between 1983 and the December 1996 Board meeting in Concepcion, Chile, with its formation of a South American Regional Council, there were a number of organizational developments relevant to WFMH. The Costa Rican mental health association, for example, achieved greater recognition and influence in early 1986 as it became part of its country's National Council for Mental Health. The 1989 Board meeting in Auckland approved WFMH co-sponsorship with the University of Concepcion in Chile of a conference held November 20–22, 1989 on the prevention of mental illness. Organized by Benjamin Vicente, M.D., Ph.D., who, in the absence of a WFMH Regional Vice President for South America was named an informal "coordinator for WFMH South American developments," its theme was "Man and Psychiatry." This remained an isolated academic activity, however, and it was not until early 1991 that the *Sociedad Chilena de Salud Mental* applied for WFMH membership.

Psychiatry and the WFMH in Mexico

A meeting with significance for the Federation's future took place in Mexico on 14 March 1984. It was arranged by Federico Puente, still a staff member of the Mexican Institute of Psychiatry, headed by, now former, WFMH Latin American Vice President, Ramon de la Fuente. It was timed to fit my scheduled presence in Mexico as Chairman for the American Psychiatric Association of its 25–29 May 1985 joint meeting with various Mexican societies. The joint meeting had been initiated by the Mexican Society for Psychiatry and Neurology. In response to the desire of the American Psychiatric Association, the Mexican Psychiatric Association was a reluctant participant.

Puente wanted me, on behalf of WFMH, to meet with the officers of the 14 societies comprising the newly formed Mexican Mental Health Association, which expected to participate in the 1985 meeting. Its membership was eclectic, including organizations of psychology, psychoanalysis, mental health, family therapy, neurology, psychiatry (and biological psychiatry), public health, and behavioral modification. Puente, the founder and President (or "Executive General Secretary") of this group, had designated it as the Mexican Committee for WFMH, which gave it special significance for me. Although I had frequently been in Mexico during the 1960s, my contacts had been exclusively with psychiatrists and psychologists. This meeting allowed me to begin a relationship with a diversified group of mental health leaders from many professions (although it included no citizen volunteers in the United States mode). In retrospect, it was evident that I was being recruited to support Puente in his long-term plans.

We met again, with the Committee now comprising 16 societies, during the 1985 U.S.-Mexico joint psychiatric meeting. Although Puente, still attached to the Mexican Institute of Psychiatry, chaired the organizing committee for the Mexican Psychiatric Association, this appears to have been his first move toward developing a base separate from de la Fuente and his Institute. It can also be seen as his first move on a trajectory eventuating in the 1991 World Congress for Mental Health in Mexico, his being named WFMH President Elect in 1991 at that Congress' Assembly and becoming President in 1993 during the Tokyo World Congress.

The first major step on this trajectory was his election by the 1985 Brighton Post Congress Board as Regional Vice President for the newly defined (in 1984) Mexico/Central America/Caribbean Region. Although he had become reasonably well-known to the Board, my support for his candidacy was obviously important to them. At that same election, Alvaro Gallegos, soon to become National Coordinator for Mental Health in Costa Rica, was named Regional Vice President for South America. The overarching Latin American Region for which de la Fuente had been Vice President had been eliminated.

On 19 September 1985, two months later, there occurred an event that stimulated Puente to intense activity and helped to consolidate his position as Regional Vice President. That was the disastrous Mexico City earthquake, which caused the death of several thousand people and widespread loss of property, including medical facilities. He was a leader in the development of crisis intervention services and a telephone hotline for victims and their families. Stimulated by these developments, the WFMH Board encouraged him to plan for a regional WFMH meeting in February 1986. He accepted with alacrity. In his first demonstration of organizing ability, he was able to arrange co-sponsorship by PAHO and support from the Faculty of Psychology of the University of Mexico with which he was affiliated, the Subsecretary of Higher Education, and the Mexican Institute of Social Security.

This first ever Mexican regional meeting of WFMH established Puente's status as an effective organizer and elevated his local stature. It was held 7–9 February 1986 at the National Autonomous University of Mexico, with the theme, "Prevention and Education in the Field of Mental Health: Implications for Latin America." His chief collaborator was Professor Juan Sanchez Sosa, Director of the University's Faculty of Psychology, and current Secretary of the Mexican Committee. Inaugural speakers included, in addition to the organizers, Committee notables, and myself, Jesus Kumate Rodriguez, M.D., the senior Mexican health official and a representative of the President. It was slightly embarrassing, although gratifying, that the second half of the inaugural morning was devoted to a "tribute" for my "international work in mental health" featuring talks by my old friends, Ramon Parres and Professor Sheppard Kellam, M.D., Chairman of the Department of Mental Hygiene of the Johns Hopkins School of Public Health. The rest of the time was occupied by workshops covering all aspects of prevention and involving U.S. as well as Mexican health leaders. During the meeting, Puente also founded the "Mexican Committee for the Study and Control of Tobacco Use," *Comite Mexicano para el Estudio y Control de Tobaquismo,* known as COMECTA. Again, he demonstrated his organizing skill, attracting a range of Mexican health and political leaders and several representatives of international organizations as founding members.

Toward a 1991 World Congress in Mexico

During that February 1986 Regional Meeting, Puente first raised the question of a possible World Congress for Mental Health to be held in Mexico in 1991, five years later. It would be 40 years after that presided over by Professor Alfonso Millan in 1951. The local sponsoring group would be the one he had founded, namely the Mexican Committee for Mental Health, now the major WFMH voting organization in the Region. He was encouraged to submit an invitation to the upcoming Board meeting in London on 10–12 June 1986 and did so. However, Mexico was still an unknown quantity to most Board members, as was Federico, himself. It was also observed by UK colleagues that the sponsoring organization was his own creation and had no history of independent achievement. Yet, while other locations were discussed with more enthusiasm, there was no sense of security about their competence to mount a Congress. Furthermore, 1991 seemed far away, and the Board was already planning for Congresses in Cairo in 1987 and Auckland in 1989. It was not until a year later, in mid-1987, that Dick Hunter, who had assumed the tasks of reviewing the facilities and finances of groups asking for Federation meetings, responded to Puente's invitation and went to Mexico City to evaluate the situation. However, he was not sufficiently familiar with the city and its culture to come to a firm conclusion about the facilities. He was also doubtful about the local Committee's capacity to finance it.

The question was raised again at the October 1987 Board meeting during the Cairo Congress, and again it was unable to come to a conclusion. The Board's final decision was that I, myself, should make a site visit. I was reluctant to do so, realizing that my relationship with the Mexican group had progressed to the point where it might be difficult to arrive at a neutral and objective opinion. At any event, funds for the trip were not available. It was not until some time later that Puente proffered a formal invitation to come to Mexico, 23–25 January 1988. Visits were scheduled with Professor Sanchez Sosa, my old acquaintance from the 1960s era of the Interamerican Council of Psychiatry, Hector Cabildo, M.D., President of the Committee and a long-time mental health leader in his country, and others. It was then that I learned for the first time that a serious conflict might be in the making: Ramon de la Fuente, it developed, was opposed to such a Congress with Puente, known as having left his Institute, at the helm. It was also rumored that the Mexican Psychiatric Association, loyal to de la Fuente, might boycott it. This opposition had a negative influence on many well-known scholars and clinicians, including several of my old friends from pre-WFMH days. When I talked with them, they were not specific in their own opposition but told me politely that they probably would decline an invitation to participate in the Congress. This was disquieting. The problem seemed to have both a personal and an institutional component. Personally, there was the possible antagonism of an older established leader and his long-time associates against a young defector from the ranks who was establishing his own power base and climbing the national leadership ladder to become a possible competitor. Institutionally, there was the opposition of the traditional establishment to an independent splinter group that could have different goals and ways of attaining them. Upon my return, I reported all of this to the 1988 Board meeting. After long discussion, in which some Board members expressed their anxiety but most emphasized the desirability of meeting in a Latin American country, the decision was taken, despite possible reservations, to have a Congress, organized by Puente, in Mexico in 1991.

Then, the problem unexpectedly became more complicated. It involved our representative to UN and WHO Geneva, Stanislas Flache, M.D., a public health specialist who, before his retirement, had been an assistant director general of WHO. Flache, then WFMH President Elect and scheduled to become President in Auckland in 1989, would end his presidency by presiding over the opening of the Mexico Congress if it came to pass. He telephoned me to report that the WHO Mental Health Division, influenced by Professor de la Fuente whose Institute was a WHO Collaborating Center, hoped that WFMH would cancel its Mexico commitment. Flache, who retained a strong attachment to WHO to which he had dedicated his professional life, was greatly affected by this information. It was also taken seriously by the rest of the Board because of our close relationship with WHO. There was no corroboration, however, until late September 1988. At that time, Puente telephoned me to announce that Flache had accepted an invitation to speak to the Mexican Psychiatric Association, which wanted him to reverse the WFMH commitment to a 1991 Congress in Mexico. I called Flache immediately in Geneva. He confirmed that he was, indeed, going to Mexico as the guest of the de la Fuente group and that he, personally, was inclined to cancel the Congress because of the opposition of Norman Sartorius, M.D., Director of WHO's Mental Health Division. Sartorius was not only a friend but a distinguished investigator and a powerful political force within international psychiatry whose opinions required serious attention. He was also committed to the success of the Mexican Institute of Psychiatry as one of his Collaborating Centers. Flache stated that if no alternative venue were available, we should simply skip a year and reschedule elsewhere in 1992.

I was certain that the Board would not reverse itself and stop preparations already well under way. Puente and I had an emergency telephone consultation. I suggested that he organize a celebration of the WFMH fortieth anniversary during the time of Flache's visit and that we all, Puente, Flache, and I, could address the celebration. That would give the three of us a chance to confer, meet with the key Mexican leaders who supported the Congress, and defuse what threatened to become a difficult conflict with international ramifications. Puente agreed and, in an optimistic mood, told me that an old acquaintance, the distinguished and widely known and respected neurosurgeon, Manuel Velasco Suarez, M.D., had agreed to be Honorary Chairman of the Organizing Committee. His support was especially significant because he was to head the National Health Council, the highest authority of the new government health services. It was also historically apposite because he had been present at the WFMH founding meeting in London in 1948, was one of the promoters of the mental health movement in Mexico, and, years earlier, had established the first Mental Health Office within the Mexican Ministry of Health.

Puente organized the celebration at top speed. I called Flache again in Geneva to let him know what was happening. We agreed that it was important for him to accept Puente's invitation and, staying in the same hotel in Mexico City, we would have a chance for further conversation. On 19 October 1988, more than 500 people, with widespread television and other media coverage, gathered in the great hall, formerly an historic church, of the Hospital Juarez de Mexico, to mark the Federation's fortieth anniversary . Its theme was conveyed in a symposium on "Mental Health in Mexico for the Year 2000". Flache and I were both there along with a host of government, medical, and psychiatric dignitaries including Ramon Parres. Dr. de la Fuente had declined the invitation to attend and speak. One of the more interesting speakers, representative of Puente's wide contacts in the business as well as the professional world, was Sr. Sylvio Garcia Patto, president of one of the major public relations firms in Latin America who spoke of the need to use all aspects of the media to educate the public about mental illness, reduce stigma, and increase access to appropriate prevention and treatment. He offered the voluntary services of his company to work toward this aim and in promotion of the 1991 World Congress.

Flache and I, together on the dais, presented diplomas in recognition of the memory of distinguished contributors to Mexican mental health. These included Alfonso Millan and one of my former close associates, Guillermo Davila, M.D., who established the mental health services of the Mexican Social Security System and for whom I had been a sometime consultant in the early 1960s.

The prospect of putting a fortieth anniversary celebration together at such short notice had been daunting and Federico Puente had met the challenge with flying colors. After seeing the skill with which he organized the celebration, under the threat of losing the 1991 World Congress, any doubts that the Board might have had about his ability in this respect vanished. The anniversary meeting also indicated the depth of his local support, despite a significant body of detractors. The Congress organizing committee under Velasco Suarez included many outstanding personalities in the mental health field, psychologists, nurses, and social workers, as well as psychiatrists and psychoanalysts, and others, comprising a very broad range of groups and disciplines. This boded well for a stated Congress aim, which was to stimulate development of a broadly based mental health movement in the Region, including volunteers, ex-patients, and survivors of illness, and the range of mental health disciplines.

The progress made toward the Congress in the face of significant obstacles, and the need to affirm Puente's leadership, still under attack, was recognized by the Federation Board. At its 3-4 December 1988 meeting in London, chaired by President Gamal El Azayem of Cairo, it took the unusual step of moving a vote of confidence in Federico Puente and his colleagues. This vote put the final stamp on the plans: the Federation's next World Congress for Mental Health was now definitely scheduled for 18–23 August 1991 in Mexico City. At the same time, the Board remained concerned with the split within Mexican mental health professional groups. This was expressed in its explicit request to Puente that a persisting effort should be made to bring all of the Mexican groups together in a supportive relationship with the Congress.

By now other ripples of Puente's activities were being felt in the Mexican mental health scene. One was the increased prominence of the Mexican Foundation for the Rehabilitation of Psychiatric Patients, *Fondacion Mexicana para la Rehabilitacion del Enfermo Mental*. Led by his friend, the dynamic Virginia Arevalo (later to become Gonzales Torres), it was a precursor of the first psychiatric user/survivor movement in the country. Another consequence was increased interest in the community mental health movement. Both of these developments evoked the distrust of powerful elements of the psychiatric establishment embodied in the Mexican Psychiatric Association, the Institute of Psychiatry, and the large state hospital bureaucracies. More "liberal" elements, notably the Mexican Society for Psychiatry and Neurology, with its President Elect, Jaime Ayala Villareal, M.D., as co-chairman with Puente of the World Congress for Mental Health, supported the community and user/survivor movements. This Society, founded in 1947, included leading professionals in education and health planning as well as in the clinical disciplines.

The new tension between what came to be regarded as conservative and liberal elements in the psychiatric community helped form the theme for the 1991 Congress. With Puente and Arevalo, I visited the largest state mental hospital in the Mexico City area, discouragingly reminiscent of many old, understaffed institutions elsewhere in the world. Then we visited a community halfway house operated by the Foundation. The contrast was dramatic. Although the physical facilities were unimpressive, the dignity and self-esteem of the chronically ill persons who helped manage it were significant demonstrations of what the new philosophy could accomplish. As we drove away, we began to talk about what we hoped the 1991 Congress might achieve. High on the list was the involvement of service users in community-based facilities and increased patient opportunities for self-determination. Arevalo, especially, felt it immensely important to put the word "people" into the official theme. Puente and I very much wanted it to serve as a reintroduction of "science" into Federation deliberations. While still in the car, driving back to the city, we agreed on an official theme: "People and Science: Together for Mental Health." It was announced in the following year, 1989, at the Auckland Congress.

With an increasingly broad base supporting the Congress, I received more requests to visit Mexico and participate in its development. One such opportunity was Jaime Ayala's inauguration as President of the Mexican Society for Neurology and Psychiatry on 6–8 April 1989. It was clear that he brought many strengths to the Federation and the Congress. In addition to the universal personal esteem in which he was held, he was on the Board of the *Asociacion Psicoanalitica Mexicana* and a founding member of the *Comite Mexicano Pro Salud Mental*.

1989 also saw a crescendo of other preparatory activities led by Puente and his loyal adherents. In May, in his capacity as President of COMECTA, he organized a "World No-Tobacco Day" in conformity with the WHO program. This was done with a host of television and radio programs through joint efforts with Dr. Rafael Camacho-Solis, General Director of Health Promotion for Mexico. After this, COMECTA was identified as a co-organizer of the Congress along with the Mexican Society of Neurology and Psychiatry.

In July, Puente convened a meeting of the Organizing Committee to discuss program themes, which was attended by representatives of 15 associations. During the 21–25 August 1989 World Congress for Mental Health in Auckland, he nominated (without opposition) Jaime Ayala to succeed him as Regional Vice President while he, himself, was elected Board Member-at-Large. On 22–24 September 1989, WFMH member association, the *Sociedad Psicoanalitica de Mexico* held its seventh Congress with Puente as an honored guest. Later, at an International Conference on Global Priorities organized by the Autonomous University of Mexico, he drew attention to the Congress by speaking on "Global Issues in Mental Health." Beginning on 14 December 1989, he initiated a weekly radio program on "Mental Health All Over the World: Present, Past and Future," under the auspices of the Congress Organizing Committee. By the beginning of 1990, the Organizing Committee was meeting monthly with an attendance of approximately 60 people representing at least 15 societies as well as the Ministries of Health, Tourism, and Education, and the National Autonomous University of Mexico. Unlike other Congresses, the Committee appointed Regional Chairpeople to bring the message and to solicit participation from different WFMH world regions. Finally, at Puente's request, I agreed to co-chair with Carlos Leon of Colombia, an Honorary International Advisory Committee, most of the members of which had to be personally recruited. With the agreement of most major world figures in the field to be on the Honorary Committee and (despite the original opposition from its Mental Health Division) co-sponsorship by WHO and other international agencies, a sense of the Congress' inevitability and its rushing momentum grew. Any thought of stopping it had evidently been abandoned.

1990, the year immediately preceding the Congress, was characterized by a fever pitch of activity involving larger numbers of people and events than in any previous or succeeding pre-Congress preparations. Although this crescendo of activity may have been initially motivated by the threatened opposition, it was now linked to Puente's expressed intention that the 1991 WFMH Congress would be the largest and most significant in Federation history. To achieve this goal, events were planned to lead up to the Congress, which would represent their culmination. In March of that year, a preparatory meeting of consumers was held in Houston, Texas. In April, Puente represented WFMH at the World Conference on Smoking and Health in Australia where he met with WHO Director General Hiroshi Nakajima, M.D., to discuss WHO participation in the Congress. In May, the Organization of American States offered its support. Puente, accompanied by Velasco Suarez and Ayala came to the May 1990 American Psychiatric Association meeting in New York where I arranged an informal meeting in the UN dining room. There, we were joined by a number of other supporters including my old friend, psychiatrist, and social scientist Marten de Vries, M.D., Professor of Social Psychiatry at the University of Limburg, the Netherlands, who was to become the WFMH President only a few years later in July 1997. By now, Puente had obtained support for the production and printing of announcements from the Governor of Mexico City, and the Organizing Committee had grown to include the President of the Mexican Red Cross Board of Directors and the Executive Secretary of the Pastoral Department of Health of the Catholic Church in Mexico. This last presaged a new development in Puente's thinking. He was aware that after decades of secularization, exemplified by the use of the former church as the great meeting hall of the hospital, many people were again thinking of Mexico as a Catholic nation. This suggested the possibility of enhancing the prestige of the Congress by forging an allegiance with the Church that might lend it some high-level sponsorship.

In the midpoint of this near-triumphal year, 1990, for Puente came the annual Board meeting. Flache, as President, chose to have it at the Geneva headquarters of WHO, his major and continuing source of support and prestige. Although the momentum of the Mexico Congress preparations had reached the proportions of a steamroller, he had not fully abandoned his ambivalence toward Puente. It was only realized later that he had included neither Puente nor Jaime Ayala in the series of invitations to his home extended to all other Board members. This was a clear affront to the pride of the Mexican colleagues who had been characteristically generous and inclusive in their own hospitality to foreign visitors in Mexico City. Although there was no comment at the time, this had later consequences.

On 27 September 1990, a planned preparatory event to the Congress, a "Symposium on Technology, Education and Health," was held in Mexico City with government support and papers by leading scientists and clinicians. Although I was unable to attend, Dick Hunter was on the scene and reviewed the developing logistics and finances. By now these included support from UNESCO, the Mexican Red Cross, American Express, and the Mexican Institute of Social Services and Social Security for Employees of the State. Seven full-time support staff members were working at several locations, including Puente's home, which had become the administrative nerve center of the effort.

In October 1990, Unicef agreed to co-sponsorship. Puente decided that this was a golden opportunity to involve European colleagues outside of ERC/WFMH and began inviting colleagues from Spain. The Spanish Ministry of Health and the government of the Spanish province of Catalunya accepted, announcing that they would send delegations as did the Mental Health Nurses of Spain (which invited him to lecture at their annual convention in Pamplona in February 1991). In November, he visited Spain, the first of a number of visits extending through his 1993–1995 presidency including several lecture tours. In each instance, the Mental Health Nurses Association was a host. Its President, Pedro Torrejon, became Puente's discretionary Board appointment in 1993, and his Association provided accommodations for the 1994 Board meeting in Madrid.

From the initial visit to Spain in 1990, Puente went to Rome where he was able to arrange an audience with Pope John Paul II who agreed to send a videocassette message to be shown during the Congress Opening Ceremony. In December, UNESCO's Director General Federico Mayor Z. visited Acapulco, giving Puente, through the Mexican government's representative, Dr. Enrique Martinez del Campo, the chance to persuade him to be Honorary Chairman of one of the thematic subcongresses then being arranged, "Social Communication Sciences and Mental Health." Somewhat later the co-sponsorship of WHO and the actual participation of its Director General, Hiroshi Nakajima, M.D., were confirmed.

Another event brought into the Congress preparations was the annual meeting of the Mexican Society for Neurology and Psychiatry held 29 January–3 February 1991, in Jaime Ayala's hometown of Monterrey. It was marked by his inauguration as the Society's President, which conferred more local prestige than his other title of WFMH Regional Vice President or even his post as the relatively silent co-chairman of the forthcoming World Congress. This meeting gave me an opportunity to support the Congress by speaking on the role of nongovernmental organizations in the formation of health policy across national boundaries. It also presented an opportunity to get to know Jaime's family, still traditional denizens of Monterrey. His wife and mine had become friends during the Geneva Board meetings in 1990, and this was a pleasant opportunity to renew our friendships.

May 1991 saw an anticipatory event in Washington DC. Puente and a considerable number of his leadership team greeted guests at the Federation's fifth Embassy Reception held at the Mexican House of Culture under the patronage of the Mexican Ambassador to the United States. By June, Congress participation had been confirmed by groups from Argentina, Belize, Brazil, Chile, Colombia, Cuba, Peru, Uruguay, and Venezuela, Central America, and the Caribbean As expected, the sponsoring Mexican group had nominated Puente for the post of President Elect, the vote to be taken by the Assembly during the forthcoming World Congress. Jaime Ayala was renominated for an additional two-year term, 1991–1993, as Regional Vice President. He would finish his term as Puente took office as President in Tokyo in 1993.

The 1991 World Congress for Mental Health and its Sequelae

Recognizing a Record-Breaking Event

The Mexican Congress had 6200 registrants. By far, the largest number, 5100, were from the host country, including many students. However, 1100, representing 45 other nations, were from abroad. The inaugural and closing ceremonies each filled the new 10,000 seat National Auditorium in Chapultepec Park to overflowing. This record attendance reflected the wide national publicity accorded it, the government's perception of its importance for the national image, and its significance for students and the range of nonmedical mental health workers attracted by the opportunity to hear, at first hand, the views of contributors from many countries. It was probably also due to the range of interests represented by the record number of 22 thematic subcongresses meeting every afternoon with simultaneous Spanish/English translation covering topics from the mental health of refugees to the rights and roles of women. The opportunity for interaction presented by these subcongresses vastly facilitated future work on the Federation mental health agenda, beginning with activities in the Region itself, which will be noted in relation to the WFMH agenda.

This Congress fulfilled Puente's ambition for a Congress of record-breaking size. It marked a peak in numerical attendance, which will probably not be matched, or even aspired to, by future organizers. It followed six biennial Congresses none of which had achieved more than 1000 attendees. After that in 1977, which brought 2000 participants to Vancouver, those in Salzburg, Manila, Washington DC, Brighton, Cairo, and Auckland had all been of modest size. Although the 1993 Congress in Tokyo approximated 4000 participants, the organizers of the 1995 Congress in Dublin deliberately opted for modesty, both in attendance and in program. Their attitude, suggesting a philosophy of "smaller is better," was reflected in their Congress theme, "Time for Reflection." The attendance, which nonetheless strained the facilities of its venue, Trinity College, was perhaps one-quarter of that in Mexico.

The Federation Board was impressed both by the exceptional outpouring for the Mexican Congress and by its rich substantive content. It was sensitive to the unusual effort that had been expended by Puente as Congress Chairman to bring the event to fruition. However, it also wished to recognize as many of the Congress producers as possible. It noted especially, out of the 300-person Organizing Committee, the contributions of Jaime Ayala, Dr. Rosalba Bueno Osawa, and Congress Treasurer Lic. Eduardo Ramirez.

The Interpersonal Context of Congress Organization, Regional Organization and Mental Hospital Reform

The Congress placed Mexico unequivocally on the world mental health stage, cemented Federico Puente's claim to the WFMH presidency, and reduced, although did not eliminate, the antagonistic gulf between him and the staff of the Institute of Psychiatry. It did not, however, extinguish the residual hostility between him and outgoing President Flache. Flache, as President, had been a figure in the opening ceremonies. Midway in the Congress, at the Assembly of voting members, in keeping with the usual custom, the presidency was transferred to incoming President, Max Abbott, Ph.D., of New Zealand. Puente, as Congress Chairman, moderated the closing ceremonies in which a role was assigned to Abbott. However, he did not include Flache, depriving him not only of his rightful place among the dignitaries but of the usual opportunity afforded the outgoing President to make some final remarks. No one on the Board or in the Secretariat was aware that the exclusion was in process until all participants had been seated on the stage and it was clear that no place had been allotted to Flache. At that point, in response to our distressed comment, Puente expressed his willingness to include the outgoing President on the program, but Flache was nowhere to be found. He only appeared at the next morning's Post-Congress Board meeting to tender his resignation. That was a most uncomfortable moment. By the end of the next day's meeting, however, he was persuaded to stay as he was needed in his role as our senior representative to the United Nations and WHO in Geneva. He also realized that he had more to gain than to lose by remaining on the Board in his new capacity as Past President and Chairman of the Nominating Committee. The immediate crisis was smoothed over. Its persisting organizational impact, however, was uncertain..

Nor did the exceptional success of the Congress, during which Puente was elevated to the position of WFMH President Elect, result in a total mending of his relations with Mexican colleagues. Continued jockeying for power within the national mental health community, even among his supporters, was reflected in the ongoing formation and dissolution of new organizations, many of which applied for WFMH voting membership. Thus, the *Comite Pro Salud Mental*, which had been organized by Puente before the Congress, was now abandoned in favor of a new group, the *Federacion Mexicana de Salud Mental* led by Jaime Ayala and Hector Cabildo. It was described as "the central mental health forum in which Mexican mental health workers all have an equal voice."

Puente took office as WFMH President during the 1993 World Congress for Mental Health in Tokyo at the same time that his nominee, Andres Gaitan Gonzales, Ph.D., succeeded Jaime Ayala as WFMH Vice President for the Mexico/ Caribbean/Central America Region. In the summer of 1994, midstream in his WFMH Presidency, as described in earlier chapters, a Board meeting and a two-day symposium on "Mental Health in the World," including many prominent Spaniards, were held in Madrid, supported by the Spanish Association of Nurses in Mental Health. Afterwards, he attended a meeting of NGOs in "official relations" with WHO and visited Dublin to learn about the organization of the 1995 World Congress. Then, upon his return to Mexico, he confronted a new challenge. On 19 June, he telephoned me to report that he had received a "legal demand" (from Sanchez Sosa and others with whom his relations had cooled) for his resignation from the University on grounds that he had not met his teaching responsibilities because of his absence from the country. Despite the fact that he was a part-time faculty member receiving minimal compensation, the appointment was important to him. Of primary importance, he held Ramon de la Fuente and his supporters responsible for the offending demand as part of their resistance to his efforts (along with those of Virginia Gonzalez Torres) to reform Mexican mental hospitals. He said that he wished to weaken Dr. de la Fuente's hold upon public officials immediately responsible for patient care and hospital standards. He would do this by fighting the accusation of neglecting academic duties "as a matter of principle" and demand an apology. He was encouraged in this decision, he reported, by student demonstrations on his behalf. If the "legal demand" were not withdrawn within a week, or if no apology was forthcoming, he would initiate a hunger strike. To my question about the possible adverse perception of a hunger strike, especially to a watching audience of psychiatrists and psychologists, he replied that it was appropriate in his culture.

The threat was evidently effective. Just five days after being confronted with the "demand," on the night of 23 June he telephoned me to report that the University had withdrawn its demands. He believed that his "successful resistance...strengthened his position in Mexico vis-à-vis those who are obstacles to mental hospital reform." Among the groups demonstrating support for his position were, he said, the Catholic Church, the Mexican Red Cross, various student bodies, and UNESCO officials in Mexico.

The Latin American Council

Puente's ascension to the post of President Elect on the 1991 Congress' wave of enthusiasm gave him confidence to press some of the controversial administrative concerns, discussed in Chapters 5 and 6. His view of regional organization and the opportunities for continued leadership that it might offer were revealed in his plans for a new regional entity. This was a Latin American Council of WFMH (LAC/WFMH) in which the South American Region would be one component, instead of an autonomous geographical unit of itself. He, himself, would head the new Council (with the exact title still indeterminate). Benjamin Vicente, M.D., Ph.D., newly named WFMH Vice President for South America, who apparently was consulted only in passing, would chair a component South American Council, and Jaime Ayala would head the Mexico/Central America/Caribbean Council. Its Secretariat would be headed by psychologist Rosalba Bueno Osawa with the title of Secretary General. Spanish organizational members of WFMH were invited to participate on an honorary basis.

The first Draft By Laws of the proposed new organization arrived in my office before the end of 1991 with the intent that they would come into force by 22 February 1992 and that the items concerned with its elected officers would become effective by January 1, 1994. At its next annual meeting in Sydney later in 1992, the Board became fully acquainted with the irregular founding of this new "Council," for which there was no place in the Bylaws. However, noting Vicente's failure to mount an objection, it accepted it on a provisional basis pending development of an independent South American Regional Council. Meanwhile, Puente initiated a series of meetings aimed at creating a structure for it with the involvement of influential high status citizens. They included, in the pattern of the Congress Organizing Committee, leaders from government institutions, the Red Cross, the Mexican Council Against Addictions, the Catholic Church, and now, for the first time—since Puente had established friendships with some of de la Fuente's junior staff members—the Mexican Institute of Psychiatry. An advisory committee of distinguished citizens, including Dr. Jose Felix-Palma, Director of the Mexican Office of the Organization of American States, was formed and the new Latin American Council was launched.

A series of regional activities, which will be described elsewhere, was sponsored by LAC/WFMH. An outstanding example was a symposium on "Wild Flora and Fauna and Emotional Well-Being," held 15–16 November 1993 with the total financial support of the Ministry of Agriculture. A group of LAC members, sponsored by the national office of Unicef, attended the International Conference on Health Psychology held in Cuba on 5–9 October 1992. Besides Puente and Bueno Osawa, they were leaders of the nascent consumer movement, Virginia Gonzales Torres and Azul de Landeros. During the next year, other projects demonstrated the new Council's strength and progressive mental health concerns.

In 1994, the Latin American Council issued a new and comprehensive list of officers. With Puente as Honorary President, it remained primarily Mexican in nature while including a place for almost every subregional constituency. Thus, while its "Executive Co-Presidents" included Keens-Douglas (Caribbean) and Vicente (South America), they also included Gaitan Gonzales (Mexico/Central America). Ayala, still WFMH Vice President for its Mexico/Central America/Caribbean Region was "Liaison Chairman," and the governing body included Mexicans Bueno Osawa as General Secretary, Ramirez Garcia as Treasurer as well as six Mexican Associate Secretaries. On the eve of its dissolution, scheduled for the December 1996 formation of a new South American Council, LAC/WFMH prospered with grants from PAHO, the Eli Lilly pharmaceutical firm, and equipment from telephone companies to maintain its hotline services.

Toward a South American Regional Council

Planning for the establishment of a South American Regional Council of WFMH (SARC/WFMH) began with the Board's decision during the 1995 Dublin World Congress to have the 1999 World Congress in Chile. This came with its acceptance of an invitation from Board Member-at-Large Vicente, a professor of psychiatry at the University of Concepcion, Chile. There were some misgivings because of the unusual nature of our representation there, with Vicente's wife, Mabel Vielma, M.D., also on the Board as Regional Vice President for South America and no other representation from that vast continent. It was, indeed, a silent area and there had been long periods of silence from Vicente, himself. On the other hand, he had demonstrated a consistent interest in the Federation and was the kind of fluently English speaking academic psychiatrist, with training in England and Europe and shared Western values, with whom Board members found it easy to communicate.

The first concrete step occurred at a PAHO conference of Latin American mental health directors in Panama in June 1996. Although they paid their own way and were only observers during much of the meeting, Past President Puente, Regional Vice President Gaitan Gonzalez, and patient's rights activist Virginia Gonzalez from Mexico were there as well as Vicente and Vielma from Chile. Without difficulty or fanfare, the Mexicans agreed to change the name of the Latin American Council headed by Puente to a Mexican, Central America, and Caribbean Council. Whether the new Council would continue to be headed by Puente or, as the Bylaws dictated, by Regional Vice President Gaitan, was momentarily deferred.

The final step was a regional congress in Concepcion. It was co-sponsored by WFMH, the University of Concepcion's Faculty of medicine, and the Chilean Society of Mental Health, which held its fifth annual Chilean Congress for Mental Health from 5–7 December 1996. This Congress was attended by approximately 350 people including nearly 50 from outside of Chile representing every South American country except Ecuador. To show support for the formal inauguration of the new Council, WFMH held its 1996 Board meeting there. This occasioned some difficulty, because poor communication led to its being scheduled very close to the same time as the Pacific Regional Meeting in Taiwan (see Chapter 10). It was, therefore, the first Board meeting that I had missed in my nearly 16 years of close WFMH involvement. It was also missed by Honorary Secretary Asai and Regional Vice President Inoue of Japan who were with me in Taiwan, as was Honorary President Lin. Board members Pirkko from Finland did not attend because of preparations for the 1997 Congress; O'Mahony was ill, and with some other absences and late arrivals, the existence of a quorum was in doubt. Nonetheless, the Board members present acted as a unit formally observing the inauguration ceremony of installation for the members of the new South American Council representing most of the countries of the continent. Some uncertainty persisted into 1997, particularly in regard to who would be the Regional Vice President and the possible roles of South Americans other than Vicente and Vielma. As the mid-year Finland Congress approached, however, with its voting Assembly, it seemed likely that Vicente would move into a definitive leadership role in preparation for the 1999 World Congress in Santiago de Chile. There was general hope that, at last, this might usher in an era of WFMH activity throughout South America.

Chapter 10

WFMH in the Eastern Mediterranean, Africa, Asia, Oceania, and North America

EASTERN MEDITERRANEAN

Egyptian Association for Mental Health

In 1946 several Egyptian psychiatrists who had been meeting monthly in Cairo were visited by John R. Rees, who spoke about the importance of supporting the anticipated WFMH. With this stimulus the Egyptian Association for Mental Health (EAMH) was formed in early 1948 before the founding of WFMH. EAMH became one of the original members of WFMH and was represented on the Federation's first Executive Board by its president M. Kamil el Kholy, M.D., of Cairo, head of his country's Mental Health Services. Four years later he became WFMH president, serving for the 1952–1953 term. At that time the only other voluntary WFMH member in the region was the Pakistan Association for Mental Health. A governmental institution, the Pakistan Institute of Mental Hygiene, was also a member.

Between 14 December 1954, and 9 February 1955, Director Rees and President Fremont Smith, during a more extensive trip, visited Egypt (Cairo), Pakistan (Karachi), Lebanon (Beirut), and Sudan (Khartoum). This trip, like others of the Rees era, was less concerned with the initiation of new voluntary mental health associations than with the simultaneous process of gaining information about psychiatric/mental health activities in a particular region and influencing them in a manner congruent with what was perceived as the WFMH mission. In all instances contacts were confined to the dominant elite. Psychiatric services were reported to be inadequate in all countries; in all Rees expressed concern with the status of women, especially in relation to purdah, and in the Sudan, genital mutilation. Sudan's only psychiatrist at the time, Tigani el Mahi, M.D., had attended the 1954 International Congress for Mental Health in Toronto. In Cairo, in addition to a press of government ministers and other notables, a previous officer of the EAMH, psychologist Dr. N. Fouad Galal, Secretary General of the Permanent Council for Services of the Government, was engaged in planning the development of village centers including services for agriculture, education, health, and child welfare. Typically Rees suggested to Galal that all these topics should be included in the program of EAMH.

Gamal Mady Abou El Azayem, M.D. (WFMH President 1987–1989), recalled a 1968 visit from then WFMH President Morris Carstairs. El Azayem was superintendent of Egypt's largest mental hospital, the Abbassya (sometimes spelled Abbassia) in Cairo, and a prominent figure in Egyptian psychiatry. As he remembered (personal communication, 1996), their discussion of Egyptian mental health programs led to the idea of organizing the first mental health congress of Arab countries to be sponsored by WFMH in 1970. Annual reports of the era confirm that after Carstairs' visit, psychiatrist Ahmed Wagdi, M.D., in collaboration with the EAMH, helped organize the first Pan Arab Congress on mental health in Cairo in 1969. It was chaired by Taha Baasher, M.D., Minister of Health of the Sudan who had been a member of the WFMH Executive Board. Dr. El Azayem was the congress secretary general. Participants included the range of mental health related professionals and Muslim religious figures. The meeting was marked by an unusual exchange between young people wanting greater freedom at the same time that they expressed adherence to the Muslim faith and older people determined to preserve traditional values. A recurrent theme was rapid social change accompanying the urbanization and industrialization of peasant populations.

One recommendation of that first congress was that the psychiatrists in the Arab region should convene biennial meetings. In 1972 Wagdi was named the first WFMH vice president for the Eastern Mediterranean region. The moving voluntary mental health force in the area continued to be EAMH, which conceived itself as the regional link to WFMH. It was essentially an organization of psychiatrists that sponsored the Second Arab Congress on Mental Health (22–24 December 1975) with the collaboration of the World Psychiatric Association and the Egyptian Ministry of Health as well as WFMH. The theme, though, was of general public interest, "Youth and Mental Health." Cairene psychiatrist, Dr. Adly Fahmy Abdou, represented the Federation at a 12–17 June 1976, World Health Organization (WHO) regional meeting on mental health and mental health legislation.

With the passage of time, EAMH gradually became more broadly based, including the range of professionals as well as (to a quite limited degree) citizen volunteers. In the 1980s and 1990s, although its main support was through membership dues, it received subsidies from the ministries of health and social welfare. These funded some of its educational efforts focused in rural areas and among the poor. They included mental health discussions and symposia at schools, clubs, and mosques. In association with hospitals and other organizations it developed clubs and camps for schizophrenic patients. In addition EAMH published its own magazine. But its special efforts have been reserved for mosques, religious leaders, and influential citizens such as police officials, teachers, and government administrators.

The Arab/Islamic World Enters the Federation: the 1987 World Congress and Beyond

Despite the early contacts of the Rees era, Islamic and Arab psychiatrists did not attempt to exert a philosophical or ideological influence on the Federation or to utilize its credentials in their work until nearly 30 years later. The central figure in the reactivation of the region and its closeness to WFMH was Dr. El Azayem, now the owner of a private psychiatric hospital in Cairo. His international experience outside the Arab world included a 1954 WHO fellowship in Europe, a 1973 WHO consultancy on drug dependency, and membership on the 1977 WHO Expert Advisory Panel on Drug Dependence. In 1978, he was principal investigator of a joint United States-Egypt project on the voluntary treatment of opium dependence. During these years he also functioned as a university lecturer and consultant to the Egyptian Ministry of Justice and continued as the long-time secretary of EAMH.

Gamal El Azayem became a member of the WFMH Board, as it existed before the new by-laws, during the Salzburg World Congress in 1979. Although I, too, became a Board member then, we did not really communicate until my first meeting as Federation president after the Manila congress of 1981. He had then been appointed regional vice president. However, he was notably silent; it appeared that he did not fully comprehend either English or the European-dominated Board process and was deliberately cautious in expressing himself.

During these meetings it became my privilege to help him deal with a medical emergency. This involved a level of intimate communication and produced a rapport between us not usually attained between Board members. During our interaction he spoke of his Islamic faith and particularly of the Sufi background that he had acquired from his father. It was these conversations that, when I was planning the 1983 World Congress in Washington, DC, led me to notice that the Mary Hemingway Rees lecture on spiritual issues in relation to mental health had dealt mainly with topics related to Christianity. I immediately thought of the contribution that Gamal might make and invited him to deliver the lecture on a topic of his choice. He agreed and spoke on "The Mosque as a Mental Health Center." His presence at the congress attracted delegates from Saudi Arabia, Pakistan, Sudan, and other Arab nations.

In the same year his well-received lecture, which gave him prominence in the congress, accelerated formation of the World Islamic Association for Mental Health (WIAMH). In addition to Egyptian groups its initial members were the mental health associations of the Gulf states, Pakistan, Bangladesh, and Kuwait; later members came from Algeria and Sudan. Its first president was WFMH Life Member Osama Al Radi, M.D., the first head of Saudi Arabian psychiatric services, with Gamal as Secretary General. Senior vice president was Mohammud Rashid Chaudry, M.D., Professor of Psychiatry at King Edward Medical College in Lahore, whom I had first met at the 1981 Manila congress where he presented me with a gold-colored toy cannon. The "advisor" was Taha Baasher, M.D., former WHO Mental Health Advisor for the Eastern Mediterranean region and Professor of Psychiatry at the University of the Sudan in Khartoum. The new organization's first General Assembly was on 9 October 1983, in Cairo, and shortly thereafter Al Radi represented WFMH at the WHO regional meeting in Jordan that was attended by the health ministers of all the Middle Eastern countries. There he gave a speech about the developing role of the Federation in regard to the region's mental health with special emphasis on the formation of WIAMH. Its first annual meeting was in Istanbul in August 1984 during an Islamic congress.

In 1983 and 1984 organizational work among the region's mental health leaders proceeded rapidly. In February 1984 Chaudry, acting for the Lahore Mental Health Association's Committee for the Prevention of Drug Abuse, helped develop a three-day seminar on "Problems of Drug Abuse." In late February my wife and I were guests of WIAMH in Cairo with Gamal and in Riyadh with Osama Al Radi. In Riyadh we were greeted at the airport by Osama and his daughter, whom we had met at the Fountain House meeting in Stockholm. She was unrecognizable, however, because she was completely covered in accordance with local custom. The veil, physical and communicative, was removed, however, at the gatherings of women attended by my wife where they wore fashionable European clothing and revealed various cosmopolitan interests. In Cairo we also met members of Gamal's family; this became first of many visits over several years.

Beyond its personal significance this early 1984 visit provided many opportunities to bring the Federation message to local institutions and leaders. Among them were interviews with the Egyptian health minister and senior mental health advisor; lectures at the departments of psychiatry and psychology of the University of Cairo; a press conference sponsored by a leading Egyptian magazine; discussions with volunteers at the Mosque Health Center in Riyadh; meetings with the vice director of the Islamic University, Imam, M. Bin Saud; the dean of the King Saud Faculty of Medicine, chairman of its department of psychiatry and several others at the King Faisal Specialty Hospital; lectures at the King Khalid Hospital of Saud University; and meetings with patients and staff on the psychiatric wards. The staff was predominantly from outside Saudi Arabia, often from Arab countries and trained in the United States, the United

Kingdom, or Canada, and fully conversant with contemporary treatments and theories. One, whose residency had been in Topeka, was especially interested in the impact on his female patients of having to remove their veils during therapeutic hours.

Gamal had accepted my invitation to speak in Washington as a mark of confidence in him and his culture. The organizing successes of these two years led him to suggest that the 1987 World Congress for Mental Health be held in Cairo. Before the May 1984 Board meeting at the Sheppard Pratt Hospital in Baltimore, Gamal spoke, along with other Board members, at a symposium on "The Prevention of Mental Illness: An International Perspective." Later, with the support of the Egyptian Health Ministry he presented a bid to sponsor the 1987 congress, and a sympathetic Board voted to accept.

At the same time, in keeping with WFMH custom, an effort was begun to find a non-European to succeed the 1985–1987 president, Edith Morgan of London. The Eastern Mediterranean was one region that had not had a president in recent years. Partly because of his experience as a Board member, partly in consequence of his new prominence at the 1983 congress, and significantly because of his role in organizing the forthcoming world congress in Egypt, Gamal was nominated for WFMH president-elect at the 1985 Brighton assembly. Overcoming some resistance from colleagues whose negative view of Egyptian capacities may have reflected remnants of the British colonialist perspective, he was elected to become WFMH president for the 1987–1989 term.

At the same time a cluster of interpersonal and political events set the stage for future complications. Chanita Rodney, founding president of ENOSH (Israeli mental health association) and a personal friend of President Morgan, was elected a Board member-at-large. Her presence lent urgency to the Board discussion when it decided-as a political gesture in support of Israel's permanence-to move Israel away from its United Nations assigned "location" in the European region to the WFMH eastern Mediterranean region. This took place at the precongress Board meeting in Brighton on 12–13 July 1985. As reported, "In recognition of geographic realities, and reflecting the Board's hope for a significant Israeli delegation to the 1987 World Congress for Mental Health in Cairo, Israel's location in the WFMH Eastern Mediterranean region was explicitly reaffirmed" (WFMH, 1985). After this, Rodney was nominated by President Morgan to be WFMH vice president for the region. The prospect of an Israeli vice president created consternation in President-elect El Azayem, who believed that Rodney's appointment to the post would destroy the possibility of a regional organization. But, with his never-failing civility, he answered "Excellent!" when asked how he felt about it. Rodney was attracted to the position and was urged strongly by some colleagues to remain as a candidate. She was politically and personally sensitive, however, and after considerable introspection and consultation with her backers, withdrew her name.

Once nominated and assured of a congenial regional vice president with the naming of his old friend, Taha Baasher, Gamal felt secure enough to expand his regional activities in the name of WFMH. He lectured on substance abuse to Saudi social workers, reported on Federation activities at WIAMH's meeting in Lahore, and participated, at the invitation of the Council of Churches in the Middle East, in a training course on substance abuse for Middle Eastern religious leaders in Cyprus in the autumn of 1985. Combining his two major interests, religion and substance abuse, he helped develop a WIAMH committee for research on the role of religious institutions in reducing the demand for addictive drugs. Baasher also increased his regional activities , becoming president of the Sudanese Association of Psychiatrists, a member of the Sudan Narcotic Control Board, and organizing a program on psychosocial and mental health issues at the university. Other Eastern Mediterranean leaders, combining their WFMH and WIAMH identities, also cultivated their liaison with organized psychiatry in the area. Thus, several participated in the Third Pan Arab Congress on Psychiatry held 14–16 April 1986, in Amman, Jordan, where Gamal distributed circulars on the 1987 World Congress and chaired a WFMH sponsored session entitled "The Organization of Mental Services in the Arab World."

As these events stimulated increased regional interest in mental health related activities, planning progressed for the 1987 World Congress. Gamal's program consultants included both the former and current WHO Mental Health Advisors for the Eastern Mediterranean, Taha Baasher, M.D., WFMH regional vice president, and R. Narendra Wig, M.D., former chairman of Psychiatry at the Universities of Chandigahr and New Delhi in India. A special issue of the WIAMH journal, *Mental Peace* entitled "Islam and Mental Health" was recommended reading for those planning to attend the congress.

In February and March 1986 I was teaching at Tel Aviv University. During this period riots involving the young Egyptian security police, conscripted from the villages, led to a reduction in tourist reservations. At Gamal's request and to demonstrate the lack of danger to visitors, my wife and I flew on the Egyptian Air Sinai line from Tel Aviv to Cairo, where he met us on the morning of 12 March 1986. Passage through airport formalities was uneventful, and street traffic was normal despite a visible military presence. This visit gave me the opportunity to confer with Ahmed Nair Kotry, M.D., the chief of the Egyptian Health Ministry's Department of Mental Health who was especially interested in the concept of community-based mental health facilities; Abdel Ashour, M.D., Secretary General of the 1987 congress during part of its preparatory period; Professor El Gawad, Chairman of Psychiatry at Cairo University and president of the Egyptian Psychiatric Association; and Omar Shaheen, M.D., president of EAMH, the primary local congress sponsor. While in Cairo we also visited the Abou El Azayem mosque—owned by the family—in an ancient, densely populated section of the city. There we participated in a youth meeting at its mental health clinic. The mosque also housed a child welfare clinic for working women, an addiction treatment center, and a library of almost 1000 books, mainly about religion and mental health. The facilities were financed partly by the Ministry of Social Affairs and partly by donations supplementing the nominal fees paid by patients.

Gamal asked me to decide on a theme for the 1987 WFMH World Congress, and we agreed on "The Many Worlds of Mental Health" as a way of emphasizing the cultural issues that were certain to be prominent. We disagreed, however, on the Margaret Mead lecturer. My choice was my long-time friend, Dr. Phyllis Palgi, Chair of the Department of Behavioral Science at Tel Aviv University Medical School where I had been a visiting professor in 1986. She seemed most appropriate as a woman, a cultural anthropologist, and a friend of Mead. However, Gamal was concerned about a negative reaction from Egyptian colleagues and newspapers and was adamant about not having an Israeli as the main speaker. Instead he selected Dr. M. Elgohary, Vice Chancellor of the University of Cairo, an anthropologist who spoke on "The Concept of Psychosis in Egyptian Folklore" with special reference to the Zar cult, which was also a particular interest of Palgi's.

Palgi introduced the session and was the discussant while I acted as moderator. She was one of only a handful of Israelis, including Chanita Rodney, willing to breach the "cold peace" and come to the congress. They were sufficiently enthusiastic about their experiences to request newsletter space to express their feelings. The February 1988 issue contained a statement from Ofra Ayalon, Ph.D., of the University of Haifa: "The interdisciplinary meetings from different countries engendered a whole new set of connections that had not occurred beforehand. This seems to be a further step toward achieving the common goal of World Citizenship" (WFMH, 1988). Indeed, Egyptian participants at this meeting with its new experiences of meeting foreigners, including students, numbered nearly 700, and there were more than 500 from other countries, many from the region. However, although both Israel and Egypt offered tours in association with the congress, the former sponsored by ENOSH (Israeli mental health association), no Egyptians came to Israel. At least one Israeli took advantage of the Egyptian trip, which included five days on the Nile with stops for major historical sites.

The Cairo World Congress, during which Gamal El Azayem became the Federation's second Egyptian president, was the first such WFMH gathering in Africa and the Middle East. Its significance for the country and region were embodied in his postcongress summation: "Now in

Egypt every one knows about mental health!" The Egyptian congress committee, in keeping with local tradition, also made many recommendations for action. Those with particular significance for the region included the importance of peaceful resolution of societal and international conflict, abolishing the torture of political prisoners, and the recognition of spiritual values and their supporting institutions.

The El Azayem presidency, 1987–1989, reflected the character of the man. He was relaxed, generous, and ecumenical. At the same time he put his personal and institutional resources, as well as his effort and talent, into our work. He truly brought a new world, that of the Arab and Islamic peoples, into our fold. But he was also organizationally ambitious. His presidency was marked both by attempts to recruit other regional associations to WFMH membership and to establish a regional council of WFMH, the Eastern Mediterranean Regional Council (EMRC/WFMH). The World Congress under his leadership did much to attract regional interest. It was also generally appreciated that the primary financial support for the congress came from the El Azayem Hospital Center. As president he carried the message of the Federation throughout the region. Examples in 1988 were a series of lectures on the mosque as a mental health center at Yarmouk University, Jordan; lectures on drug addiction and rehabilitation at the Ministry of Interior Affairs in the Gulf Emirates; and a regional conference in Cairo on mental health services for victims of community violence. The emphasis on substance abuse was carried forward by EAMH, which took the lead in celebrating the United Nations' "International Day against Drug Abuse and Illicit Trafficking" on 26 June and by El Azayem, who participated in the closing ceremony of the First Arab Congress for Confronting the Problems of Substance Abuse (Cairo, 13–16 September). He also traveled widely outside the region, participating in an international congress on rehabilitation in Stockholm and coming to Washington DC, for a Federation fund-raiser at the Turkish embassy.

An activity attracting both regional and general WFMH participation was a conference and Nile cruise on 17–21 January 1989, to celebrate the Federation's 40th anniversary (21 August 1988) as well as that of EAMH. It was conducted with the cooperation of EAMH and New York Medical College where Gamal's son, Ahmed Gamal Abou El Azayem, M.D., clinical director of his hospital, had been taking courses on new technology for brain mapping. The El Azayem hospital financed the attendance of several Board members, including Past President Edith Morgan, President-elect Stanislas Flache, Treasurer Robert Gibson, Honorary Secretary Isaac Mwendapole, EMR Vice President Taha Baasher, and Board member-at-large and EAMH President Omar Shaheen. The days on the Nile offered a mixed cultural and political experience. Culturally the contrasts were endless between the technology of the ship and the primitive settlements along the shore with occasional camels and donkeys and villagers often seen bathing and washing clothes in the river. Politically, there were endless conversations with Palestinians, Egyptians, and others in the Arab world who favored the establishment of a Palestinian state and decried the Israeli occupation of the West Bank and Gaza.

Gamal also had a particular agenda. As noted in Chapter 13, he wanted to crown his anniversary celebration with a WFMH Declaration on the rights of the mentally ill. In October 1988 I had drafted such a declaration, after an initial version had been rejected by a small working group convened at the beginning of August in London. Dominated by U.K. colleagues, the group felt that it was not yet suitable for general adoption. That opinion was reiterated after I circulated a second draft by mail. Part of the problem related to its differences from a manifesto prepared by Chris Heginbotham, then director of MIND (the national mental health association of England and Wales). I had set it aside. Then Gamal asked me to bring the draft to Cairo to present for adoption at his 40th anniversary conference. I realized that he wanted to steal a march on the Europeans by being the first to sponsor such a declaration. Nonetheless, I presented it to the conference audience during a meeting on shore in Luxor. It was no surprise that the conference, without discussion, adopted it by acclamation as the "Luxor Declaration of the Rights of the Mentally Ill." Although Gamal knew that it would be subject to further discussion at the coming Board meeting before the congress in Auckland, New Zealand (21–25 August 1989), he regarded this as a triumph that might pave the way for an Arab regional council of WFMH. In his Message from the President in the June 1989 newsletter, he wrote of the "positive messages [which] have come to the office in Cairo from the four corners of the world hailing the Federation's efforts in this field" (WFMH, 1989).

Another source of strength for El Azayem's ambitions was WIAMH, in which he exerted great influence. With its founding of an Arabic language newsletter, *Mental Peace*, he concluded that an Arab working group or an Arab regional council might be possible, perhaps as a precursor to a later EMRC/WFMH. This because the countries listed in the region were Arabic-speaking although not all in fact were "Eastern Mediterranean." In addition to Egypt, early expressions of interest came from associations, mainly of psychiatrists, in Algeria, Morocco, Pakistan, South Yemen, and Sudan. All were members of the Arab League (registered as an intergovernmental organization with the United Nations and some of its affiliated agencies including WHO). The League had only recently placed mental health on its agenda, stimulated by the attendance of WFMH members in a conference after a meeting of its national health ministers.

A major advocate for the embryonic Arab Council was Sheena Dunbar of the United Kingdom who had been a public information officer for MIND as well as correspondent for an Arabic language daily in London. More recently she had moved to Cairo, married an Egyptian psychiatrist, and become an assistant for Federation matters to President El Azayem. In April 1989 she assisted in the preparation of the first Arab Council Newsletter. It presented an inclusive list of clinical and socioeconomic problems affecting mental health in the region, with special reference to drug addiction but including terrorism, aggression, and victims of war. It also included an announcement soliciting membership in "Amaan," the minuscule Palestine mental health association, which emphasized "the profound effect of the Israeli occupation and intifada on the mental well-being of the Palestinian people." In May 1989 Dunbar drafted working rules for an Arab regional council of WFMH so that they might be ready for the first meeting of its steering committee in the fall during the conference of the Arab Federation of Psychiatrists in Yemen. Optimistic plans were made for preparatory meetings of a steering committee for a WFMH Arab working group during psychiatric meetings in Athens in October 1989 and Yemen in December, but these did not materialize. The WFMH Executive Committee, meeting in May 1989 in time to receive the working rules, concluded that because WFMH had no "Arab region," neither an Arab working group nor an Arab Council was possible as part of its structure. However, to show good will and facilitate the development of EMRC/WFMH and after consultation with Chanita Rodney-who said that the WFMH move although good-hearted had not been effective in integrating the region-it "sadly and reluctantly" agreed to move Israel back to the European region where it was still located in the WHO schema. This move also recognized the continuing resistance of Egyptian WFMH members to real integration.

The issue finally came to the Board meeting on 26 August 1989 after the Auckland World Congress for Mental Health. By that time, after considerable discussion, the designation of regional council was abandoned in favor of the more informal notion of an Arab "working group" of interested member associations. The Board approved this, specifying that their approval did not mean obviating the WFMH Eastern Mediterranean region that included non-Arab countries. The terminology was understood to refer to a cultural grouping and to avoid confusion with the concept of a regional council which was so far used only by the European region.

Although a WFMH Arab regional council did not finally materialize and there was an inevitable slow-down after the peaks of the 1987 World Congress and the 1987–1989 El Azayem presidency, regional activities continued. These were mainly in the areas of religion and drug abuse and, beginning in 1991, on conflict resolution. WIAMH also continued to increase in size and vigor, both as an independent entity and as a member organization of WFMH. In 1991 President Al Radi made the first proposal in the Arabic Gulf region for a mental health law, "putting in consideration our Arabic Islamic cultural aspects." Its fifth biennial meeting (6–10

February 1994) with a Nile cruise carried forward its focus on Islamic issues: the role of Islam in conflict resolution and preventing substance abuse and the status of the mosque as a social organization. Its growing resources permitted an increase in publication frequency of *Mental Peace* from quarterly to monthly.

Meanwhile, organizational activity continued on other fronts. In mid-1989, before the Auckland World Congress, a letter came from Taha Baasher transmitting an application from the Palestine Red Crescent Society (equivalent of the Red Cross), headed by Fathi Arafat, M.D. (brother of Yasir Arafat), for membership in WFMH. It had come to him in his role as regional vice president; he had been nominated by Gamal El Azayem after Chanita Rodney had declined. Although Baasher realized that the mandate of the Red Crescent Society did not fit the WFMH membership requirements, he was especially concerned with how WFMH might react to the Cairo-based Palestinian mental health association (Amaan) "being established by" it. In fact Amaan had been founded the year before, in June 1988, with the encouragement of Dr. Arafat. The secretary of its steering committee was Sheena Dunbar, who actively promoted its membership in WFMH.

By 5 July 1989, Amaan had held seven meetings. Its minutes indicate that they were attended by the same five or six people and that they were primarily concerned with administrative organization. The minutes of the fifth meeting (May 1989) noted Arafat's report of "a positive response from those in the occupied territories on the establishment of Amaan." The minutes of the seventh and last meeting referred to the group's application for WFMH membership. This application required WFMH Board discussion beyond the usual membership scrutiny, because there was no Palestinian state with general international recognition (just as there was no "Arab region") within the WFMH purview. The matter was quickly resolved on grounds that WFMH was a Federation of associations, not political entities, and Amaan was invited to submit a formal membership application. Arafat, apparently in pursuit of this goal, attended the assembly of voting member associations moderated by President El Azayem at the August 1989 Auckland World Congress. However, he had no message for the assembled members, nor did the completed application ever arrive.

The Auckland Board's confirmation of the executive's May 1989 decision to remove Israel from the WFMH eastern Mediterranean region and return it to its United Nations position in Europe made a regional council (EMRC/WFMH) politically feasible. However, psychiatrist Omar Shaheen, M.D., who succeeded Taha Baasher as regional vice president from 1989 to 1993, was a politically conservative, intensely anti-Israeli member of the Egyptian medical syndicate who was also skeptical about regional organizations. It was necessary for movement toward regional organization, a precursor to council formation, to be carried forward by Gamal in the United Arab Emirates and Saudi Arabia. During 1993, in particular, he sponsored or participated in Cairo meetings cosponsored by the EAMH, which had the effect of building an interdisciplinary network of mental health related groups. They dealt with such diverse topics as the role of faith in mental health (in collaboration with Islamic clergy), social workers and community mental health (at the High Institute of Social Work), and the relationship between mental health and general medicine (with the participation of the head of the often hostile medical syndicate and under the patronage of the Grand Sheik of El Azhar University).

An Eastern Mediterranean Regional Council: the Role of Ahmed El Azayem

Rapid organizing movement began in 1993 when Omar Shaheen was succeeded in the regional vice president's post by Gamal's energetic oldest son, Ahmed. Before the formation of a council he established a "WFMH Regional Office" for the Eastern Mediterranean. He dealt with the lack of funding and of a legal status for a council under Egyptian law by working through the WIAMH office in Cairo, depending on the Abou El Azayem Hospital for secretarial support. This permitted for the first time a monthly letter to actual and potential individual and organizational members in the region that took advantage of all available organizing and networking opportunities.

It soon became clear that Ahmed's vision of mental health did not focus on the conditions of mental hospitals in the region. Perhaps that was realistic considering his professional tasks as a hospital director. Without doubt, however, it also reflected his awareness of the difficult life circumstances of his countrymen, especially those in rural areas. At any event his view was closer to that of the 1948 Federation founders because it was much more concerned with social issues with preventive significance than with mental hospital reform.

Although his conferences on conflict resolution, especially that held 3-5 February 1994, on "building tolerance for diversity," drew some condemnation from the medical syndicate and more militant Muslims, Ahmed braved their criticism and invited the mental health and psychiatric associations in the area to participate; in time an increasing number attended. The censure was further minimized by his astute arrangement of sponsorship for the conferences by the Grand Mufti of Egypt and of the Dar Il Eftaa', the Islamic center of the country, as the venue. This last was attended by several Israeli psychotherapists as well as Shimon Shamir, former Israeli Ambassador to Egypt, who described it as a trust-building process, laying building blocks for future cooperative ventures. Dr. Arafat held a lunch at the Red Crescent Hospital for international, including Israeli, visitors, accompanied by a performance of traditional Palestinian folk dance and music. These conferences led in time to the development of the WFMH Joint Program on Conflict Resolution by Ahmed and Dr. Leila Dane of the Institute for Victims of Violence in McLean, Virginia..

Ahmed's new WFMH regional office soon developed extensive communications with Amaan and mental health professionals in Gaza and Arab East Jerusalem, aiming at plans to protect and promote mental health after completion of the Israeli-Palestinian peace process. It also sponsored free training for Palestinian mental health nurses in the Abou El Azayem Hospital and lent the name of the WFMH region to mental health activities in Qatar and the Arab Emirates, the last regarding the prevention of substance abuse. The offices, groups, and institutions with which Ahmed made contact in the name of the WFMH Eastern Mediterranean region during 1993-1994 included some in Libya, Afghanistan, Kuwait, Oman, and Jeboti as well the Egyptian Health Ministry, the new Egyptian Human Rights Association, the Islamic World Medical Association (through Dr. Gamal), and the United Nations International Drug Control Program. It helped stimulate the formation of an Arab Association for Combat of Alcohol and Drugs and an Arab Association for Care of the Handicapped.

Ahmed continued to take advantage of opportunities to bring interested colleagues together in anticipation of a regional council. Although it was not intended, many of the opportunities furthered the original WFMH aim of facilitating the ability of people to live together in one world. A preliminary regional meeting was held on 7 February 1994, at the time of the conference on "Building Tolerance for Diversity." In September 1994, preparatory to the United Nations Population and Development Conference, the EAMH sponsored a regional meeting with Dr. Henry David, WFMH Board member-at-large and chairman of our Committee on Responsible Parenthood who was our official delegate to the conference. The meeting, organized by Ahmed and chaired by Gamal El Azayem, endorsed David's emphasis on the mental health value of gender equality. In terms of the conference goals this meant giving women expanded access to higher-level economic and political positions, resources to control their own fertility, and a major voice in determining policy about family planning in relation to development.

While awaiting the resolution of formalities of Egyptian law necessary to form a council, Ahmed organized a regional general assembly in Lebanon (6–10 October 1994) during the congress of the Lebanese Association for Mental Health. It elected a slate of officers, with him as head, approved by-laws, and established groups to concentrate on special programs. This enhanced the visibility of the nascent council in the region and the expectations of others regarding it. For example, Dr. Hassan Kassem, a prominent member of the Yemen Mental Health Association, came to Egypt to consult with him on the development of mental health services for war victims, especially children, in his country. He also designated Dr. Moza El-Malky of Qatar University to represent WFMH at the WHO regional meeting in Bahrain, 2–5 October 1994. This gave her an opportunity to stress the importance of mental health in improving the quality of life and the need for an appropriate distribution of funds in relation to this issue. Ahmed and Leila Dane, acting as co-chairs of the WFMH Committee on Trauma Victims in the Middle East, also worked in East Jerusalem on 10-11 November and presented papers at the Pan Arab Psychiatric Association meeting in Cairo on 16–18 November 1994.

The actual founding of the Federation's EMRC/WFMH took place in February 1995 at a third WFMH cosponsored conference on nonviolent conflict resolution in Cairo. The founding group was dominated by psychiatrists. It included Ahmed el Azayem and Drs. M. El Nabolsky of Lebanon, A. el Hamad of Saudi Arabia, and Mohammud Rashid Chaudry of Pakistan, as well as psychologist Moza El-Malky. It next met as a formal entity in 1996 at the same time as the sixth meeting of WIAMH, organizing itself to include a division of substance abuse and one on conflict resolution. Meanwhile it strengthened its position through Ahmed El Azayem's founding role in other organizations intended to work in cooperation with EMRC/WFMH. Leading were the Egyptian Association for Family and Social Conflict Resolution and the Egyptian Association for the Disabled. Along with EAMH, and the Giza Mental Health Association, they organized a program called "Mobilizing a Community Toward Mental Health" in one of the poorest rural areas of the country. With the assistance of the Egyptian Women Physician's Medical Association, training covered primary mental health issues for schoolteachers, women village leaders, social workers, and general practitioners.

I sent the draft of this description to Gamal, wanting to be certain that I was not omitting items he considered essential or including some that he felt were not accurate. His reply, in a letter of 14 August 1996, was both welcome and touching as he expressed his pleasure at having been "honored" by my friendship: "Among the precious achievements I managed to carry out," he wrote, "was to revive mental health programmes in the Arab region. I am grateful to you for having opened the way for me to explore the treasures of the Religious High Road and the Old Mental Health writings to integrate them with modern approaches. Your draft considers a piece of my life in which trust and love have been major presences in our mutual work."

The growth and development of the Eastern Mediterranean Region continued under Ahmed's leadership in autumn 1996 and spring 1997.

AFRICA

Republic of South Africa

In the Beginning

In the early 1900s when the national mental health associations of the United States and Canada and the International Committee for Mental Hygiene (ICMH) were being formed, most countries of sub-Saharan Africa had neither the tradition of voluntarism nor the communications and health infrastructures to support a national mental health association. The exception was the Republic of South Africa, at that time the Union of South Africa. (South Africa became a Union within the British Empire in 1910 through the amalgamation of four separate British colonies. In 1961 it became a Republic and withdrew from the Commonwealth.) A thesis by Lage Vitus reviews the mental health movement in South Africa before 1920 (Vitus, 1987). It arose not from the work of Clifford Beers but from the perception that mentally handicapped girls were behaving in an undesirable way and needed to be controlled. A 24 June 1913 meeting in Cape Town under the auspices of the Child Life Protection Society confronted the problems of vagrancy and prostitution in this population. An almost immediate consequence was the formation of the South African Society for the Care of the Feeble Minded, later to become two committees, one for mental defectives and one for "mental hygiene." They later combined to form the Cape Mental Health Society. These were the first community service organizations in South Africa to negotiate for funds from the central government.

By 1916 Dr. J. T. Dunston, the national Commissioner for Mentally Disordered and Defective Persons initiated the country's first Mental Disorders Act. In 1917 he made working contacts with the United States National Committee for Mental Hygiene. Taking his cue from the mental health reform movement in America, Dunston was the driving force behind the formation in 1919 of the Johannesburg Society for Mental Hygiene and in 1920 of the South African National Council for Mental Hygiene and for the Care of the Feeble Minded. The National Council (today's South African Federation of Mental Health) was the third national association to join the International Committee for Mental Hygiene after those in the United States and Canada. With the Committee's transformation into WFMH the South African association continued as an active member.

In 1922 the council, responding to Dunston's recommendation, changed its name to the National Committee for Mental Hygiene. This was an attempt to conform to Clifford Beers' feeling that it would be easier to establish an international body if all national societies were named in the same fashion. However, in 1929 the name was changed back to National Council for Mental Hygiene.

Early WFMH documents include an occasional reference to individual South African mental health leaders, but not to the actual state of clinical services in the country. The report of its Second Mental Health Assembly held during the second WFMH annual meeting in Geneva, 22–27 August 1949, lists as one of its working papers, "A Survey of Mental Health Services in South Africa and an Account of the Progress and Development of Mental Nursing in South Africa" by Iris Marwick, Matron of the Tara Hospital in Johannesburg.

There is no record of a South African representative at the third annual meeting in Paris in 1950 or the fourth in Mexico in 1951. However, the list of discussion groups for the 1952 meeting in Brussels contains the name, Mrs. I. E. Gericke, as a participant in the group on "Education of the Public in Principles of Mental Health." In 1953, at the sixth annual meeting in Vienna, Marwick was named a consultant and elected to the WFMH Executive Board for the 1953–1954 term. That year also saw affiliate Federation memberships by the Cape Mental Health Society and the Mental Health Society of the Witwatersrand. Marwick continued her consulting role until 1957 in regard to WFMH's advocacy for enlightened mental hospital practices. In 1954 a South African mental health pioneer, Netta Levine, was elected by the Executive Board to be part of a permanent Committee of Honor of world leaders in the field. In 1957 Marwick chaired a plenary session, "Growing Up for Cooperation or Conflict," with Otto Klineberg as the main speaker at the 10th annual meeting in Copenhagen. The 1960 annual report lists 47 individual WFMH members from South Africa. This sudden rise, after years when the South African WFMH individual membership varied from a low of zero to a high of two, was a consequence of the WFMH designation of 1960 as "World Mental Health Year." Much publicity was given to the Federation and members recruited in preparation for the country 's first national mental health congress (Lage Vitus, letter of 11 July 1996). The increased membership was not sustained after the national congress of 1963 attended by WFMH Director General Cloutier.

The Period of Exclusion

The South African presence in WFMH was threatened when the United Nations and most of the world's nations imposed sanctions upon it to force the abandonment of its official policy of apartheid. Despite WFMH's stance for world citizenship it was late in its condemnation of apartheid on mental health grounds and because of its accompanying human rights violations. This was a matter of some embarrassment to me in contacts with the American Psychiatric Association, which had been so supportive during my tenure as WFMH president. The American Psychiatric Association passed a resolution in January 1985 that I reprinted in the WFMH newsletter: "It is the belief of the American Psychiatric Association that when discrimination is practiced by governments in an organized fashion, the mental health of all of its citizens is affected, not only those against whom discrimination is directed." The resolution urged both the Society of Psychiatrists of South Africa and the World Psychiatric Association to "voice opposition to the policy and…launch a vigorous protest against all aspects of discrimination in that country" (WFMH, 1985a).

The WFMH problem was its Board's concern for colleagues in South African member associations. But a move was made inevitable by the 1985 refusal of U.K. labor groups to prepare the Brighton World Congress facilities with a South African organization as a member of the sponsoring body. On 13 July 1985, the Board, was concerned about the congress' threatened viability. Upon the recommendation of incoming President Edith Morgan it suspended all WFMH memberships from within the Republic of South Africa until a review two years later during the 1987 World Congress. This was the beginning of a prolonged debate on the issue. The initial suspension was voted with some reluctance in the knowledge that the mental health association was a force against apartheid; its leaders were opposed to the National Party government, and it would have less influence if it were no longer an active WFMH member. Lage Vitus, Director of the South African Federation National Council for Mental Health, presented his case for continuing membership to the Board. Its sympathetic response to his presentation recognized the antiapartheid activities of existing South African members. However, it could not "offer any kind of support to the regime within which these organizations and individuals must operate, or support a kind of discrimination which is totally antithetical to the basic principles to which the Federation is committed" (WFMH, 1985). It noted that its decision was for "suspension" rather than expulsion from the Federation. During the period 1985–1987 the Board committed itself to remain in touch with members by correspondence and possibly by a fact-finding visit and to review its position in 1987. It was understood that the suspension might be lifted if a committee of WFMH concluded, on the basis of personal inspection, that the South African mental health organization was in fact acting as an aggressive opponent of apartheid and an advocate of equal treatment of black and "colored" mentally ill individuals. This proviso was never put into effect because the Board felt that a valid visit of inspection could not be financed from South African sources. When, in the late 1980s, I was invited in a private capacity as a professor of psychiatry to do a lecture tour of the country's major medical schools, the Board member from Zambia, Isaac Mwendapole (with a Master's degree in Social Work from a Welsh university), made arrangements, with South African agreement, to accompany me. However, the Board requested that I not accept, fearing that my visit as a lecturer rather than solely as an inspector would be taken as WFMH condoning of apartheid.

The 1988 Board meeting in London reconfirmed the decision to suspend the membership of South Africa's National Council for Mental Health and its affiliate bodies. This was done on the grounds that current government policies made it impossible for associations within South Africa to comply with the policies and practices of WFMH. However, after prolonged discussion, including a presentation by Rene Dembo, Executive Director of the Witwatersrand Mental Health Society, the Board voted to revise its policy concerning individual memberships. It was decided that applications for readmission to membership from suspended individuals should be sent to the WFMH Secretariat that would then forward them to the office of the WFMH vice president for the African region for review and possible action. The matter was discussed again three years later at the mid-year 1991 Board meetings associated with the World Congress for Mental Health in Mexico. Although the Board voted to continue the suspension, to be reviewed again in 1992, it planned to begin a study of the South African Council's 19 component societies regarding whether they practiced apartheid. The intention was to admit some to WFMH membership if they seemed suitable. The study was never carried out because "independent funding from a neutral source" was not obtained for the requisite study mission. However, it became moot, because a scant six months later, in December 1991, the United Nations General Assembly passed a resolution presenting guidelines for readmission to United Nations affiliation of nongovernmental organizations (NGOs) characterized as anti-apartheid. They were also to be identified as favoring affirmative action and community development of a sort that would advance disadvantaged persons in South Africa.

Reacceptance

The WFMH Board lifted the suspension of South African memberships at its meeting in Sydney, Australia, 9–11 April 1992, with the possibility of an inspection tour still under consideration. This preceded by a year the final 1993 lifting of sanctions against South Africa by the United Nations.

At its biennial conference on 28 August 1992, the National Council for Mental Health changed its name to the South African Federation for Mental Health. It noted that five representatives of user support groups could be co-opted onto its board. Isaac Mwendapole also announced the formation of a Secretariat in Lusaka, Zambia, for an African regional council of WFMH to include the South African Federation and eight other member organizations south of the Sahara.

In October 1994, Pretoria, South Africa, was the site of the first conference of the newly formed African Regional Council of WFMH (see below). In spring 1996, supported by an independent organization and with a schedule arranged by Lage Vitus, I finally visited a series of mental hospitals and clinics in the country. Lage was our escort in Johannesburg, Pretoria, and environs. In the Durban area, Tim Ntombela and colleagues of the Durban and Coastal Areas Mental Health Society accompanied us. In the Cape Town area Director Toni Tickton of the Cape Mental Health Society and her colleagues were our constant companions. The country was in the throes of a difficult transition from a repressive police state-where security forces were engaged in abduction, murder, and torture-to a government of national unity, which some called a "healing society" and others a "human rights culture." One mechanism to effect the transition was the Truth and Reconciliation Commission, which was prepared to grant amnesty to perpetrators of atrocities if they applied and came forth with full confessions. This was a compromise between the desire of the former security forces for blanket amnesty and the wishes of victims and their families for revenge and compensation. The process was vastly complicated by the fact that approximately three-quarters of the South African population that was black was semiliterate and heavily unemployed and had been forced to live for years with inadequate resources. In no sector were health, housing, or education resources sufficient to care for the entire population. As one observer put it, it was naive to think that "everything would be alright with the end of apartheid...the period of euphoria is over." In these circumstances the mental health associations emerged as forces for the protection of civil rights for all minorities in the country.

Africa South of the Sahara

The Rees Era

The first African to become WFMH President was Chief Sir Samuel Manuwa, a distinguished jurist from Nigeria who was First Commissioner of his country's federal public service commission in Lagos. He served for the 1965–1966 term. In his foreword to the 1966 annual report he wrote of racial riots and intraethnic quarrels resulting in "genocidal holocausts" and 20 coups in three years "on one continent alone" but did not identify that continent. Nor did he specifically mention Africa elsewhere in his remarks.

In succeeding years several academic psychiatry leaders served as regional vice presidents for Africa. They functioned as individuals whose presence added stature to the Federation, but did not engage in organization building or sponsor activities in the name of WFMH. WFMH also enjoyed the support of Thomas Lambo, M.D., former professor of psychiatry and later dean of the medical school in Ibadan who was Deputy Director General of WHO in Geneva for several years.

In the middle 1950s Director Rees, in consultation with the WHO regional office for Africa, began contemplating a mental health conference as a way of initiating systematic work in the region. It finally took place in March 1958 in Bukavu, Belgian Congo, at the headquarters the Commission for Technical Cooperation in Africa South of the Sahara with the strong backing of WHO. This was late in the colonial era, and non-African professionals, predominantly from the colonizing countries, still exerted major influence. Before the conference Drs. Paul Sivadon (French-born professor of psychiatry at Brussels who acted as conference chairman) and Brock Chisholm visited Senegal, Ghana, Nigeria, French Equatorial Africa, Belgian Congo, Portuguese West Africa, and Ruanda Urudi. After the meeting Sivadon visited Uganda and the Sudan. Rees visited the Union of South Africa, Rhodesia, Kenya, Tanganyika and Ruanda Urudi. Fourteen territories were represented at the meeting by African, Belgian, British, and French psychiatrists, anthropologists, educators, nurses, and administrators. The senior African psychiatrist was Dr. Tigani El Mahi of Sudan who was vice president of the conference. The gathering was notable for establishing contacts between previously isolated workers, the activity later known as "networking.

There were two follow-up meetings: a seminar on mental health organized by WHO in Brazzaville at the end of 1958, and a meeting of specialists planned by the Commission for Technical Cooperation in Africa on the Basic Psychological Structures of African and Madagascan Populations in Madagascar in August 1959. A meeting was also held at United Nations New York in 1959, and its report entitled "Africa: Social Change and Mental Health" was advertised among WFMH publications. Records of WFMH work in Africa in that period note "representation" at three meetings in Dakar, Senegal, formerly French West Africa. One from 8–22 February 1966, attended by Professor Henri Collomb, a French academic psychiatrist who was a resident of Dakar, was a United Nations seminar on human rights in developing countries. A second meeting was an African psychiatric colloquium (16–20 January 1967) attended by Dr. Taha Baasher. The third meeting (27 March–1 April 1967) on "The Evolution of Familial Relations in Black Africa" was also attended by Professor Collomb. On 14–17 April 1969, after a joint initiative by WFMH President Carstairs and Professor Alan German of Makerere medical school in Uganda, the Commonwealth Foundation in collaboration with WFMH held a workshop on the administration of mental health care in Kampala, Uganda. Participants came from Nigeria, United Kingdom, Ghana, Mauritius, Zambia, Tanzania, Kenya, Sudan, and Ethiopia, with two observers from the United States. Lady Norman, characterized widely as a "peripatetic mental health worker," spoke on the role of voluntary workers, stimulating interest in the recently formed Uganda National Association for Mental Health. She persuaded WFMH and the Epilepsy Association to support a social worker from Hong Kong to help the association organize itself, including the building of a home for mentally handicapped children (WFMH, 1970c).

On 18–19 and 28 August 1972, I organized the first United States-Kenya Mental Health Conference (in Nairobi) with sponsorship from WFMH, the Kenyan health ministry, and the University of Nairobi. Because this came at a time of severe political unrest, scheduled participation by the Department of Psychiatry at Makerere University was canceled at the last moment. However, we had significant discussions regarding such locally important issues as relations with witch doctors and native healers, the education of clinical assistants, and implications for mental health of rapid social change and national development.

Voluntary Mental Health Associations

The Mental Health Association of Zambia was established in 1969 as a service organization for patients discharged from mental hospitals and for mentally retarded children. This service was extended to community education through schools, clubs, and other groupings. It gradually grew to include branches in different parts of the country but enjoyed only limited and intermittent support from the mainly hospital based government psychiatric services.

What was billed as the Federation's first regional meeting in the African region took place 4–7 November 1975, in Mauritius, an island in the Indian Ocean (WFMH, 1976). Organized by the Mauritius Mental Health Association on "Racism in Mental Health" (with additional workshops on mental health in relation to malnutrition and to economic growth) it drew delegates from Liberia, Ghana, Niger, South Africa, Uganda, and Nigeria as well as representatives from the United Kingdom, United States, Denmark, Thailand, and Canada. It was attended not only by Deputy Director General Thomas Lambo of WHO but by WFMH Honorary President Otto Klineberg and the WFMH regional vice president for Africa, Professor Tolani Asuni, M.D. of Nigeria.

Organizing Africa: the Role of Western Countries and the United Nations

In May 1977 WHO established its African Mental Health Action Group to foster technical cooperation among African countries in the field of mental health. It eventually grew to encompass representatives from 29 countries, but there was little, if any, grassroots participation.

In the 1980s there were renewed efforts to stimulate voluntary mental health association activities in various parts of Africa. Funding and ideas came from United Nations agencies; European sources, particularly the former colonial powers; Britain and other parts of the British Commonwealth that retained their interests in former colonies; and Canada. In keeping with Canadian interests in Africa the executive secretary for the Vancouver Secretariat, Roberta Beiser, was in touch with academic psychiatric leaders on the continent. A 1980 letter from Asuni replied to Beiser's inquiry about possible WFMH recruits. He was not optimistic: "It is sad to observe that the psychiatrists who should be loudest in their support for mental health associations have not been as active as one would wish them to be. The African Psychiatric Association is experiencing the same lukewarmness. Perhaps what is needed is a traveling salesman/public relations officer to stimulate local interest among lay people" (Asuni, 1980). He did not suggest a formal linkage of the African psychiatric group with WFMH.

However, a direct approach with the promise of financial support was welcomed by lay people in some quarters. In August 1984 former WFMH Board member George Rohn, general director of our member organization, the Canadian Mental Health Association, visited mental health services in Zimbabwe. This was preparatory to an intercountry workshop organized by the Zimbabwe Health Ministry and the Zimbabwe Mental Health Association in Harare, Zimbabwe, 10–13 September 1984. Isaac Mwendapole could not attend but sent a message from WFMH.

In 1986 the U.K. Commonwealth Medical Office planned a workshop on mental health and youth in Africa. Owing to the efforts of President Edith Morgan, WFMH was a cosponsor. The meeting took place 15–19 June 1987, in Lusaka with Mwendapole in attendance. It was attended by representatives from Zimbabwe, Swaziland, Botswana, Malawi, Kenya, and Zambia.

The Canadian connection continued to be valuable. On 23–27 January 1987, Mwendapole and Rohn met in Harare with local colleagues to review the proposed subregional project, "Establishing and Strengthening Mental Health Associations in Africa"; funding had already been submitted to the Canadian International Development Agency (CIDA). On 4–13 March 1987, Stanislas Flache, our United Nations Geneva representative, was funded by the Christian Medical Commission to be part of a group of governmental and NGO consultants for developing a mental health program in Kenya. This was the culmination of a pilot project initiated by discussions in 1984 between WHO's Mental Health Division and others, including Flache and Morgan for WFMH. The focus was how to incorporate mental health components into primary health care.

Another opportunity presented by the United Nations was a national workshop on problems of childhood and adolescence held in Zambia with the assistance of UNICEF, 13–16 April 1987, where Mwendapole presented a paper. In early 1989 Rohn visited us in the central Secretariat for a discussion of WFMH involvement in CIDA's efforts to assist in the organization and strengthening of mental health associations in southern Africa. At that time he reported that the branch development project in Zambia had reached its goal with the establishment of 18 community branches. In Zimbabwe CIDA funds had allowed the local mental health association to acquire a 100-acre farm for rehabilitation of discharged hospital patients, and several other projects were being formulated. The Tirivanhu Farm opened in February 1991. CIDA had also been involved in the formation of the new mental health associations in Botswana and Swaziland, and plans were underway to form one in Lesotho. A goal for later 1989, never achieved, was to hold the first regional conference of mental health associations in southern Africa. However, Executive Director Mwansa of the Zambian association accepted a Canadian Mental Health Association invitation to attend its general meeting in September and to tour its branches. This allowed a first-hand exchange of information. At the same time WHO's African Mental Health Action Group was revived, and in 1985 Flache, newly appointed as our Geneva representative, addressed the group on behalf of WFMH.

The United Kingdom also maintained its long-standing interest in former colonial possessions. In 1988 the Kensington and Chelsea Mental Health Association formed a "twinning" relationship with the newly formed mental health association of Botswana.

In February 1990 George Rohn, having retired from his post as General Director of the Canadian Mental Health Association, was appointed a consultant to the organization and a WFMH volunteer coordinator for Africa. In that capacity he again visited Botswana, Zimbabwe, and Zambia, meeting with Isaac Mwendapole and Ministry of Health officials. While there he announced a CIDA grant of $65,000 to the Zimbabwe Association for Mental Health to support its executive director, some part-time positions, and money for travel. He also submitted other projects to various agencies for funding in Zimbabwe and Zambia.

The African Mental Health Action Group continued to meet occasionally, and when feasible WFMH attended as an observer. On 11 May 1993, our representative to its meeting in Geneva was Douglas Deane. Its agenda encompassed community programs, refugees, and the neuropsychiatric consequences of HIV infection.

African Leadership and Continental Organization

In the mid-1970s regional vice presidents included two Nigerian professors of psychiatry, Tolani Asuni from Abeokuta and Oye Benite from Benin. Considerable hope was invested in Asuni because of his international stature and academic reputation. Educated in medicine at Trinity College in Dublin, he served in various capacities in Nigeria for several years before going to England to study psychiatry. But, at the time of his being named to the WFMH vice presidency he was overcommitted, both professionally and extracurricularly. As medical superintendent of Aro Hospital in Abeokuta , he taught psychiatry at the University of Ibadan and was professor of psychiatry at the University of Ife. He was also president of both the Association of Psychiatrists in Nigeria and the Association of Psychiatrists in Africa. As WFMH vice president he attended a 1975 regional meeting in Mauritius on racism and mental health and appeared at world congresses. He was an impressive figure dressed in the flowing robes of his native country, but the anticipated organizational efforts did not materialize. He took a United Nations assignment in Rome and was succeeded at Salzburg in 1979 by Benite, who again held the vice president's position with élan during the congress, but contented himself with the local distinction that it brought him.

Several years elapsed before WFMH began the ambitious task of creating a continent-wide organization with local leadership in this vast and culturally diverse area. The key figure in connecting Africa's isolated mental health workers and giving them a sense of communal identity, and eventually in establishing an African regional council of WFMH, was Isaac Mwendapole of Lusaka, Zambia. As housing administrator in his country, he had some local political influence and persisting drive. This was not evident when we first met in 1981 in Manila during my initial Board meeting as WFMH president. He was then beginning his first term as vice president for the African region. At that time, confronting the Federation's fragile financial situation, it was necessary to make a decision whether to have a congress in 1983. Mwendapole did not appear to be a future leader as he spoke in favor of conserving our scarce funds and simply trying to stay alive through a Secretariat in the new president's office. However, with discussion, a Board consensus was reached that we should work toward a 1983 congress in Washington, DC. The strongest voice in this regard was that of Tsung-yi Lin, who believed that to do otherwise would be to doom the Federation to a permanently ineffective state.

That 1983 congress gave Mwendapole a chance to adopt a more progressive perspective. In fact his staying powers were such that he achieved a record for continuous Board representation, holding positions for four years each as WFMH vice president, honorary secretary, member-at-large, and again vice president. During this period he was the essential, stable contact point for African NGOs interested in mental health. The designation of an interested and responsive individual to serve as a focal point for communications was essential in beginning the long slow process of development. At the same time, however, non-African countries were also doing mental health related development work on the continent. Although their efforts were independently motivated, conceived, and financed they provided support for the intra-African leadership embodied in the WFMH officers from the region. In many instances the efforts of WFMH, represented by Mwendapole and his colleagues in local mental health associations and those of the international agencies of non-African countries, were thoroughly intertwined-although the latter always supplied the needed funding.

Toward an African Regional Council for WFMH: the Role of Isaac Mwendapole and Colleagues

As early as 1983 Mwendapole corresponded with the Kenya mental health association, which reported a new emphasis on decentralized community support systems for patients discharged from mental hospitals. Some of this followed a Unicef sponsored seminar in October 1981. A newly reorganized Kenya mental health association was represented at the first subregional mental health conference convened by Mwendapole in Lusaka, Zambia, 22–25 June 1983. It also initiated a Good Practices in Mental Health study led by social worker Remi Aruasa of Mathari Hospital (Nairobi), who brought the idea after a visit to London with President-elect Edith Morgan.

Between 12 and 24 August 1984, Mwendapole visited Botswana to promote a national mental health association there and met with the health minister and local psychiatrists

At the Brighton precongress Board meeting in July 1985 he reported that he had succeeded in establishing concrete communications with mental health associations in 12 countries: Botswana, Kenya, Lesotho, Malawi, Mauritania, Nigeria, Rwanda, South Africa, Swaziland, Tanzania, Zaire, and Zimbabwe in addition to his own country of Zambia. Beyond this he developed contacts with interested individuals in Angola, Congo, Ethiopia, Gambia, Ghana, Madagascar, Mauritius, Mozambique, Senegal, Sierra Leone, Cameroon, Zaire, Sudan, and Eritrea. He also established himself as a presence in the United Nations, attending, as a WFMH observer, the 35th session of the WHO regional committee for Africa meeting 11–18 September

1985, in Lusaka. He reported that as a result of this meeting he developed contacts with African ministers of health to advance mental health advocacy work on the continent. He established communication with the regional WHO director for Africa in respect to its African mental health action group and was invited to be an observer at the 36th session of the regional WHO committee in Brazzaville, September 1986.

By the summer of 1986 Mwendapole announced a major reorganization of his region. Its mental health associations were divided into three geographic groups: eastern and southern, central, and western. The eastern and southern group, working with Dr. Nawa Lifanu, had already had its first planning meeting in October 1985, aided by financial support from CIDA arranged through the Canadian Mental Health Association. It included the Zimbabwe National Association for Mental Health, with its able honorary secretary, Sandra Morreira, as a significant force holding it together.

The central group, assisted by former WFMH vice president for the European region, Stijn Jannes, M.D., of Belgium and Mukama Matthieu of Rwanda, was gathering information on mental health needs from Rwanda, Burundi, and Zaire as well as other francophone countries in central Africa.

The western group was coordinated by Yemisi Agunbiade, Director of the Nigerian Mental Health Association. Trained as a nurse in Nigeria and with advanced training in social work in England, she was also principal social welfare officer of the Department of Psychiatric Social Work at the WHO Training and Research Centre of the Aro Neuro-Psychiatric Hospital in Abeokuta. An energetic, optimistic woman of considerable presence, she organized the 1986 National Mental Health Humanitarian Week (15–21 December) around the theme, "Coping with Stress: Which Way Nigeria?" Major symposia focused on the need for voluntary mental health services and the status of women in developing countries. Of special note were social events for psychiatric patients and handicapped children as well as Muslim and Christian prayer services.

During the elections at the 1987 World Congress in Cairo, Mwendapole, having completed two terms as regional vice president, was nominated to be president-elect. This was an auspicious moment for him because several Africans were present at the congress and he had achieved a degree of prominence. However, retiring President Edith Morgan nominated Stanislas Flache, M.D., our Geneva representative, and he won the post. As a form of consolation and to help retain his local leadership role, Mwendapole was named by the Board as honorary secretary. The new African regional vice president, Dr. Nawa L. Lifanu of Zambia, was also an active promoter of WFMH activities. One of his interests was in developing mental health groups and individual volunteers in Ethiopia. In this endeavor he was joined by colleagues from the Rehabilitation Agency for the Disabled and assisted by Yemesi Agunbiade (now Agun-Wole) through her correspondence with individuals involved in mental health activities in Sierra-Leone, Ivory Coast, Ghana, Gambia, and Senegal.

Despite the election disappointment, Mwendapole continued his network building. On 23–24 September 1987, he attended the workshop in Gaberone that established the first mental health association in Botswana. Basic resource information was provided by Executive Director Mwansa of the Mental Health Association of Zambia. In October 1988 Mwendapole delivered the keynote address at a Swaziland mental health society (founded in 1982) seminar on "Mental Health and Family Life."

At the Auckland World Congress for Mental Health in August 1989 Yemisi Agun-Wole was elected regional vice president for Africa. The meeting of African regional members during that congress, chaired by Mwendapole, included leaders of the mental health associations in Botswana, Swaziland, Zimbabwe, Zambia, and South Africa. Dr. Lifanu, having completed his term as vice president, noted the formation of a new mental health association, in Tanzania. As vice national chairman of the Zambian association, led by Justice Ernest Sakala, he helped organize a week of activities, 21–28 September 1989, on the theme, "Mental Health: A Concern for

All," which focused on the need for community involvement. By 1990 Agun-Wole, who had retired from her other posts, concluded that without an office or financial support it was impossible to manage the responsibilities of vice president and announced her resignation in 1991.

Without question the strongest WFMH member association on the continent remained that in South Africa. However, it was still under suspension. But the preeminent mental health association in the continent's southern region, and the one receiving most help from foreign sources, notably Canada, was that in Zimbabwe. Founded in 1981 it was an active advocacy, education, and service organization. In later years it profited from its association with the Canadian Mental Health Association and CIDA. From 30 October to 1 November 1991, it affirmed this status with a national symposium on mental health, bringing together volunteers and professionals including social workers and psychologists as well as psychiatrists. In March 1992 it presented its report to the minister of health, who concluded that the national mental health plan of 1985 had not been implemented effectively. A major recommendation was that an NGO network and a national advisory Board on mental health be created under the direction of the mental health association to collaborate with government services. By June 1992 nine Zimbabwe organizations had joined the network, and it was devoting increasing time to public education in high schools and training primary care nurses in mental health issues.. Its first new major advocacy initiative was a program to mark the International Day on Alcohol and Drug Abuse on 26 June. At Mwendapole's urging the Zimbabwe National Association for Mental Health newsletter was to serve as the newsletter of a new WFMH African regional council until funding became available to publish a separate one.

In 1992 Mwendapole appointed an interim committee of nine members from countries with national mental health associations to form the initial Boardof an African regional council. The members came from Nigeria, Rwanda, South Africa, Zambia, Swaziland, Zimbabwe, Tanzania, and Kenya. The Zimbabwe National Association for Mental Health was the most effective in developing inter-association communications. Due in part to its efforts, the broader membership of the council included organizations from all countries south of the Sahara. The African regional council was formally inaugurated in Harare, Zimbabwe, on 3–5 April 1993. It was incorporated as an NGO in Zambia on 2 July 1993. Its charter was adopted on 25 October 1994, at its general assembly meeting during its first regional congress in Pretoria, South Africa.

The African regional council (ARC/WFMH) spelled out its mission at its inaugural meeting in 1993. In addition to the features common to all mental health associations it included the provision of "information and advisory services to organizations working on behalf of people with mental health problems in the African continent south of the Sahara." Its short-term goals revealed the vast organizational problems confronted by any group attempting to deal with Africa-wide issues. They included establishing contact with interested persons and organizations working in mental health services; strengthening existing and establishing new national mental health associations; determining mental health needs in the region and providing information and education relevant to them; and holding an all-Africa regional conference.

Detailed reports came from Sandra Morreira of Zimbabwe, Dr. Thandi Malepe of the Swaziland National Mental Health Association, Frere Mukama of Rwanda, and Irene Mutabiku of Zambia, who was the African contact person for the WFMH women's network. Organizing this meeting was a significant achievement. The obstacles of distance and lack of funds were overcome with some help from the WFMH Secretariat and the Zimbabwe National Association for Mental Health.

The First Regional Conference

The first African regional conference, sponsored by the new council in cooperation with the South African Federation for Mental Health, was held in Pretoria, South Africa, 24–27 October

1994. Its theme, "Africa Now: The Mental Health of Families," recognized 1994 as the United Nations International Year of the Family. A major challenge, met by assistance from the South African Federation and other sources, was to ensure adequate representation from countries in Africa. More than 200 people eventually attended with representation from Botswana, Eritrea, Kenya, Malawi, Nigeria, Swaziland, Zambia, and Zimbabwe. Registrants also came from Australia, India, Israel, Sweden, and Taiwan. Several WFMH Board members including President Federico Puente, who spoke on family mental health in informal settlements, President-elect Beverly Long, and Dick Hunter from the Secretariat also attended.

The meeting was organized around eight major tracks: displaced families; sustaining mental health in families; violence; AIDS/HIV; crisis intervention; mental retardation; treatment of mental illness; and rehabilitation. A highlight was the keynote address by Professor Kwaki Osei-Hwedie of the Department of Social Work at the University of Botswana on "A Holistic Approach to Family Mental Health in Africa." An entire day was devoted to human rights issues for persons with mental illness, or mental retardation and in relation to mental well-being.

This first international WFMH congress within Africa stimulated membership interest in the Federation as a whole. The 1995 World Congress for Mental Health in Dublin was attended by professional and lay mental health advocates from Kenya, Nigeria, Sudan, South Africa, and Zambia and provided an opportunity for face-to-face discussion. Additional opportunities were present at a conference on mental health policy at the University of Cape Town in November 1995 focused on a Harvard "report" on mental health issues in low-income countries. These experiences led Mwendapole in January 1996 to propose a "networking project for mental health in Africa." He noted that of 46 countries in the sub-Saharan region, 21 were French-speaking, 20 English-speaking, and 5 Portuguese-speaking. Only 21 had national mental health services, and only 26 had allocated funds for mental health budgets in 1994–1995. There were only 100 psychiatrists serving a population of 600 million people. The exception was South Africa with 300 psychiatrists for its population of 43 million (most of whom served the 13% of the population defined as white). Where there were mental health services the central preoccupation was with diagnosable, usually chronic, disease with no focus on prevention or health promotion. Mwendapole concluded that "there is absolutely no political will among the various governments of Africa and they capitalize on their own ignorance and that of their nationals by not providing mental health services." In the absence of government collaboration he proposed a center headquartered in Lusaka for collecting and disseminating information, with a focus on influencing national governments. However, because it did not include a funding plan and depended on financial support from the WFMH exchequer, its activation in more than an elementary sense was to await continuing WFMH efforts at fund raising. We discussed the matter in great detail during my March 1996 visit to South Africa, but several approaches to funding sources were not productive.

ASIA

Overview

Geography and Culture

The WFMH Asian regions have been those specified by WHO: (*a*) southeast Asia, for which a WHO regional office was established in January 1949; and (*b*) western Pacific, for which a regional office was established in 1950. Over the years, however, WFMH, while retaining the overall regional names, made several changes in their components. At the beginning of the 1980s Australia, New Zealand, and the Pacific Islands were removed from the western Pacific to form a newly designated Oceania region of WFMH. The 1989 Board meeting in Auckland moved the Philippines from the western Pacific to the WFMH southeast Asian region. But they, along with Australia, New Zealand, and the Pacific Islands, remained in WHO's original western Pacific region.

Communication between the culturally similar countries in this revised region was facilitated by their shared features. In a 17 January 1994, letter the 1993–1997 western Pacific regional vice president, Shimpei Inoue, M.D., Professor and Chairman of Neuropsychiatry at Kochi Medical School in Japan, noted that although this sharing could be beneficial it could also lead to difficulties. In similar cultures similar stigma is associated with mental illness: relatives are forced to sacrifice their own lives; there is similar neglect of the human rights of mentally ill people; and similar underdevelopment of NGOs in favor of governmental institutions.

During the half century since WFMH was founded, Asian associations, public and private institutions, and governments worked actively to promote positive mental health and the care of the mentally ill, sometimes with the stimulation of WHO. However, only a fraction of this activity was related directly to WFMH. This reflected a combination of factors: the state of industrial development in the countries of the region; the dominant influence of Western European values in the articulation of WFMH priorities; and the fact that the global WFMH held its meetings mainly in Europe and the Americas. Exceptions were the 18th annual meeting in Bangkok, Thailand, from 15–19 November 1965; the 1981 World Congress for Mental Health organized by the Philippine Mental Health Association in Manila; and the 1993 World Congress for Mental Health sponsored by a consortium of societies in Tokyo. WFMH western Pacific regional meetings were held in Tokyo in 1988 and in Taipei, Taiwan, in 1979 and 1996, in addition to that associated with the 1993 Tokyo World Congress.

Recruiting Influential Individuals and Associations

The earliest links between Asia and the embryonic Federation were forged, as in the case of other regions, through the recruitment by Jack Rees and his colleagues of influential, internationally active professionals, predominantly although not exclusively psychiatrists. Many of these people were noted in Chapters 2–4, which cover the Federation's founding and the years of the London and Geneva Secretariats. In many instances their contributions were not specifically regional.

Perhaps the most significant WFMH figure around whom Asian developments occurred was Tsung-yi Lin, M.D., descendent of an influential Taiwan (then called Formosa) family, founding chairman of the Department of Psychiatry at Taiwan National University in Taipei (1947), and long-time scientist at WHO. With his medical education in Japan and fluency in Japanese, Mandarin, and English, he was an important bridge between professionals, particularly academic investigators and clinicians and volunteers belonging to the three language groups. Although his early involvement with WFMH as an Executive Board member came while he was still professor of psychiatry in Formosa, his major contributions to the Federation's survival were during his long tenure as a "working president" from 1974 to 1979, while he was on the faculty of the University of British Columbia in Vancouver, Canada. These, as well as his continuing contributions after being named honorary president upon his retirement as president during the 1979 World Congress in Salzburg, have been described in Chapters 5 and 6, which describe recurrent Federation organizational and financial themes, and Chapter 11.

Another significant Asian figure was Dr. Estafania Aldaba-Lim of Manila. In contrast to Lin she did not maintain a consistent focus upon the Federation. She added to its reputation instead through the host of other international roles and activities in which she was identified, as a past WFMH Board member and later president. In these activities she was always willing to assist the Federation in achieving its goals. She was an early member of the WFMH Executive Board in the Rees era, and her later role in regard to the establishment of the Baltimore-Washington Secretariat during her tenure as WFMH president from 1983 to 1985 is described in Chapter 5.

Aldaba-Lim obtained a doctorate in clinical psychology from the University of Michigan in Ann Arbor in 1942, but although she was responsible for student mental health at Women's University in Manila for several years after 1947, her career was mainly in governmental, inter-governmental, and voluntary work. At the time of her WFMH regional vice presidency (1975–1977) she was Minister of Social Service and Development in the Philippines, chairman of its governmental commission on population, member of the UNESCO Executive Board and chairman of its Credentials Committee, as well as president or chairman of several other national groups. In addition she had represented her country, leading its delegation to various international conferences. In October 1977 she was appointed the United Nations Secretary General's Special Representative for the International Year of the Child. By May 1978 in this capacity she had visited 15 countries in Asia, Africa, Europe, and Latin America. As noted in Chapter 5 it was my privilege, following Tsung-yi Lin's request, to get to know Fannie Aldaba-Lim (as she asked me to call her) during the 1981 Manila Congress and to nominate her as WFMH's president-elect to suceed me as president in 1983.

During and after her WFMH presidency she continued to transfer her personal prestige to the Federation in numerous national and international roles. A special interest was the well-being of children. On 12–14 November 1984, during her WFMH presidency, she chaired a meeting of experts on the "Exploitation of Children" cosponsored by LAWASIA (a regional volunteer organization of 47 bar associations with prominent groups in the Philippines, India, Malaysia, Pakistan, Thailand, and Singapore) and the Asia Foundation in Singapore. Particular attention was paid to the legal aspects of child labor and child prostitution. She chaired a follow-up LAWASIA conference of ministers, investigators, and policy makers entitled "Child Exploitation, Child Labor and Child Prostitution" 21–24 February 1986, in Kuala Lumpur. This line of advocacy was pursued by her in the mid-1990s as a member of the WFMH Committee on Preventing the Commercial Sexual Exploitation of Children and, simultaneously, as a WFMH and Philippine government representative to the Stockholm world meeting on the topic.

Another outstanding Asian woman of the early Federation was Khunying (Lady) Ambhorn Meesook, D.Ed. (Harvard), President of the Thai Mental Health Association, and Senior Inspector General of the Thai Ministry of Education. In her long and active career Mesook was on the Thailand National Commission for UNESCO, a member of the UN Commission on the Status of Women (of its Economic and Social Council-ECOSOC), and headed delegations at several United Nations conferences on women. When we first knew each other in 1985 she had the unusual distinction of being president of both the Thai Mental Health Association and Thai Planned Parenthood Association. In 1995 as president of the International Council on Social Welfare she represented WFMH as well as her own organization at several mental health relevant meetings. Some of her activities are noted below under "WFMH in Southeast Asia."

With these and other notable exceptions, however, representatives of Asian mental health and professional associations have been less involved in the WFMH Board and Secretariat than those from Europe and North America. Some areas have been largely silent. Vast regions of southeast Asia, for example, have not been significantly involved in Federation work. Although the leading Indonesian psychiatrist, Kusomonto Setyonegoro, M.D., accepted Board membership for a time during the Lin presidency his participation was brief and limited.

Nor, despite the occasional Board presence of colleagues from India, was a continuing WFMH presence ever established on that subcontinent. K.R. Masani, M.D., of Bombay represented his country on the first Executive Board in 1948–1950 and again, although he had relocated to London, in 1963–1965. In those years the Indian Council for Mental Hygiene with which he was affiliated was among the 62 member associations listed from 33 countries. But his presence on the Board was not marked by corollary Federation activity in India, although by 1966 the Indian Council for Mental Hygiene and the Indian Psychiatric Society became members for a time.

The only other Asian group on the initial membership list was the Chinese National Association for Mental Health from the People's Republic of China. However, its name disappeared from the list after the first year.

In 1951 the Philippine Mental Health Association became a WFMH member, and its president, Dr. M. V. Arguelles, was elected to the Executive Board. In 1953 Phon Sangsingkeo, M.D., Director, Thailand's Division of Hospitals for Mental Diseases in Bangkok, was elected a substitute member of the Executive Board. He was also president of the Psychiatric Association of Thailand, which, along with the Japan Association for Mental Health, joined 80 member associations from 41 countries. By 1954 Dr. Arguelles had completed his term, and Dr. Sangsingkeo moved to the Executive Board proper. He became WFMH president for the 1962–1963 term. During his term the Mental Health Association of Thailand Under Royal Patronage became a WFMH member.

WFMH Outreach to Asia

Director's Trip

A breakthrough for Asian participation in WFMH came, as it did for other parts of the world remote from the Federation's European center, when Director Rees personally visited many countries in the region. The invitation to do so came in 1954 during the Fifth International Congress on Mental Health at Toronto. It was issued by member associations in the four Asian countries (Thailand, Japan, the Philippines, and India), suggesting that he visit them as part of a trip already planned to meet with colleagues in the WFMH eastern Mediterranean region. The trip also included visits to Burma, Hong Kong, Ceylon, and Singapore, none of which, at that time, had individual or organizational WFMH members. Despite the extensive period devoted to this journey, Rees declined invitations to visit Israel, Formosa, Indonesia, and Iraq. The exact reasons for his selectivity in these respects are unclear, but they may have stemmed from the regional WHO Directors for Asia and the western Pacific who helped plan the itinerary. The trip included various eastern Mediterranean countries and lasted from 14 December 1954, to 9 February 1955. Contributions toward travel and housing were made by the governments of the countries visited. Some support was also obtained from the Josiah Macy Jr. Foundation whose medical director, Frank Fremont-Smith M.D., the 1954–1955 WFMH president, accompanied Rees on the journey. Rees' report on the visit began with a meticulous detailing of financial arrangements. As he put it: "In so major an undertaking, for a Federation so hard up as ours, a word about the financing is indicated" (WFMH, 1954, p.45)

The foray into hitherto unexplored Asian territory began with Rangoon in Burma where the pattern for the rest of the trip was set. It involved detailed visits to general and mental hospitals and training institutions, lectures to students and practitioners, interviews with high governmental health officials, travel to outlying areas, and warm hospitality. The visitors were impressed by a Burmese school for health assistants but were made aware that some countries had resisted the concept because of fear of creating "second-class doctors." Rees recommended, as always, the development of stronger support for mental hospitals, spoke of the importance of their being part of the community and near university or other teaching centers, and supported the idea of psychiatric wards in general hospitals. Later it occurred to the visiting group that "staff visiting between hospitals in Burma and Thailand might be interesting" and that it might be profitable to study "the social, economic and cultural reasons that may underlie the [hospital admission] figures" (WFMH, 1954, p.47).

In Thailand the visit was facilitated by Executive Board member Sangsingkeo. In addition to the responsible government officials and medical specialists, the visitors encountered UNESCO and WHO health projects and a Cornell University anthropological team from the United States.

Their major policy recommendation was to support a move, already formulated by the Thai government, to create a Department of Mental Health in the ministry instead of a Division of Mental Hospitals. They also recommended that the resource-rich Thai solutions to interrelated health and social problems be shared with less endowed neighboring countries.

In Tokyo the WFMH visitors were hosted by the Ministry of Health headed by Dr. Yamaguchi. Ministry representatives met them at the airport with detailed briefings on psychiatric hospitals, programs, and patients in the country. They also visited the National Institute of Mental Health set up by the ministry in 1952 with some WHO assistance. Dr. Tsuneo Muramatsu, Professor of Psychiatry at Nagoya, was with them throughout, representing the Japan Association for Mental Health. A new organization, not yet a Federation member, was the Japanese Federation for Mental Health, which brought together several societies involved in various aspects of education and social welfare. Their officers included a considerable number of leading Tokyo businessmen interested in such matters as mental health in industry and the care of defective children. Another society, which later developed a WFMH affiliation, was the Japan Mental Hospitals Association. Rees and Fremont-Smith left Japan impressed with the forward looking attitude of its psychiatrists and left no special recommendations.

The Philippine Mental Health Association, headed by its president, Aldaba-Lim, and accompanied by visiting Professor of Psychiatry, Dr. Karl Bowman of San Francisco, greeted the travelers at the Manila airport. Again there was a detailed review of the national psychiatric situation and meetings with high ranking officials including the nation's president and the president of the University of Manila. But this visit was distinguished first by the ubiquitous presence of the Philippine Mental Health Association and second by the large number of foreign specialists associated with UNESCO, WHO, Unicef, and various universities, mainly from the United States. The Philippine Mental Health Association itself was unique among the associations encountered in its volunteer orientation and multidisciplinary makeup. It included nonprofessional citizen volunteers, educators, jurists, lawyers, social workers, and child development specialists as well as psychiatrists and other physicians-still true at my first personal encounter with them during the Manila WFMH World Congress of 1981. Much of its high status and wide acceptance was due to the position and work of Aldaba-Lim. Rees and Fremont-Smith urged, as they had elsewhere, the development of psychiatric units in general hospitals. They also recommended that the training, so badly needed by hospital and clinic staffs, be arranged by visiting teachers in the Philippines rather than having students sent abroad.

The fourth country was India. Visits were made to Bombay, site of the single Federation member association, Bangalore, and Delhi. The WFMH visitors urged that officials responsible for constructing mental hospitals become familiar with others in Asia and that more attention be paid to the place of psychiatry in medical education. They identified the lack of interest by educated citizens as a primary factor in the failure to develop adequate resources for the care of mentally ill people.

In Hong Kong the Federation had no member society, but a recently started mental health association had benefited from WFMH help. The visitors engaged in thorough inspections of clinical and training facilities there and in Singapore, where there had been no Federation influence (a Singapore association for mental health was established on 17 December 1968, and later became a WFMH member). Many of the Hong Kong medical administrators with whom they met were British expatriates. Colombo, Ceylon, was the site of a similar visit. The remainder of the trip was devoted to Egypt, Sudan, and Pakistan. In the closing comments of his report, Rees noted the potential impact of cultural change on mental health and recognized the possibility of reciprocal contributions: "We need to be concerned with what the West can contribute to the East, and the East to the West" (WFMH, 1954, p.71)

By 1955, perhaps in consequence of the visit, the Mental Health Association of Hong Kong had become a WFMH member, and its founder, Dr. Irene Cheng, Senior Woman Education Officer of Hong Kong, was elected to the Executive Board. The Psychiatric Association of

Thailand remained a member, and its president, Dr. Sangsingkeo, continued as an Executive Board member. However, there were no other Asian member groups.

Asian representation slowly increased in 1956. The reconstituted Chinese Mental Health Association (of Taiwan), first founded in Nanking on the mainland in 1936, became a member organization, joining members from Japan, the Philippines, Thailand, and Hong Kong. New, nonvoting, affiliate member organizations included groups in Ceylon and the Philippines. Aldaba-Lim was one of four new members elected to the Executive Board. This made her, along with Chen of Hong Kong, Margaret Mead of the United States, and Eileen Younghusband, Lecturer in Social Science at the London School of Economics, the fourth woman on the Board.

The Seminars on Mental Health and Family Life

This long anticipated seminar took place at Baguio, Philippines, 6–20 December 1958, under the sponsorship of the Philippine Mental Health Association and the government sponsored National Family Life Workshop (WFMH, 1958b). Its main financial support came from the WHO Regional Committee for the western Pacific and from the Asia Foundation. Although it was attended by 66 people from 11 different disciplines from 13 Asian countries, it was less an Asian regional activity than one put together jointly by WHO and WFMH. Thus, it was directed by WFMH Scientific Director, Kenneth Soddy, with Margaret Mead as an official WFMH representative. WHO appointed both Aldaba-Lim and Dr. Margarethe Stepan of Vienna as consultants. Along with Tsung-yi Lin, Stepan was coeditor of the seminar report, "Reality and Vision," published by the Philippine government in June 1960 as a contribution to World Mental Health Year (Stepan and Li, 1960).

The Tokyo Conference on Community Planning

The advent of the 1958 International Conference on Social Work in Tokyo permitted WFMH to organize a continuing discussion group on this topic. The presiding officer was Helen Speyer of New York. One large public meeting for the discussion of mental health issues was held under the chairmanship of Professor Tsuneo Muramatsu, but the main speakers were Mead and Professor Hendry of the Institute of Social Work in Toronto. Again, although Rees' report indicated that the discussions "were extremely useful for our Japanese colleagues" (WFMH), 1958b, p.14), they clearly could not be viewed as constituting a meeting of Japanese mental health workers organized to pursue WFMH goals. Instead they were organized by North Americans for the presumed benefit of Japanese professionals.

An important stimulus to systematic WFMH-Asian involvement was the outreach activity of Tsung-yi Lin during his period as "working president" for 1974-1979, combining the functions both of WFMH president and Director. He continued the Rees tradition of "parish work," emphasizing Asia in frequent visits from his base in Vancouver, Canada . A major trip, with his wife, social worker Mei-Chen Lin, was from 25 October to 19 November 1976, in part to stimulate interest in the forthcoming 1977 Vancouver World Congress for Mental Health. This took them to the Philippines, Thailand, Singapore, Hong Kong, and Japan. A highlight was the Asian Psychiatric meeting organized by the Thai Psychiatric Association with participation from Hong Kong, Indonesia, Malaysia, the Philippines, Singapore, South Korea, Sri Lanka, and Taiwan. The "Far East" seminar stimulated by Carstairs in Hong Kong in 1968 had encouraged precursor gatherings to this meeting (WFMH, 1977).

The WFMH Southeast Asian Region

Thailand and 18th Annual Meeting

The first annual meeting of WFMH in Asia, its 18th, occurred in Bangkok, Thailand, on 15–19 November 1965, under the presidency of Alan Stoller, M.D., of Australia. However, because of its distance from Europe and North America and the expense of travel it was not attended by a sufficient number of Board members to constitute a quorum. For those who did attend it offered an initial opportunity for first-hand acquaintance with an Asian culture. A highlight was the Fifth Mary Hemingway Rees Memorial Lecture given by Sana Dharmasakdi, Chief Justice of the Thai Supreme Court and President of the Thai Buddhist Association, who spoke on "Buddhism and Mental Health."

The annual meeting hosts were the approximately 10-year-old Mental Health Association of Thailand Under Royal Patronage and the Psychiatric Association of Thailand. Meesook chaired the national organizing committee and thus became well-known to many Federation leaders as "Amy." Along with Past President Sangsingkeo (1962–1963) she convened the first formal gathering of Asian delegates during the meeting to emphasize the growing opportunities for mental health work in the region. In consequence she was named to the Executive Board for the 1966–1969 term (along with Dr. Jesus M. Tan of the Philippine Mental Health Association).

The Mental Health Association of Thailand continued as an active entity with a program focusing as much on positive mental health as on services for mentally ill persons. Its main work was promoting the general public's awareness of the importance of mental health through television programs, public lectures, and discussions. Among its special continuing projects were the rehabilitation of convicted prisoners with members of its Board of Directors trained as volunteer probation officers, activities for out-of-school children and slum dwelling youth, and, in particular, a drive to promote better mental health in schools through the involvement of teachers (WFMH, 1979a). Amy Meesook, while not diminishing her efforts for mental health and education, achieved international distinction as a leader of the family planning effort in her country, maintaining close touch through Henry David with the WFMH Committee on Responsible Parenthood. When she spent an evening with my wife and me during a 1994 visit to Bangkok for the Harvard Program in Refugee Trauma (when I also lectured to the Department of Psychiatry at Chulalonghorn University) she was still an icon in her country, vastly respected and physically and mentally vigorous.

Meesook was a force on the Board, in several capacities, until 1977 when she was succeeded as WFMH vice president for the region by Professor Jaswant Singh Neki, M.D., Head of the Department of Psychiatry at the All-India Institute of Medical Sciences in New Delhi. He served quietly until 1981 and then for a time as honorary secretary. From 1981 to 1985 the regional vice president was Dr. Setyonegoro, by that time Director of Mental Health in the Ministry of Health of Jakarta, Indonesia, as well as a professor in the medical school there. However he attended no meetings. In early 1981 he was named the first president of the new Association of South East Asian Nations (ASEAN) Federation for Psychiatry and Mental Health, but the organization did not survive. Despite the nominal presence of regional leaders on the Board during this era there was no corollary development of WFMH work in Indonesia or India, and the lively connections between the global Federation, the Thai, and other national associations in the region became less vibrant. The later years were complicated for Dr. Neki by the persecution of Sikhs in some parts of India, which made it necessary for him to abandon his academic posts. During this period I devoted much time to helping him find a suitable residency for his son in a hospital affiliated with a U.S. medical school.

The 1981 Manila World Congress for Mental Health

The Federation's Asian focus was renewed through the efforts of the Philippine Mental Health Association that, encouraged by Tsung-yi Lin, hosted the 1981 World Congress for

Mental Health in Manila (see Chapter 5). At that time I was not sensitive to the history of WFMH in Asia and paid little attention to the site of the upcoming congress until becoming WFMH's president-elect in late 1980. Then I realized that I would succeed to the presidency during the 1981 congress in Manila

On one hand this was a matter of pride. I quickly learned the reputation of Philippine Mental Health Association as a senior, active, and influential body, established in 1950 and a longtime member of WFMH. It had initiated the first National Mental Health Week in the country in 1951 and since then had been an active supporter of community mental health services. It was, perhaps, unique in its region as a major source of information and training for mental health professionals. The high status of the Philippine Mental Health Association and its broad-based membership were indicated by the fact that during the period of the congress its president was Roberto Concepcion, WFMH vice president for the region (then WFMH western Pacific region) and the distinguished chief justice of the Philippine supreme court. The steering committee for the congress was chaired by Judge Eduardo C. Tutaan and cochaired by WFMH Past President and Honorary President Lin.

On the other hand I was afraid that the Federation's presence in Manila could be construed as condoning the Philippine dictatorship, which was palpably incompatible with our principles. However, the die was cast, and with some discomfort I accepted the inevitable. Official dealings with the Marcos regime, indeed, involved some strain, requiring, for example, searches for firearms as we entered the auditorium for Marcos' welcoming speech and a feeling among some WFMH leaders that they should not be photographed with the dictator. During the official reception at the Malacanang Palace (again with tight security precautions) I was expected to join the three person receiving line, which included Imelda Marcos and Gowan Guest, the 1979–1981 WFMH president. By then I had come to know Estafania Aldaba-Lim and -at Tsung-yi Lin's request-had obtained her consent to be nominated as president-elect to succeed me as president. Fannie, as we had been asked to call her, came through the line with my wife. Mrs. Marcos turned her head away and did not greet her; we later learned that Fannie, in protest against Marcos' actions, had resigned as secretary of social services. After the congress I received a photograph from Marcos' office of Mrs. Marcos in an idealized, backlighted, beneficent pose with a beggar in a wheelchair. It was accompanied by a request to publish it in the newsletter, which still emanated from the Vancouver Secretariat. I vetoed its publication, despite warnings that refusal to publish might have adverse consequences for us. However, there were none.

The congress itself was held 27 July–2 August with the theme, "Mental Health, Values and Social Development: A Look into the '80s." It was summarized in the WFMH newsletter (WFMH, 1981b) by Edita Martillano, National Executive Director of the host organization. According to her report it was attended by representatives of 33 WFMH member associations, including 313 foreign participants from 31 countries and 370 from the Philippines. The United Nations was represented by WHO and Unicef, and NGO representatives came from the World Psychiatric Association, the International Council for Women's Clubs, the International Council of Nurses, and World Vision. Major themes addressed in lectures and workshops included socioeconomic factors in mental health, mental health in the Third World, school mental health, rehabilitation of the disabled, mental health in primary health care, age-related concerns, transcultural issues, strategies for interventions, and substance abuse.

The Manila congress brought several Philippine jurists and lawyers to prominence within the Federation. From 1985 to 1989 Judge Eduardo Tutaan of Manila, President of Philippine Mental Health Association, was WFMH vice president for the southeast Asian region. This strengthened his already strong influence on mental health work in his country, facilitating the creation of a National Coordinating Committee for Mental Health and a task force to pass a constitutional amendment, a Bill of Rights for Children. He also developed a joint regional meeting on mental health for WFMH member and nonmember groups in both the southeast Asian and western Pacific countries. There was no southeast Asian vice president from 1989 to 1993. In

1993 another Philippine Mental Health Association president was nominated. He was Oscar A. Inocentes, a lawyer whose career had combined professional practice with government service and business interests. He had been active in a range of volunteer activities, including the international Rotary Club. Unfortunately his varied responsibilities led to his relative inactivity as a vice president; he rarely attended Board meetings. In his absence, the interests of the Philippine Mental Health Association were competently represented by its Executive Director, Regina de Jesus. The Board members welcomed her comments but did not agree to let her vote as a substitute for Inocentes or act as the official Board representative to the region.

Other Southeast Asian Regional Activity

From time to time individual mental health associations in the region, occasionally in concert with WFMH, held significant meetings. On 21–22 January 1971, for example, a workshop cosponsored by WFMH was organized under the auspices of the Indian Psychiatric Society by Professor Venkoba Rao in Madurai. With the inclusive theme of "Priorities in Mental Health Care" it attracted participants from Ceylon, Singapore, Australia, the United Kingdom, and what was then called the United Arab Republic encompassing Egypt and Syria (WFMH, 1971). However, although its recommendations were transmitted to responsible administrators and plans made, successive symposiums were not held.

The next effort was four years later, on 6 January 1975, when the Mental Health Association of Kera, India, and the Indian Psychiatric Society organized a meeting under WFMH auspices on training medical auxiliaries for mental health care. Among other conclusions was the view that healers and religious leaders should be given formal training in the basic principles of mental health care. This gathering was attended by former WFMH presidents Morris Carstairs and Michael Beaubrun (WFMH, 1975). In September 1975 Dr. Neki, then WFMH vice president for southeast Asia, urged WHO's Mental Health Division to engage in more intimate collaboration with WFMH (WFMH, 1980).

Local and regional political disturbances often interfered with international collaboration. During the 1977 Vancouver congress Board meetings Meesook reported that political and social unrest restricted mental health activity in southeast Asia, making it impossible to hold regional workshops. She also felt, following Eduardo Tutaan's meeting of representatives from the two regions during his vice presidential term, 1985–1989, that it was impossible to separate their work, and there should be a closer relationship between the western Pacific and southeast Asian regions. Suggestions for closer collaboration were also made at the western Pacific regional meeting in Taiwan on December 1996.

An independent stream of Federation activity in southeast Asia has been carried on, mainly in Cambodia, by the WFMH collaborating center, the Harvard Program in Refugee Trauma. However, this work has not involved local mental health associations. There was an overlap on 16–20 August 1993, when I accompanied Drs. Richard Mollica and Kathleen Allden of the Harvard group to consult at the Institute for East Asian Refugees of Chulalongkorn University in Bangkok, regarding Burmese student refugees. I spoke, too, in the university's Department of Psychiatry under the auspices of its chairperson, Professor Birom Sukhonthabirom, on "Human Rights in the Practice of Psychiatry." Owing to the good offices of Amy Meesook, my wife and I also met with officers of the Thai Mental Health Association.

The WFMH Western Pacific Region

Hong Kong

The Mental Health Association of Hong Kong founded in 1955 soon became a WFMH member. Its first major regional meeting of record, however, with active sponsorship from the global WFMH, did not take place until 8–10 April 1968. At that time, WFMH President Carstairs joined mental health leaders from eight countries to meet with the Hong Kong Mental Health Association (President, Dr. P. M. Yap) in a "far eastern" seminar, "Education for Mental Health." This anticipated the WFMH World Congress scheduled for London in August of that year. Major attention was paid to Dr. Setyonegoro's program of educating general physicians in Indonesia, Dr. C. L. Wong's program for lawyers in Hong Kong, and Aldaba Lim's education of parents in the Philippines. The meeting ended with the resolve to hold further meetings aimed especially at exchanges of views and experiences among Japan, Korea, Malaysia, and Indonesia (WFMH, 1968b).

The association observed its first Mental Health Week (30 May–5 June, 1970) with the theme "Mental Health and the Community" (WFMH, 1970c). Hong Kong was the site of WFMH's 24th annual meeting , its first major conference in the region in 1971 with the theme of "Mental Health and Urbanization." Although there were Asian contributors to the program, other names, some familiar within the Federation, were prominent: Beaubrun from Jamaica, Carstairs from Scotland, Christmas from the United States, Miller from Israel, Klineberg from France, Pilowsky from Australia, Lazure and Gelinas from Canada, Ahmed from Egypt, and Morgan from Great Britain. Asians from WFMH included Takeo Doi from Tokyo, Aldaba-Lim from Manila, Jhabvala from India, and Meesook, who had helped with preparations, from Thailand.

In 2–7 November 1975, WFMH cosponsored the fifth pan-Pacific conference for the Society for the Rehabilitation of the Disabled in Singapore. This meeting drew 700 delegates from all over the world and included papers on community psychiatry and psychiatric rehabilitation in Malaysia, Hong Kong, and Indonesia as well as Singapore and elsewhere (WFMH, 1976). At the same time the Singapore Association for Mental Health acquired new premises to develop a mental health center with a social club for discharged psychiatric patients.

In late 1980 the president of the Malaysian Mental Health Association, Professor Deva Dass, reported to the WFMH Secretariat on a meeting in Kuala Lumpur where 300 participants explored the theme, "Mental Health: Family and Society." A major focus was role of the mental health association and mental health services.

The vice president for this region in 1975–1977, before the Philippines were redesignated in the WFMH southeast Asia region, was Aldaba-Lim. However, she had to resign because of her new responsibilities as United Nations NGO leader for the international year of the child in 1979. She was succeeded at the 1977 Vancouver elections by psychiatrist Lourdes Ladrido-Ignacio, M.D., Chair of the Department of Psychiatry at the College of Medicine in Manila and a former president of the Philippine Psychiatric Association. At the time of her appointment she was chief investigator of a WHO study on strategies for extending mental health care.

WFMH Growth in Japan

Perhaps the major stimulus for Federation development in Japan was the attention paid to the Pacific area by the 1977 Vancouver World Congress and the sponsorship of elements of that congress by Japanese organizations. President Tsung-yi Lin's educational background in Japan and his command of the language were significant in this development.

A major Vancouver Congress activity was the workshop on "Work, Leisure and Retirement" sponsored by the Leisure Development Center in Tsukuba, Japan. This led to a December 1978 follow-up conference in Tsukuba under the center's sponsorship that brought many WFMH participating in the initial workshop to Japan. An important contribution was made by psychologist Akira Hoshino, Professor of Clinical and Social Psychology at Tokyo's International Christian University, who chaired a Japanese Coordinating Committee for the 1981 Manila congress where he was later named vice president for the western Pacific region. There he joined Board member-at-large from Japan, Professor Takeo Doi, perhaps the most internationally known psychiatrist-psychoanalyst in his country. Hoshino, who had served his university in several administrative positions, was also an international scholar; he had worked in the Philippines and Hawaii. His excellent command of English along with experience with academic colleagues in other countries made him an especially congenial presence on the Board. He opened a WFMH regional office in his university and initiated printing of WFMH bylaws and application forms as well as the "Declaration of Rights and Responsibilities of Children in Residential Centers" (in Japanese) adopted in Manila. In addition he represented WFMH at such meetings as a regional symposium of the World Psychiatric Association and meetings of Japanese groups. His efforts were accelerated by a month's visit from Honorary President Lin in late 1981 after I began my term as president. This was part of Lin's two-month trip, including the People's Republic of China, as a WHO advisor on psychiatric education. In addition to presenting WFMH certificates of life membership to several distinguished colleagues, Lin helped recruit the Japanese Association of Private Mental Hospitals into WFMH membership.

Hoshino could not attend my second Board meeting as president in 1982. In that year he formed a Japanese Coordinating Committee for WFMH, including representatives of mental health associations as well as noted professionals. The committee was chaired by Masaki Kato, M.D., Director of the National Research Institute for Mental Health. Hoshino also met with Lin and many colleagues in various fields to discuss the future activities of WFMH's western Pacific region. To build a sense of regional interconnectedness, he visited WFMH and WHO colleagues as well as psychiatric centers in Manila, Taiwan, and Hong Kong in 1983. In his own country he recruited the Japanese Federation for Mental Health, which included 12 national organizations. One of these organizations was the Japanese Association for Mental Health, already a WFMH voting member. He and his staff twice edited and published information about Federation activities in Japanese language newsletters and by 1984 had stimulated sufficient enthusiasm among Japanese colleagues for them to discuss among themselves the possibility of holding the 1987 World Congress for Mental Health in Japan. He used funds from his university to make a study trip to the United States, permitting his participation in the 1984 Board meeting and symposium at Sheppard Pratt Hospital in Baltimore.

At the Brighton World Congress elections in 1985, psychiatrist Tsuguo Kaneko, M.D., Vice Medical Director of the Metropolitan Matsuzawa Hospital in Tokyo, became western Pacific vice president, succeeding Hoshino who had completed his second two-year term. He reported the parliamentary passage in September 1987 of the Reformed Mental Health Act, for which Japanese WFMH members had advocated. It became effective in April 1988. Among other items this act provided for the establishment of a Mental Health Review Tribunal to which cases of presumed wrongful detention could be appealed. On 25–30 September 1988, my wife and I were guests of Japanese colleagues at an international rehabilitation seminar for mentally ill people cosponsored with WFMH in Osaka. Our earlier discussions led to a focus on issues surrounding patient autonomy and participation in the clinical decisions that affect them, a major departure from the established clinical, administrative, and cultural tradition of Japan. This was organized by the National Federation of Families with the Mentally Ill (ZENKAREN), which, led by its secretary general, Takehisa Takizawa, sponsored my travel. They also invited Board member-at-large Hilda Robbins, whom I had recommended to speak about first-hand experience of clinical depression and its treatment.

After the Osaka activities the international seminar reconvened on 1 October 1988 as the first regional meeting of WFMH's western Pacific region in Tokyo. This was also a meeting of the Japanese Association for Mental Health under the auspices of ZENKAREN and the Japanese Association of Psychiatric Hospitals. It provided my first contact with Kunihiko Asai, M.D., of the Asai Hospital who chaired an international forum on mental health along with Masahiko Saito, M.D., of the Matsuzawa Hospital, both WFMH life members. I delivered the keynote address on "Human Rights and the Rehabilitation of the Mentally Ill-An International Perspective." The only other WFMH officer present besides Akira Hoshino (no longer vice president), was WFMH vice president for the Oceania region, Dr. Max Abbott, then executive director of the Mental Health Foundation of New Zealand, its equivalent of a national mental health association. A handful of other invited foreigners represented Canada, the United Kingdom, and the People's Republic of China.

The two meetings of ZENKAREN, in Kobe and Tokyo, attracted approximately 500 persons; each meeting featured much audience participation. I spoke extemporaneously from the floor on my own experiences with my mother's psychotic behavior, eliciting audience approval for my willingness to share my personal history. These meetings with their emphasis on self-revelation-a departure from traditional cultural norms-were regarded as successful major efforts toward reducing the stigma associated with mental illness and promoting positive knowledge of mental health in the country.

The international forum in Tokyo had an audience of approximately 200 psychiatrists, psychologist, social workers, other professionals, and volunteers. It was aimed at increasing Japanese knowledge of treatment and rehabilitation in other countries and cultures and how to integrate the concept of universal human rights of patients with that of legitimate cultural differences. Former U.S. First Lady Rosalynn Carter, who was visiting Japan with her husband, addressed the audience briefly and joined my wife and me at lunch with several Japanese leaders.

This was our first visit to Japan, and our first experience of the exceptional hospitality tendered to visiting dignitaries. It was especially pleasant to renew our friendship with Akira Hoshino, who was generous with his time in showing us historical sights not on the usual tourist itinerary. After the meetings we were sent for a few days of rest, as guests of the sponsoring associations, to the resort area of Nikko which is distinguished by beautiful shrines and mountain scenery. In retrospect the visit did much to develop mutually respectful and warm relationships with colleagues there, facilitating their interest in hosting the 1993 WFMH World Congress.

Toward a WFMH Congress in Japan

At the Auckland world congress elections in August 1989, the soft-spoken but organizationally influential Kunihiko Asai was nominated to succeed Kaneko as western Pacific regional vice president. Through him the Board accepted the invitation tendered by a consortium of Japanese societies to hold the 1993 World Congress for Mental Health in Japan. Asai was vice director of his family-owned private hospital, consultant to the Chiba Prefectural Child Guidance Center and several other public units, an officer in several professional associations, and a director of the Japanese Society of Mental Health. He was clearly an active, exceedingly well-connected representative for WFMH. By the end of 1990 he had attended on our behalf two seminars, six months apart, on community health in Seoul; a World Psychiatric Association regional symposium in Hong Kong; a meeting of the Association for Child and Adolescent Psychiatry and Allied Professions; the congress of the Collegium International Neuro-Psycho-Pharmacologicum; a congress on mental health law in mainland China (People's Republic of China); and several WHO meetings. He also promoted the 1991 World Congress scheduled for Mexico and held the initial meeting (January 1990) of an organizing committee for the 1993 congress with the older, distinguished Yasuo Shimozono, M.D., as chairman and himself as secretary general. By May 1991 Dick Hunter had accepted Asai's invitation for the WFMH Secretariat to review Tokyo congress facilities and meet with the committee. An impressive list of Japanese organizations had already agreed to cosponsor, and the committee had produced a Japanese language WFMH newsletter promoting the congress. On 17-20 September 1991, at a WHO sponsored public health meeting in Japan, Asai met with his fellow countryman, WHO Director General Hiroshi Nakajima, who confirmed WHO cosponsorship of the congress.

From this point on, like other organizational leaders who had accepted WFMH Board membership, Asai continued his heavy schedule of meetings and speaking, now adding to his other responsibilities that of representing WFMH. In addition he had to be concerned with some of the intramural chauvinism that occasionally arises within international organizations. Some European regional council leaders had been much concerned with what they perceived as neglect by the 1991 Mexico congress of regions other than the Americas (especially Europe), including concerns with mental health services and patients' rights. They were not reassured by the location of the forthcoming 1993 congress, again outside the European sphere of influence. Asai was especially careful therefore to see that Europeans participated in the program. He also drew on the potential strength of the psychiatric survivors and users movement, organizing a seminar on the subject in November 1992, which anticipated the world congress. Entitled "Mental Health: Rehabilitation and Social Participation of Psychiatric Users," the speakers included New Zealander Mary O'Hagan, Chair of the World Federation of Psychiatric Users, which WFMH had helped create. Asai's main problem in the English speaking world was his limited mastery of English, but this did not stop his being nominated for the position of WFMH honorary secretary in the assembly of voting members during the 1993 Tokyo World Congress. The nominee for regional vice president was Professor Shimpei Inoue, of the Kochi Medical School, who had received training at the University of British Columbia.

Tokyo World Congress, 23–27 August 1993

WFMH's decision to hold its 1993 congress in Japan recognized Japan's change in status since the end of World War II, nearly half a century earlier. The Japanese hosts also recognized the historical significance of the occasion in the pomp and circumstance of the opening and closing ceremonies involving not only government and United Nations figures but members of the Japanese royal family.

The congress theme was "Mental Health: Toward the 21st Century-Technology, Culture and Quality of Life." Cosponsors with WFMH included, besides the Japanese Federation for Mental Health and WHO, the Japan Foundation for Neuroscience and Mental Health. Asai had succeeded in impressing governmental authorities with the importance of the congress as a presentation of a democratic Japan entering the new century, and he received extensive support from the Prime Minister's office; the ministries of Foreign Affairs, Labor, Health and Welfare, and Education; the Tokyo metropolitan government, the Chiba prefectural government, and the Chiba municipal government.

The congress was remarkable for its size, efficiency, and the elegance of its entertainments, including exquisite food at the opening reception and other lavish buffets to which all registrants were welcome. There were aesthetic displays of music and dance at major receptions, and the "Chiba Night" presented by the government of the prefecture was marked by exceptional performances of historic as well as artistic merit. The congress attracted more than 4600 registrants from 67 countries, 550 of whom were from nations other than Japan. These last included 30 from the People's Republic of China and 12 from Eastern Europe and the countries of the former U.S.S.R.

The setting was the modernistic Makuhari Conference Center in Chiba Prefecture, with excellent simultaneous translating facilities. The congress amply justified its theme with keynote addresses followed by tracks emphasizing the concerns of the keynotes. More than 1015 presentations covered a range of mental health relevant issues. They included population technology and stress, religion, childhood and adolescent education, primary prevention, women, aging, and cultural change. Perhaps half dealt with essentially psychiatric matters: substance abuse, community care, vocational rehabilitation, mental health law, patients' families, nursing, and the concerns of survivors of psychiatric illness and users of psychiatric services. Users were heavily represented including 600 from Japan; the WFMH Secretariat along with congress organizers had helped obtain funds to facilitate the attendance of users from overseas.

Especially favorable comments noted the value of bringing clinicians and scientists to the front lines of new knowledge, together with users, administrators, volunteers, family members, and others. Booths manned by Japanese colleagues during the congress drew the enrollment of more than 900 new members to the Federation. A statement of aims, the Makuhari Declaration, was formulated by the congress organizing committee, read at the closing ceremony on 27 August 1993, and printed in the August/September 1993 issue of the WFMH newsletter (WFMH, 1983).

After the congress Former Regional Vice President Kaneko, now president of the Tokyo Metropolitan Matsuzawa Hospital, the oldest and largest in the country, organized a symposium at the hospital intended to promote a renewal of interest and activity in community mental health services in Japan. I accepted his invitation to present the keynote address. My focus was on the importance of promoting overall community well-being as a basis for reducing the prevalence of psychiatric disorders and less than optimal function, and facilitating community-based treatment. The four other speakers came from Great Britain, Germany, India, and Japan. This was another occasion for increasing our knowledge of each other as persons and professionals, which I think was much appreciated by all participants, including an audience of several hundred.

WFMH in Japan after the Tokyo Congress

A major consequence of the Tokyo congress was the increased confidence of Federation leaders in the capacity of Japanese colleagues for overall leadership. It was inevitable that Kunihiko Asai, the chief architect of what many regarded as the uniquely outstanding WFMH congress to date, was asked to be a candidate for president-elect to run in the 1995 Dublin elections. Although he did not refuse immediately, his reluctance was apparent from the beginning. Many factors seemed to determine his eventual irrevocable refusal. One was the pressure of work at home, especially because he was succeeding his father as the senior leader of the family owned Asai hospital. Another was the sheer number of posts that he held in other organizations. Unclear to non-Japanese Federation associates was the role of his self-perception; he possibly felt too junior in comparison with other Japanese colleagues for the elevated position of WFMH president. Also unclear was the significance of his lack of command of English and his perceptions of the potential difficulty in leading the organization from a place so distant from its other seats of power.

Regional Vice President Inoue, though, was active. He organized a mental health symposium sponsored by his university's Department of Neuropsychiatry and the local mental health association in Kochi on 19–20 October 1994, cosponsored by WFMH and the Japan Association of Mental Health. It covered among other issues regional mental health activities at the NGO level with special reference to stigma, neighborhood objections to group homes and other facilities, and users' concerns. Foreign speakers included Tsung-yi Lin, at that time a visiting professor in Kaohsiung Medical College, Taiwan, social work professor Dr. Agnes Chew-Chung Wu of the Mental Health Association in Taiwan, and colleagues from Korea, the People's Republic of China, and Hong Kong. Of particular interest regarding the possibly impaired autonomy of mental health associations which operate services for their governments was a discussion by Veronica Pearson, Senior Lecturer in the Department of Social Work and Social Administration of Hong Kong University, about the Hong Kong government's ability to control NGOs through the use of subsidies.

An unexpected catastrophe that influenced the Japanese perception of needed services was the Kobe earthquake on 17 January 1995, in which more than 5000 people died and thousands more were left homeless. My office responded to requests from Japan for information on psychological assistance for earthquake survivors and sent materials for distribution to our officers there as well as others. Both Drs. Asai and Inoue were involved in consultations about providing services to survivors, including telephone hotline services, some based on the experiences of former WFMH president Federico Puente with the 1985 earthquake in Mexico. The involvement in Kobe of our collaborating center the Harvard Program in Refugee Trauma, led by Dr. Richard Mollica is described in Chapter 13.

Taiwan and the People's Republic of China

Membership for the Chinese Mental Health Association?

In 1985 the opportunity arose for me to lead a group of U.S. WFMH members, mostly professionals, to inspect psychiatric institutions in the People's Republic of China (PRC) under the auspices of a university based agency. During the journey we visited hospitals and clinics, gave lectures, and held discussions with Chinese colleagues in Xian, Shanghai, Beijing, and later Hong Kong. In Beijing we visited the An Ding Hospital associated with the Capital City Medical College. The professor and director of psychiatry was Chen Hsueh-Shin, M.D., who was also president of the Chinese Mental Health Association, a government approved 5000 member, multiprofessional organization. We talked about his association becoming a WFMH member, and he seemed genuinely interested . Upon my return to the United States I took this up with our Board. It, too, was interested in bringing the contemporary Chinese Mental Health Association back into the Federation, even though it was essentially an arm of the government, so I invited Chen to apply. However, months passed with no definitive reply. It seemed likely that the Chinese Mental Health Association was unwilling to join an international organization that included representatives of Taiwan. That would have been tantamount to recognizing Taiwan as an independent nation rather than a PRC province.

Taiwan was in a difficult position. Occupied by the Japanese from 1895 until after the second Sino-Japanese war in 1937, the nationalist government of Chiang Kai-shek withdrew to the island from the Chinese mainland after its defeat by the communist forces in 1949. It was expelled from the United Nations in 1971 when the PRC took its seat in the Security Council. That meant that it could have no voice in WHO or in any United Nations specialized agencies and that NGOs, such as WFMH, enjoying official relations with these agencies risked losing those relations if they collaborated with Taiwan. Although it was not mentioned, PRC colleagues were probably aware of the fact that in January 1985 WFMH President Aldaba-Lim had initiated the observation of International Youth Year in Taiwan, as well as the 75th anniversary of the World Association of Girl Guides and Girl Scouts. Also in that year WFMH Honorary President Tsung-yi Lin was invited to the celebration of the 40th anniversary of the Mental Health Association on the island, which still called itself the Republic of China, in contrast to the PRC on the mainland.

Organizers of the 1989 World Congress for Mental Health in Auckland, New Zealand, tried hard to encourage PRC attendance. Despite repeated invitations, however, neither Professor Chen, nor a representative of the Chinese Mental Health Association, attended. Tsung-yi Lin, Stanislas Flache, who became WFMH president for 1989–1991 at that congress, and I met several times with child psychiatrist, Professor Wei-Tsuen Soong, M.D., president of what was still called the Republic of China Mental Health Association. It agreed, after some deliberation, to change its name, omitting the designation "Chinese," to the "Mental Health Association in Taiwan." This fitted what I understood as Professor Chen's requirement for inclusion of his Chinese Mental Health Association. The postcongress Board in Auckland voted to accept this change of name and further resolved that no association had the right to dictate the name of another member association. To make a reply more likely I sent Professor Chen a telegram with this information. In response he sent the following fax on 28 August 1989: "I am very delighted to receive your telegram. We think Mental Health Association, Taiwan, China, is more appropriate than Taiwan Mental Health Association. I am showing appreciation at your great efforts. Thank you once again."

The situation remained unchanged despite visits to PRC by Lin, accompanied on one occasion by Asai. However, we remained optimistic and decided to use the approaching 1991 World Congress in Mexico as another opportunity. In a letter to Chen of 14 February 1991, I once more noted the change of name of the Taiwanese association, saying "It is our understanding that this action removes one barrier to the inclusion of your organization as an active partner in our efforts in the field of mental health." I again invited the Chinese Mental Health Association to apply for membership and expressed the hope for his personal participation in the congress. Eventually on 31 May a reply dated 16 May arrived. In it he informed me that the China Association for Science and Technology, of which the Chinese Mental Health Association was a component member, suggested "in order to remove any barrier that the name of the Taiwanese group would better be changed to 'China Taipei Mental Health Association' or 'China Taiwan Mental Health Association'." If one of these changes were effected, he wrote, the Chinese Mental Health Association's application for WFMH membership would be approved. He also expressed his intention to come to Mexico.

The exchanges persisted for a while longer, but it seemed evident that the PRC colleagues, while they wished to maintain communication if possible, could not join us within the constraints imposed by their overseeing bodies. A letter of 17 June 1991, from Tsung-yi Lin, with whom I shared all correspondence on this matter, strongly supported the idea that WFMH should stick with its resolution about the renaming of its member association in Taiwan: "This resolution," he wrote, " should, in my view, satisfy Beijing since the association in Taiwan no longer claims that it represents all of China...this is not the time to engage in a meaningless, futile and political game surrounding the issue of name." Just two days later, on 19 June 1991, I received another telegram from Chen Hsueh-shin. In it he said, "We prefer Association for Mental Health, Taiwan China, or Taiwan Association for Mental Health of China." After another week a letter (dated 27 June 1991) arrived from Soong in his capacity as president of the Mental Health Association in Taiwan. While recognizing that the WFMH board's Auckland resolution meant that "the Chinese Mental Health Association has no right to request my association to change name," he indicated that he would raise the issue at his association's next Board meeting, and if any new decision emerged he would notify me. This was the end of the affair. We did not hear from him again.

The Mental Health Association in Taiwan

The Mental Health Association in Taiwan has a long history. It was described in a letter to me from its president, Dr. Agnes Chew-Chung Wu, in the summer of 1994. I printed a condensed version in the Summer 1994 issue of the WFMH newsletter (WFMH, 1994).

The association had its ultimate roots in the Chinese National Association for Mental Health founded in Nanking City, China, on 19 April 1936. This association began with more than 200 distinguished professionals including prominent figures in psychology and education. Its aim was "to promote nationwide mental health and to develop treatment and prevention strategies academically and progressively for the mentally ill." On 20 March 1955, an association with the same name was formed in Taipei with members including "psychiatrists, psychologists, educators, social workers, nurses, public health professionals, students and the public interested in mental health." Two years later, under the presidency of Tsung-yi Lin, it became a member of WFMH during the 1957 World Congress in Copenhagen. As of 1996 it had approximately 1200 members. Its major interests were in integrating mental health concepts into the programs of schools and other community institutions, providing training programs to improve the mental health care system, using the media for mental health promotion, and working with other organizations regarding mental health legislation. As Dr. Wu put it, in Taiwan today "more and more people know how to take collective action" to effect change. They included a users group, the Organization of Mentally Ill in Taiwan, which had become an effective public advocate.

Shortly before coming to Dublin for the 1995 WFMH World Congress I received an invitation from Dr. Wu to participate in a meeting of the WFMH western Pacific region in Taiwan in December 1996. After meeting with her, Dr. Soong, and other colleagues during the Dublin congress, I agreed to come with my wife, whose passage they also offered to support. At the Dublin Board meeting, President Inoue made a point of obtaining approval for the Taiwan meeting, specifying the dates 16–19 December 1996, so as not to conflict with a Board meeting scheduled in Chile to coincide with a South American congress that would found a new South American council for WFMH.

This was the beginning of a long period of intermittent correspondence punctuated by Taiwan's first democratic election in spring 1996 resulting in the reelection of President Lee Tseng-hui to a second term. This election was disturbing enough to the PRC leaders, but their concern peaked when he was admitted by the United States to attend a class reunion of Cornell University. They showed their displeasure by sending missiles close to the island's shipping lanes, to which the United States reacted by dispatching battleships to the area. In this atmosphere the forthcoming international meeting gained special significance.

By this time I was corresponding about the matter with Tsung-yi Lin. It was clear that he attached significance to the meeting with its international representation. It implied professional if not political recognition of Taiwan's status as an entity independent of the PRC. It seemed especially important that a major NGO would be willing to risk its official relationships with United Nations agencies by sponsoring a meeting in Taiwan. For this reason efforts were also initiated to bring Norman Sartorius, M.D., former director of WHO's Mental Health Division and current president of the World Psychiatric Association to the conference. Unfortunately, the Chile Board meeting, originally scheduled for November, was moved to early December without prior consultation. I decided because of previously scheduled appointments en route to Taipei, not to go first to Chile and to rush from there to the western Pacific. Therefore, for the first time since serving as a member of the WFMH Board and Secretariat I missed a Board meeting. Drs. Inoue and Asai also decided that Taiwan demanded their primary allegiance, and they also decided to forgo the Chile meeting as did two European Board members. The Board, in fact, did not achieve a quorum until its second day.

Western Pacific Regional Conferences of WFMH in Taiwan

The December 1996 conference was the second WFMH western Pacific regional meeting in Taiwan. The first was a workshop on "Family, Child and Mental Health" in Taipei nearly 20 years earlier on 4–10 February 1979. On that occasion WFMH was represented by Regional Vice President Ladrido-Ignacio and Milton Miller, M.D., Chairman of the Department of Psychiatry at the University of British Columbia in Vancouver, who had been a key figure in organizing the 1977 WFMH World Congress for Mental Health. That Taiwan gathering, attended by 76 people from 12 countries, was in preparation for the Salzburg congress later that year organized around the United Nations' International Year of the Child.

The 1996 Taiwan conference, lavish and carefully planned, was organized by Professor Soong in his capacity as Secretary General, and chaired by the Mental Health Association President Chueh Chang, Sc.D. (with her doctorate in public health from Johns Hopkins). It was supported and sponsored by the range of national and Taipei ministries and departments, as well as professional associations and private businesses on the island. It was held, and visiting speakers were housed, in the Academia Sinica, a prestigious collection of research institutes, with origins dating back to 1927 on the mainland. Colleagues in Taiwan, under constant pressure from the PRC to return as a province, were eager for the success of this international meeting that symbolized their independent status. It was a particular pleasure to attend the 50th anniversary celebration of the Department of Psychiatry of the National University of Taiwan of which Tsung-yi Lin had been the founding chairman in 1947 at the tender age of 26.

The importance attached to the regional meeting was indicated by a visit with Taiwan's President Lee, arranged by Lin who had attended the same college three years ahead of him. The aim was to demonstrate the interest of international NGOs in the country. In addition to my wife and myself and Sartorius and his wife who had arranged to come at the last minute, the group included Professor and Mrs. Lin and Dr. Soong. We were surprised and impressed when the president kept us for nearly an hour, talking mainly about the mental health aspects of education, a particular interest of his. It was clear that he appreciated the presence of international mental health leaders who were unafraid of United Nations repercussions as a possible consequence of their involvement with Taiwan. We were also complimented at the meetings by the presence of Po-Ya Chang, M.D., Director General of the national health services, who was part of the opening ceremonies. At the reception that followed she used a traditional sword to cut a cake along with my wife (whose 75th birthday came during our flight over the Pacific) and was the guest of honor at the conference banquet.

Although most of the 750 participants were from the island itself, there were visitors from mainland China, Hong Kong, South Korea, and Singapore, and a sizable contingent from Japan. Several people suggested (as Amy Meesook had in the late 1970s) that it would have been logical for Philippine Mental Health Association members to participate as well, even though they were in another "region." Many Asian-Americans, mostly natives of Taiwan, were present. Board members John Henderson, M.D., from the United Kingdom and Max Abbott, Ph.D., from New Zealand, both having rushed home from Chile, and turned around, arrived in Taipei somewhat the worse for wear. A handful came from elsewhere in the world, including Caeser Korolenko M.D. from Siberia, and Professor John Copeland, Director of the new WFMH collaborating center, the Institute of Aging at the University of Liverpool. It was especially good to see Milton Miller again, now on his way to receive an honorary degree from Hunan University on the mainland. Having lived for a time in Taipei, he was delighted to practice his Chinese on the available audiences!

The conference theme was "Mental Health for All: Regional Dialogue." My assignment was to address this theme as keynote speaker, with an emphasis on global mental health. It gave me an opportunity to speak of the Federation's history with special reference to its initial concerns with mental health and world citizenship. The other conference themes were health policy, health promotion, and mental health in daily life. They were addressed enthusiastically by the mainly young participants who took evident pleasure in describing their own initiatives and exchanging information with colleagues from elsewhere in and out of the region. In addition we made a special effort to acquaint them with the roles of NGOs, especially their capacity for advocacy.

OCEANIA

Australia, New Zealand, and Pacific Islands

Early Representation in the WFMH

In 1949 the 62 WFMH member associations representing 33 countries included the Australasian Association of Psychiatrists (of both Australia and New Zealand) and the New Zealand Council for Mental Health. They were classified, following WHO, as part of the WFMH western Pacific region. Although the newly formed WFMH Executive Board did not yet include regional vice presidents an effort was made to achieve a more or less equable geographic distribution. Thus if a person from a particular area resigned, he or she was replaced by another from the same part of the world.

At the 26 August 1949, plenary session of the Second WFMH Mental Health Assembly in Geneva, National Health Director John Russell, M.D., of New Zealand, who had represented Australasia on the original Federation Executive Board, did not stand for reelection. He was replaced by psychiatrist Alan Stoller of Australia, then with his country's repatriation commission (A few years later the repatriation department psychiatric services joined the Federation, remaining for one or two years). In 1950 another New Zealand organization, the Family Guidance Centre, became a member, heralding an emphasis in that country on voluntary associations and mental health rather than professional psychiatry. For the next several years these memberships remained static, supplemented by a handful of individual members from the two countries. But in 1954 Dr. Stoller, who had become Chief Clinical Officer of the Mental Hygiene Authority of the Australian state of Victoria, attended the annual meeting in Toronto. There on 17 August 1954, he was elected to the Board for another one-year term, bringing with him as a new member organization the Victorian Council of Mental Hygiene. By 1956 the New Zealand Council for Mental Health had dropped out, and the Family Guidance Centre had shifted status to the less expensive affiliate membership. As New Zealand professionals began to differentiate themselves from Australasia, they formed a New Zealand branch of the Australasian Association of Psychiatrists and joined the Federation. Affiliation with a major international organization was an accepted way for an association in a small country to bolster its identity, and because the World Psychiatric Association before 1961 was yet to be an established body, WFMH was perceived as a plausible affiliation for professionals.

Meanwhile, through Stoller, who by now had become director of the Mental Health Research Institute of the Health Commission of Victoria, the region was developing a presence at the overall leadership level. He was reelected to the Board at the 15 August 1956, annual meeting in Berlin. With him another Australian organization, the South Australian Association for Mental Health, Inc., gained voting membership. Despite the welcome membership from Australia, however, there was no significant local WFMH linked activity. The Federation ethos of the period did not require accelerated regional development at home to justify election to the board. High value was attached rather to the recruitment of influential individuals. In her address as outgoing WFMH president at the 11–17 August 1957 annual meeting in Copenhagen, Margaret Mead was explicit, "As each new member comes on the Board we know that we are adding one more person committed to responsibility for the well-being of mankind; as each member leaves .[ths].[ths]. we know that we have added to the number of the responsibly wiser men and women who will be a resource for their own countries, for the United Nations, for other international nongovernmental agencies" (WFMH, 1958b, pp. 8–9).

At this Copenhagen meeting Stoller chaired a panel on the prevention of juvenile delinquency. His last Board attendance at the annual meeting in Barcelona (30 August–4 September 1959) brought another voluntary organization from his home state, the Victorian Council for Mental Hygiene, as well as one from Sydney, the New South Wales Association for Mental Health.

By now mental health associations from Canterbury and Otago in New Zealand had joined as affiliate members. At the annual meeting in Amsterdam (22–26 July 1963), Stoller, after a three-year absence from the Board, was elected WFMH vice president and succeeded to the presidency for 1964–1965. Despite his welcoming attitude toward voluntary nonprofessional associations, his fundamental orientation was reflected in his foreword to the 1965 WFMH annual report in which he characterized the preparatory commissions for the 1948 London congress as "some 5000 social scientists," and the Federation as constituting "a wide group of professions." Even though he described these professions as seeking "solutions for a wide range of human problems," he emphasized that the mental health movement "has decades of work ahead of it to bring recognizable mental health needs under control" (WFMH, 1965, pp. 7–8).

As Stoller joined the ranks of past presidents, there had still been no major Federation events in his area. "Australasia" had been abandoned, but an Australian and New Zealand College of Psychiatrists was a full member organization.

Oceania in the Era of Working Presidents

The Carstairs presidency (1968–1972) saw no Federation activity in the Australia-New Zealand area. Local associations, however, continued to grow in size and scope. The New South Wales Association for Mental Health founded a new journal in 1967; the summer 1968 issue of the WFMH bulletin reported the construction of a mental health center as part of the headquarters building of the Western Australia Mental Health Association. In July 1967 the Australian National Association for Mental Health was inaugurated to coordinate the work of state associations active at least since the founding of the Victorian Council for Mental Hygiene in 1930.

ANAMH

By 1971 the Australian National Association of Mental Health felt strong enough to invite WFMH to mark its 25th anniversary with a world congress in Sydney, Australia, on 8–13 October 1973. The mental health association in New South Wales accepted organizing responsibility for the congress, and Professor Issy Pilowsky, the first vice president of the WFMH western Pacific region to which Australia and New Zealand then belonged, agreed to play a leading role. In 1972 the executive committee for the congress was named with Dr. Beryl Hinckley, President of the Australian National Association for Mental Health, as president. It attracted more than 400 participants, 228 from Australia and 175 from other countries including the United Kingdom, continental Europe, the United States, Canada, Israel, Ceylon, Singapore, Japan, Hong Kong, India, the West Indies, Malaysia, Mauritius, New Zealand, the Philippines, Nigeria, and South Africa. This despite the Sydney airport being shut down by an air traffic control strike. Delegates had to arrive via Fiji or New Zealand, land in Melbourne or Canberra, and get to Sydney by whatever transport they could find (WFMH, 1973–1974). The main speaker at the opening session was Dr. Khunying Ambhorn Meesook, WFMH vice president for southeast Asia, by then Deputy Under Secretary of State for Education in Thailand. Her topic was "Cultures in Collision," the focus of the congress' main plenary session (Pilowsky, 1976). The other panels included the topics of family, community, education, law, migration, religion, social stress, and migration.

The main administrative move of the Executive Board meeting on 13 October 1973, in Sydney was occasioned by WFMH President Michael Beaubrun's announcement that he was moving to Trinidad in June 1974. He was scheduled to be reelected for two more years but suggested that it would not be in the interests of the Federation to move the Secretariat to Trinidad for one and a half years. Under these circumstances it was decided that Dr. Tsung-yi Lin should assume the presidency in mid-1974 after Dr. Beaubrun's move and that the Secretariat would be relocated to Vancouver at the end of that year.

Establishing an Oceania Region

New Regional Representation

The separation of Oceania out of the WFMH western Pacific region became more likely with the election as Board member-at-large (at the 1979 Salzburg congress) of Basil James, M.D., an émigré from Wales who was professor and chairman of psychological medicine (psychiatry) at New Zealand's University of Otago. Not long before he had resigned as the first chairman of the newly established Mental Health Foundation of New Zealand (MHFNZ), having been an unsuccessful candidate for the post of executive director. Clinical psychologist Max Abbott, Ph.D., was subsequently appointed to the director's position in 1981. At that time MHFNZ was heavily dominated by professionals, mainly psychiatrists. Indeed, all four of the country's chairs of psychiatry were required by its constitution to serve on its board. Several years passed before the constitution was amended to limit the role of academic psychiatry. Although the process began shortly after Abbott's appointment with the naming of a clinical psychologist, Andrew Hornblow, to a six-year term as chairman, he was, in fact, on the Board in his capacity as professor and head of one of the academic departments of psychiatry (at Christchurch). He later became dean of that medical school, one of the world's few nonphysician heads of an institution of that type (Abbott, Max, personal communication, 1997).

At the time of James' 1979 election to the Board he had just completed a term as president of the New Zealand branch of the Royal Australian and New Zealand College of Psychiatrists. His vigorous speaking style and strong interest in administrative matters made the existence of Australia and New Zealand with a language and culture quite different from the rest of the western Pacific more real to the Board than before. Without fanfare the 1979 board meeting at Salzburg decided that New Zealand along with Australia and some of the Pacific Islands should be separated from the western Pacific region to form a region of their own.

This development was almost lost in the hurly-burly of that meeting, with some 40 members vying for attention. It was my first as an elected member-at-large and the last before the new by-law changes (recommended at Vancouver in 1977 to be ratified in Salzburg) went into effect. They first went into force at the 12–13 April 1980, board meeting in Mexico where they were reflected in the smaller and more manageable group. There, once the existence of Oceania was accepted, Basil James, after having served less than a year, was moved from member-at-large to become the Federation's first regional vice president for Oceania. This also marked a break with the WHO classification since Australia, New Zealand, and the several Pacific Islands including Micronesia remained in the WHO western Pacific region.

The new 1980 Board was small enough so that we all became rapidly acquainted. The process was accelerated as we participated in the Mexico meeting. Basil was outstanding as the only man in that intensely urban and formal setting to wear a bush jacket. He invited me to be a visiting professor in his University of Otago Department for six weeks in February and March 1981. New Zealand was an unknown area for us; and after some thought I accepted, understanding that he would provide travel and accommodations in Otago for both my wife and me. By that time I had become WFMH president-elect, so in addition to teaching psychiatry and behavioral science to medical students and residents I could represent the Federation on various semiceremonial occasions both in association with the medical school and at local mental health associations. On one occasion I overlapped with Roberta Beiser, the recently appointed WFMH executive director, who had been sponsored to visit a range of groups in New Zealand and Australia to advertise the August 1981 Manila World Congress for Mental Health.

Early Activities

En route to New Zealand my wife and I stopped for what was expected to be a week in Sydney, Australia, but it was extended for several days by an airline strike. There I learned that an Australian mental health foundation had been established with the initial task of fundraising to support projects by state mental health associations. I had little contact with them (leaving that to Bertie Beiser) except to meet the foundation's first president, WFMH Life Member Graham Burrows, M.D., Professor and Chairman of Psychiatry at the University of Melbourne.

Most of my work was at the University of New South Wales where I gave some lectures and consulted with my old friend Professor John Cawte, a specialist in cultural psychiatry and aboriginal life. An honorary member of at least one aboriginal tribe, Cawte had helped form an aboriginal mental health association and arranged for me to meet with some of its leaders affiliated with the university.

We finally reached New Zealand. The University of Otago is located in Dunedin, a charming town on the South Island carrying the ancient Scottish name for Edinburgh. Its quietness and the civility of its residents reminded me of the Columbia, Missouri, of my childhood in the 1920s and 1930s. But the beauty of its sea-rimmed surroundings, the presence of such exotic creatures as albatross and black swans, and other indications of its nearness to the South Pole were a constant reminder of its vast distance from the United States. Basil James turned out to be a solicitous host as well as a stimulating and thought-provoking colleague. His department would have been rated superior by any standard. One conclusion was quick in coming: all New Zealand professors were adept at carving lamb. The stay there also gave me the opportunity to speak about the virtues of the Federation and to teach and consult at the outlying two-year medical schools, Christchurch and Wellington, whose students finished their work elsewhere.

At the 1981 elections in Manila where I became WFMH president, Basil moved to the position of honorary secretary while Graham Burrows, Australian National Association of Mental Health president (nominated to the WFMH Board by his council), replaced him as vice president for Oceania. On 6–7 August a postcongress symposium was held in Melbourne to celebrate the 25th anniversary of the Mental Health Research Institute there. Dr. Stoller, then retired, was one of the guest speakers. With Burrows in its top leadership post, the Australian association became more active and visible on the world scene. The proceedings of its 1980 workshop on "Aboriginals in Mental Health" were edited; it hosted a national workshop on "Stress and Anxiety in the Community" in July 1981; and accelerated its seminars for the Australian NGO sector project on the roles and resources of voluntary agencies. The Australian National Association of Mental Health began publishing a newsletter in 1984, a year that saw a national mental health week (30 June–7 July), a national workshop on families in August, and plans for a national forum on the future of mental health services.

Abbott, Director of MHFNZ, attended the 1983 Washington, DC, World Congress where we got to know each other. Afterward, with the establishment of the Baltimore-Washington Secretariat, WFMH became even more closely connected with Oceania with two Board members: Regional Vice President Burrows and Honorary Secretary James who had left academic life to become Director of Mental Health Services for New Zealand. I asked Abbott to represent us at a symposium during the August Congress of Anthropological and Ethnological Sciences in Canada. With its newly strengthened identification with the Federation, the MHFNZ with the sponsorship of WFMH held a reception for long-time mental health volunteer, former U.S. First Lady Rosalynn Carter in Auckland on 16 February 1984.

The representative triad from Oceania was especially interesting because all were able, highly educated, and sophisticated leaders yet with differing points of view. Abbott, the professional executive of MHFNZ, the leading voluntary mental health organization of his country, was most closely connected to the grassroots with a strong concern with patient's rights. He was, almost structurally by virtue of his MHFNZ leadership, in a chronically adversarial position vis-à-vis James. The latter, after the relative tranquillity of academic life, had become the national mental health director and was besieged by the kinds of problems that are endemic in public mental health systems, including criticism from the voluntary sector. Burrows, himself a native of New Zealand who had escaped to the "big world" of Australia, was safely ensconced in a professorship. He continued as the elected leader of his national mental health association as well as our regional vice president. Some years later, when he had accumulated more presidencies, I asked him how he did it. His reply was, "Never volunteer, never refuse, and never resign!"

James participated in the WFMH Board meeting in Baltimore (23–25 May 1984) and spoke at a symposium at the Sheppard Pratt Hospital where it convened. At this meeting he presented the election plan that persisted in basic outline through 1987. MHFNZ, under Abbott's leadership since 1981, saw an intensification of activity. It broadened its purview to include political advocacy and mental health law, studies of television violence, the relation of unemployment to mental health, good practices in mental health, rape, and child abuse prevention. Abbott became a member of the New Zealand Planning Council's "Social Monitoring Group," analyzing and commenting on issues relevant to social development in New Zealand. He was also active in various other issues, including the bicultural nature of New Zealand society (with whites of English descent and Maori), racism, and refugees. James, in his official governmental capacity, participated in the 1985 MHFNZ conference on 5–8 June on "The Future of Mental Health Services in New Zealand," focusing on deinstitutionalization, primary prevention, mental health promotion, and Maori perspectives on mental health matters.

At the 1985 Board meeting in London, Abbott became Oceania vice president, replacing Graham Burrows. Most significantly his bid for the 1989 World Congress to be held in Auckland, New Zealand was approved, contingent upon the confirmation of adequate support facilities. This put the previously peripheral Oceania region at the center of global WFMH concerns.

Abbott's wide ranging social concerns led him in 1986 to foster a collaboration of MHFNZ with the New Zealand Foundation for Peace Studies considering "entertainment violence." At the Board meeting (11–13 June 1986) in Windsor Park, England, he reported on this as well as plans for regional development including a membership drive. His perspective on the geographic and cultural entities in the region, which he conceptualized as "Oceania/South Pacific," foresaw new linkages between the area's indigenous ethnic groups interested in mental health issues. I joined him in viewing the 1989 congress as an opportunity to foster the development of transnational and intercultural mental health initiatives within the region. This fitted my own perspective on a unique mission for WFMH.

At Windsor Park, then President Morgan recognized Abbott's administrative bent and reliability by asking him to organize a meeting of regional vice presidents to produce a job description for the position. This he did with dispatch, and it was published in the newsletter. However, most of the other regional vice presidents, less dedicated and persistent, did not conform to the description or engage in the expected reporting about their regions, which required the description to be republished on several occasions.

In 1986 Oceania's new prominence was reflected in the nomination of Basil James for president-elect by Judge Eduardo Tutaan of the Philippine Mental Health Association. Other candidates for the election during the Cairo World congress assembly (20 October 1987) were Stanislas Flache, M.D., Board member-at-large and WFMH representative to United Nations Geneva, and Isaac Mwendapole, M.S.W., regional vice president for Africa from Lusaka. James lost to Flache who became President while Mwendapole was named honorary secretary. Abbott was continued for a second two-year term as regional vice president, making him the next logical presidential candidate from Oceania.

Oceania Comes of Age

The Mental Health Foundation of New Zealand

With the separation of Oceania from the western Pacific region, the already existing mental health organizations in the area became more visible members of the WFMH family. Among them MHFNZ had, perhaps, the dominant role. In 1987 I refreshed my first-hand acquaintance with the region largely through the support of a Fulbright grant arranged through Abbott and MHFNZ. Our first stop, dictated by the airline schedule, was Sydney, Australia. This permitted additional meetings with John Cawte at the University of New South Wales concerning the mental health of the aborigines. Cawte was also an expert on the psychology and social adaptation of the Pacific Island populations, such as those from the Torres Straits between Australia and New Guinea and more recent immigrants especially from southern Europe. The university apartment where we stayed was, in fact, on Coogee Beach (sometimes spelled Cougee) in a neighborhood heavily populated by Greek and Italian immigrants. He arranged for my attendance at case conferences in an outlying hospital that illustrated some of the problems of Pacific Islanders living in Australia. Later, at his request, I wrote to Australian Prime Minister Robert Hawke in support of his proposal for an "Aboriginal Healing Service" to train aboriginal healers in both traditional and contemporary methods. The healing service was also intended to examine the parameters of aboriginal community dislocation and, especially, the deaths of aboriginal detainees who more often than expected by chance committed suicide while in police custody.

The next stop was in Melbourne to deliver the E. Cunningham Dax Lecture of the Victorian Association for Mental Health in conjunction with the Australian National Association for Mental Health and the University of Melbourne. With long-term WFMH concerns in mind I spoke on "Behavior in New Environments: Migration and Ethnicity," with commentary by the country's outstanding expert on the subject, Jerszy Krupinski, Ph.D., Professor Emeritus of Epidemiology in the University of Melbourne's Department of Psychiatry headed by Graham Burrows.

The final stop in Australia was the 27–28 August 1987, annual meeting of the Australian National Association of Mental Health in Canberra, where I delivered the keynote address, "Mental Health and World Citizenship." Under Burrows' presidency the meeting was held in government headquarters with the presence of the governor general and attended by representatives of member associations from New South Wales, Victoria, Queensland, South Australia, Western Australia, Tasmania, and the Territories. It was an impressive event and the governor general seemed well informed about mental health and illness issues.

Late in the afternoon, after the final session, we discovered that our Canberra hosts had been unable to book a scheduled flight back to Sydney in time for us to make the connection to Auckland on New Zealand's North Island. Instead they had chartered a four-seater, which was waiting for us with its single engine warming up as we drove onto the airstrip. The young pilot gave us a spectacularly scenic trip low over the Snowy Mountains with my wife in the copilot's seat and I looking over their shoulders. It reminded us of earlier flights in South America, especially from the Costa Rican Pacific coast over the mountains to a grassy landing field in San Jose. But we were spared the disconcerting downdrafts generated by the hot Central American mountain jungles and made it smoothly to the Sydney airport-although with little time to spare, taxiing right up alongside of the huge Boeing aircraft ready to depart for Auckland.

Our major goal for this trip was the 1–4 September 1987, annual conference of the MHFNZ in Auckland, which, with approximately one million inhabitants, was the largest urban center in New Zealand, also called the "largest Polynesian city in the world." This outstanding meeting focused on advocacy and consumer issues, the prevention of mental ill health, and the relation of social circumstances and social policy to ill health and disease. Its concerns with the problems of biculturalism and multiculturalism with special reference to the Maori people stimulated some heated debates. The meeting opened with an address by the MHFNZ's patron, the Most Reverend Sir Paul Reeves, the nation's governor general and former Anglican Archbishop (later Chairman of the United Nations' NGO Committee on Indigenous Peoples), who had the added distinction of being a Maori.

The Maori, constituting approximately 12 percent of the population, occupied a range of social statuses. On one hand they consumed the largest proportion of the welfare budget, were disproportionately represented in the criminal record, and were perceived by some of the white population not only as economic burdens but as threats, with their "black power" agenda and motorcycle gangs. On the other hand, many had achieved high positions, and a touch of Maori blood carried a certain social status. One woman psychiatrist with blue eyes and light brown hair introduced herself at the beginning of a public lecture as a Maori woman. The legal battle for half the national budget, based on the 1852 Treaty of Waitangi, was just beginning.

Welcoming and introductory addresses were given by Abbott as well as other local officials, most beginning with a few Maori words of greeting. The opening keynote address by Mason Durie, M.D., a member of the Royal Commission on Social Policy, gave an account of hearings currently being held throughout the country on "Mental Health Through Social Policy," with frequent references to the Maori situation. I delivered a keynote address on "International Developments in Mental Health," emphasizing issues regarding the mental health of minority and indigenous peoples common to various settings. Elsewhere in the conference I spoke on the scientific, historical, and clinical aspects of patient's rights movements in relation to other civil rights movements.

This experience was quite different from the earlier ones in New Zealand, particularly the leisurely, contemplative perspective of the University of Otago in tranquil Dunedin. Basil James, with whom we met on several occasions, was no longer a WFMH Board member and no longer academically focused. He was a political figure under fire (sometimes from Abbott's MHFNZ) in his capacity as national director of mental health services. Unlike the South Island where Maoris were a distantly abstract presence, here they were physical and political realities. We were met at the meeting's opening by a circle of leaders with whom we touched noses in ceremonial greeting. After one leader gave a passionate speech with threatening facial gestures and protruding eyes and tongue, a Maori member of the government who sat next to my wife explained to her that this was a customary way of expressing respect for a "visiting chief."

Perhaps most significant for the future of the Federation was the opportunity to get to know Max Abbott. It became clear that he was ready to work hard for the organizational health of WFMH and that he saw himself as a future president.

The 1989 Auckland World Congress for Mental Health

Only a year later, in early 1988, we had progressed sufficiently for the newsletter to carry notices of a World Congress for Mental Health to be held in Auckland on 21–25 August 1989, sponsored by the MHFNZ under the organizing leadership of Executive Director Abbott, our WFMH regional vice president. The issues to be emphasized included the mental health of indigenous peoples, minorities, and refugees; patient's rights; prevention; consumer rights; and advocacy. Attention was to be paid to mental health issues throughout the Pacific, with special reference to Oceania.

In August 1989 my wife and I arrived in Auckland via Sydney and Melbourne. In Sydney we visited again with John Cawte. We were in Melbourne at the invitation of psychiatrist Lorraine Dennerstein, M.D., Director of the Key Centre for Women's Health in Society, under whose auspices I was scheduled to speak and conduct a seminar on ethical issues in artificial reproduction. These activities sponsored by UNESCO and the International Social Science Council are described in Chapter 8. The main organizational consequence was Dennerstein's agreement to have her organization designated a WFMH Collaborating Center. The formalities took some time, but this move was accepted by the Board at its 1991 meeting in Mexico.

The 1989 WFMH World Congress for Mental Health was held at the University of Auckland, cosponsored by WHO, the International Council of Psychologists, the International Social Science Council, the International Academy of Law and Mental Health, and the university's School of Medicine. Its inclusive theme was, "Mental Health-Everyone's Concern." Abbott's personal hand could be seen in almost every aspect. Eight major tracks were laid out in great detail so they could be followed throughout the congress. This was excellent for in-depth immersion in an issue but made it difficult for those who wished to sample the broad range of discussions. The major themes began with "global issues." These included the nuclear threat, a matter of great concern to New Zealanders, conflict resolution and peace, environmental change and hazards, population growth, demographic and rapid social change, poverty and unemployment. Other major themes, with equally detailed subthemes, included new public health, mental health services and alternatives, drug dependence and disorders of impulse control, cross-cultural and minority issues, and victimology and trauma studies.

Maori citizens of New Zealand, including Governor General Reeves, were prominent contributors to the event that opened and closed with Maori rituals. The Honorable Helen Clark, Minister of Health and Deputy Prime Minister, delivered the opening address. Norman Sartorius, M.D., Director of WHO's Division of Mental Health, and Herbert Pardes, M.D., who had been a long time director of the U.S. National Institute of Mental Health (NIMH), were the opening keynote speakers. Several special lectures were delivered by global dignitaries including Dr. Kinhide Mushakoji, Rector of the United Nations University in Tokyo who spoke on "Mental Health as a Unifying Concept."

The congress attracted approximately 1000 persons, almost half of whom were non-New Zealanders coming from 44 different countries. The largest "foreign" contingent was from Australia and the next largest from Japan. Morning and afternoon tea breaks included in the registration fee and reasonably priced lunches in the University of Auckland gymnasium facilitated informal exchanges among the participants. A consequence of the heavy attendance of consumers or "users" of mental health services-with those from the United States and the U.S. Pacific Trust Territories supported by the NIMH-was a proposal to form a new users organization affiliated with WFMH (see Chapter 7).

Mary O'Hagan, a patient activist and employee of MHFNZ who was a member of the congress organizing committee, played a leading role in organizing and coordinating the consumer sections throughout the congress.

The event saw the consolidation of a new center of Federation power in Oceania. The assembly of voting members elected Max Abbott, nominated both by Hilda Robbins and the MHFNZ, as president-elect to take office in 1991. The candidate for vice president for the Oceania region, also nominated by MHFNZ, was also elected. He was a friend of Abbott's, Trevor Elligett, Chief Executive of the Psychiatric Rehabilitation Association of Sydney, former National Director of the Australian Hospital Association, and former president of several societies of association executives. As founder and National Convenor of the National Association of Psychiatric Rehabilitation and Support Services he had led a successful campaign to have national disability legislation amended to include psychiatric disability. The WFMH agenda also began to have a noticeable effect on the regional associations. Thus a major theme for the Australian National Association of Mental Health congress in Tasmania, addressed among others by former Regional Vice President James, was human rights issues for the mentally ill.

In New Zealand national and local seminars held with WFMH cosponsorship concerned the changes necessary to move the mental health system toward community-based services. Among the prominent issues were refugee mental health needs and services. With the upsurge in WFMH activity, Abbott's more central position in the organization may have been one of the factors influencing his being awarded a 1990 national 150th anniversary commemoration medal for service to the New Zealand community. When he moved to the WFMH presidency on 21 August 1991, during the Mexico congress he was the youngest person to have occupied that post. At the same time he left the MHFNZ to become dean of the faculty of Health Studies at the Auckland Institute of Technology, effectively changing his professional role from that of an advocate for patients and minorities to an academic administrator.

Trevor Elligett, who was elected for a second term as regional vice president, marked the occasion by announcing a WFMH regional conference (billed as a Pacific rather than an Oceania meeting) for spring 1992. It took place in Sydney on 12–15 April with the official title, "Mental Health on the Pacific Rim." Emphasis was laid on the health of indigenous peoples of the region, sparking some heated remarks by advocates of both the Australian aborigine and the Maori. In addition discussions dealt with the more usual topics of mental health services, human rights, the family, and the future. At the instigation of local members the congress passed a resolution expressing concern at the existence of a detention center in a remote section of Northwestern Australia used principally for people of Indochinese background seeking asylum as refugees. The center's isolation, the lengthy process of determination, and the unavailability of counseling for torture and trauma victims were at variance with the United Nations conventions under which Australia had signatory responsibilities. President Abbott informed the prime minister of this resolution in a 6 May 1992, letter urging the development of humane approaches to asylum seekers.

From Sydney my wife and I proceeded to Townsville in far North Queensland where Basil James, who had left New Zealand to become Director of Mental Health for Northern Queensland and a Professor at James Cook University, had invited me to be a consultant and visiting lecturer. Townsville had been the staging area for the Battle of the Coral Sea, a turning point in the Allied struggle against the Japanese early in World War II. It was intensely tropical with land covered by jungle and seas containing jellyfish capable of inducing cardiac arrest. We visited on Magnetic Island, which had disoriented the compass of Cook's ship during his exploration of the area. Although the unfamiliar surroundings threatened to divert attention from the work, the quality of the university was high; the professionals whom we met were knowledgeable; and informed concern about the indigenous inhabitants-including Pacific Islanders as well as aborigine-was prominent. Basil and his wife Gerri—a geriatric nursing specialist—were well-integrated, highly useful members of the community, but aware of the distance from the rest of their family on the temperate South Island of New Zealand.

After the 1992 Board meeting, the idea of an Oceania regional council for WFMH began to emerge but was not acted upon. Trevor Elligett visited Auckland on 11 October 1992, to discuss the matter with immediate Past President Abbott, Board member-at-large psychiatrist Peter McGeorge, M.D., and psychologist Dr. Barbara Disley, who had succeeded Abbott as director of MHFNZ. An ad hoc body was formed but acted mainly as a nominating committee for regional vice presidents at the biennial voting assemblies.

Despite the presence of WFMH officers, most Federation related activity in the region came from its member organizations and visitors from abroad. Thus, Richard Mollica, M.D., chair of our committee on refugees, and director of our collaborating center at Harvard, spent November and December 1994 as a Fulbright professor working with Derek Silove, M.D., of Sydney. Silove was the consultant to our collaborating center there offering services to torture and trauma victims. Mollica had spent some weeks in 1988 working with the MHFNZ to promote mental health services for refugees resident in New Zealand and to train clinicians to work with refugees and victims of trauma in general. Similarly, there was intermittent WFMH activity in relation to our collaborating center in Melbourne (see Chapter 13).

In 1995 and 1996 a WFMH committee for New Zealand met on several occasions and established contact with colleagues in Australia. The possibility of a regional council was again discussed. The core group included Abbott, WFMH Board member-at-large Mary O'Hagan, Chris Jane, Jim Crowe, President of the New Zealand branch of the World Schizophrenia Fellowship, and Dr. Barbara Disley (before her appointment as Mental Health Commissioner for New Zealand). Contact was also maintained with Richard Redom in Australia. A major annual event was the Mental Health Services Conference of Australia and New Zealand held in Brisbane on 18–20 September 1996. The WFMH profile was also raised by the group's support of other conferences, mainly of professionals. Despite these efforts, though, no lasting structure was developed, nor was meaningful contact established between the mental health societies and such key WFMH collaborators in Australia as Dennerstein and Cawte. Even though Abbott himself was now an academic administrator, the gulf between research and teaching oriented professionals and service and advocacy oriented voluntary organizations seemed to persist.

As in the days of Basil James, the state of the national mental health services in New Zealand continued to be controversial. After a long legal and professional inquiry, Barbara Disley was appointed commissioner with powers to monitor and evaluate services and expenditures. In pursuit of this aim a conference on education, training, and supervision of mental health workers, organized by McGeorge and Abbott, was scheduled under WFMH Oceania auspices for May 1997. A major landmark scheduled for Sydney in September 1997 was the Mental Health Services Conference of Australia and New Zealand. This conference, established in 1991, has grown rapidly in size and influence since its inception. Like the WFMH congresses it has attracted a diverse range of people from consumers to professional clinicians, managers, and researchers.

The Pacific Islands

Although the WFMH Oceania region nominally included a range of Pacific Islands, there was been little formal recognition of them. One exception was a Honolulu conference at the University of Hawaii on mental health in the Pacific sponsored from 12–15 August 1985, by the NIMH Minority Affairs Branch under James Ralph, M.D. Social scientists, health planners, and clinicians, many from the islands, examined problems in policy making, personnel training, and mental health services delivery for citizens of the U.S. Pacific states and territories. I was invited by Ralph with whom I shared concerns about minority rights as a WFMH representative and, along with Senator Daniel Inouye of Hawaii, addressed the opening plenary.

Another exception was the occasional NIMH sponsorship, worked out by Dick Hunter with Ed Kelty, Ph.D., of NIMH, of some consumers from the islands to WFMH world congresses in the late 1980s. In 1995 Dr. Annette Zimmern of the Department of Health Services of the Federated States of Micronesia wrote about the situation there (WFMH, 1996.)

From his Auckland base in 1996 Peter McGeorge began the process of contacting the Pacific Islands to discuss their interest in mental health issues and in WFMH. A Pacific studies expert in New Zealand considered Oceania to include the Polynesian islands such as the Cook Islands, Tonga, and Tahiti to the northeast, Papua New Guinea and Micronesia to the north, with Fiji sitting geographically, culturally, and ethnically between Melanesia and Polynesia. In January 1997 McGeorge visited the Undersecretary of Health for the Cook Islands group. Support groups and advocacy for people experiencing domestic violence and substance abuse had been established there. But general services, even in Fiji, were rudimentary.

NORTH AMERICA

In the Beginning

Geography

As noted in Chapter 9, the WHO and the PanAmerican Sanitary Organization were integrated on 24 May 1949, with the latter becoming the PanAmerican Health Organization of WHO (PAHO/WHO). In 1950 it was given stewardship of the "Americas" as a single unit. As the twentieth century drew to a close WHO still alloted responsibility for the health of populations in this massive, socioculturally and geographically diverse area to PAHO, considered its hemispheric branch. Because its headquarters was in Washington, DC, the PAHO staff had easy access to U.S. colleagues. Since 1962 I worked with its mental health advisors, Jorge Velasco Alzaga, M.D., of Mexico, Rene Gonzalez, M.D., of Costa Rica, and Itzhak Levav, M.D., of Argentina and Israel, all on the basis of mutual trust and friendship. But with a small staff, including one "mental health advisor for the Americas," PAHO attention was almost exclusively focused on the Latin American and Caribbean regions.

WFMH, after what its boards have considered more realistic from the geopolitical, social, and cultural standpoints, has divided the Americas into smaller units. At first, as noted in Chapter 9, North and Central America were lumped together. In 1951, influenced by the site of its congress in Mexico and the election of Alfonso Millan as president, Central America and several island nations were reclassified as the "Caribbean region" of WFMH. This designation persisted until the 1974 resignation of President Michael Beaubrun of Trinidad and Jamaica (1972–1974). Since then the Americas south of the United States have been subject to continued reclassifications, stimulated largely by the wishes of regional WFMH leaders. The area classified as North America, stable since 1951, was defined in approximately 1978 to include Bermuda as well as the United States and Canada. Some remaining uncertainty referred to politically related, but socioculturally and geographically differing, entities such as Puerto Rico and Hawaii. The North American players in WFMH history have been largely voluntary mental health and professional associations and individuals in the United States and Canada.

Early North American Involvement, 1908–1975

Chapter 1 briefly reviews the story of Connecticut's Clifford Beers and his Canadian colleague, physician Clarence Hinckley in founding the International Committee for Mental Hygiene. Chapter 2 describes the Federation's origins in the ideas immediately after World War II of such North American visionaries as psychiatrists Harry Stack Sullivan of the United States and Brock Chisholm of Canada and the 1946 recruitment by Britain's Jack Rees of other U.S. physicians such as George Stevenson and Frank Fremont-Smith. It also describes the International Preparatory Commission at Roffey Park and the crucial participation of such Americans as anthropologist Margaret Mead and Canadian, social scientist Otto Klineberg, then with UNESCO's Paris based project on the reduction of international tensions.

Chapter 3, on the Rees era, and Chapter 4, on the Geneva Secretariat, describe the New York based funding arrangements for the Federation of that era. Chapter 9 describes the New York roots, particularly in the work of psychiatrist/psychoanalyst Bertram Schaffner, of much of the Federation's initial involvement in the Caribbean. During the nearly quarter century from 1948 to 1972 programmatic and financial support from North America were essential to WFMH's growth and survival.

The first North American to become WFMH president was Canadian psychologist Dr. William Line, Professor at the University of Toronto who served for 1950-1951. His view of mental health, socially rather than clinically oriented, was expressed as "a responsibility and a challenge to every citizen of the world" demanding a "progressive social policy…[and] a deep sense of history." The key disciplines in his view were social, and looking back over his presidency he noted, "during the past year…the Federation has begun to take seriously the importance of social science to the movement itself" (WFMH, 1951b, pp.7–8).

The first U.S. Federation president was Frank Fremont-Smith, M.D., elected for the 1954–1955 term. He had been responsible, as the New York Macy Foundation's Medical Director, for the generous grants that enabled the initial organization of the new WFMH. Rees, concerned from the beginning about organizational financing, was sensitive to Fremont-Smith's contributions and the essential role of the United States behind-the-scenes leadership in general. He wrote, "It may not be realized that our colleagues from the United States who have provided more than their share of support, both in ideas and finance for the Federation during the past six years, have very modestly insisted that the Presidency should not in its rotation go to anyone from their country, though the matter has been raised on several occasions previously" (WFMH 1954, p.12)

After Fremont-Smith, subsequent U.S. presidents in the Rees era made no effort to interfere with the administrative status quo, despite the continuing financial and programmatic leadership of North Americans. The Secretariat and most administrative meetings remained tied to the United Kingdom and Europe. The brief location of the Secretariat in Jamaica, from 1972 to 1974, was in retrospect a transition to the first North American Secretariat located in Vancouver under the leadership of President Tsung-yi Lin (1974–1979). The story of this transition is told in Chapter 5.

It was in relation to the Jamaica Secretariat that I first developed some sense of the Federation: its achievements, ambitions, and chronic funding difficulties. Morris Carstairs had appointed me a member of the Executive Board in 1969 after an invitation so casual that I had forgotten it. It came as a surprise, therefore, when Michael Beaubrun asked me in 1972 to join his administrative committee for WFMH. However, because I was curious, was informed that I was already a Board member, and was already on the scene as a visiting professor in his department at the University of the West Indies, I agreed. The other two North Americans were Tsung-yi Lin and the Treasurer Sol Steinwurtzel of New York, a genial banker with an interest in mental health.

1975–1983

Vancouver, 1975–1983

After Beaubrun's resignation as WFMH president in mid-1974, and his move to Trinidad, the Secretariat remained at the University of the West Indies for the balance of the year. As described in Chapter 5 it moved to Lin's office at the University of British Columbia at the beginning of 1975. The establishment and evolution of the Vancouver Secretariats, and the gradual shift of their functions to my University of Maryland office in Baltimore for the two years of my WFMH presidency beginning in 1981, are also recounted in Chapter 5. So is the story of establishing a definitive Baltimore-Washington Secretariat in 1983.

The first Vancouver Secretariat was Lin's departmental office at the University of British Columbia in 1975. As funds became available, especially after the 1977 World Congress, and the Federation's activities expanded, the responsibility for its operation became heavier, and Roberta Beiser who managed it was designated executive director. With the 1979–1981 presidency of Gowan Guest its support by the University of British Columbia diminished, and the cost of maintaining it led Guest to recommend its immediate closure in his unexpected and hurried 1982 telephone resignation from the Board and from the Canadian Corporation, i.e. the incorporated body of WFMH (described in Chapter 5). In this administratively disturbed period, though, WFMH continued to regain its momentum and capacity lost during 1979-1981. Among other positive events, the WFMH vice president for North America received a significant scholarly honor. He was University of British Columbia Professor Morton Beiser, M.D., who was named National Scholar by Canada's National Health Research Directorate.

The Vancouver Secretariat was finally closed in September 1983. This came after many months of gradual change as plans were made to move the Secretariat to a new location "on the Eastern Sea board of the United States." The final step was the August 1983 vote by the Washington, DC post-congress Board chaired by my successor as president, Dr. Estafania Aldaba-Lim of Manila, to reestablish the Secretariat in new quarters, mine as Secretary General in Baltimore and Dick Hunter's as Deputy Secretary General, in Alexandria, Virginia. The files went to Alexandria. Dick leased storage space for the massive boxes of papers, and most have remained in storage, unopened.

Baltimore-Washington, 1981–1983

During this period Baltimore (and Alexandria, Virginia) became hotbeds of Federation activity with astonishing rapidity. Planning for the 1983 World Congress could not be delayed. I also took advantage of the opportunity to use WFMH cosponsorship of university activities to advertise its existence and mission. Two major lectures within the University of Maryland Institute of Psychiatry and Human Behavior were especially appropriate for Federation sponsorship. On 11 September 1981, Helen Caldicott, M.D., of Australia, founder of Physicians for Social Responsibility, spoke on the medical consequences of nuclear war. On 20 November Dr. Yael Danieli of New York, formerly of Israel, spoke on the problems of psychotherapists working with survivors of the Holocaust and their families.

During the fall of 1981 a flurry of other high profile activities advertised our existence and mission. Among them were a U.S. National Mental Health Association reception at the home of recent World Bank President Robert MacNamara; an award ceremony for public service to former governor and ambassador Averell Harriman along with former President Jimmy Carter, Rosalynn Carter, and former United Nations Ambassador Andrew Young; a Washington reception, attracting the government, university, and voluntary mental health community (which I organized in honor of President-elect Aldaba Lim for the International Affairs Committee of the American Psychological Association); a talk at the opening plenary of the Canadian Psychiatric Association meeting in Winnipeg; and meetings in Toronto with officers of the Canadian Mental Health Association. We also arranged a symposium for the spring 1982 meeting of the American Psychiatric Association.

1983 Washington, DC, World Congress for Mental Health

The discussion at the 1981 Boardmeeting in Manila preceding the decision to hold this congress is noted in Chapter 5. Dick Hunter's and my concerns about financing are described in Chapter 6. I finally came up with a theme that, while cumbersome, expressed my concerns at the time: "Personal and Social Responsibility in the Search for Mental Health: Collaboration between Volunteers, Professionals and Governments in the Formation of Mental Health Policy and the Delivery of Services." The congress was intended to celebrate the 75th anniversary of the world mental health movement begun in 1908 with the publication of Clifford Beers' book, *A Mind that Found Itself* (Beers, 1908). By December 1981, the Board of the U.S. National Mental Health Association, after several preliminary meetings and much thought, had agreed to be the local host organization. Their hesitation reflected concern about congress funding, and they required assurances that they would have no financial obligation. Important was their official designation of Dick Hunter, already operating informally in the role, as head of the congress operations committee. The American Psychiatric Association and American Psychological Association had already given me agreements of close support, and I had begun negotiations to involve the American associations of anthropology, social work, sociology, and nursing. The interest in nursing in particular yielded unexpected results. Owing to the efforts of Grace Roessler of the United States, nurses met in an international convocation during the congress for the first time in our history. The gathering chaired by Roessler explored the potential role of nursing within the Federation and in mental health work in their respective countries. A nurses convocation was planned for every future WFMH World Congress. Unfortunately, this plan, supported by the International Council of Nurse,s did not materialize.

WFMH, 1983–1997

Overview

This period was the era of the Baltimore-Washington Secretariat from the time of its September-October 1983 relocation from Vancouver to the spring of 1997. It has been detailed in Chapter 5. Once the August 1983 Washington World Congress was behind us, Dick Hunter and

I began to think about building a regional organization for North America. We were too busy establishing the newly transplanted Secretariat to be personally involved, but we were both concerned. However, although this concern was present and sometimes voiced over the next 14 years, none of the North American vice presidents or North Americans in other Board positions were sufficiently motivated to build a committee for WFMH in the United States, Canada, or Bermuda. Nor, despite the efforts of Vice President Beverly Long (1987–1991), did an active regional council develop. Under these circumstances the global Federation did not become a significant or visible influence on mental health developments in the region. In some ways this is not surprising. Within their own countries, each larger than Western Europe, the U.S. and Canadian mental health associations, both voting members of WFMH, have been major influences on mental health legislation and to a lesser degree practices. They have served the unifying function in their countries that the European Regional Council has attempted in Europe. In addition national professional organizations, especially the American Psychiatric and Psychological Associations and their Canadian counterparts have acted increasingly as mental health promoting organizations spanning the continent.

The same is true for other mental health professional organizations such as those for social workers and nurses and for research oriented organizations of patient's families such as the National Alliance for the Mentally Ill. North American leaders of WFMH emerging from these organizations, primarily the National Mental Health Association, have not felt the need for an overarching regional council. There have been no moves toward developing a common U.S. and Canadian agenda, and the relationships between U.S. and Canadian organizations, while amicable, have not led to significant collaboration. In fact, as noted earlier, the Canadian Mental Health Association led by George Rohn, a WFMH Board member, had refused (apparently because it feared financial responsibility) to become a sponsor of the 1977 World Congress for Mental Health in Vancouver.

Despite the lack of organizational development, individual officers resident in the United States and members of the Secretariat have carried the WFMH agenda and philosophy into their varied professional and volunteer activities in both the United States and Canada.

Two other elements have also been significant regional influences. One is the presence of United Nations headquarters in New York. The WFMH representatives to United Nations New York have been U.S. citizens (since the mid-1980s primarily psychologists), and their presence has constituted a visible WFMH presence in the region as well as in the United Nations. The work of WFMH in relation to the United Nations, including that carried on in New York, is described in Chapter 8.

The other force sustaining some Federation visibility in the region has been the Secretariat's location in the Baltimore-Washington area, preceded by the placement of my office in Baltimore from 1981–1983. With the Secretariat in place, an era of WFMH administrative meetings in the United States began. They were either at Sheppard Pratt Hospital in Baltimore, which supported my offices after my final retirement from the university in 1986, or at the National Mental Health Association headquarters in Alexandria, Virginia, where Dick's office was located. An early meeting, accompanied by a symposium on the prevention of mental illness and alternatives to hospitalization, was at Sheppard Pratt on 23–25 May 1984, where I had already relocated my *Journal of Nervous and Mental Disease* offices from the university. At this meeting the Board adopted the new by-laws and articles of incorporation that allowed WFMH to operate as a U.S. corporation.

1984 was also the first year in which the North American region formed a regional committee. Under Vice President Hilda Robbins this was a North American Committee on Prevention chaired by former National Mental Health Association President Beverly Long.

Our proximity to the nation's capital also made it possible for WFMH to become known to many government figures from the United States and other countries (stationed temporarily in Washington, DC). as well as headquarters offices of most U.S. professional associations. As described in Chapter 6, awareness in the Washington area was also stimulated by WFMH annual fund raising receptions at various embassies, started at Dick Hunter's initiative in 1986. These have been significant ways of bringing the Federation to the attention of the U.S. political and mental health community.

WFMH Influence through Involvement with North American Organizations

As indicated earlier the American Psychiatric and Psychological Associations had not been part of the WFMH network before 1981. My term as WFMH president gave me the opportunity to recruit the psychiatric association, of which I was a life fellow, into Federation membership. This was accomplished through the goodwill of its medical director, Melvin Sabshin, M.D., as well as that of a series of friends who were or had been its presidents, beginning with Bob Gibson. Unfortunately, with the passage of time and the increasingly biological orientation of psychiatry, as well my own diminishing participation in the association's affairs, the interaction with organized American psychiatry has lessened. Although our relations with organized American psychology remain friendly, and psychologists are more interested in Federation agenda items than psychiatrists, here too our connection is less close and personal than it was for some years beginning in 1981. My status as personal liaison from the American Psychoanalytic Association and the International Psychoanalytic Association, beginning in 1979, was reaffirmed several times between 1981 and 1997.

The National Mental Health Association was outstanding in its sponsorship of projects compatible with the aims of WFMH. In 1984 it developed a commission on the prevention of mental and emotional disability chaired by WFMH Board member Beverly Long with the participation of North American Regional Vice President Hilda Robbins. On 20 June 1986, Robbins presented a statement on catastrophic insurance for mental illness to the U.S. Department of Health and Human Services, calling for parity in the treatment of all illness, including mental illness. In her WFMH capacity she also participated in the 12–15 November 1986, national conference of the Canadian National Mental Health Association.

In 1986 my appointment to the international advisory Board of our member organization the Simon Bolivar Foundation of the University of Illinois, based on my earlier work in Latin America, allowed me to introduce WFMH to the foundation. We cosponsored its meeting on the mental health of Hispanic Americans on 15–17 May 1987. WFMH affiliated speakers, in addition to myself, included former Executive Board member Professor Carlos Leon, M.D., of Cali, Colombia, and Federation member Jose Arana, M.D., of Lima (Peru) and Baltimore, one of my former residents.

Another opportunity to bring the WFMH perspective to work in the United States came with my participation beginning in 1987 in the NIMH committee on AIDS research centers, for which I chaired site visits to the University of California and Columbia University.

The Federation's 40th anniversary year, 1988, was marked by several events in the region. On 16–18 February 1988, our collaborating center on prevention at Johns Hopkins University, headed by Professor Sheppard Kellam, M.D., an old friend whose unit I had recruited as our first WFMH collaborating center in 1986, was inaugurated as a WHO collaborating center for the study of epidemiology and the prevention of mental illness and addictions. That event brought many WFMH friends from WHO to Baltimore, including former Board member Gaston Harnois, M.D., Director General of the Douglas Hospital Centre in Montreal, which was also a WHO center.

In 1988 WFMH began to cosponsor the annual scientific symposia of the National Mental Health Association. In that year the National Mental Health Association formed a coalition of NGOs from the mental health, health, education, and business communities, chaired by WFMH

Regional Vice President Beverly Long to provide visibility to the prevention field and develop consensus for recommendations to policy makers and agencies.

On 10 May 1988, Gaston Harnois organized a commemorative celebration of the 40th anniversaries of both WFMH and WHO at the Douglas Hospital, which he headed during the meeting of the American Psychiatric Association in Montreal. I spoke on behalf of WFMH to an audience that included representatives of many national and international NGOs as well as members of the Canadian and Quebec governments and United Nations agencies. The next day I attended the gathering when Bill Beaty, some of whose story is recounted in Chapter 4, was honored by members of the American Academy of Child and Adolescent Psychiatry for his contributions to their field in his role as Executive Director of the Ittleson Foundation of New York City (which was a financial supporter of WFMH in its early days). In 1988 I also joined the Board of our new member association-the Institute for Victims of Violence, headed by psychologist Dr. Leila Dane who, after presenting a symposium at the 1987 WFMH congress in Cairo, had rapidly initiated collaborative work with Dr. Ahmed El Azayem and other WFMH members in the eastern Mediterranean.

The education of mental health and health care workers has always been among our concerns. Thus Dick Hunter and I were glad to accept an invitation from the Carrier Foundation for a 26 January 1989, meeting to learn about a proposed behavioral science and television series for worldwide distribution to health care workers. Convened by WHO and the World Psychiatric Association this meeting brought together representatives from a significant number of professional groups in the United States.

In 1989 the American Psychological Association reconstituted its Committee on International Relations and appointed Dr. Henry David, Chairman of the WFMH Committee on Responsible Parenthood, whose earlier work with WFMH is recounted in Chapter 4, to be the official liaison to WFMH. At its 7–8 April meeting David reported on a range of WFMH activities. The committee voted to take a positive position on the WFMH 1988 Declaration of Luxor on Human Rights and Mental Health as modified and accepted by the Board in Auckland in 1989 and its Board of Directors later endorsed it.

In 1986 I had begun a three-year term as a member of the National Advisory Council of our member organization, the Hogg Foundation for Mental Health of the University of Texas. Professor Wayne Holtzman, its president, was a longtime personal friend and a friend of the Federation. At its meeting on 2–4 February 1989, the council began preliminary planning for a North American regional meeting on the mental health of refugees and migrants that Beverly Long had suggested to Holtzman after we had had some informal conversations. After the council adjourned our steering committee for the regional meeting met, chaired jointly by Holtzman and Long. A key Federation addition was Richard Mollica, M.D., chair of the WFMH committee on the mental health of refugees and other migrants. Other influential participants were Leonel Castillo, former Commissioner of the Immigration and Naturalization Service under President Jimmy Carter, and Dr. Thomas Bornemann of the section on refugee mental health programs of NIMH.

A special WFMH opportunity for international and United Nations advocacy took place in Canada on 10–13 October 1989. In her capacity as vice president for the region, Long represented us at the "European and North American Conference on Urban Safety and Crime Prevention" in Montreal. Sponsored by mayors from the United States, Canada, and the countries of Western Europe, it focused on the need for community action in "social prevention." A key conference organizer was Professor Irvin Waller, a member of the WFMH Committee on the Mental Health of Victims of Violence who had also conducted a seminar on crime prevention at the August 1989 WFMH congress in New Zealand. The recommendations from that conference, which was attended by more than 900 representatives from more than 20 countries, went to federal and local levels of governments as well as to the 1990 United Nations congress on crime.

Dr. Yael Danieli, our senior representative to United Nations New York, presided over the annual meeting of the Society for Traumatic Stress Studies on 27–30 October 1989 in San

Francisco. She created a special significance for WFMH by arranging an opening ceremony in Union Square commemorating victim survivors "of all nations, all cultures, all groups and all faiths." This was in the tradition of WFMH's founding document, "Mental Health and World Citizenship." Her Association, through a task force chaired by John H. Krystal, M.D., of the Yale Department of Psychiatry, also produced a report on curriculum, education and training for workers with victims of violence and collective abuse. It was received by representatives of different professions and groups. I received it for WFMH, noting its potential as the basis of a cross-culturally useful training program for health workers in the developing world. Our WFMH representative to Unicef, Nancy Dubrow, M.Ed. (who had not yet finished her Ph.D.), chaired a symposium on "Children Exposed to Chronic Violence." Other WFMH participants included Maurice Eisenbruch, M.D., of Melbourne, then a member of our committee on the mental health of southeast Asian refugees. I spoke on the prevention of homicide through gun control. Federico Puente, M.D., then one of our Board members-at-large, was also present, distributing information about the forthcoming 1991 WFMH congress in Mexico.

In 1990 Regional Vice President Long, as chair of the National Mental Health Association's National Prevention Coalition, continued to foster the WFMH concern with prevention. She and President-elect Max Abbott arranged for WFMH to collaborate with the Vermont Conference on Primary Prevention, Inc., a nonprofit educational foundation, and cosponsor an international conference in Burlington, Vermont, on the range of issues associated with prevention (25 June-1 July 1990). These included family planning, parenting, prenatal and perinatal nutrition, health care, education, reduction of economic and social distress, sexism, racism, delinquency, AIDS, and drug abuse.

Long also activated a new relationship with our Johns Hopkins Collaborating Center on Prevention, which had not become fully involved with us since its 1986 affiliation. She and the center's director, Sheppard Kellam, M.D., were panelists at the National Institutes of Mental Health Prevention Research Conference on 19 May 1993. This stream of activity will be discussed in Part III.

Toward a North American Council for WFMH

The refugee meeting organized by the Hogg Foundation with our collaboration-described in Part III-was held in Houston, Texas, 22–25 March 1990, with approximately 240 registrants, mostly mental health workers and members of the U.S. and Canadian refugee communities. Regional Vice President Long took advantage of the opportunity to invite representatives of 22 WFMH voting member organizations to convene during the meeting on 24 March with the aim of founding a North American council of WFMH. The handful who appeared included representatives of the Canadian and U.S. National Mental Health Associations, the American and Canadian Psychological Associations, and the American Psychiatric and Orthopsychiatric Associations. I represented the American Psychoanalytic Association. Despite inadequate representation there was general enthusiasm for a council, and, in time, after polling the North American voting membership, a council was declared formed. It drew a planning group from the Houston meeting to form a regional committee on the mental health of refugees and immigrants. This group, identified as a North American regional committee, met occasionally until 1992 with outside funding. However, the lack of continued funding and a clear mission led to the project's evaporation.

Long decided to hold a first annual meeting of the infant council in conjunction with the annual meeting of the American Orthopsychiatric Association in Toronto on 23–26 March 1991, where I was already scheduled to speak as part of a panel on violent behavior. Each of the 27 advocacy, professional, and consumer WFMH member organizations (with national or international scope) was invited to designate a voting representative to serve as a liaison with the

Federation. The response was minimal, and those who attended confronted the fact that both the United States and Canada had continent-spanning mental health associations that made the organizational challenge much different from that in Europe or other multinational regions. The feeling was that programmatic emphasis should be on the development of mutual agendas that the existing associations could promote.

A second annual meeting of the North American council, its final one, was convened by Long on 18 August 1992, during the Centennial Convention of the American Psychological Association. Mary Oordt, a former Canadian Mental Health Association President who was Long's successor as WFMH regional vice president, organized a significant program comparing financing and related mental health program issues in Canada and the United States. Unfortunately, there was no systematic organizational follow-up, and the council did not become established as a viable entity.

In 1997 the North American regional vice president was L. Patt Franciosi, former president of the U.S. National Mental Health Association and former chair of the U.S. National Prevention Coalition. She was elected during the 1995 World Congress in Dublin. Competent and experienced, she was doubtful about the suitability of the regional council model for North America but discussed future possibilities with the Canadian Mental Health Association and U.S. National Mental Health Association leadership.

Chapter 11

WFMH in Europe and Its Regional Council

1948–1981

The story of the European Regional Council of WFMH (ERC/WFMH)parallels in many respects the political development of the European Community. The story begins with more than a half century of inconclusive attempts at cooperation among mental health related organizations interrupted by world war. The late 1970s and early 1980s saw more systematic efforts at increased communication and unified action that were at first difficult and then became increasingly successful. Finally, in the late 1980s and with a rush in the 1990s, an ERC emerged with a program of action and an efficiently organized bureaucracy. During this evolution a certain transformation had occurred. Its agenda was no longer the broad, philosophical one of preserving world peace and promoting good human relations, but was focused on the provision of services for mentally ill and emotionally distressed persons and protecting their rights. This reflected a shift in the Board membership from professors and investigators to include more citizen volunteers, activists, and mental health association staff members.

In Retrospect: the London Congress and the New WFMH

The roots of ERC/WFMH in the European League for Mental Hygiene (ELMH) have been described in Chapters 2 and 9. It was ELMH that proposed a Third International Congress of Mental Hygiene to succeed the two earlier congresses that had been held under the auspices of the International Committee for Mental Hygiene (ICMH) in the United States in 1930 and in France in 1937. The idea was to resume the contacts among mental health related groups, both lay-voluntary and professional, in different countries that had been interrupted by World War II. The date for the proposed congress was tentatively set for the summer of 1948. The National Association for Mental Health of England and Wales agreed to the League's request to organize it. The distinguished psychiatric consultant to the British Ministry of War, Dr. John R. Rees, was nominated to be chairman, and the ELMH then obtained his consent to assume that responsibility (Morgan, 1996b).

As indicated in Chapter 2 the idea of a new nongovernmental organization (NGO) to succeed the International Committee for Mental Hygiene arose independently, although within the context of preparations for the London Congress. Rees had gone to New York in 1946 to search for collaborators immediately after accepting responsibility for the congress. The idea arose during his conversations with a small group of longtime friends in the New York office of George S. Stevenson, M.D., Medical Director of the U.S. Committee for Mental Hygiene. It came from George Brock Chisholm, M.D., the Canadian idealist and visionary who was just beginning to create the new arm of the intergovernmental United Nations, the World Health Organization (WHO). By 1947 the articles of association for the new WFMH had been circulated, and in August 1948, during the London Congress, it was officially founded.

Although significant leadership and funding for the new WFMH came from the United States, European activities and concerns were dominant in its early years. This reflected in part the location of its headquarters in London and Geneva from the time of its founding in 1948 until the final closing of the Geneva Secretariat at the end of 1967. The organizational work of this era is described in Chapters 3–6.

After the closing of the Geneva Secretariat the WFMH headquarters or Secretariat was peripatetic, residing in the offices of its now "working" presidents. These were all university professors of psychiatry: George Morrison Carstairs, M.D., in Edinburgh from 1968 to 1972; Michael Beaubrun, M.D., in Kingston, Jamaica, from 1972 to 1974; and Tsung-yi Lin, M.D., in Vancouver, British Columbia, Canada, from 1974 to 1979.

Keeping the Federation Alive in Europe

Carstairs assumed the WFMH presidency in November 1967 and retained the post through 1971 (with Beaubrun assuming responsibilities and moving the Secretariat to Jamaica at the beginning of 1972). Faced at the outset with a massive lack of funding, deficits, and the loss of the central Geneva Secretariat, he had to reestablish the Federation's financial viability. His ultimately successful struggle to manage these difficulties is described in Chapter 5.

Next was the need to set up a new WFMH headquarters in his Department of Psychiatry at Edinburgh University. The new Edinburgh Secretariat was managed by Mrs. S.M.C. Kreitman. An influential colleague was Thomas L. Pilkington, M.D., who directed the Gogarburn Hospital for mentally retarded persons in Edinburgh. Pilkington, known for his interest in mental health and films, developed a relatively short-lived WFMH project in the area of mental health films. Another Executive Board member, psychiatrist Ralph Hetherington, M.D., lived in Liverpool and was a sometime Edinburgh faculty member. Deputy Treasurer Russell Cook, Director of Administration for the International Telecommunication Union, was located in Geneva , whereas the actual Treasurer, Dr. Roland Burnstan, lived in Washington, DC.

Carstairs, "Morris" as he was widely known, used his academic and hospital facilities at Edinburgh to host various psychiatric and mental health events under the WFMH auspices, bringing participants from all over Europe and the rest of the world. This fitted the mission of his department that he had previously conceived as specializing in the training of physicians from countries other than the United Kingdom. It also fitted his view of how the Federation should operate that was expressed in a May 1971 letter to the Board: "We have found in Edinburgh that one does not need to wait for an ambitious Regional or International meeting in order to promote a WFMH-sponsored International Forum-interested and motivated participants are already here in our midst, and respond readily whenever we invite them to join in discussing one of the many challenges to mental health with which we are confronted both in the developing and in the richer countries." He specified that activities which qualify for the WFMH sponsorship should be international and multidisciplinary and concerned with mental health (Carstairs, 1971).

He also traveled indefatigably to meetings elsewhere. For nearly four years these meetings dealt with many aspects of mental health. One of the more unusual, reflecting the broad social heritage of Brock Chisholm and Harry Stack Sullivan described in Chapter 2, took place in Edinburgh 3–5 September 1969. A group of 160 social psychiatrists, architects, health planners, sociologists, jurists, and religious figures discussed the difficult relationship between society and mental health.

Another multidisciplinary event heavily weighted with social scientists was a WFMH Regional Seminar in Amsterdam on 13–15 September 1972. With the topic, "Strategies of Change in Mental Health Care and Other Social Systems," it was described by its participants as "stormy and extremely unpredictable due to the intense involvement of all participants with the scene and with each other. Some leading personalities…walked out in protest." This may have been precipitated in part by an attempt to replace the traditional lecture format with a group process involving the speaker seated on a low stool and the attendees on the floor in concentric circles about him. Although this arrangement was reported as being common and effective in the United States, "some of the European participants objected" (WFMH, 1972–73). The storm may have also been associated with a developing split in the Netherlands Association for Mental Health between groups advocating scientific research and those more interested in care and service delivery (Morgan, 1996b).

Carstairs presided over the 21st WFMH Annual Meeting that, with its associated 20th Anniversary World Congress, was held in London in 1968 under the sponsorship of the National Association for Mental Health (NAMH) of England and Wales. The brunt of the organizational work for the congress was handled by Edith Morgan who was then social worker and Deputy General Secretary of the NAMH. She was able to achieve funding independent of the support being slowly accumulated to operate the Federation after the financial collapse in Geneva. Held at the Holland Park School in London, and presided over by Lady Priscilla Norman, the congress was attended by nearly 2000 people.

Although most speakers came from Western Europe and North America the perspective was international. The congress proceedings (Freeman, 1969) indicate its broad scope with the overall theme: "Keys to Progress: Education for Mental Health." Among the notable themes was that of conflict and conflict-resolution, with Dr. Johan Galtung of the International Peace Research Institute in Oslo speaking on "Conflict as a Way of Life" and Dr. Anatole Rapaport of the University of Michigan speaking on approaches to large scale theories of human conflict.

In Carstairs' presidential address, he tried to define the Federation and in so doing foreshadowed some of its later areas of concentration: "WFMH is an association of a wide diversity of groups and individuals united by the belief that human mental life whose development has made possible the proudest achievements of our species also holds the key to its future triumphs and disasters…In the relatively short recorded history of mankind we have seen the rise and fall of a number of major cultures…Each…had its characteristic world-view, its own interpretation of man's nature." He went on to note that in the contemporary era the most significant development was "the forward surge of technology" and to express the already prevalent view that "In man the evolutionary process is no longer merely biological, but is increasingly taking the form of the evolution of learned behavior" (Freeman, 1969).

The 1969 annual meeting in Washington, DC, was organized by the WFMH Vice President Paul Lemkau, M.D., Professor of Mental Hygiene at The Johns Hopkins University School of Public Health in Baltimore. It was a low-key affair with minimal advertising and a small attendance. The 1970 annual meeting was again in the WFMH European region. Its site, Jerusalem, was officially classified as European in keeping with WHO and United Nations practice. Held at Hebrew University with the theme, "Mental Health in Rapid Social Change" (Miller, 1971), it attracted 350 Israelis and another 150 participants from seventeen other countries. Many did not come because of the continuing political crisis involving Israel's relationship with the Arabs and Muslims. Many presentations concerned the stresses of war, and attention was devoted to the impact both on Arabs, including Palestinians in refugee camps, and Israelis. Carstairs emphasized the similarities in the hardships experienced by all populations involved. As he wrote, "Until…free communications are reestablished between Jews and Arabs, the WFMH will continue to collaborate with our members in both communities" (WFMH, 1970b). This led him to stimulate the organization of a December 1970 WFMH Workshop in Cairo to encourage members from Arab countries to discuss their problems.

New Executive Board members from Europe elected for 1970–1974, in Jerusalem, included Edith Morgan, Dr. Claude Veil of Paris as fourth vice president, and psychiatrist Louis Miller, M.D., Director of Israeli Mental Health Services who had organized the 1970 annual meeting. In 1971 when Miller came to the United States on a lecture tour I invited him to my Institute at the University of Maryland, and the faculty and students there found him a compelling speaker. Sometimes, though, his personal charm threatened to eclipse his message. One of our senior social workers put it graphically when she said: "I was so busy listening to the music that I sometimes didn't hear the words!"

In the 1970s under the presidencies of Carstairs, Beaubrun, and Lin, WFMH bulletins (later called newsletters) reported many member association meetings. Meetings of other European groups that dealt with matters of the WFMH interest were also brought to the attention of the membership. Although only a few of these were cosponsored with the WFMH, many were attended by Federation members who could be designated as official representatives. Thus Irma Tobing, Administrative Committee member from Surinam, was the WFMH representative to the August 1972 International Conference on Social Welfare at The Hague, Netherlands.

The WFMH participated in or had representatives at United Nations agency conferences in Europe that were concerned with the range of life cycle and clinical psychiatric issues. Among them was a 24–30 May 1972, forum on psychiatric services in developing countries led by President Carstairs during a WHO conference on comprehensive psychiatric services and the community in Scotland. Another example was a meeting on prevention of drug abuse at UNESCO headquarters on 11–20 December 1972. There the WFMH representative participated in discussions on drug education for pupils, teachers, and adults.

Sometimes the WFMH organized its own meetings, bringing in WHO and other relevant United Nations agencies. For example, Dr. Henry David, whose work as the WFMH Associate Director was described in Chapter 4, organized a meeting in Geneva 28–30 April 1970. Sponsored jointly by the WFMH and the International Planned Parenthood Federation, it dealt with psychosocial factors in family planning and psychological aspects of reproductive health. I participated, along with David, as an official WFMH representative and served as rapporteur. The broad interdisciplinary and international nature of our group, and the social and preventive mental health emphases of our discussions, led me to realize the potential of the WFMH as a significant influence upon WHO and as an international advocacy group for a broad range of mental health related issues. Indeed, our points of view were expressed in a WHO joint consultation between its Divisions of Mental Health and Human Reproduction held two months later.

Some European conferences in this period were organized by the Federation in collaboration with other groups. A WFMH-International Committee for Occupational Health seminar on "Stress in Industry," was held at Windsor Castle on 29 June–2 July 1970 with participants from nine European nations plus the United States. In view of the disquiet expressed in the 1990s by European members regarding pharmaceutical company funding, it is interesting to note in retrospect that the official WFMH representative, Dr. Alistair Weir, was partly supported to the meeting by an earlier grant from Interpharma of Switzerland (minutes of the Executive Board, 8–9 August 1970).

The WFMH also co-sponsored what was essentially a psychiatric congress on the "Mental Health of the Elderly" in Dresden that was organized by several East German psychiatric groups. Speakers came from East Germany, Bulgaria, Poland, Czechoslovakia, Switzerland, Austria, and Great Britain. Although the content was important for the WFMH, at least equal importance was attached to the gathering of people from behind the Iron Curtain with those from Western Europe.

The WFMH in Europe after 1974

President Tsung-yi Lin, who had been a member of the Federation's Executive Board in its early years and was sensitive to its potential fragility, was concerned from the beginning of his tenure in 1974 about the future location of the Secretariat which, possibly, could be in Europe. This concern was intensified by the decision of the Canadian Mental Health Association not to be the responsible organizer for the next World Congress for Mental Health planned for 1977. It was among the factors leading him to form the Task Force on the Future of the Federation noted in Chapter 5. The task force was headed by George Rohn, General Director of Canadian Mental Health Association, and included Edith Morgan and Mary Chase Pell, a former president of the U.S. National Mental Health Association and the Federation's vice president for North America. As Morgan recalled, the task force concluded that the long-term health of the Federation required a permanent location and that London might be a favorable place (Morgan, 1996b). Explorations in various parts of Europe, particularly the United Kingdom, confirmed the preference for London. The process went so far as inspecting possible premises and drafting job descriptions for personnel. However, WFMH Treasurer Gowan Guest of Vancouver traveled to London to check the progress of negotiations and announced that a final decision could not be made because he had not been authorized to pay the first quarter's rent on the new offices (Morgan, 1996b). This seems to have been the end of the matter for the time being.

Lin though, remained concerned with the status of the Federation in Europe. While the 1977 congress in Vancouver under his leadership was a major substantive and financial success-doing much to effectively resuscitate the faded image of the Federation-there were no bids for a 1979 congress, the first such biennial gathering projected in the new by-laws discussed by the 1977 Federation Board. Lin hoped especially that the 1979 congress might intensify the WFMH presence on the continent. In May 1978, therefore, he encouraged the Board's Honorary Secretary, Gaston Harnois, M.D., of Montreal, to address the United Kingdom and Eire Committee for Mental Health, chaired by Mary O'Mahony of the Mental Health Association of Ireland. Harnois also visited Tony Smythe, Director of MIND, the renamed British National Association for Mental Health. Although this resulted, he reported, in "valuable contacts" for future collaborative work between the Federation Board, Secretariat, and European members, there were still no bids for the 1979 congress. Lin asked the Belgians if they would host it, but they felt that a single year was insufficient for preparation. Finally an arrangement was made to hold it in Salzburg, Austria, 8–13 July with the major planning to be performed by Lin and Peter Berner, M.D., of the Austrian Mental Health Association.

Perhaps because of the rushed preparations this was regarded by some observers as an atypical and somewhat disorganized meeting (Morgan, 1996b). It was the second WFMH congress in which I was a full participant (the first being 1977), having organized a symposium for it on "preventing unwanted children" with the support of the Pathfinder Fund, and I also found it somewhat confusing. This judgment was confirmed by a friend, a high-ranking U.S. mental health administrator, who said that he hoped that I was not planning to tie my future career to such an inept organization. However, it was a cross-culturally interesting experience; perhaps because of its location in the home of the world-famous Mozart and Salzburg Festivals, it attracted a paid attendance of 728 people from 51 countries.

That congress also had some special features. Because 1979 was the United Nations Year of the Child, its topic was announced as "Mental Health of Children and Families." Former Executive Board member Dr. Estafania Aldaba-Lim, who had been appointed by Unicef as the United Nations leader of the Year of the Child, gave a major address. The United Nations was also involved through WHO. Lin made a particular effort to interest Halfdan Mahler, M.D., Director General of WHO, and Norman Sartorius, M.D., of its Division of Mental Health. In consequence this became the first time that WHO cosponsored the WFMH World Congress. Finally, Lin had organized a postcongress meeting with Unicef, WHO, and other United Nations officials to discuss possible WFMH involvement in the various children's programs in which the United Nations had an interest. So, despite its problems, I was impressed by the Federation's advocacy potential.

EUROPE AS A BASE FOR WFMH ACTIVITIES

The WFMH Regional Vice Presidents and Early Subgroupings

As noted in Chapter 9 , there were no formal regional vice president positions before 1971, although Board members were chosen to give broad regional representation to the WFMH. In that year, during the WFMH Annual Meeting in Hong Kong, revised by-laws introducing the new offices of regional vice president were approved. This was a first step toward recognizing the concept of regions as geopolitical areas including a cluster of national mental health associations that, by virtue of shared social organization, culture, and geography might have common goals and problems. The first vice president for Europe, psychiatrist Kurt Palsvig, M.D., of Denmark served from 1971 until 1974 when he was succeeded by psychiatrist Marianne Cederblad, M.D., of Sweden.

The 1970s, especially after the creation of the vice president positions, saw accelerating numbers of meetings sponsored by individual mental health associations in Europe, some of which were attended by representatives from the WFMH Board or Secretariat. A few made deliberate efforts to tie their meetings to the central organization. For example, the Austrian Society for Psychic Hygiene held a meeting on 14–15 December 1973, to celebrate the 25th anniversary of the WFMH that coincided with its own anniversary. The topic, "Planning of Psychiatric Services," was addressed by invited psychiatrists from five non-Austrian countries. In May 1975 European Vice President Cederblad sent the WFMH Bulletin a report on "study days" of the "United Kingdom and Eire Committee for the WFMH" (Edith Morgan, Secretary)" on migration in relation to mental health, a topic chosen in part because it was the subject of general Federation interest.

Topic oriented meetings with no official connection to the central organization, but sponsored by WFMH member (including affiliate) groups, were reported from Greece, Ireland, Scotland, Switzerland, Belgium, Portugal, Germany, France, and Sweden. However, there was no integration of these meetings, and although various attendees were designated by the presidents as Federation representatives, there was no organizational advocacy at them or based upon them. The main point seems to have been to "show the flag" of the WFMH with an occasional opportunity to influence the program or to intervene as it unfolded. The U.K. Committee for the WFMH had organized a joint conference with the National Society for Mentally Handicapped Children in Dublin in March and April 1971. Carstairs was involved, but although retardation had once been part of the WFMH international agenda, he let it be dropped, much to the distress of Pilkington (Morgan, 1996b). Closer to his interests were the issues discussed at an international forum in Edinburgh on cultural factors that might prevent the development of mental illness.

Most significant for the future, were continuing efforts to take advantage of the developing institutional ties among the nations of Europe. Thus the WFMH sent a representative to the Council of Europe's Multidisciplinary Symposium on Drug Dependence in March 1972 in Strasbourg. He was Professor Helmut E. Ehrhardt, M.D., Ph.D., of the University of Marburg, who also represented West Germany at the symposium.

The United Kingdom and Eire Committee for the WFMH, noting the growing importance of the European Economic Community, organized a workshop in London (30 July–4 August 1973) to study the ways in which different European societies show their concern for the mentally ill and handicapped. Emphasis was placed on personal responsibility, voluntarism, self-help, and advocacy. A later example, noted below, was the April 1980 effort to improve the representation of mental health issues before the European Parliament.

The Nordic countries were most prominent in forming their own regional subgroupings. In March 1971 and April 1972 the "Scandinavian Mental Health Seminars", sponsored by the Swedish and Danish Associations for Mental Health, with participation from all of the region's countries, produced five-day WFMH cosponsored seminars on "The Therapeutic Community" and on "Family Therapy" led by professionals. The following month (13–14 May 1972) the Danish association hosted a joint Nordic conference (Denmark, Finland, Iceland, Norway, and Sweden) that fit the initial vision of Rees and his colleagues for the WFMH conferences. Representatives from each country reported on their mental health association activities and then divided into discussion groups. Special attention was devoted to international cooperation in mental health services and education and the production of a multilingual journal.

The European League for Mental Hygiene and the WFMH

This organization, founded in 1926 to bring together national mental health associations and groups with similar interests, achieved formal status with the adoption of a constitution in 1939 (Morgan, 1988). Its relation to the European Reunion on Mental Hygiene and Prevention is not completely clear. The Reunion met in Paris on 30–31 May 1932, immediately after a meeting of the European members of the International Committee for Mental Hygiene, to which many if not all belonged (see Chapter 2). The purpose of the meeting was to plan a second international congress on mental hygiene for Paris in 1935 (which eventually happened in 1937). Although the Reunion had officers including a president, secretary general, and an executive committee, the 30–31 May meeting, held at the Henri Rouselle Hospital, was marked by further structural formalization. This involved a council including "a representative of each participating country in Europe who should act as Corresponding Secretary for his own country .[ths].[ths]. chosen by their own national mental hygiene organizations." The list of British delegates to this Paris meeting included two future founders of the WFMH: psychiatrist Doris M. Odlum, M.D., Joint Honorary Secretary with psychiatrist Professor R.D. Gillespie, M.D., of the National Council for Mental Hygiene, and Jack Rees, then Honorary Deputy Director of the Institute of Medical Psychology, member of the Committee of the National Council for Mental Hygiene, and future first president and Director of the WFMH. "European Reunions" were expected to meet annually in different countries, with the next scheduled for Rome in 1933 at the invitation of the Italian League for Mental Hygiene (News and Notes, 1932, p. 23).

The establishment of the WFMH did not result in the final demise of the ELMH. Rather, there was a limited intertwining on the continent of elements of the two organizations. For example, NAMH was simultaneously the British member organization of the ELMH and a component of what became the U.K. Committee for the WFMH. The ELMH "still retained its role of promoting mental health within Europe, though now in cooperation with the WFMH. Its annual meetings were held in conjunction with meetings of the Federation whenever these took place in Europe. In other years a European conference was organized by the League" (Morgan, 1988).

Despite the collaboration there were hints of nascent conflict between the global WFMH and its components with more limited regional concerns. As noted in Chapter 9, the 18 February 1954, minutes of the U.K. NAMH's International Committee expressed "concern with the relationship of the WFMH to various regional bodies," noting that "regionalization might be undesirable" from the global WFMH viewpoint but that "the European League was an established body whose existence must be reckoned with and whose part in world affairs must be recognized." More evident ambivalence was expressed after psychiatric social worker Robina Addis' report on 13 May 1954 of her attendance at the 7–11 April 1954, meeting of the ELMH in Rome. At that time the International Committee agreed to support the ELMH, "provided that it limits itself to European problems and a satisfactory relationship with the WFMH is reached." On 25 September 1955, Rees, pursuing a greater appearance of unity, asked that the name of the International Committee of the National Association for Mental Health be changed to either the British or the U.K. Committee for the WFMH. After some debate this change to a "U.K. Committee," specifying that it was "for the WFMH" rather than "a part of the National Association for Mental Health," was accepted as of 31 May 1956.

ELMH's annual meeting on 17–20 August 1971, was only its 21st, reflecting missed meetings caused by wartime conditions and other problems. As time went on, although it did not invite official WFMH representation, it was fully reported in the WFMH quarterly bulletin (WFMH, 1972b). The continuing reality was that the same people, including such figures as Odlum who had been a National Association for Mental Health representative to the 1932 reunion, were involved in supporting both ELMH and the WFMH. Thus there was no actual need for official reciprocal representation (Morgan, 1996b).

That 1971 meeting of ELMH was in Helsinki, chaired by the President of the Finnish Association for Mental Health, psychiatrist Professor Kalle Achte, M.D., who at the end of the meeting became its new president, succeeding Ehrhardt. Approximately 250 persons, described as "professionally associated with the domain of mental hygiene," attended from 20 European countries. Two major issues were discussed: (*a*) essentially professional, "suicide prevention from the point of view of several disciplines," and (*b*) more in keeping with the concerns of voluntary associations, "attitudes toward people with mental illness."

The WFMH Attempts a Rapprochement with the European League for Mental Hygiene

The level of the WFMH related European activity during the Carstairs presidency diminished when he left office in December 1971. However, Beaubrun, his successor as the WFMH president in 1972, was ready to do more because he had inherited an organization significantly healthier than Carstairs had at the end of 1967. As noted earlier Beaubrun was professor and chairman of the Department of Psychiatry at the University of the West Indies in Kingston, Jamaica. His university level and postgraduate education in Canada, England and Scotland made him sensitive to what seemed to be a reduced the WFMH profile in Europe. Having already announced his premature retirement late in 1973 and as one of the last acts of his presidency he organized a joint meeting between the leaders of the WFMH and the ELMH at WHO in Geneva, 11 March 1974. It had three stated objectives: "(1) to revive world mental health activity in Europe under regional Vice President Cederblad; (2) to re-establish links with ELMH and to define the roles and lines of communication between [ELMH and the WFMH]; and (3) to assist Dr. Cederblad in enlisting European support for the 1975 World Congress to be held in Copenhagen" (WFMH, 1974). The groundwork for the meeting had been laid by Administrative Committee member Paul-Marcel Gelinas of the Quebec Mental Health Association who had been dispatched by Beaubrun to Europe for that purpose, in part because he spoke French. In November and December 1973 he met with the ELMH members in Paris, London, Vienna, and Copenhagen.

Primarily because of Gelinas' efforts, the Geneva meeting, moderated by Beaubrun with incoming WFMH President Tsung-yi Lin in attendance, was a success. It was attended by 27 representatives of the leading European mental health associations. They came from France, Switzerland, Sweden, Germany, Portugal, Norway, Belgium, Austria, Greece, the United

Kingdom, Denmark, Ireland, and Finland. Beaubrun pointed out that the last major European WFMH activity had been the 1968 World Congress, which was itself in London rather than on the continent. He acknowledged that with the move of the Secretariat to Jamaica there had been "a slight shift of emphasis to the West" and that "there may have been a tendency for the image projected by the WFMH in Europe to fade a little." Furthermore, with the coming move of the Secretariat to Vancouver under Lin (preceded by the apparently disrupted agreement to bring it back to London), "there would very likely be a Pacific focus." In view of this Beaubrun felt that "it would be important to the WFMH to have its efforts in Europe supported by the ELMH, either as a Transnational Branch or independently, though in close collaboration." Dr. Lamarche, the ELMH Secretary General, agreed but with reservations. ELMH would limit itself to collaborating with the WFMH in European meetings and projects, and there could be a joint congress between the two organizations. He felt, however, "that it was important that the League maintain its independent identity" (WFMH, 1974).

Continued Efforts to Develop WFMH in Europe

Although the Geneva meeting did not result in cooperation with the ELMH, it offered an opportunity to continue planning for the WFMH activity in Europe. The August 1975 WFMH Congress in Copenhagen was a central concern. Incoming President Lin was particularly interested in its potential impact on the status of the WFMH within Europe because it would be the first such gathering on the continent during his tenure. The person immediately responsible was Cederblad, Palsvig's successor as European vice president for a three-year term beginning in 1974. After Geneva, her organizing and representational activities accelerated. They involved many conferences in different cities, and, in retrospect, it is not totally clear that the activity of European WFMH affiliates was, in fact, waning to the degree described by Beaubrun. However, it is true that most conferences were national rather than international, and relatively few, aside from those attended by Cederblad herself, had official WFMH representation. The most active European mental health associations were in Switzerland, the United Kingdom, Ireland, Belgium, Portugal, West Germany, Sweden, Luxembourg, Yugoslavia, and Greece. Their meeting topics ranged from migration to community mental health, psychiatric team work, preventive psychiatry, social psychiatry, and the education of field workers. Some were inspirational and social in nature. Thus the Danish Mental Health Association, anticipating the 1975 WFMH congress, arranged five lectures, each attended by about 500 people, on "The Human Being in the Growth Society."

Cedarblad, in her role as the WFMH European vice president, was key in the August 1975 World Congress. Organized by the Danish Mental Health Association headed by Palsvig, it attracted about 800 participants from 51 countries to consider issues associated with "Mental Health and Economic Growth." The congress issued a broad-ranging idealistic position statement far removed from the narrowly focused psychiatric services reform concerns of most mental health associations. It called "for an alteration in the consumption patterns of the affluent countries and strenuous efforts to construct a new global system of production, distribution and consumption." However, there is no evidence that it was formally approved by voting delegates as an official Federation resolution.

One new step toward regional development was taken at the Copenhagen Congress. Daily regional workshops were scheduled to give the regional vice presidents opportunities to work with colleagues from their own regions and discuss regional plans and activities, including fundraising and member recruitment. It was later recommended that these workshops be "structured in such way as to encourage development of regional programs in respective parts of the world" (WFMH, 1976). Since that time regional workshops have been regular parts of the WFMH world congresses, but their effectiveness has varied.

Despite the functional success of the Copenhagen Congress it produced a financial deficit; the sponsoring association was pushed into bankruptcy and died. Carstairs and Lin issued appeals for assistance, but were ineffective. The old Danish association was succeeded by the Danish National Society for the Welfare of the Mentally Ill, called SIND. Its perspective was less broad, and it was more oriented to the work of citizen volunteers including survivors of mental illness and users of psychiatric services.

During this period Cederblad continued to maintain her contact with the ELMH, attending what appears to have been its final meeting in Paris on 2 January 1976. In response to Beaubrun's urging she also tried to mount a WFMH regional activity, inviting all European member associations and individual affiliates to a continuing seminar on "The Planning, Organization, and Management of Mental Health Services" under the WFMH sponsorship. Unfortunately the response was insufficient. She also suggested themes for other regional or European seminars or workshops. Among them were mental health acts, patient organizations, unemployment, strategies for reaching political leaders, better care for mentally ill prisoners, preventive mental health, and "ideology and values for the further well-being of man" (WFMH, 1976).

The only WFMH activity of 1976 identified as a European regional meeting was an "International Congress on Transcultural Psychiatry," on 27–31 July. It was organized by psychiatrist Philip Rack, M.D., who had it cosponsored by and held at the University of Bradford. Its topics were "diagnosis" and "psychopharmacology," along with "migration and mental health," a topic of enduring interest to the Federation. Although it appeared, superficially, to be an essentially academic conference, Edith Morgan notes that this was not the case and that its "main purpose was to get ethnic issues on the map" (Morgan, 1996b). In her capacity as Secretary of the United Kingdom and Eire Committee for the WFMH, she was also helping to prepare an international seminar for the spring of 1977, in anticipation of the Vancouver Congress. It was to follow the Copenhagen theme on some aspects of employment and mental health. She was also working on a project with the International Hospital Federation entitled "Health Care in Big Cities."

At the Executive Board meetings during the 1977 Vancouver Congress, Cederblad was not optimistic about the concept of a unified, proactive European Region of the WFMH. Summarizing her impressions, she said that she would have liked to see the WFMH European office acting as "a switchboard" for communicating ideas among people in different countries. In other words it would be a communications headquarters for the mental health associations in Europe. However, she had not been able to succeed even in this limited aim because so little information had reached her.

TOWARD A EUROPEAN REGIONAL ORGANIZATION FOR THE WFMH

The Role of Edith Morgan

Edith Morgan, who succeeded Cederblad in 1977 as the Federation's European vice president, was deeply interested in strengthening cooperation between nongovernmental mental health bodies in Europe. She had perceived the ELMH's 1974 Geneva declaration of independence from the broader mental health movement as a harbinger of its extinction. In any event, as she wrote some years later, it had been becoming "more difficult for the same people to sustain two separate international organizations" (Morgan, 1988). She felt that the "time had come" and that there was no longer room for two overarching mental health associations in Europe. In her view the "European effort [should be] incorporated into the world movement," a development that would require her and her European colleagues "to give priority to WFMH" (Morgan, 1996b).

Morgan brought to this task not only energy and persistence but a significant background in theory and practice. She had received a scholarship that enabled her to take an honors degree course at Oxford University entitled "Politics, Philosophy and Economics." After further study in social administration at the London School of Economics she began her career with four years as a Child Welfare Officer with the London County Council. In 1954 she joined the staff of MIND and rose to the position of deputy director. During this time she organized a new community program. In 1977, seconded from MIND, she accepted an invitation from the International Hospital Federation (IHF) to set up and direct the "Good Practices in Mental Health" project that became a model throughout much of Europe. For many years she was secretary of the United Kingdom Committee for the WFMH, and in 1968, as noted above, she was chief organizer of the World Congress for Mental Health.

She was the leader who changed the effort to create a European mental health linkage from an ineffective to a systematic and highly effective one. This was begun by stimulating interest in several mental health relevant topics. It was facilitated during 1979–1981, after the Salzburg World Congress of 1979 and before the Manila Congress in 1981, by her direction of "Good Practices in Mental Health," collecting and disseminating information on effective European programs and promoting their implementation. Her summary of the WFMH activities in Europe in this period outlines the precursor of a coherent European mental health entity. It was a tying together, not only of the WFMH member associations but their ideas, in a form that could be useful within the rapidly evolving political and social organization of the new Europe (WFMH, 1981a). Regional workshops and meetings for which different organizations took primary responsibility were outstanding. All of these activities, funded from within Europe, were made possible by generous individual gifts of time as well as organizational gifts of money. Their aim was producing "practical results in terms of increased knowledge and understanding, [and] development in work and activity" (Morgan, 1996b) as well as spreading interest in the Federation. Taken together they constituted the functional initiation of what later became the ERC of the WFMH. They mark a pattern of mental health association sponsored, topic-oriented meetings aimed at discernible outcomes that has continued in Europe to the present day.

The first of these regional activities was a September 1979 study visit to England by mental health association volunteers from 14 countries including Israel. Organized in cooperation with MIND and IHF, it aided, as noted below, the further development of ENOSH, the Israeli mental health association comprised mainly of the relatives of mentally ill people that had been founded in 1978.

In March 1980 nearly 300 people attended a workshop on alternatives to mental hospitals organized for the WFMH by the Flemish section (headquartered in Ghent) of the Belgian League for Mental Health, the latter founded in 1923. It had the additional sponsorship of WHO's European Region, IHF, the Belgian Ministry of Health, and the State University of Ghent. The proceedings were published in book form and are still available (Nationale Vereniging voor Geestelijke Gezondheidszorg, 1980). Many papers also appeared in a special issue of the IHF journal, *World Hospitals*, in a report by MIND and one by the Belgian Association (WFMH, 1982). The single dissonant note was heard in *Nursing Times* (17 April 1980): "Of 250 delegates" to the conference, "only a handful were nurses." The local organizer most responsible for the workshop was the association's executive director, Josee van Remoortel (future WFMH European vice president 1989–1993), whose ideas are credited with being a major influence on the mission of the developing European regional grouping of the WFMH associations (Morgan, 1996b). After van Remoortel, retired from her salaried post she became the volunteer executive director of the ERC with its offices in Brussels.

In April 1980 a meeting on mental health and social policy in the European parliament was held in London. Two European parliament members from the United Kingdom took part in this meeting that aimed to increase understanding of ways to more effectively represent mental health interests.

In May 1980 Gaston Harnois was again in the United Kingdom under WFMH auspices, this time to speak on alternatives in the provision of mental health services. The meeting was organized for the WFMH by John Jenkins, Senior Nursing Officer at Exeter, Devon, United Kingdom (Morgan, 1981b).

In September 1980 at the annual congress of the Danish National Society for the Welfare of the Mentally Ill in Randers, Denmark, Morgan joined representatives of several Scandinavian mental health associations in a special meeting convened to discuss international collaboration.

March 1981 saw a conference organized by the Netherlands Center for Mental Health in Amsterdam on "Mental Health Development in Europe." Six countries were represented, and a resolution defining several mental health issues was passed (see under "Formal Planning Begins").

Finally, in May 1981 the Finnish Association for Mental Health headed by its first director, Irja Rantanen, working with Morgan organized a symposium in Helsinki on mental health and old age for the WFMH. Rantanen and van Remoortel were among Morgan's strongest supporters in her effort to achieve a union of mental health associations within Europe (Morgan, 1996b). Some 150 people attended this Finnish symposium with the opening paper given by WHO's mental health advisor for Europe. Again, it ended with unanimous approval of a resolution "outlining important areas where more attention should be given to the mental health of elderly people" (Morgan, 1981b). This resolution was submitted both to the WFMH Board and to WHO. The European regional director for WHO acknowledged its usefulness because the theme of World Health Day 1982 was to be "Add Life to Years." Both Drs. Halfdan Mahler, WHO Director General, and Norman Sartorius, Director of the Mental Health Division, welcomed the resolution. Among the programmatically relevant contacts with WHO was attendance at the July 1980 congress in Copenhagen on the United Nations Decade for Women where the WFMH was represented by Mrs. Bente Nygaard Jensen.

Conferences planned for 1982 and 1983 wereconcerned with deprived children (a study visit at the University of Newcastle organized by MIND); schizophrenia and employment (in York, England, organized by the National Schizophrenia Fellowship); and the role of the consumer in mental health planning.

Morgan's international organizing effort was greatly enhanced by the production of a newsletter, *Rapport*, edited by a medical student volunteer, Graham Thornicroft (who became a professor at the Institute of Psychiatry in London), with the assistance of IHF. In addition to European mental health news, each issue included original articles and a letter from the vice president. It included the first systematic effort to elicit candidates for the election of the next European vice president who could truly represent the regional constituency and comments on the WFMH policy and program in Europe (Morgan, 1996b). Also significant was her maintenance of a useful working relationship with WHO in Europe. This involved both discussions with key staff members and formal WFMH observer representation at WHO regional meetings by key staff of nearby WFMH member mental health associations.

Formal Planning Begins

Early in Morgan's second term as European vice president, the workshop on Alternatives to Mental Hospitals in Ghent, Belgium, on 30 March 1980, provided the opportunity for a first formal "exploratory meeting to consider plans for development of European cooperation in mental health" (Morgan, 1980). It was attended by representatives from the U.K., Finnish, Dutch, and Belgian (Flanders) mental health associations as well as by WFMH honorary secretary, Harnois. There was general agreement that the goal was "a European voluntary movement similar to movements led by national mental health associations" (Morgan, 1980). Among the issues demanding clarification was the relationship of a new European mental health alliance to the WFMH. "There was some feeling amongst those present that the WFMH had in recent years been over dominated by North America. Nevertheless the aims of the WFMH embraced those that had been identified...or a European mental health group, and there was undoubted value in being part of a worldwide movement" (Morgan, 1980). Thus it was agreed that the new European group should be organized under the umbrella of the WFMH. Much of the succeeding discussion concerned logistics and finances, including the possibility of contributions from the WFMH dues received from Europe and that of a "European Section of the WFMH." Harnois was asked to convey a report from the meeting to the WFMH Executive Board that was convening in Mexico on 12 April 1980 (chaired by President Gowan Guest). Meanwhile, Morgan would begin to consult groups in other European countries about the proposed European organization. Looking back at the sequence of events 15 years later, Morgan recalled: "Informal consultations from 1977 had led a handful of European WFMH members to meet during a historic conference on 'alternatives to mental hospitals' in Ghent, Belgium, to explore possibilities for a European mental health movement. The page was blank; there were no resources or funding. But the group refused to be daunted" (WFMH, 1995).

The next step was the 20–21 March 1981 meeting in Amsterdam organized by the Netherlands National Institute for Mental Health. Again chaired by Edith Morgan in her role as European vice president, it was the first gathering of people designated as representative "delegates" with decision-making power from their associations. As reported by Morgan it included representatives from six organizations: MIND in the United Kingdom, the National Association for Mental Health (Flanders) of Belgium, the national associations in Finland and Denmark, the Mental Health Group of the National Institute for Sport Medicine in Hungary, and the National Institute for Mental Health of the Netherlands (Morgan, 1981). These six were the yield from the 48 WFMH member bodies in Europe that had received invitations. The aim was to form a systematic linkage between the WFMH member mental health associations within Europe. Its main recommendation was to establish a geographically stable "European Desk for the WFMH" to share with the European vice president the responsibility for building a strong mental health movement, in effect "a mental health alliance" in Europe. As reported both by Morgan and by the WFMH Newsletter (WFMH, 1981a), it would support planning a long-term program of workshops and meetings, facilitate an exchange of information and personnel, and create a partnership and information channel on mental health matters among governmental and intergovernmental bodies such as WHO's European office, the Council of Europe, and the European Community. The November 1980 meeting of the WFMH Board in Vancouver was attended by Morgan and me, first in the role of Board member and then of president-elect; it had expressed strong interest and support for the idea of a European desk and had offered an initial grant of up to $5000 to get it started.

The Amsterdam group produced a resolution indicating several areas of preferred future action: the rights of mental patients and the need for legislative reform; the involvement of consumers, including patients and their families, in the planning and functioning of mental health services and agencies; and the primary prevention of "mental breakdown and illness." In addition the resolution included a list of concerns relating to the adequate delivery of psychiatric services. "It was decided in particular to invite the European Office of WHO to provide funds to investigate the progress and experience of primary prevention in a number of countries throughout the European Region [in view of] the WHO intention to launch a major program of activity on prevention in 1984...in welcoming this it was agreed to encourage member organizations to engage in preliminary action which could lead to involvement by the WFMH in the plans of WHO" (Morgan, 1981).

The expansion of the Federation's educational and advocacy activities through the European seminars, at the same time that a regional structure was being explored, appears in retrospect to have accelerated a return to the goals of Clifford Beers' hospital reform movement and away from the post-World War II concerns with peace and human relations. The new orientation emphasized the practical contributions of citizen volunteers to the well-being of persons identified as mentally ill and foreshadowed a later emphasis on the contributions of survivors of mental illness themselves. The major concerns were such issues as alternatives to conventional psychiatric care, particularly that in hospitals, and the civil/human rights of people diagnosed by professionals as psychiatrically ill, particularly those detained against their will. In the 1980s, and 1990s first as president and then as Secretary General, I was happy to support the inclusion in planning and discussion of persons who, themselves, had survived mental illness or serious emotional distress.

The opportunity unexpectedly arose to bring Morgan and her interests back into the center of Federation planning. During the summer 1982 Board meeting in Washington, the second which I chaired as president, I was taken aback, as described in Chapter 5, by Gowan Guest's unexpected resignation by telephone from the Board. We had all wondered about his absence, especially because he had promised his unstinting support. But the facts were different. Fearing bankruptcy proceedings after leaving a cash-starved organization-and with no optimism about our ability to resuscitate it-he hurriedly resigned from his positions as past president and member of the Canadian corporation of the WFMH.

I had to take quick action to repair the loss of an experienced supporter. Morgan, with her long involvement with the Federation, was my immediate choice to replace him on the Executive Committee, and-with the Board in session-I called her in London from a pay phone near our meeting room within minutes of Guest's phone call from Canada. Fortunately I reached her. Her unhesitating acceptance was a relief because she was not only a knowledgeable WFMH veteran but a "take charge" person within an organization that I was just coming to know from the inside. Before the year was out I had placed her name in nomination for president-elect to be voted on at the 1983 assembly during the congress in Washington, DC. She was elected there to take office as the WFMH president for the 1985–1987 term.

In time her work was honored from many sources including, in 1982, the medal of the Finnish Mental Health Association. Her return to the WFMH Board added advocacy force to MIND in its campaign for the new October 1983 Mental Health Act in England and Wales. The Act created new safeguards for psychiatric patients who were compulsorily admitted, detained, or treated in mental hospitals, i.e., without their express consent. A new interdisciplinary visiting and standard setting group of mental health commissioners included Morgan, who also joined its Central Policy Committee. Later, her position as the 1985–1987 WFMH president reinforced her influence in the final formation of an ERC/WFMH. In 4–5 May 1990, it awarded her the title, "Founder President." In 1995 she was awarded the Order of the British Empire.

THE EUROPEAN REGIONAL COUNCIL OF THE WFMH: 1983–1997

By May 1983 the Board meeting of what was informally called the European Mental Health Council felt that a formal organization of mental health associations on the continent was inevitable. This confronted the WFMH Board with the need to take action regarding the general question of regionalization at its next meeting less than three months later during the 1983 World Congress in Washington, DC. It was my privilege as president to chair the precongress meeting of the WFMH Board of Directors in July 1983 which formally decided that regionalization should become a Federation priority.

The new policy was greeted with optimism by European leaders present at the congress. An immediate consequence was endorsement of the earlier Amsterdam proposals by the European regional meeting held in midcongress. An action group formed to take them forward was led by Stijn Jannes, M.D., Professor of Psychiatry at the University of Ghent, who in 1981 had succeeded Morgan as regional vice president for Europe. As president of the consumer-oriented National (Flemish) Mental Health Association, he was acceptable to the mental health activists who tended to be uncertain about the true interests of academic professionals. In his continuing capacity as the WFMH vice president for Europe, reelected for the 1983–1985 term during the congress in Washington, he became the first chairman of a still not formally organized European Mental Health Council. A genial, scholarly person, he was an especially appropriate choice for the post, having just been appointed chairman of the Belgian government's Advisory Committee for Ambulatory Mental Health Care.

Jannes' reelection and the Board's unanimous decision in Washington to move toward regionalization opened the way for a meeting on 25 November 1983, at the offices of the National Association for Mental Health in Ghent. There a cross-national linkage of European mental health associations was established entitled the "European Regional Mental Health Council," to which later was added the qualifier, "of the World Federation for Mental Health"; its official abbreviation was ERC/WFMH. This emphasized its intention to operate within the framework of the WFMH with the WFMH vice president for Europe acting as its chairman for his or her term.

The Ghent meeting was noteworthy for the character of those attending it. Traditional citizen volunteers representing their mental health associations were outnumbered by mental health association staff persons. This was not only a marked difference from the make-up of the Federation Board as it had existed during the Rees and Cloutier periods; it also presaged the increasing influence of mental health association staff during the coming years. Those present included van Remoortel, still executive director of her association and later to become the WFMH vice president for Europe and ERC/WFMH chairperson; Mary J. O'Mahony, Chief Executive of the Mental Health Association of Ireland, later to become a member of the WFMH executive committee as membership chair; Pirkko Lahti, Director of the Finnish Mental Health Association and later to become a WFMH Board member-at-large; Bent Pederson, Executive Director of SIND; Christopher Heginbotham who had succeeded Tony Smythe as executive director of MIND; Alan Ferguson, Director of the Northern Ireland Mental Health Association; and Huw Richards of the Scottish Mental Health Association. In addition there were the WFMH President-elect Morgan, once a staff member of MIND; psychologist Dr. Inge Schock of the West German Mental Health Association; psychologist Brian Glanville, President of the Mental Health Association of Ireland; and two psychiatrists, Drs. Wout Hardeman of the Netherlands and Pini Pino of Italy, who were also social activists with particular affiliations with emerging groups of people who themselves had survived mental illness. These people constituted a steering committee with the additions of Peter Clarke, Jean Engelen, Thaddeus Galkowski, and Nikki Ingelopoulous from their own mental health associations.

The operating office of the new council, then called the European Desk of the WFMH, was to be located in MIND headquarters in London, "contingent upon the Council's ability to meet the costs involved" (WFMH, 1984). However, the Irish were more generous, and, with expected support from their government, a temporary Secretariat for the new ERC was arranged for the next two years in the head office of the Mental Health Association of Ireland in Dublin, with Chief Executive Mary J. O'Mahony serving as honorary secretary.

With the help of this steering committee, Jannes and colleagues held workshops, surveyed European mental health associations, collaborated with WHO in Europe and other nongovernental organizations (NGOs), and attempted to increase European membership in the WFMH, especially among individuals. This was the group that later sponsored the summer 1984 Copenhagen meeting on compulsory hospitalization and the rights of psychiatric patients and, in autumn 1984, helped organize the Ben Gurion University meeting on mental health and primary care described below.

The next organizational step took place at the Board's annual meeting on May 1984 that I had arranged through the generosity of Robert Gibson at the Sheppard Pratt Hospital in Baltimore. This was the first Board meeting at which ERC was represented as a reality. The Board approved its proposed rules of operation, expecting that they would be presented again in revised form by the ERC on 15 July 1985, with a provision for review no later than 1990.

The establishment of ERC/WFMH was quickly followed by an announcement from Knud Jensen, M.D., Professor of Psychiatry and Neurology at the University of Årrhus and Director of Psychiatry and Neurology at the Odense Hospital in Denmark. In his capacity as president of SIND he organized a regional conference of European mental health associations affiliated with the WFMH in Copenhagen, 12–15 August 1984. Also including jurists and lawyers, it focused on involuntary commitment to mental hospitals and the civil rights of the mentally ill. The idea was to carry the theme forward to the 1985 World Congress in Brighton as part of a WFMH initiative toward formulating a model mental health code that could ultimately be referred to the United Nations. This conference, with its emphasis on the human rights of people defined as mentally ill and vulnerable to coerced hospitalization and treatment, foreshadowed ERC's advocacy emphases during the following decade.

Jensen, a graduate of the University of Åarhus medical school, was an unusual combination of academic administrator, investigator, and dedicated mental health volunteer. His research interests included problems of cannabis use that had involved work over many years with cannabis users in Pakistan. Since 1976 he had arranged postgraduate training programs for Pakistani social workers, psychologists, and laboratory personnel in conjunction with the Danish International Development Agency. In 1984 he became a member of the Danish National Committee, which dealt with the revision of legislation affecting the welfare of people defined as mentally ill.

During the meeting of the WFMH European region members at the Brighton World Congress on Mental Health in August 1985, the Action Group converted itself into an ERC that then elected additional members. It adopted its first working rules, and Jensen succeeded Jannes as chairman. He chaired its first formal meeting three months later in November 1985 in Copenhagen.

From this point on the ERC/WFMH council (of voting delegates elected by country) held regular annual meetings and topic-oriented conferences, sometimes together and sometimes separately. Its meeting of 11 April 1986, was hosted by Josee van Remoortel at the National (Flemish) Association for Mental Health in Ghent. Six months later its second annual conference was held 28 September-1 October 1986, at Trinity College, Dublin, by the Mental Health Association of Ireland. It drew 262 participants from 13 European countries in addition to visitors from the United States and South Korea. The focus was societal with a keynote address by a Dutch sociologist. Major sessions dealt with attitudes toward mental illness and the mentally ill, patient and family education, prevention, the education of health professionals, and European governmental policies for health education.

The ERC was now in a position to formally articulate the program that had been evolving during the years of its formation. One decision at its February 1987 meeting was to organize a project on women and mental health in several European countries, encouraging women's involvement in the WFMH and office holding in general. By 21 February 1988, the group had been formalized as the "WFMH/Europe Project on Women," chaired and coordinated by Morgan. Information about women's mental health in several European countries, along with possible preventive solutions, was gathered by a staff of three Danish women psychiatrists and the data studied at a residential workshop 18–19 May 1989, on the "European Situation of Women in Mental Health." Limited to 30 invited female participants it now added to its goals that of considering how women could become more involved at senior levels in United Nations agencies as well as NGOs relevant to mental health. A high point was a celebration dinner at the House of Commons sponsored by the shadow minister of the "Opposition Party" for "Women's Affairs."

In early May 1988 in Middlefart, Denmark, ERC began the process of inventing its mature structure and operating mechanisms. It met under the chairmanship of then WFMH vice president for Europe, Knud Jensen. Several working rules, prepared largely by Morgan and van Remoortel, were adopted. They specified that ERC, its committees, working groups, officers, and members, all operate within the overall structure, policy, and by-laws of the WFMH. There would be no membership independent of the WFMH. Furthermore, the president and Secretary

General of the WFMH together with members of the WFMH Board located in Europe were to be, during their period of office, members of the council-a suggestion that was never activated. The general purpose of ERC would be to further the objectives of the WFMH. More specifically it aimed to give practical encouragement to European WFMH members, both individual and organizational, in improving mental health care in their own countries and protecting the rights of persons affected by mental illness. A particular goal was to affirm a right of those who use the mental health services to have a voice in planning and managing them.

By this time the main thematic line of ERC conferences and projects was crystallizing. It was, essentially, psychiatric services reform with special reference to vulnerable or unrepresented groups. This focus reflected the contemporary state of European psychiatry that, still based mainly in large mental hospitals, was significantly dependent on physical and chemical restraint and tranquillization. An ERC project, "Mental Health and Children," was initiated in early 1988 by the WFMH member organization, Federal Conference for Family Counseling, in Furth, West Germany, under the leadership of Dr. Klaus Schutt. The intent was to evaluate existing European services for children, adolescents, and families. Ultimately the data would be used in a symposium on mental health questions in Europe with an emphasis on developmental crises and prevention.

Meeting in Bologna, Italy (19–20 October 1988), ERC considered the problems of Greek mental hospitals, particularly institutions on the island of Leros, and a new project on the mental health of children. At the next meeting (20–21 May 1989) in Torbay, England, the topic was the pre-and posthospitalization care of mentally ill people in the community, continuing the 1980 theme of alternatives to hospital care.

Another leadership transition took place during the 21–25 August 1989, World Congress for Mental Health in Auckland, New Zealand. Josee van Remoortel was elected vice president for the WFMH European Region, thus becoming chairman of ERC/WFMH. She set up an advisory group consisting of current or retiring ERC officers: Drs. Knud Jensen, Wout Hardeman, and Stanislas Flache (who had taken office as the WFMH president in Auckland), Mary J. O'Mahony, and former president Morgan. At the ERC annual meeting in Warsaw on 5 November 1989, Jensen was elected Honorary Secretary and O'Mahony Honorary Treasurer. By this time ERC included representatives from 14 countries: Czechoslovakia, Denmark, England, Finland, Ireland, Israel, Italy, Northern Ireland, Poland, Scotland, Sweden, the Netherlands, Wales (independent of the United Kingdom), and West Germany.

The ERC's 1990 annual meeting was held on 4–5 May in Bremen, West Germany. On that occasion Edith Morgan was appointed to a new lifetime office of Founder President of ERC in recognition of her work.

A significant event was the adoption of the "ERC Manifesto" in Prague in 1991 that had been drafted in the context of "Charter 2000" from the 1985 World Congress in Brighton and of the WFMH Declaration of Human Rights adopted by an Egyptian Congress in 1987 and, with revisions, by the Board meeting in Auckland in 1989. It spelled out the ERC "philosophy and priorities...an identity for the ERC and a framework for the development of its work programme through projects, campaigns, conferences, offers of practical help, and negotiating at every NGO and governmental level" (Morgan, 1994). It did this by asserting the ERC commitment to a range of goals, most of which concerned the delivery of psychiatric services. These included community mental health services; the involvement of service users in planning, developing, providing, and monitoring those services; stronger legal rights for people diagnosed or treated as mentally ill; publicity and promotion of good practices; and support of the development of national mental health associations. In addition the ERC Manifesto included the goals of "working for better socio-economic conditions for all citizens" and "combating discrimination."

ERC took another step toward maturity with its initiation in August–October 1991 of a newsletter, the *Mental Health Observer*, published in both French and English. In June 1992 it relocated its Secretariat into a building in Brussels that it later purchased. It printed a booklet on the functions of national mental health associations and the steps needed to establish one.

In 1992 the ERC Executive Committee met in London on 8–10 May and its annual conference, focusing on poor conditions in Greek mental hospitals, especially on Leros, was held in Thessaloniki, Greece, on 7–10 October. On 13–15 November 1992, after an earlier London seminar on seclusion, a joint conference between the Flemish Association for Mental Health and the French Speaking Confederation of Mental Health Leagues of Belgium was held under van Remoortel's leadership. The topic, again reflecting the state of institutional psychiatry on the continent, was "The Hidden Power in Psychiatry," referring to "the disparity between declared policies and the reality of practice in restraining mentally ill people."

In 1993 the ERC held its general assembly in Brussels (26–27 March), which was attended by 70 delegates from 20 countries. Its annual conference on the theme of "Reform of Mental Health Services: New Perspectives of Mental Health Care in Europe" was held in Portugal, 25–27 November.

At the elections during the assembly of the August 1993 WFMH World Congress for Mental Health in Tokyo, John Henderson, M.D., became the new regional vice president for Europe, succeeding van Remoortel who had served two terms, 1989–1991 and 1991–1993. He was a former WHO regional mental health advisor who had been based in both Europe and India. His presence significantly strengthened ERC/WFMH as he continued to attend the WHO regional meetings, especially in Europe, but now as an ERC/ WFMH observer. Van Remoortel was honored in her own country by being named Grand Officer in the Order of King Leopold II, an award recognizing significant humanitarian activities abroad. The citation noted her contribution to mental health care in Europe and on a worldwide level.

The next annual conference of ERC held at Queens University in Belfast, Northern Ireland, 1–4 September 1994, was organized by the Northern Ireland Association for Mental Health with the theme "Conflict and Mental Health." It was closely supported by the Centre for the Study of Conflict at the University of Ulster, Coleraine. That was a special moment because it coincided by chance with a cease-fire by both the Irish Republican Army and the loyalists. Its content, thus, was unexpectedly timely as well as unusual for the WFMH, although sessions on peace and nonviolent conflict resolution had been in the 1968 World Congress program. It was also a special moment for me because this was the first ERC meeting that I had been able to attend since the first a decade earlier in Copenhagen, and I was especially pleased to be able, along with WHO's Dr. Jose Bertolote, to address the closing session.

1994 was an important organizational year for ERC/WFMH. Its newly elected Board convened in Brussels on 21-22 October and confirmed procedures for the nomination and election of a new executive committee. In January its statutes had been lodged in Brussels in accordance with Belgian law, and regulations for application of the statutes were confirmed in April 1994. In the Winter 1994 issue of the *Mental Health Observer*, ERC Chairman (now designated "President") Henderson wrote of "the emergence of a potent and claimant Regional structure within the nations of the European Union." Morgan, in a March 1994 annual report entitled "European Section for the WFMH," summarized the past achievements and current status of ERC. She noted that "there was much early skepticism to overcome about what was feared could become another 'talking shop'" and the consequent emphasis on "activities linked to practical mental health development [contributing] to the mental health of people and societies" (Morgan, 1994).

By this time, with the fragmentation of the Soviet Empire, ERC was active in 50 East and West European countries. Its "quality and effectiveness are acknowledged by governmental, intergovernmental and non-governmental organizations throughout Europe. It is designated the European Community's lead European mental health NGO and has consultative status with the Council of Europe and the European Office of WHO. It provides specialist and consulting services to all of these. Two Executive Committee members serve on the seven-person Independent

Team of Experts that evaluates progress on the European Community's Regulation 815 for Greek psychiatric reform, and one member serves on the council of the European Committee on torture and degrading treatment. The ERC is a member of the European Community Forum and the European Community Liaison Committee for the Integration of Disabled People (Helios Programme). Jose van Remoortel chairs the committee of NGOs in consultation, coordinating more than 100 NGOs in the field of disability" (Morgan, 1994).

In 1995 ERC cosponsored three major meetings in Paris, Federicia (Denmark), and London, respectively, and purchased the house in Brussels that provided increased office space. The 1 April 1995, council meeting in Brussels was celebratory, attracting 25 of its more than 40 elected members. Stijn Jannes represented Belgium; Knud Jensen was on the executive committee and editor of its quarterly, the *Mental Health Observer*. As Edith Morgan wrote for the July 1995 WFMH Newsletter: "The mood was not complacent or self-congratulatory…But there was a feeling of celebration for an efficient and effective body making a real difference to mental health in Europe, operating from its own building, albeit with a bank loan…The ERC has earned the respect not only of non-governmental mental health associations which are its lifeblood, but of all relevant European national and international bodies with interests in mental health" (WFMH, 1995).

The ERC's annual report for 1995, organized by Executive Director van Remoortel, describes its contemporary structure and policies. Noteworthy is its reiteration of a mission statement enunciated by Vappu Taipale of Finland at the Dublin World Congress: "She declared that the greatest challenge to us all was to raise the prestige of mental health in our communities, in our countries and on the international scene. Together, alongside our fellow NGOs, we can rise to this challenge in Europe."

From 18–21 January 1996, ERC and ERAGINTZA, the Basque region's voluntary organization for mental health, sponsored the European Conference on Multidisciplinary Activities in Community Care in Bilbao, Spain, and allowed the ERC executive committee to meet in conjunction with it. There representatives from the Spanish Autonomous Communities came together for the first time in a decade to share developments on community care for the mentally ill.

Integrating the European Regional Council of WFMH within the European Community

The context provided by the European Community became increasingly the major determinant of the vigor and activities of ERC/WFMH. By 1995 its Annual Report listed ERC participation in a series of European agencies. Within the European Union were the Helios Programme, with special reference to the European Disability Forum, the Helios II Conference on Trade Unions and the Rights of Disabled People. Within the Council on Europe were groups on Health, Aging and Disability, Bioethics, and Psychiatry and Human Rights. The Autumn 1996 issue of the *Mental Health Observer* announced the new European Disability Forum of which ERC-WFMH was among the founding members.

Much of this began in April 1988 when the European Council of Ministers resolved to promote the full social integration of all disabled people in the European Community. Subsequently on 11–12 January 1989, the European Commission convened a meeting (expected to recur annually) of representatives of 28 NGOs. Attended by Josee van Remoortel on behalf of the WFMH, it focused on direct NGO involvement in activities by and with disabled people in the region under the "Second Community Action Programme for Disabled People" (Helios II). In the same year the ERC meeting on 20-21 May 1989, in London chaired by Knud Jensen included the topic of closer collaboration with and funding possibilities from the European economic community. This was followed actively by van Remoortel who, on 20 November 1989, in her role as the WFMH regional vice president succeeding Jensen, spoke to the European Parliament's all-party group meeting in Strasbourg and sent WFMH brochures to all of its members. On 6-8 December 1989, in Brussels she represented the ERC (and the Federation) at the First European Conference of Helios for the Promotion of Independent Living for Disabled People.

1991 was a year of exceptional movement toward ERC integration within the intergovernmental European framework. It was accepted by the European Community as its NGO liaison body (i.e., the leading one) for mental health. The Helios II program would now provide links between the European Community and European NGOs including ERC with a new office for NGO liaison assisting in the coordination of European NGO activities. Helios II included ERC as a partner with eight European NGOs: European Network of Users and Ex-Users in Mental Health; European Association of Multidisciplinary Practices for Mental Health Care of Children, Young People and Their Families (AESMEAF); European Federation of Relatives of Mentally Ill People (EUFAMI); European Committee for Law, Ethics and Psychiatry (CEDEP); International Federation of Settlements, European Group (IFS Europe); Foundation for European Cooperation in Psychiatric Reform and Cultural Integration of Mental Health (FERMENT); EuroPsy Rehabilitation; and Alzheimer Europe. In fall 1991 ERC also became eligible to apply for funds from the increased European Community budget for NGOs in the region. Van Remoortel represented ERC at the European Community's Committee of Member States on 29 October 1991. On 14 November 1991, another major milestone was when ERC was given consultative status on mental health matters with the Council of Europe.

The year also saw the individual recognition of ERC/WFMH workers. Josee van Remoortel retired from her 30-year post as executive director of the Flemish Association for Mental Health and was honored by a special "academic day" in her honor in Stijn Jannes' department at the University of Ghent. Not long thereafter she was reelected for a second two year term as the WFMH European vice president at the 1991 World Congress in Mexico.

In 1991 the Council of Europe granted unusual recognition in her private status to Pirkko Lahti, Director of the Finnish Mental Health Association, who was also a member of the ERC Executive Committee. It appointed her to membership on the European Committee for the Prevention of Torture and Inhuman or Degrading Treatment or Punishment. This 19-person committee, based in Strasbourg at the Council's headquarters, was the world's first multinational body of inspectors assigned to examine the treatment of detainees.

With the support of the European Community, ERC could now move on several projects, including some close to the WFMH goal of improving positive mental health. Notable was an ERC Standing Committee on Women's Issues, which met in Utrecht on 13–15 February and was funded by a European Community grant. The project "Consumer Evaluation of Community Mental Health Care" was closer to ERC's service delivery theme.

The Thessaloniki, Greece, conference of ERC on 7–10 October 1991, marked yet another advance in the integration of ERC into the developing political structure of the continent. It had the official support of the European Community (and its Hospital Committee) and the Council of Europe as well as the European Regional Office of WHO and the Greek government. Entitled "The Changing Scene in Mental Health Care in Europe-the Reforms of Practice, Policy and Structures," it was organized jointly with the psychiatry department of the local hospital and the Association for Mental Health and Social Integration of Thessaloniki. During this conference ERC organized the first coordinating meeting of European NGOs working in the mental health field. In addition to ERC and the European Community's Hospital Committee, conference participants included the European Association of Child, Adolescent and Family Mental Health, the European Society for Mental Health and Deafness, and the Foundation for European Cooperation in Psychiatric Reform. The result was a recommendation to ERC to organize a formal network of interested European associations that could organize annual meetings with a broader membership aimed at joint advocacy efforts.

The European Community also increased its funding for the mental hospital program in Greece with which ERC was concerned. In August 1987 Edith Morgan, after discussions within the U.K. Committee for the WFMH, began correspondence with the Greek Minister of Health, Welfare, and Social Security concerning mental health services development in Greece. The expertise of the ERC/WFMH volunteers was offered to assist in the Greek national plan for reform, especially in seeking solutions to the problems of large mental hospitals in Athens, Leros, and Corfu. But the Greek response was reluctant, despite continued face-to-face discussions with academic and government representatives, including Costas Stefanos, M.D., of Athens, President of the World Psychiatric Association.

In 1991 Morgan and John Henderson were appointed to the European Community's independent team of experts to visit Leros and other Greek facilities. The team's last visit, led by Henderson, was from 28 January to 4 February 1996.

In 1995, along with the Dutch Prevention Fund and the Province of Limburg, Helios II helped support a conference initially organized by the Department of Social Psychiatry at the University of Limburg headed by then WFMH President-elect Marten de Vries. Held from 31 August–1 September 1995, it brought together more than 300 users of psychiatric services ("voice hearers") and service providers. Among the cooperating sponsors was "Resonance," an organization of users, and ERC/WFMH.

The ERC leadership's perception of its status as part of the European Community was dramatized in its annual report for 1995 where its organizational philosophy was announced as "breaking the mould of the past whereby national associations accredited by the central office of the WFMH carried the primacy of managing the Federation throughout the world" to recognize "international alliances of different kinds among nation states and…a Regional structure within the nations of the European Union." (p. 3).

The WFMH and ERC/WFMH in Eastern Europe

With the passage of time since the formation of ERC and since the opening of Eastern Europe, an increasing number of countries have revived or begun mental health associations, and many of these have been visited by ERC members. This account is sketchy and does not continue past 1995. Some organizations, not all of which belonged to the WFMH, later joined its ERC. An example was the Polish Society of Mental Health founded in 1939. It was concerned less with hospital reform and mental health service delivery than with broad philosophical aspects of health and world peace. By November 1989 it was sufficiently integrated to hold a symposium on "Universalism, Mental Health and Co-Existence" with the cosponsorship of ERC and Warsaw University's "Philosophy of Peace Research Project." However, after this project, developing interests in more practical mental health service reform issues led to the formation of another voluntary organization, Coalition for Mental Health, that applied for ERC membership. Its goals were to develop public education and advocacy systems for the mentally ill, sheltered employment, community care, and several mental health promotion projects. In 1990 the new Coalition took advantage of its formal affiliation with ERC to ask its assistance in obtaining publications and journals and arranging exchange visits. The mediating organization in this case was MIND. On 16–19 June 1995, the Coalition held a symposium on "Mental Health and Human Rights," its fourteenth such activity. Its chief organizer was Dr. Elzbieta Bobiatynska, along with Professor Andrzei Piotrowski, who was on the ERC/WFMH board. Its aim was to consider the Polish mental health act of 19 August 1994, in the context of the new Europe. The only speaker from abroad was ERC/WFMH representative Knud Jensen who compared Polish legislation with laws in other countries.

A significant development took place in Czechoslovakia. In June 1987, before the nonviolent revolution that overthrew the Communist regime, the Family Therapy section of the Czechoslovak Medical Society held a conference in Prague organized by Dr. Petr Bos. Under general WFMH auspices it attracted 1700 participants from many countries. WFMH President

Morgan and 1985–1987 WFMH Vice President for Europe Jensen were official Federation representatives. Henry David, Chair of the WFMH Committee on Responsible Parenthood, a long-time consultant to the Prague Psychiatric Research Institute, also participated. The congress president was charismatic family therapist Virginia Satir who had spoken at the Vancouver WFMH World Congress of 1977. In November 1987, Morgan, in her capacity as the WFMH Past President, returned to Prague to pursue earlier discussions on strengthening links with the WFMH. She also lectured there at the invitation of the British Embassy, focusing on the role of voluntary and consumer organizations on mental health development. When she proposed the idea of a voluntary mental health association most Czech colleagues thought it impossible because there had never been a tradition of voluntary community involvement in health and social welfare (Morgan, 1996b). Despite these doubts, a Czechoslovak-WFMH committee was formed as a nucleus from which plans for participation in the ERC could be considered, and on 20 January 1990, a Czech Society for Mental Health was established to take part in the health ministry's new Committee for Reform of Psychiatry and Mental Health. An ERC symposium in Prague in spring 1991 allowed Morgan to initiate an information exchange project with it. ERC now had two Czech members, Hana Junova, Ph.D., and Kamil Kalina, M.D., Ph.D., who in 1987 had been in charge of rehabilitation in psychiatric hospitals and was now a member of the newly formed advisory Board to the Czech Ministry of Health. At their invitation Morgan had spent a week in Prague (23 April–1 May 1990) to discuss mental health developments and the overall restructuring of the country's mental health services. Her program included meetings at a large range of mental health services, hospitals, and projects and one with Mrs. Olga Havel, wife of the Czech president. She also met with the senior mental health official at the Ministry of Health who volunteered help for the translation of documents from abroad for the new Czech mental health society.

The Czech Society worked closely with the Fokus Kolegium-Association for the Development of Mental Health. This was a multiprofessional group interested in the enlightened treatment of psychiatrically ill patients. It had sponsored a Czechoslovakian "Week for Mental Health" for several years and did so again 24–30 September 1990, to promote the destigmatization of mental illness in the country. Its activities included concerts, theatrical performances, exhibits of art work by mentally ill individuals, and tours of the state psychiatric hospital in Prague.

A major project organized by the Society for Psychotherapy, Family Therapy Association, and Psychiatric Society (all components of the Association of Czechoslovak Medical Societies and now cosponsored with ERC/WFMH) revealed the enthusiasm of Czech colleagues for broad collaboration with Europeans. A congress on "Mental Health in European Families: Family System Health-A New Concept in Mental Health" was held in Prague on 5-8 May 1991. Coorganizers included the new Czechoslovak Society for Mental Health, Institute of Health Promotion, Family Therapy Institute of Prague, and European Foundation for Family Studies in Prague. ERC/WFMH met in Prague just before the congress (4–5 May), and its annual meeting was held on 7 May in conjunction with it. The immense good will of the Czechs was seen in the designation of the WFMH European Vice President and ERC/WFMH Chair Josee van Remoortel as congress president. Among the vice presidents were Edith Morgan and Knud Jensen; honorary Board members included current WFMH President Flache and ERC/WFMH Honorary Treasurer Mary J. O'Mahony. I was pleased to receive an invitation from the Czech organizers in my capacity as the WFMH Secretary General but could not accept.

In September 1992 I led a group of U.S. WFMH members, mental health professionals, and volunteers to visit societies and institutions in Poland, Hungary, and Czechoslovakia. At that time, based on prolonged discussion with Dr. Kalina, it became possible to trace the roots of the contemporary mental health movement in the Czech Republic. They were in what was called the "Working Group for Comprehensive Therapy of Psychoses" that was part of the Section of Psychotherapy of the Czech Medical Society. The working group was founded in 1975 by several young psychiatrists, psychologists, and philosophers. During its first five years of existence it had to overcome police harassment; some of its members lost their jobs, and others were imprisoned, partly because they were monitoring the political misuse of psychiatry and other human rights issues. Nonetheless, by 1982 the climate had changed sufficiently for a unit in psychotherapy, social therapy, and family therapy at the Charles University teaching hospital in Prague to become established. This unit was linked with a small day treatment center. In 1983 the first social club for former patients was begun. By 1987 a new sensitivity was developing in public and professional attitudes toward people with psychological and emotional problems, especially those defined as mentally ill. In 1987–1989 the dominant mental health movement called "Therapists Seek Allies" was a broad network of professionals along with consumers and volunteers. From it emerged the Prague Mental Health Programme, which pointed the way to modern health care; this was the precursor of various groups taking advantage of the new postrevolutionary freedoms. All worked together to produce Mental Health Weeks in September 1990, 1991, and 1992.

Although the Czech Association for Mental Health founded in 1990 was originally intended as a common umbrella for everyone involved in the previous movements, it had developed into what was described by several commentators, including Kalina, as "basically a consumers' organization." Among its members who greeted our group in 1992 were engineer Jan Gottwald, a survivor of mental illness, and psychiatrist Jan Pfeiffer, M.D., a leader of the Czech health ministry's program for reforming psychiatry. Pfeiffer was an elected Czech representative to the ERC Board and a member of its executive committee.

Kalina left the health ministry in 1992 to become a member of the Czech parliament. He was part of a group working to develop three major mental health projects: community mental health care in Prague, an independent committee for mental health reform to continue the reform process, and a committee with the Filia Foundation for Mental Health concerned mainly with drug abuse prevention.

Beginning in autumn 1994 the Danish mental health association, SIND, has worked in Albania with the support of the Danish government to establish an Albanian mental health association. By 1995 it had its own office and executive director and was working closely with relatives of mentally ill people. Groups of Albanians including professionals, politicians, and relatives paid educational visits to Denmark. However, it had not yet forged a relationship with ERC.

As other formerly closed countries of Eastern Europe became more accessible with the demise of the Soviet Union, the WFMH members in Europe became more active in visiting them. One of the most active was Knud Jensen. In September 1990 he lectured at the University of Tartu, Estonia, and took part in discussions on the founding of the Estonian mental health association. A leading figure, Henno Ligi, M.D., was already in contact with the WFMH Secretariat concerning the new association's possible membership in the WFMH. In 25–27 September 1991, Jensen represented ERC at the first meeting entitled "Mental Health Cooperation in the Baltic Region." Held in Finland, it included participants from Leningrad, Estonia, Latvia, and Lithuania as well as Poland, Denmark, Germany, Norway, and Sweden.

In 1991 the Romanian Mental Health League was formed as an NGO open to all persons interested in mental health issues. In the same year the Hungarian psychiatric association applied for the WFMH affiliated membership. Josee van Remoortel visited Romania in March 1992 where she obtained interviews with the Prime Minister and Minister of Health to seek their support for the League. In 1995 Knud Jensen addressed the mental health association of Sofia.

OTHER WFMH MENTAL HEALTH ACTIVITIES IN EUROPE

General Considerations

The ERC, even as it became well established in the mid-1980s and was appointed the lead mental health NGO for the European Community in 1991, was never the sole regional conduit to the WFMH Board and central Secretariat. Various independent and significant mental health activities as well as three WFMH World Congresses for Mental Health (1985, 1995, 1997) took place in Europe during the 14 years after the founding of ERC from 1984 to 1998. These included conferences of member associations that preferred to relate to the global rather than the regional office. In some instances an effort was made to compromise. An example was the 10–11 October 1996, World Mental Health Day conference of the French Federation for Mental Health held at UNESCO headquarters in Paris. The topic, "Ethics and Psyche," was developed independently of ERC with my office and the collaboration of UNESCO, which was a sponsor and consultant. However, as a matter of form, ERC was listed among the sponsors, and Josee van Remoortel was invited to chair the session at which I spoke.

There were also conferences organized by nonmember groups for which the WFMH became a cosponsor and sent a representative. For example, 1–6 July 1984, saw meetings on mother/infant mental health in Greece cosponsored by the WFMH under the immediate auspices of an international group of child psychiatry organizations. I brought the WFMH greetings from President Aldaba Lim at the opening ceremonies and also spoke on a personal research topic of WFMH interest.

Other activities represented interests of members not fully taken up by ERC. Thus, the WFMH, independently of ERC, pursued its concerns about international collaboration and community services with a conference, 4–7 September 1986, on "Community Related Psychiatry" in Germany. Initiated and chaired by the WFMH member Dr. Klaus Schutt, it was cosponsored by the WFMH with the German Association for Mental Health to bring together professionals from the German Democratic Republic and West Germany. An important result was to establish that there were few differences between the two German states concerning practical work in "community psychiatry and the anthropological philosophy of psychiatry." According to Dr. Schutt this represented a major difference from 20 and even 10 years earlier.

On 12–14 June 1991, with the participation of Dr. Dorothea Maria Simon (WFMH representative to United Nations Vienna), the Austrian Association of Families and Friends of the Mentally Ill, of which Simon had been president, marked the ending of the United Nations Decade of the Disabled. It was active in a symposium that assessed the impact of the 10-year effort to end all discrimination against the disabled. The association held its first national congress in Vienna on 24–25 April 1992, with cosponsorship from neither ERC nor the WFMH. However, before the 1993 Tokyo World Congress I facilitated the inclusion of Diane Froggett, Executive of the World Schizophrenia Fellowship (WSF), on the program, and there was more family representation at the Dublin Congress where I had the chance to get to know Jim Crowe of New Zealand, later to become a vice president of WSF. Simon, still feeling somewhat discouraged by the lack of interest of ERC/WFMH, spoke on the tension between users, i.e., survivors of mental illness, and their "carergivers" i.e., parents or other relatives concerned with their safety and well-being at the annual meeting of another organization. This led me to greater efforts, including a Secretary General's message in the Newsletter, and by the time of the 1997 Finland World Congress, a place had been assured for WSF and related speakers on the program.

Finally, a parallel stream of the WFMH related activities, noted below, was conducted for the most part by professional, scientific, and clinical organizations in which Federation leaders were involved.

Parallel Streams of WFMH Linked Professional Activity and ERC Volunteer Activity

Some European meetings of scientific-clinical organizations in which the WFMH members or concerns were prominent were cosponsored by the global Federation without ERC involvement. They exemplified a continuing stream of parallel activities by Federation members. On one side were professionals, often non-European; on the other were European citizen volunteers and occasionally some professionals.

Work with the global agencies of the United Nations (in contrast to its regional divisions) required the global WFMH rather than one of its regional councils as the collaborator. The activities of Europe based United Nations agencies with WFMH representation also proceeded independently of ERC. The WFMH, for example, had four accredited representatives from the United States and Canada to the 7th United Nations Congress on the Prevention of Crime and Treatment of Offenders in Milan (August 1995). Although the regional divisions of global United Nations agencies were free to deal with our regional councils, only in Europe and only between ERC and the European office of WHO was this actually formalized.

Occasionally an ERC member would be appointed by the WFMH president as a global WFMH representative to participate in non-ERC activities. Thus on 20–22 April 1989, the World Psychiatric Association organized a symposium marking the closure of a large Victorian hospital in the United Kingdom with the participation of WHO's mental health division. Edith Morgan chaired a session and represented the WFMH, which was one of the cosponsors.

Another example was our cosponsorship of the 9th Congress of the International Society of Psychosomatic Obstetrics and Gynecology (ISPOG) in Amsterdam on 28–31 May 1989. Other congress cosponsors included WHO, the Commission of European Communities, and the Royal Dutch Academy of Sciences. Our relations with ISPOG were close because its president and congress chairman, Eylard van Hall, M.D., Professor and Director of the Department of Obstetrics and Gynecology of the University of Leiden, had been a member of my 1987 WFMH-UNESCO working group on "New Reproductive Technologies and Human Rights" (see Part III), and I was a member of ISPOG's Board of Directors as well as a plenary speaker at the congress. In addition the ISPOG congress program included a major WFMH sponsored symposium on ethical issues in reproductive health involving several members of the WFMH Committee on Responsible Parenthood as well as our WFMH representative to United Nations Vienna. With the theme "Women's Health in the 1990s," it overlapped some of the concerns of the ERC group on women's' health.

The Second International Conference on Medicine and Migration in Rome, sponsored by the Diocese of Rome, the Chair of Mental Hygiene of the University of Rome, and the Harvard University School of Public Health (11–13 November 1990), was interested in a tie to the global WFMH but did not request official cosponsorship from ERC. Its prime mover and major contributor was our Federation's Committee on Southeast Asian Refugees. Richard Mollica, M.D., its chairman as well as director of our collaborating center, the Harvard Program on Refugee Trauma, and I were among the speakers, so the WFMH was prominently displayed as a major collaborator.

In Prague the longtime collaboration of the WFMH's Committee on Responsible Parenthood member Zdnek Dytrych, M.D., of the Prague Psychiatric Research Institute with the committee's chairman, Dr. Henry David, proceeded independently of ERC. In 1991 David, in the context of the Institute's 30th anniversary, was presented by the rector of Charles University with the University Medal and Citation in recognition of his years of international scientific cooperation. In the same year Edith Morgan, in her ERC role, was presented with the Jan Purkyne award for her contributions to community mental health.

From 6 to 11 October 1991, the First International Working Conference on the Mental Health and Psychosocial Adjustment of Refugees and Displaced Persons was organized by the Karolinska Institute in Stockholm. The WFMH was one of the global cosponsors along with WHO, UNHCR, and the International Organization of Migrants as well as the U.S. National Institute of Mental Health and several Swedish organizations. Invited speakers included Richard Mollica, chair of our WFMH International Committee on Refugees and Other Migrants, and myself. The WFMH was a prominent participant especially because it held and disbursed the funds for the Conference which were supplied by the U.S. National Institute of Mental Health.

At the same time that the ERC women's program was becoming more active, the Fifth International Congress on Women's Health Issues, organized by the International Council on Women's Health (a WFMH member organization), took place in Copenhagen on 25–28 August 1992. The Council inquired about possible speakers, and although I referred the inquiry to the ERC women's program, no participation ensued, nor did the Council request sponsorship from either ERC or the WFMH.

One of the more interesting cultural linkages was between Spanish speaking colleagues in Europe and Latin America. In February 1993 Federico Puente, the WFMH president-elect, gave a series of lectures sponsored by the Mental Health Nurse's Association of Spain in Madrid, Valladolid, Seville, and Barcelona. While in Madrid he received the Amafe Honor Prize from the Spanish Association of Friends and Families of Schizophrenics. As president (1993–1995) his discretionary appointment as member-at-large of the Board was Pedro Torrejon, president of the association of Spanish mental health nurses. This was followed by the 1994 Board meeting in Madrid with the support of the nurse's association, and in autumn 1995, as immediate past president, he keynoted the 16–18 November National Conference of the mental health nurses and renewed his ties with a range of Spanish colleagues. At this time, although there was no Spanish participation in ERC, its officers made no attempt to recruit member associations from the country and noted Puente's involvement with Spanish colleagues without comment. When Torrejon's two-year term ended during the 1995 Dublin Congress, Puente nominated him for an elected position as Board member-at-large, but he did not receive enough votes to be elected.

Another globally oriented European meeting that did not seek ERC affiliation was the follow-up to the 1990 WFMH sponsored Jerusalem conference on children of war (noted below in relation to Israeli events). This major international gathering, entitled "Children-War and Persecution," was held from 26–29 September 1994 in Hamburg, Germany. Organized by the Department of Child and Adolescent Psychiatry at the University of Hamburg, it was cosponsored by the WFMH in addition to Unicef and several German organizations. As a member of its international scientific committee I brought WFMH greetings to the opening ceremonies and moderated the closing three-hour session, "Where Do We Go from Here?" The only other WFMH speaker was Dr. Gillian Walker of the Republic of South Africa who had also been present at the Jerusalem meeting.

The WFMH in the Former Yugoslavia

Although ERC maintained occasional contact with some individuals it did not have a systematic presence either in the intact Yugoslavia or during or after its civil war, and its interest in the area was not clearly defined. However, Knud Jensen visited Slovenia on 24–25 February 1995, as an expert member of the European Committee for the Prevention of Torture and Inhuman and Degrading Treatment or Punishment (of the Council of Europe) and spent time with two mental health associations.

The work of one Yugoslav colleague, psychologist Nila Kapor Stanulovic, Ph.D., on our WFMH Committee on Responsible Parenthood and my UNESCO-WFMH working group on the new reproductive technologies (see Part III), stimulated me to urge the formation of a Yugoslavian mental health association to work with ERC. This was not successful, however, and instead, as a Professor at the University of Novi Sad , she was only able to form a Novi Sad psychological association that, not being national in scope, could only be admitted to the WFMH membership as a nonvoting affiliate. It did not maintain its membership beyond the one-year initial period. In autumn 1991, before the outbreak of hostilities, the Novi Sad colleagues arranged for me to visit Yugoslavia where I spoke and consulted with the Institute for Mental Health at the University of Belgrade School of Medicine and lectured at the Center for Comparative Studies on Technological and Social Progress in Novi Sad. Despite my recommendation they seemed uninterested in applying to ERC for membership, although they were pleased to announce that my lectures were held under WFMH auspices.

In early 1993, after the civil war began, our WFMH collaborating center, the Harvard Program in Refugee Trauma, sent Elizabeth Murphy, M.D., as one of a United Nations Committee of Experts to be part of a professional team interviewing alleged victims of rape and assault in the Bosnia/Herzogovina region. From 1993 through 1995 my office received many requests for the names of North American mental health personnel who might be willing to work for a short term with institutions in the area. In response we identified several Yugoslav expatriates working in the United States and sent requests to various WFMH member organizations. In consequence of this correspondence, and meetings with Yugoslav colleagues at other European gatherings (e.g., the Hamburg meeting on children of war), we carried occasional reports from former Yugoslavia in the Newsletter. Prominent was "War-time Rape: Coping Behavior of Women in a Concentration Camp," an account from the director of a medical rehabilitation center for torture victims.

Arshad Husain, M.D., Co-Chair of the WFMH Committee on the Commercial Sexual Exploitation of Children, visited Sarajevo in February and April 1994 to train teachers to work with traumatized children. His visits were funded by the Coordination Council of Humanitarian Agencies, a coalition of 20 relief agencies working in Bosnia under United Nations auspices from a base in Croatia.

During 1995–1997 our Harvard Collaborating Center carried on a program in Croatia described in Part III.

Israel and the WFMH

The Society for Mental Hygiene in Israel, in its infancy and surrounded by hostile Arab states, was among the 62 member associations from 33 countries listed in the initial WFMH roster (September 1949). Later, as the United Nations system developed, the hostility within the countries designated as its Eastern Mediterranean Region (division adopted by the WFMH) continued. Israel asked WHO to designate it as a member of its European region. The WFMH did so, although as noted earlier there was a short-lived attempt in 1985-1986 to place it in the geographically appropriate Eastern Mediterranean Region. This attempt was a corollary to the 1985 election as member-at-large to the WFMH Board (during the Brighton WFMH Congress) of Chanita Rodney, National Chairperson of ENOSH (Israeli mental health association). She had helped found ENOSH, the successor to the old Society for Mental Hygiene, in 1978. Rodney was a distinguished addition to our Board, having received many national awards including that of Israel's Woman of the Year ("Beautiful Israelite") presented by the Knesset. However, her interests were more congenial with the biomedically oriented research programs of organizations such as the Alliance for the Mentally Ill and with the World Schizophrenia Fellowship's emphasis on families than on the Federation's philosophy of patient autonomy and user participation in their own care. Although she continued to attend the WFMH congresses and remained a friend of the Federation she did not continue to participate actively in its programs or administrative interactions.

This different orientation may have contributed to the nonparticipation of Israeli mental health groups in ERC activities. The degree of this nonparticipation may also have been due to ERC neglect, or other sources of Israeli resistance. But an early effort at support and involvement was made by members of the nascent ERC led by its first president, Stijn Jannes. From 30 September–4 October 1984 Jannes and others participated in that year's only regional meeting in Europe as it was defined by WHO with the WFMH following suit. With the theme of mental health in primary care, it was held at Ben-Gurion University of the Negev in Beersheva, Israel. However, it was not cosponsored by ERC, which had no official role. This occasion revealed an apparent preference by Israeli colleagues for closer association with the WFMH rather than ERC, and succeeding Israeli activities were sponsored, at their request, by the global WFMH.

An unusual episode took place in a workshop at the 1984 meeting. It was led by Dr. Yael Danieli, an Israeli with American citizenship and one of our representatives to United Nations

New York. There, for the first time, Rodney spoke publicly about her childhood experiences. She had to cope with potentially overwhelming stress at age 10 when she was sent out of Germany by her parents to escape the Holocaust. They and her brother, all of whom remained behind, perished at the hands of the Nazis. Like so many who have devoted themselves to mental health, she was motivated by personal experience. Her interest in schizophrenia, its etiology and treatment, began when her daughter (now living independently and working productively) suffered a severe mental breakdown after serving in the Israeli Defense Force.

In early 1986 an opportunity arose for me to become more familiar with the mental health situation in Israel, including that encountered during everyday life in an apartment in Ramat-Aviv, not far from the Tel Aviv medical school. My wife and I lived there from 16 February to 18 March after I was appointed a fellow of the Sackler Institute of Advanced Studies at Tel Aviv University. The invitation came through my old friend, Professor Phyllis Palgi, Ph.D., former chief anthropologist of the Israeli Mental Health Services and current chair of the Department of Behavioral Sciences at Tel Aviv University. In addition to university lectures and consultations regarding behavioral science teaching and research I worked with Palgi on Israeli mental health policy issues with particular reference to the nation's immigrant population. This involved meetings with many government health officials and revealed the significant influence of ENOSH in the country.

This trip made it possible to spend time in Cairo with President-elect Gamal El Azayem to help in planning the 1987 World Congress. It also allowed me to attend two Board meetings of ENOSH. ENOSH was then and remains the single voluntary organization in the country that deals with all aspects of education and promotion for better mental health and the prevention of ill health, including both advocacy and the operation of facilities for the rehabilitation of mentally ill persons. Some of its fundamental interests were revealed in the presence of its active Scientific Committee for Research on Schizophrenia and Allied Illness headed by a distinguished Hebrew University biologist.

At the Assembly of Voting Members during the Auckland World Congress in August 1989, another Israeli, Emanuel Chigier, M.D., a pediatrician and adolescent psychiatrist from Tel Aviv, was elected a WFMH Board member-at-large. He was nominated by Rodney, and I supported his nomination. This was partly because of his cross-cultural orientation and partly because of his high level of organizing activity. I had spent some time with him in his capacity as the consultant for the depressed and suicidal Ethiopian Jews in Israel known as Falasha. Many were teenagers. A few months earlier, from 8–12 January 1989 he had organized the fourth International Conference on Stress in War and Peace in Tel Aviv, with WFMH cosponsorship. He went on to organize many meetings of general interest to the WFMH but made little effort to obtain ERC sponsorship, feeling that it might be disinterested.

Perhaps the most important WFMH cosponsored conference in Israel took place 24–28 June 1990. Entitled "Children in War" it was organized by the Sigmund Freud Center of Hebrew University in Jerusalem. Its organizers did not request ERC involvement but were specifically interested in sponsorship by the global WFMH,. This was granted, placing us with the Israel Psychoanalytic Society and Harvard Medical School. Several individual WFMH members, including myself as a keynote speaker on public mental health policy for children traumatized by war, were on the program. This activity is described in greater detail in Part III as it bears on the WFMH international mental health agenda.

The WFMH and the Former Soviet Union

Although there were occasional discussions about mental health in the states of the Soviet Union and the possibility of Soviet societies becoming WFMH members, no action was taken until the dissolution of the Soviet Union. On 14–27 August 1990, I led a group of U.S. WFMH members, mental health professionals, and volunteers to visit six U.S.S.R. institutions. These, with clinical and investigative goals, were in Moscow, Leningrad, Tbilisi (Georgia), and Kharkov (Ukraine). At each institution we talked with the staff about the nature and aims of the WFMH and the possibility of establishing a voluntary mental health association in the area. Hilda Robbins, a WFMH Board member-at-large, its former vice president for North America, and past president of the U.S. National Mental Health Association, was effective in presenting the nature and role of voluntary mental health associations as well as discussing the participation of families in patient care. But the concepts involved in the WFMH, and the voluntary mental health movement seemed unfamiliar and not well understood, even at the Bekhterev Institute in Leningrad, known for its community orientation. Considerable stigma was still attached to mental illness, despite some new media openness consequent to the return of Afghan war veterans and increasing awareness of the emotional impact of the Chernobyl disaster.

There was considerable curiosity and some amazement among U.S.S.R. professionals when they learned that volunteer nonprofessionals and consumers were actively involved in many areas of the mental health field in the United States. Two members of our group, Dr. Agnes Hatfield, one of the founders of the U.S. National Alliance for the Mentally Ill, and Hilda Robbins described the advocacy work of their organizations. The only positive response was from Tbilisi, where movement toward a new mental health association began. This was also the single site at which there was familiarity with world literature on psychotherapy with schizophrenic patients including some of my work and notably that of another group member, Professor Theodore Lidz of Yale University. On 29 November 1991, inspired by our 1990 meeting and led by Simon A. Surguladze, M.D., of the Institute of Psychiatry of the Georgian Academy of Sciences, the founding meeting of the Georgian National Association for Mental Health took place. The new association was based upon the principles of the WFMH Declaration of Human Rights and Mental Health proclaimed in 1988 and 1989 (see Part III).

Two WFMH leaders participated as WHO Temporary Advisors in a WHO regional office consultation on mental health legislation in Europe held in Moscow on 3–5 June 1993. They were Knud Jensen, also in his role as a representative of ERC/WFMH, and psychologist and former dean of the Vienna School of Social Work, Dr. Maria Simon, who was the WFMH main representative to United Nations Vienna.

WFMH WORLD CONGRESSES FOR MENTAL HEALTH: 1985, 1995, 1997

1985 World Congress for Mental Health in Brighton, England, and Sequelae

A major activity of the global WFMH, with the active participation of the still embryonic ERC, was the WFMH World Congress for Mental Health in Brighton, England. It took place 14-19 July 1985, organized by MIND, led at that time by Christopher Heginbotham, a housing specialist. The theme was "Mental Health 2000: Action Programmes for a World in Crisis," and its aim was to create a forum for debate on national and international issues in mental health for consumers, volunteers, and professionals. This aim led to the formulation of Charter 2000, a set of declarations on the rights of mentally ill people and the promotion of mental health to provide a philosophy and policies to serve as a foundation for global mental health and WFMH activities into the 21st century. A document was written, edited, printed, and formally presented to the Board and then distributed by the end of the congress. By August 1988 a revised document was ready to be reviewed by a working group in London. I participated in that group along with President-elect Stanislas Flache, M.D., Past President Morgan, and Chris Heginbotham. Charter 2000. Its significance for the WFMH international agenda is discussed in Part III.

Brighton saw the second WFMH Mental Health Association Day organized and chaired by Hilda Robbins, U.S. WFMH Vice President for North America. More than 100 delegates, representing Mental Health Associations in 24 countries participated. Robbins was subsequently appointed by President Morgan to chair a WFMH committee on mental health association affairs.

An especially poignant occasion was a dinner organized by three founding members of the WFMH—Lady Priscilla Norman, Robina Addis, and psychiatrist Dr. Doris Odlum, a friend and colleague of Clifford Beers. Odlum died on 14 October 1985, at age 95. Addis, one of the world's first psychiatric social workers, died one year later on 5 September 1986. Aside from her professional eminence she was an organizational activist who, along with Lady Norman, had pressed for the inclusion of the Child Guidance Council as one of the three organizations joining to form the National Association for Mental Health of England and Wales, forerunner of MIND. Later, working with Rees at Tavistock, she became part of the Association's organizing committee for the 1948 London congress.

Most participants sensitive to the differences in the Federation goals and those of international professional unions such as the World Psychiatric Association were pleased with the 1985 congress and its philosophy. However, some attending from other countries felt that it was too predominantly a British activity in terms of themes and participants, and some psychiatrists perceived it as antiprofessional. This perception, voiced to me by some colleagues from the American Psychiatric Association, was shaped by the prominence of such themes as citizen advocacy, the voluntary sector, and hospital closure in pursuit of community-based services. It also reflected the prominent role of ex-patient or "user" and other organized consumer groups. This last was epitomized in an evening debate, "Should Mental Health Services be De-Medicalized?" moderated by Lord Colville, Chair of the British Mental Health Commissioners. As noted in Chapter 7, a group of mental health service users led by United States activist Judi Chamberlin, who had been sent to a 1982 Federation meeting by the American psychiatric, psychological, and mental health associations, circulated a statement asserting that there was no such thing as mental illness. Although Board members along with others were asked to sign it, none did so. Judi took the refusal with good humor, as though she had expected it.

The presence of a WFMH president in Great Britain offered, as it had in other countries, opportunities for Federation sponsorship of and international participation in locally initiated activities. A postcongress seminar was organized by the Torbay Health Authority and South Devon Services in England and entitled "Providing a Local Mental Health Service: The Process of Change." It dealt with universal issues, reflecting the state of European and U.K. psychiatry, such as how to replace large outdated institutions by local services. Special attention was paid to such issues as accountability regarding patients' rights, quality of care, and staff mental health during periods of transition. A follow-up conference under WFMH auspices entitled "Coming Home: Meeting Mental Health Needs Locally" took place in London in 1986.

Edith Morgan, who took office as president during the August 1985 congress, succeeded an almost unbroken 37-year string of male professionals (Margaret Mead and Estafania Aldaba-Lim, both with doctorates, were the exceptions). In her first WFMH Newsletter message in September 1985 she signaled her enduring commitment to citizen volunteers, including survivors of serious mental and emotional distress: "As a former staff member of a national mental health association" she believed in the work of voluntary bodies "where ordinary citizens and people who have had personal experience of mental illness work in partnership with… professionals…on an equal basis and with mutual respect" (WFMH, 1985).

The 1986 Board meeting began in London where Morgan had arranged a visit to the Sigmund Freud Museum before its official opening sponsored by the International Psychoanalytic Association, a WFMH member. This was of particular interest because in 1953 the WFMH was the first international organization to place a plaque on the building at 19 Bergasse Street in

Vienna where Freud had lived and worked. On 9 June MIND also hosted a daylong symposium, "A World Focus on Mental Health and Human Rights." The Board meeting at Cumberland Lodge (Windsor Park, England), 11–13 June had many visitors. They included John Orley, M.D., of WHO's Mental Health Division; Dr. Stephen Mills of the International Social Science Council; Drs. Yael Danieli, Elena Millan Game, and Maria Simon, WFMH representatives to United Nations New York, Paris, and Vienna; and Mary J. O'Mahony, ERC Honorary Secretary.

Although national committees for the WFMH seemed a logical route for organizational development, the only one formed in Europe was that in the United Kingdom for which minutes are available from 1949 to 1959. In 1985 a small United Kingdom and Ireland working group was cochaired by Edith Morgan and Lady Juliet Bingley, Chairman of MIND. Aside from developing national interest in the WFMH , and many projects on mental health resource development for less developed countries, it held open meetings in 1985 on mental health services in Japan and in 1987 on conditions in the mental hospital on the Greek island of Leros, later to become a cause celebre for the European mental health reform movement. It met in March 1988 to discuss ways of strengthening links with the WFMH. Afterward was an open meeting for U.K. members of the WFMH, featuring mental health in Italy with a discussion led by Paolo Crepet.

With the Board's agreement to hold its 1988 meeting, chaired by President Gamal Abou El Azayem in London, it became certain that the United Kingdom would be the site of one of several 40th anniversary observances expected in the year. Held after the 3–4 December Board meetings with support from the King Edward's Hospital Fund for London it was billed as "An International Symposium on Quality in Community Mental Health Care." Speakers from Europe, as well as Board members from Egypt and the United States, focused on the identification of key components of quality service. Unfortunately, attendance was minimal.

The 1995 World Congress for Mental Health in Dublin, Ireland

This meeting was held in historic Trinity College, 13–18 August 1995, sponsored by the Mental Health Association of Ireland under the direction of Chief Executive Mary J. O'Mahony. It attracted nearly 1600 people, many more than expected. By far the largest contingent came from the host country, although geographic proximity ensured a large turnout from the United Kingdom with a substantial number from Northern Ireland. Large groups also came from the United States and Japan; 67 countries were represented. With its theme, "A Time for Reflection," the program committee headed by John Connolly, M.D., produced a packed schedule of 194 meetings, workshops, and poster sessions. The opening on 14 August at the National Concert Hall was addressed by Irish President Mary Robinson, former U.S. First Lady Rosalynn Carter, the acting head of the European commission's office in Ireland, and many of us from the Board, the Secretariat, and the Mental Health Association of Ireland. In my report to the assembly I reviewed Federation growth since establishing a stable Secretariat in 1983, noting that with more than 300 national, international, and local organizations we now represented several hundred thousand people. With approximately 3500 individual members and representation in 101 countries, WFMH was larger and more active than at any period of its 47-year history, with highly concentrated activity in Europe. The substantive issues addressed at the congress, insofar as they carried forward the international mental health agenda, are noted in Part III. The newly prominent activities of psychiatric user/survivor groups are described in Chapter 7.

An aftermath of the Dublin Congress was the naming on 27 November 1995, of O'Mahony as the Irish Laureate (national candidate) for the 1995 Woman of Europe award. The selection was based on both her national and international work as a mental health advocate. The citation praised her contribution to the health and welfare of persons suffering from mental illness in Ireland and Europe.

The 1997 World Congress for Mental Health in Lahti, Finland

Although it was understood that world congresses should be rotated around the world, the Board decided to accept Finland's application because it would mark the 100th anniversary of the organization that had preceded the Finnish Association for Mental Health. That organization, aimed essentially at the welfare of patients being discharged from mental hospitals, is described briefly in Chapter 1.

THE FUTURE OF THE WFMH IN EUROPE

By 1997 ERC/WFMH has moved toward an identity more resembling that of a national mental health association with a single set of goals and a single source of financial support than an identity as a union of separate organizations from the politically and culturally separate nations. It seems likely that, already strong, growing, and well integrated into the European Community, it will expand as the dominant mental health NGO in Europe.

Part III

THE INTERNATIONAL MENTAL HEALTH AGENDA

Chapter 12

A Purpose and a Program

THE REES ERA: 1948–1962

Peace, Mental Health, or Hospital Reform? Science, Service or Advocacy?

In 1945 and 1946, Brock Chisholm and Harry Stack Sullivan articulated an overall purpose for a new nongovernmental organization to succeed the International Committee for Mental Hygiene. It was to achieve harmonious relations among nations, groups, and individuals. This was compatible with Chisholm's definition of health in the World Health Organization (WHO) constitution: "a state of complete physical, mental and social well-being" (World Health Organization, 1946). Including well-being as a goal permitted attention to all of life's circumstances and legitimated efforts at social change. Although the Federation's official statement of purpose in its articles of incorporation referred specifically to health, it was congruent with an international perspective, and subject to interpretation: "to promote among all peoples and nations the highest possible standard of mental health in its broadest biological, medical, educational and social aspects" (WFMH, 1947).

These initial stirrings and post-World War II enthusiasm and idealism resulting in the WFMH founding document, "Mental Health and World Citizenship," are described in Chapter 2. That document was a major departure from the usual service delivery goals of mental health associations as it defined an international mental health movement aimed primarily at "helping people live with their fellows in one world." The preservation of peace and the prevention of war were regarded as the overriding mental health issues of the era. A more general aim, listed in the 1952 annual report, was "to further the establishment of better human relations in all possible ways." By this time, four years after the 1948 founding congress, the Federation's "aims and purposes" included goals that could also be regarded as tools for achieving mental health and good human relations. These were working with United Nations agencies, helping member associations to improve mental health services in their own countries, and promoting communication and understanding through meetings and international congresses (WFMH, 1952).

The resolutions submitted by discussion groups to the Executive Board at the end of the 1950 annual meeting in Paris indicate the perspectives of the meeting delegates. Among their recommendations, two in particular reflected the dominant ethos of the moment. One was a resolution to establish a "Chair or Lectureship of Human Relations in all Schools of Medicine, Education and Social Work." The other was to establish "a Committee which will be active in the prevention of war and the propagation of peace." Its functions would include collecting evidence about "the pathology of war-mindedness" and ways to combat it. Its proposer, Dr. Giuseppe Mastrangelo of Italy, reminded the group of a 1935 resolution by the Netherlands Medical Association aimed at the world's statesmen. It resolved that the principles of psychology should be applied to human relations everywhere. He felt that "scientists," as embodied in WFMH, had the responsibility of bringing "the great moral principle of the unity of the human race to the notice of nationalistically minded people who relied on force…social psychiatry should expose the pathological nature of the current war fever and undertake its treatment" (WFMH, 1950, pp. 99–100.).

A high minded view of the Federation's goals was also embodied in the remarks of Toronto Professor of Psychology Dr. William Line, who was WFMH president in 1950–1951. He referred to mental health as a "responsibility and challenge to every citizen of the world" who was concerned with "progressive social policy." It followed that "to be a widespread people's movement must, therefore, be one of the objectives of the Federation." And he expressed satisfaction that during the past year the Federation began "to take seriously the importance of social science to the movement itself." A seminar on infant development scheduled for July 1952 was regarded as an initial step "to broaden and deepen by research the foundations of knowledge on which, ultimately, our work must rest" (WFMH, 1951, pp. 7–8).

Psychiatrist Alan Stoller of Australia, who had a strong, conventionally medical bent, also felt that the Federation's aim should be reviewed from a scientific standpoint. Consequently the Interprofessional Advisory Committee composed of core members of the original International Preparatory Commission that had composed "Mental Health and World Citizenship" met from 24 March to 2 April 1951, in Dublin to consider the problem under the chairmanship of social anthropologist Professor T. S. Simey of the United Kingdom. The committee's considered view was that "WFMH should be regarded essentially as an international instrument for the application of scientific knowledge to the problems of promoting better mental health." These problems included "the treatment and prophylaxis of mental illness" as well as "the improvement of basic conditions of living and human relations" (WFMH, 1951c). Treating and preventing mental illness fitted the original goals of the International Committee for Mental Hygiene as well as the conventional missions of mental health associations. Improving the "basic conditions of living and human relations" constituted a link to the founders' initial brave goal of internationally diverse peoples harmoniously sharing the planet. During the Rees years this view legitimated Federation attention to a range of psychologically significant issues: poverty, childrearing, education, employment, racial prejudice, status of women, political oppression, urbanization, and technological change.

Migration, especially the involuntary dislocation of those uprooted by war, was another recurrent theme requiring both scientific research and the provision of service. In 1952, when Director Rees surveyed the four years of WFMH work since 1948, "studies of refugee problems" led the list of topics considered "of central importance" by the Interprofessional Advisory Committee. After this came concerns with the social consequences of technological change (a special interest of Margaret Mead), tensions and problems in international conferences, international institutes for education and research in mental health, seminars for high level personnel in international work, and mental health of children. There were also regional concerns: mental health issues in Africa, Germany, and Latin America (WFMH, 1952, pp.10–11).

Despite the apparent acceptance of both the psychiatric service reform and world peace goals of the Federation, the first U.S. WFMH president, Frank Fremont-Smith, M.D. (1954–1955), felt compelled to reassert its primary global peace mission. He wrote in the foreword to the 1955 annual report, "Have we indeed lost the enthusiasm generated in London in 1948 and are we today less concerned with world peace and the promotion of harmonious relations among all peoples? Or is it rather that we now recognize more fully that these central aims of the Federation constitute our long range goals and that many intermediate and more modest goals must be achieved before we can hope to contribute effectively to the prevention of war?" (WFMH, 1955a).

Speaking as a physician and foundation head who was accustomed to reviewing grant proposals, he attempted to reconcile the long range and intermediate goals of the organization. "Our Federation must have concrete, immediate and achievable goals based as firmly as possible upon scientific findings and pursued as far as possible by means of the scientific method, but we must never lose sight of our ultimate goal, the only goal that fully justifies our continued existence, that the insights of physicians, psychiatrists, social scientists and religious leaders be integrated and brought to bear upon the problems of social disharmony and human conflict, for the prevention of war; and upon the promotion of mental health for the fulfillment of the spiritual aspirations which are common to all mankind" (WFMH, 1955a).

The same effort at reconciling their own views was apparent in the utterances of various leaders who continued their efforts to clarify the Federation's mission for themselves. In every instance they linked public societal with private psychological concerns. Thus, at the August 1952 annual meeting in Brussels, Professor Auguste Ley of Belgium, a founder of the Belgian League for Mental Hygiene, described WFMH as "engaged on a continuous peace mission" with members working "for the improvement of human relations"(WFMH, 1952, p. 31). The introspective William Line, reflecting on the 1954 international congress in Toronto, felt that "to have symbolized the fundamental hope that honest partnership among the nations, among the humanistic disciplines, among the serious moral intents of people, can be addressed effectively to the pressing problems of human society, is—if real—a remarkable achievement." He spoke of "a re-awakened faith not only in the value of science…particularly in the science of man-but also in the dignity of the partnership between the scientist and the layman, the citizen…a renewed faith in the solidarity, spiritually, philosophically, scientifically and practically, of the design for living that the Mental Health Movement is seriously endeavouring to explore by *all* of the means at man's disposal" (WFMH, 1954, pp. 28–29).

Hans Hoff, M.D., Professor of Neurology and Psychiatry at the University of Vienna, concluded at the end of his 1958-1959 presidency that WFMH "in reality must play the role merely of a sociological catalyst whose primary function it is to stimulate and direct man's thinking toward the ultimate solution of his problems"(WFMH, 1959, p. 10).

The next president, Paul Sivadonna Professor of Psychiatry at Brussels, described the creation of WFMH as "an act of faith…by a few socially-minded men of science." He noted that while it grouped together in a world movement most who work "for the protection of mental health and the full development of human personality," it had accomplished something else. This was "the recognition of the gravity and vast scale of mental and social problems in the world of today" (WFMH, 1960, p. 12).

Director Rees, who had chaired the Third International Congress for Mental Hygiene during which WFMH was founded and had been its first president (1948–1949), maintained his eclectic pragmatic outlook without difficulty. He was ready to take advantage of any opportunity that presented itself to engage in advocacy for a mental health goal. Always integrating and compromising in the service of getting something done, his vision was not confined by a single "ultimate goal" for the Federation. Instead, in his tenth year with WFMH (noted in Chapter 8), he reiterated the inclusive view of its goals with a more modest reference to international relations. Thus, he viewed the "critical tensions in the world situation" as emphasizing "the need for better relationships and greater wisdom in the affairs of groups and nations as well as in individuals," with the Federation having a "responsibility…to try to add to the sum of wisdom available for those who govern." At the same time he noted the importance of ensuring "some steady progress in the care of the mentally sick and some advance in our comprehension of the basic facts about mental illness" so "succeeding generations might avoid mental illness and disability" (WFMH, 1957, p. 10). By this time advances in psychiatric knowledge and interest were also influencing the programs of Federation meetings. The 1957 annual meeting in Berlin, for example, included for the first time a conference on genetics and mental health, as well as sessions dealing with adolescence, crime, and juvenile delinquency.

The struggles of early Federation leaders to agree on appropriate and feasible goals for their new organization were all compatible with the perspective of the founding document. Especially as viewed through Rees' pragmatic eyes, a mentally healthy world was one in which people of differing beliefs, ethnicity, nationality, appearance, or other characteristics could live together in a peaceful and mutually constructive manner. The founding document based on a concept of supranational, nonpolitical allegiance to the human race made little reference to psychiatry or psychiatric illness, confining itself to references to "mental health." However, its encompassed such issues as access to care, standards of care (with special reference to patients' rights), and community based care before, after, or instead of, hospitalization.

The special conferences and WFMH projects of the Rees era are listed in Appendix I. They were often oriented toward studying a problem or gathering data. The topics, following Rees' own interest in human relations and group process, included the conduct of international meetings, the effective functioning of discussion groups and small conferences, and the behavior of international administrators. They also dealt, as noted above, with mental health in relation to general social and cultural problems such as prejudice, race relations, urbanization, infant development, migration, and family life. Aside from discussing the feasibility of psychiatric units in general hospitals, however, there was little of the contemporary mental health association focus on hospital practice and patients' rights.

The ethos of an annual meeting during these early years was that of an international study group with high value attached to research and science. This reflected the Board's inclusion of many scholars and university professors for whom scientific investigation and the exploration and integration of ideas had high value. Indeed, in his retrospective view of the recommendations of the International Preparatory Commission regarding the organization of national mental health services, Rees noted that they were addressed significantly to "universities" as well as "other institutions properly concerned with mental health" (Rees, 1966).

Rees also recognized that much of what the Federation did depended on its capacity as an international information disseminating body: "There has never been any serious doubt that the Federation as a channel of communication—by the written word and through personal contacts, in Annual Meetings, by visits and on other occasions—is fulfilling a valuable function in the transmission of ideas, the spread of knowledge and the maintenance of a sense of corporate interest in the problems of mental health as they affect the major part of the world" (WFMH, 1959a, p.11). What Rees described as "a sense of corporate interest" has also emerged in my own thinking about the Federation's emblematic function. Much of its information clearinghouse function supports its status as the emblem of a unique global entity, the international voluntary mental health movement.

The Search for a Method

Over the years WFMH has used many methods to further its aims. In 1948 the International Preparatory Commission recommended that the new Federation encourage the formation of associations "concerned with mental health problems ." According to Rees it succeeded in establishing "some 30 or 40" of these in the 1950s, most of which became Federation members. The seeding of new organizations has continued as a major Federation activity. Rees also understood that advocacy and education directed to the new United Nations was an important means of achieving Federation goals. United Nations advocacy has continued as one of the most important WFMH activities. For this reason Chapter 8 is devoted to WFMH-United Nations relations.

An important element of the Rees program was sending consultants to speak to governments engaged in developing mental health services and to national mental health associations. Most paid their own expenses and felt amply recompensed by the opportunity to see new places, make new friends, and contribute their knowledge in a helpful way.

The Federation's founders placed great faith in the creative potential of small group discussions involving professionals of many disciplines. Confidence in small group discussions of people with diverse training and backgrounds grew in part from the determinedly interdisciplinary UNESCO conferences on "tensions which cause wars." Social scientists such as Mead and Klineberg, and socially oriented psychiatrists such as Sullivan and Chisholm, were especially inclined by education, experience, and sentiment to agree with the value of this kind of discussion. Most were familiar with the generation of ideas in conversation, and enjoyed the process.

During the Federation's first year (1948–1949), the small group method was further refined. A report of discussions during the third annual meeting of WFMH in Paris in 1950 acknowledged the "cross-national, cross-professional nature of the participants" as "a major stimulus for productive discussion." At the same time doubts were expressed: "The Federation has a great deal at stake in relying on interprofessional and international discussion groups as its main working method at annual meetings. This is a new technique which is not yet highly developed. There are problems in efficiently selecting and briefing the participants" (WFMH, 1950).

Klineberg, one of the major proponents of the small group approach to problem solving wrote "WFMH has the very interesting procedure...of not merely holding annual meetings, but of getting a lot of people working on problems in preparation for these meetings." In preparation for the December 1951 meeting in Mexico (later designated a world congress) four areas of mental health study were defined: education, industry, the transfer of populations (migration and immigration), and problems of leadership, both local and general. "This is being set up through local groups and societies in various parts of the world in the form of research studies, the pooling of information across disciplinary lines...so that there will be a body of data ready for international discussion at the time of the next Congress" (WFMH, 1951b, p. 252).

An interest in the small group approach was inherent in Rees' own Tavistock background in "human relations." He put the idea into action in 1946, calling for interdisciplinary "preparatory commissions" (i.e., working groups) in as many countries as possible to explore ideas related to mental health that could form the basis for a new international, interdisciplinary, nongovernmental, and voluntary mental health organization. He also managed the process of distilling ideas from their reports and organizing the International Preparatory Commission that, meeting in Roffey Park two weeks before the Third International Congress on Mental Hygiene, produced the Federation's founding document, "Mental Health and World Citizenship." The details of the process and the content of the document are described in Chapter 2. This experience among others instilled an optimism about the approach that he later felt had been confirmed by the enthusiastic response to the discussion or study groups that were part of every annual meeting as well as special conferences or seminars: "Our belief in the value of work in small free discussion groups seems to be justified. and this is particularly true in relation to the Seminars which have been organized" (Rees, 1966).

Despite this enthusiasm, however, Rees was, as suggested above, less tied to the particular technique than to the overall importance of communication in the service of advocacy and education. "Although we are by no means satisfied with the techniques we employ for running international meetings or congresses we have the conviction that some real purpose is served by such meetings. Members of our member societies make new contacts and exchange ideas, and consequently get considerable stimulus for their work. The societies of the country where the meetings are held benefit considerably by the enlarged interest that is created and despite their shortcomings there seems little doubt that the interprofessional international working groups which assemble on these occasions provide an experience which is valuable and which is reflected in the later work of many people in different countries" (WFMH, 1953a, pp. 11–12).

The 1951 Interprofessional Advisory Committee proposal that WFMH should be an international instrument for the application of scientific knowledge to mental health problems carried its own methodological agenda: "In order to deal effectively with these problems it [is] necessary for WFMH to collect and assess all existing scientific knowledge in the field of mental health, extend it through research, and subsequently disseminate it by all possible means" (WFMH, 1951c). A fundamental means of achieving these aims would be the establishment of an international institute for mental health. This ambitious idea interested several members, notably anthropologist Margaret Mead. Eventually a formal proposal for an institute at McGill University in Montreal "for research and training in the field of world mental health" was considered by a joint planning committee convened by George S. Stevenson, M.D. The committee included Klineberg, William Line Ph.D., Professor of Psychology at Toronto who became WFMH president in that year, and McGill University representatives headed by D. Ewen Cameron, M.D., Chairman of the Department of Psychiatry . Detailed plans were formulated but eventually abandoned because adequate funding could not be obtained. Nonetheless, the call for increased attention to science continued to recur depending upon who was president. At the end of the decade Hoff still called for an extension of the Federation research program "to fortify our scientific foundations" (WFMH, 1959, p. 9).

THE ERA OF "WORKING PRESIDENTS"

Rees retired at the end of 1961. After this the systematic use of small-group preparatory discussions was largely abandoned, although it was revived in principle for occasional conferences, mainly in Europe. During the years beginning with 1962, especially after the final financial collapse and 1967 closure of the Geneva Secretariat (see Chapters 3–5), the focus of WFMH leaders was largely on ensuring the organization's survival. From 1968 to 1979, as the "working presidents" struggled to keep the organization alive, their programmatic emphases varied with available opportunities. These included linking WFMH with nationally or regionally sponsored professional and voluntary organization conferences, piggybacking WFMH onto United Nations conferences, and finding other opportunities in their personal professorial capacities (see Chapter 5). Carstairs, who assumed the presidency at the end of 1967, maintaining it in his Edinburgh University offices until 1972, wrote that in the new circumstances, "the main roles of WFMH are communication and mutual aid between associations in many countries which share its aims and which are confronted with similar problems and similar practical tasks.... One important task is to identify areas of special need. When this is done there are resources of financial and practical know-how within its membership which will help to meet these needs, one by one. It is my hope that in the next few years when people ask us: 'What does WFMH stand for, anyway ?' we can point to deeds and not volumes of words as our best answer" (WFMH, 1968a).

In 1972–1974 under President Michael Beaubrun in Jamaica (see Chapter 9), the agenda was primarily carried forward by showing the WFMH flag at Caribbean events and his occasional attendance at meetings elsewhere in the world. He also presided at the 1973 World Congress in Australia from which he issued an early statement condemning Soviet abuse of psychiatry to stifle the utterances of political dissidents.

In his opening address to the August 1975 World Congress in Copenhagen President Tsung-yi Lin listed as his "First Law of Mental Health" the traditional commitment "to make mental health services of quality available to the greatest number of people in all lands." A former WHO scientist, his major emphasis (as indicated in Chapter 8) was influencing United Nations agencies to include mental health in their programs. In addition he promoted regional programs and the importance of WFMH vice president's offices. Although Lin could not convince WHO or Unicef, the agencies of greatest interest to him, to create joint programs with WFMH, the success of the 1977 World Congress in Vancouver under his leadership with that of Professor Milton Miller, M.D. (Chairman of the Department of Psychiatry, University of British Columbia), restored much of the Federation's international visibility (see Chapter 10). From 1979–1981 under lawyer-businessman President Gowan Guest of Vancouver the programmatic agenda was largely static (see Chapter 5).

1981–1983 AND BEYOND: PROGRAM DEVELOPMENT IN THE CONTEXT OF A STABLE SECRETARIAT

Transition

After the Manila World Congress in August 1981, the Federation's nerve center shifted rapidly away from Vancouver. Although the Baltimore-Washington Secretariat was not formally established until autumn 1983, Dick Hunter and I were already at work in our geographically divided headquarters. My office as WFMH president was first at the University of Maryland medical school and then at the Sheppard Pratt Hospital, both in Baltimore. Dick's office was at the United States National Mental Health Association first in Arlington, then in Alexandria, Virginia, just outside of Washington, DC. Although we still depended on the Vancouver office, the future was already with us. As president I functioned as chief executive while Dick chaired the arrangements committee for the 1983 World Congress for Mental Health.

Inevitably, he devoted more time to organizational processes and fundraising, while I was more concerned with the content of the congress and its relation to future Federation programs. I believed that our international character should determine our agenda. In my inaugural speech in Manila, entitled "An Agenda for the 1980s," I followed my predecessors of the Rees era in recognizing the Federation's role as advocate for the "socially deprived, disenfranchised, chronic mental hospital patients and their families" (Brody, 1984, pp. 331–332). While remembering the goals of prevention and protecting the rights of access on an international basis, I also emphasized the concern with social conditions that would promote the optimal growth and development of individuals in all societies and cultures. This, too, was compatible with the philosophy of the Rees era. Although I was aware of the Federation's capacity for independent action, I stressed the relationship with the United Nations agencies as our major operating modality.

Two issues, both with human rights and prevention aspects, impressed me as especially relevant to international mental health concerns. One was the mental health of minorities, however defined. This included the problems of migrants, refugees, and interracial, intercultural, and interethnic relations. The second was the failure of communities to provide equitable health care and developmental and educational opportunities for all their citizens. Finally I stressed the "symbolic and emblematic importance of a worldwide Federation of mental health associations—one which includes both volunteers and professionals" (Brody, 1984, pp. 333–334).

It seemed clear that "as a multicultural, multinational organization WFMH should have a special interest in how mental health at various points in the life cycle is influenced by socioeconomic, cultural, and other factors" (WFMH, 1981a, p. 63). In an article for the American Anthropological Association newsletter these and several related themes were noted among our continuing interests to be addressed at the 1983 congress. They included "the problems of minority groups, migrants and refugees, women with special reference to fertility-related behavior, pregnant mothers and those with very young infants, and victims of violence" (AAA, 1981). The article reminded readers that I was the second Federation president (after Margaret Mead) to belong to the anthropological association.

Defining the relationship between mental health and mental illness required repeated clarifying messages (Brody, 1981a, 1987, 1995). This was partly because changes in the membership of the WFMH Board of Directors influenced its climate of opinion. A welcome consequence of establishing a stable Secretariat in 1983 was that for the first time since the closing of the Geneva Secretariat, people without institutional support could serve as elected members of the Board. This resulted in change. Although university professors remained as leaders and contributors, they were replaced as major sources of influence by mental health association executives and volunteers who had held elective office in their national mental health associations.

The change in the culture of the Board was manifested in the substantive content of its discussions. In comparison with the Rees era it became less focused on international relations and the mental health of the world understood in terms of peaceful global relations, less interested in research, and less explicit regarding issues relevant to prevention. The Board became more concerned with typical mental health association issues such as the humane care of hospitalized people, aftercare, community based services, and the role of consumers—or "users" (term preferred in Europe)—of mental health services (see Chapter 8). Practicality and immediate action, utilizing already available knowledge, became more important. "Good practices" was a watchword put forward by Edith Morgan (president 1985–1987), who had headed a group promoting good practices in mental health for the International Hospital Federation in London. Those European groups making up the European Regional Council of the WFMH (ERC/WFMH) recognized the value of research but felt that it was not the proper focus of Federation interest. In 1996 the ERC/WFMH chairman and WFMH regional vice president, John Henderson, M.D., and its executive director, Josee van Remoortel, wrote me expressing their view that WFMH should abandon its program of university based, research and service focused, collaborating centers because they were irrelevant to our mission.

Although these exclusionary views were not shared by the rest of the Board it became necessary to indicate the interconnections of the various aspects of mental health. The WHO definition of health formulated by Chisholm, its first Director General and a founder of WFMH, proved useful in this respect. It is "more than the absence of disease or infirmity…a state of complete physical, mental and social well-being" (World Health Organization, 1946). Prevention, as a link between the broadly social and international and the more narrowly clinical, became a leading advocacy issue.

Reformulating the Agenda after 1983

In my first message as Secretary General, in the first issue of the revived and reformatted newsletter after a lapse of approximately two years, I continued to define the Federation in traditional mental health association terms. This was as an advocacy and educational organization with "efforts directed mainly toward enhancing the rights and welfare of the mentally ill and their families, and toward preventing mental disorder, deficit and disability" (WFMH, 1984). However, our presentations to foundations and other potential donors required a new, more comprehensive, mission statement. A step in this direction was taken on 25 April 1984, when, largely at Dick Hunter's initiative, we convened a group that met for nine hours in Arlington, Virginia. A lawyer, five psychiatrists including myself, an academic social worker, and three nonprofessional volunteers including Dick were members of the group. They were our treasurer, lawyer Joel Klein (counsel for the American Psychiatric Association) and American Psychiatric Association Medical Director Melvin Sabshin, M.D., both of whom I had appointed to our Board. Also with us were Thomas Bryant, M.D., Director of the Carter administration's Commission on Mental Illness, Herbert Pardes, M.D., former director of the National Institute of Mental Health who chaired Columbia University's Department of Psychiatry, Dr. Herman Stein, Distinguished Professor of Social Work at Case Western Reserve University, Shirley Starr of the U.S. National Alliance for the Mentally Ill, Harold Visotsky, M.D., Chairman of the American Psychiatric Association's Council on International Affairs, and Ellie Kohn, former officer of the U.S. National Mental Health Association.

It took all day to reach consensus on a mission statement sufficiently comprehensive to satisfy potential donors, our members, our beneficiaries, and our Board and, at the same time, to maintain some semblance of specificity. It was disappointing that the Board did not examine it closely and seemed to take the effort for granted. The statement was approved with minimal discussion at the Board meeting at Sheppard Pratt Hospital in Baltimore on 24–25 May 1984.

The statement focused on four major aims, all of which reflected our international, multidisciplinary, and voluntary status: (*a*) advocacy for increasing the knowledge base essential to understanding the causes, treatment, management, and prevention of mental disorders and disability; (*b*) advocacy for applying current knowledge about these matters with special emphasis on prevention; (*c*) identification, discussion, and support of the mental health issues inherent in all public policy debates; and (*d*) encouragement of the development of mental health associations and WFMH support groups in as many of the world's regions as possible.

One of these four aims was accepted in principle but not put into action. That was the aim of identifying relevant mental health issues in all public policy debates (*c*). It has been largely ignored, partly because of lack of necessary staff support. After the 1991 World Congress in Mexico, President-elect Federico Puente, M.D., unaware of the 1984 statement, deplored the Federation's failure to take positions on major issues with mental health relevance. Again the Board recognized the potential importance of this goal but accepted its inability to act upon it because of the lack of an adequate Federation infrastructure. Another, sometimes compelling, reason for not pursuing it has been the fact that many public issues are national or regional rather than global and can be more effectively addressed by national or regional organizations. In Europe the task has become a responsibility of ERC/WFMH. In North America this aim has been effectively carried out by organizational coalitions led by the U.S. and Canadian voluntary mental health associations and the national professional associations in psychiatry, psychology, social work, nursing, and other health disciplines. In other regions leading national mental health associations, or to a limited degree the new regional councils, have published policy statements about issues relevant to mental health.

Two of the four aims have remained central to WFMH work. First, advocacy for primary prevention (*b*), always recognized as a logical Federation aim, has assumed increasing emphasis with the passage of time. Second, there has never been any question about the importance of stimulating the development of local and national mental health associations (*d*) that would then become affiliated with WFMH.

As noted in Chapters 5, 7, and 13, two types of associations have not been recruited to WFMH membership. One type has been associations of relatives and families. They were not recruited because their concern with supervising and controlling the behavior of psychotic family members, especially chronically ill young adults in the community, has conflicted with the emphasis on individual autonomy espoused both by the U.S. National Mental Health Association and the various users' groups. The association most interested in participating in our meetings was the World Schizophrenia Fellowship, and I facilitated the inclusion of Diane Froggett, its executive director, in our World Congress programs, beginning in 1993 in Tokyo. However, close collaboration has not yet developed.

Dr. Maria Simon, our WFMH senior representative to United Nations Vienna and a one-time president of the Austrian Association of Relatives of the Mentally Ill, did not find WFMH a sympathetic forum for her concerns and in 1995 delivered a major lecture on the subject at the annual meeting of another nongovernmental organization.

There has also been controversy about supporting research, a principle that would seem to warrant no conflict. As noted above, ERC/WFMH expressed serious reservations about whether this is an appropriate Federation activity. Particularly negative feelings have emerged about supporting studies on the pharmacological treatment of mental illness, partly because this might create conflict with its increasingly influential consumer/user constituency.

In 1987 at the precongress Board in Cairo, just four years after establishing the new Secretariat, I noted that under the presidencies of Estafania Aldaba-Lim (1983–1985) and Edith Morgan (1985–1987) our goals had become more sharply focused on preventing mental illness and ill health in vulnerable populations (women, very young, elderly, refugees, and victims of trauma) and promoting the therapeutic care and protection of the human rights of those already ill. Beyond these patient oriented aims, special efforts were made "to renew our commitment to the hope of our founding members: that the promotion of mental health might be used as a route to building a world community" (Flugel, 1948a and d) Much of this community building was carried out through telephone, fax, and face-to-face communication as well as through the newsletters and WFMH sponsored conferences. Major opportunities for informal advocacy and recruitment to our cause arose with increasing frequency during meetings and professional contacts.

Some of these contacts led to increased interest in the mental health of indigenous peoples, a seemingly natural issue for WFMH. This was a long-time professional concern of North American Regional Vice President Morton Beiser (1979–1983) and was addressed in many sessions at the 1977 Vancouver World Congress. In succeeding years social and political conflicts involving North American indigenous peoples, especially in Canada, kept the issue alive. It became a focus at the 1987 meetings of the national mental health associations in Australia and New Zealand and the 1989 World Congress for Mental Health in Auckland because of the aborigines in Australia and the Maori in New Zealand. There was recurrent recognition of the issue, e.g., by psychiatrist-anthropologist Maurice Eisenbruch, M.D., in regard to minority groups in Cambodia and elsewhere in Southeast Asia. A brief flurry of interest in a nongovernmental organization committee on indigenous people emerged at United Nations New York. A committee was formed, headed by former New Zealand Governor General Sir Paul Reeves. However, specific WFMH activity in this area did not continue, although it resurfaced in the context of advocacy for minority groups in general or concerns with human rights of particular populations such as women subject to genital mutilation.

Increasing Specificity of Subgoals

The deliberations of the April 1984 group had no discernible effect on Federation programmatic activity. Instead, the mission gradually became specified in terms of potential target or client groups. This was partly a matter of availability and partly the consequence of the continuing WFMH philosophy of caring for the "human family," this last stemming both from the WFMH founding document of 21 August 1948, and the 10 December 1948, United Nations Universal Declaration of Human Rights that referred to "the inherent dignity and...the equal and inalienable rights" of all human beings. Both implied a cross-cultural and international perspective concerned with reconciling the universal with the particular. This perspective became clear in discussions in the late 1980s and 1990s with leaders of our collaborating centers. Possible public mental health programs and advocacy involving supranational goals were described with an emphasis on understanding "the relation between the universal value of scientifically informed health care on one hand, and, on the other, the particular values rooted in the long family and tribal traditions of individual societies and cultures" (Brody, 1991, p. 8). The emphasis was on access to basic, dignified, humane, and competent health care as a human right, understanding that to be effective it could not be perceived as damaging to the particular societies concerned.

In a later Secretary General's annual report this view was elaborated to indicate that "our emphasis, whenever possible, is on socially and culturally appropriate initiatives carried out by members of the community in which the work is done. However, it is sometimes necessary to make difficult discriminations between goals and ideals presumed to have universal validity... and those which are accepted and can be implemented in particular settings" (Brody, 1993c). In this report, I summarized what we had actually been doing. It was apparent that our service and consultation functions were largely through collaborating centers and regional councils (see Chapters 9–11). Our advocacy and education functions were carried out by all Federation components, the Secretariat, Board, committees, and collaborating centers. They included "improving the quality of mental health services and the life circumstances of those who suffer from mental illness, distress and disability all over the world; promoting and protecting the human rights of persons defined as mentally ill; and preventing mental/emotional illness, distress, disability and less than optimal function in vulnerable groups at risk as well as general populations" (Brody, 1993c). In every year the most pressing international mental health challenge was that presented by the swelling streams of traumatized refugees and other migrants.

In spring 1997 the goals were restated twice with slightly different emphases. First, the distillation of conference calls preparatory to an early May strategic planning retreat (see Chapters 5 and 13) led to a mission statement emphasizing public and legislative awareness of mental health issues and advocacy for primary prevention, mental health promotion, and improved delivery of mental health services.

Second, my Secretary General's report for 1996, issued after the May 1997 retreat, also described WFMH as an advocacy and educational organization with major efforts aimed at the United Nations, government agencies, public and private institutions, and the general public. I noted that some clinical, personnel training, and research activities were performed by the collaborating centers and regional councils. Advocacy and education goals were pursued, as in earlier years, through regional conferences, biennial world congresses, individual discussions, consultation on request, and, since 1992, the yearly World Mental Health Day cosponsored by WHO. Additionally, local groups were empowered by regional organizations that helped establish new mental health associations; efforts continued to build networks or coalitions with other organizations to exert maximum advocacy leverage. International collaboration in regard to these activities was so routine that it did not warrant special mention.

The vulnerable groups identified by WFMH as possibly in need of advocacy for issues related to mental health (especially prevention and service access) included women of reproductive age (especially those who were pregnant), infants and children, elderly, socioeconomically disadvantaged, refugees and other migrants, child victims of war, and those subject to discrimination for any reason as well as "persons defined as mentally ill who constitute a minority in every society" (Brody, 1993c, p. 10).

To address these issues a series of committees or working groups came into being. Their performance and effectiveness have been variable and some were destined to have a short life. They dealt with substance abuse, commercial sexual exploitation of children, community care, emergency mental health, human rights and legal affairs, prevention of mental and psychosocial disorders, refugees and migrants, responsible parenthood, smoking and mental health, and women's issues.

The process of forming committees began at the Washington World Congress in July 1983. It was obvious that the committees had to be self-financing and self-propelled. Because WFMH could offer no money and only minimal advice we looked for people whose lives and professional trajectories were already focused on issues that concerned us and who had something to gain from acquiring WFMH credentials, connections, and advice.

Collaborating Centers

In 1981, shorlty after becoming president, I decided to borrow an idea from WHO and initiate a system of university based, research and teaching oriented collaborating centers for

WFMH. There were two reasons for this. First, neither the Board nor the Secretariat nor our committees or working groups had the resources or expertise necessary to move our broad agenda forward. This required, in my view, a group of university based entities that could provide a scientific/technological basis for our advocacy and give us a connection with the scientific/professional world.

The second reason was the difficulty in forming advocacy and perhaps service coalitions with professional organizations which could supply resources and expertise that we did not have. It was this hope that led me as president to bring members of the American Psychiatric Association and American Psychological Association onto our Board. Unlike WFMH these have relatively homogeneous bases, are well funded with economically bound constituencies, tightly organized and, most importantly, have a clear agenda. Some organizations of which I had been president, such as the Association for Behavioral Science in Medical Education, or a Board member, such as the International College of Pediatrics, became WFMH members for a time—mainly in response to my personal urging. However, even with goodwill and the best intentions we could not find a common focus for continuing joint programmatic activity.

It took a while to implement the idea, but the possibility of recruiting collaborating centers was facilitated by the establishment of the new Secretariat in September 1983. Some time earlier Sheppard Kellam, M.D., had come to the Johns Hopkins University School of Public Health, easily accessible from my Baltimore office, as chairman of its Department of Mental Hygiene, the only formally organized mental hygiene department in a school of public health in the world. Under its previous chairmen, including Professor Paul Lemkau, M.D., a former North American vice president of WFMH, it had a distinguished record of research and applications in psychiatric epidemiology and the relationship of social environment to mental illness. "Shep" Kellam, who had been the last resident I hired at Yale before leaving for Maryland in 1957, was an old friend, and I was pleased, after retiring from the University of Maryland, to accept an appointment to his faculty. This gave me a chance to become acquainted with his Center for Prevention that had already been designated by WHO and the National Institute of Mental Health as a collaborator with them. In 1986 the Johns Hopkins Prevention Center in Baltimore became WFMH's first collaborating center. However, the process of converting this relationship into a genuine collaboration was slow. In 1988–1989 we worked with Professor Morton Kramer of its faculty to develop information relevant to stimulating the formation of new mental health associations in Africa. But it was not until 1990, when North American Vice President Beverly Long began to engage in regular consultations with Kellam regarding the development of a WFMH Committee on Primary Prevention, that the vision of true collaboration was achieved. Long's suggestion that collaborating centers have a designated point of contact with the Federation, perhaps a related committee, was adopted as an operating principle. In 1992 the Prevention Committee in conjunction with the center agreed on a detailed plan of work, focusing on childhood and adolescence. This fitted a major element of the center's agenda dealing with precursors of later illness and deviance in school-age children and developing and initiating appropriate preventive interventions. In 1993 Kellam resigned as chairman of mental hygiene to devote his full energies to research on prevention.

The next group to become a collaborating center was the International Institute for Psycho-Social and Socio-Ecological Research (IPSER) of the University of Limburg in Maastricht, The Netherlands, headed by Professor of Social Psychiatry Marten de Vries, M.D. IPSER's research program focused on training mental health counselors in many African countries with special reference to refugees and other traumatized migrants. De Vries was a longtime student of problems in the borderland between psychiatry and anthropology. I had known him since the 1970s when, as a graduate student in cultural anthropology at Harvard, he had visited me in Baltimore to discuss the problems of field work in relation to mental illness. We had renewed our acquaintance at various meetings, and he expressed a strong interest in WFMH as a possible facilitating mechanism for the research and training being conducted by his institute in several countries, mainly Africa. IPSER was recommended as a collaborating center at the 1989 Auckland World Congress after several visits to Maastricht by WFMH President Stanislas Flache (1989–1991).

The third group to become affiliated was the Key Centre for Women's Health in Society, a unit of the Department of Community Health at the University of Melbourne in Australia. Psychiatrist Lorraine Dennerstein, M.D., its director, had been a colleague for several years when we were both on the Board of International Society of Psychosomatic Obstetrics and Gynecology, and it had been my pleasure to write a supporting letter for the Key Centre's establishment as the first formally organized university department of women's health in the world. Since then it had earned international acclaim for its work and, as described in Chapter 8, had been useful in the work of our UNESCO contract on new reproductive technologies and women's rights and roles. After my visit there in 1989 I recommended it as a WFMH collaborating center, and it was approved on 15 February 1990.

A fourth center was formed at the suggestion of Richard Mollica, M.D., chair of our WFMH Committee on Refugees and director of the Harvard Program in Refugee Trauma (HPRT). This was the Service for the Treatment and Rehabilitation of Torture Survivors (STARTTS) associated with the University of New South Wales in Sydney, Australia. The colleague best known to us was consultant Derek Silove, M.D., Professor of Psychiatry at the university. The actual director was Margaret Cunningham, M.S.W. STARTTS was recommended for collaborating center status to the July 1990 Board meeting in Geneva by Trevor Elligott, Vice President for the WFMH Oceania region and was later approved after a presentation by Cunningham at the 1992 Board meeting in Sydney.

The fifth group was HPRT itself. I had known Mollica for many years because of shared professional interests, and he was a student at a summer course on "Humane Aspects of the British Health System" that I had codirected in Oxford and Cambridge. More recently I had served as a consultant to the Indochinese Psychiatry Clinic that he founded and directed under the auspices of the Harvard School of Public Health in Boston. I was a frequent teaching consultant to the clinic and used WFMH credentials to facilitate its work with the United Nations Border Relief Organization on the Thai-Cambodian border. When Mollica established HPRT in 1987, therefore, it was natural for me to became its "Senior Advisor." At that time and at my request he formed a WFMH Committee on Refugees and other migrants that, with various regional concentrations and its nucleus at HPRT, was the Federation's primary service, research, and advocacy arm aimed at alleviating the mental health problems of refugees. In 1992 HPRT was designated as a WFMH collaborating center. James Lavelle, M.S.W. remained as its executive officer, and Kathleen Allden, M.D., continued as medical director of the Indochinese Psychiatry Clinic.

In response to the Federation's need for a center of work on aging to promote our global concerns in this area, the 1995 President-elect Marten de Vries recommended an affiliation with the University of Liverpool's Institute of Ageing directed by Professor John Copeland. I attended the session at the 1995 Dublin World Congress in 1995 at which he and Professor Tsung-yi Lin presented their work on aging in Taiwan, and we later initiated correspondence. By the time we met again at the Western Pacific regional meeting in Taiwan in December 1996, the application for his unit to become a collaborating center had been approved at the Concepción, Chile, Board meeting earlier in the month.

As time went on it was apparent that many benefits flowed from these affiliations. Federation concerns sometimes stimulated elements of their work. They in turn could benefit not only from our credentials but from the opportunity to become part of our worldwide network of professionals, consumers, and other volunteers. In our turn, we benefited not only from their consultation and technical advice but from the opportunity to influence their work, the favorable publicity that they could afford us, and the benefits of associations with strong institutions rooted in particular world regions. It was especially gratifying to note the effective mental health advocacy of the Centers' scientist-clinician leaders.

RECURRING QUESTIONS AND AMBIGUITIES

Two overlapping questions about the WFMH program or, as I conceptualized it, the "international mental health agenda" (Brody, 1987a) have recurred during our half century of existence. Both involve the way in which mental health is defined and its relation to the definition of mental ill health, illness, or disease. They have arisen with sufficient frequency to warrant repeated clarifying letters and newsletter messages (Brody, 1995).

The first question concerns the relation between mental health and mental illness. I remember being bemused by this long before I had given thought to an international mental health movement. It was after the Boston Psychopathic Hospital, where as a Harvard medical school student I had had a psychiatric clerkship in 1943, changed its name to the Massachusetts Mental Health Center (Brody, 1981a). There was no discernible difference in the kinds of people who arrived there for help after it was called a "mental health center" rather than a "psychopathic hospital" nor was there a difference in the kinds of techniques employed to assist them. Most important, perhaps, the institution's designation as a "mental health center" was not accompanied by a new effort to promote positive mental health, however defined, or to promote primary prevention of disorders of thinking, acting, or feeling. Efforts at secondary and tertiary prevention in the sense of early diagnosis and treatment leading to diminution in the severity and chronicity of disorders fitted the former psychiatric-medical model and continued.

The uncertain relation between mental health and illness appears to have been an issue for the founders of WFMH. As described in Chapter 2, along with their "one world" focus at the International Preparatory Commission in Roffey Park, their later articles of incorporation included a clinically oriented mission statement to guide future activities. Still valid, it encompasses both the positive health of all human beings and the need to deal with illness. Its reference to "the *mental health* of *all* of the world's peoples" supports the goals of the founding document, "Mental Health and World Citizenship." That is, it promotes the idea of the world's diverse peoples living together harmoniously. It reaffirms the need to construct international and intercultural bridges. However, its specification of the "medical" as well as the " biological, social and educational" aspects of mental health implies a concern with treating mental illness. It reveals the Federation's twin roots: the oldest in Clifford Beers' International Committee for Mental Hygiene first conceived to "protect the insane" and the more recent in the idealism of the post-World War II era.

The second question about the WFMH program deals with its effectiveness in relation to its breadth. Are we more likely to lose our leverage, to obtain support for, or to achieve our goals through the inclusive mental health message contained in the broad range of Federation initiatives? Or would we have greater leverage, a greater likelihood of success, if we concentrated on one or two well defined programs and focused our efforts on obtaining support for them? There are no data to substantiate any view because there has been no Federation attempt to evaluate the outcomes of its initiatives. In spring 1997 this was one of the topics that emerged in a strategic planning retreat called by President Beverly Long (see Chapter 5). However, the four goals that emerged from a scrutiny of the Federation's present and future programmatic focus were neither significantly different nor significant narrower than those of the past.

The first goal, as WFMH faced the 21st century, was prevention, with an implicit focus on its primary aspects. A second goal was closely related but difficult to define: promoting positive mental health. The third was traditional in scope: improving the care of the mentally ill, which could include anything from service delivery to protection of human rights, including a right of access to a universally acceptable level of care. The fourth goal, conceptualized as raising the public awareness of issues related to mental health, was aimed in part at the internationally influential agencies of the United Nations, especially WHO and in part national health ministries. It was also recognized as the aim of the Federation's world congresses and the many regional meetings to which it lent its name and influenced their programs as a cosponsor.

As WFMH's first 50 years are completed, its mission and goals, with their strengths and ambiguities, have proved their resilience and value.

Chapter 13

Persisting Programmatic Themes:
The International Mental Health Agenda

WHAT COMES UNDER "THE BIG TENT"?
Mental Health Reform and International Harmony

During its 50 years of existence WFMH has been a unique global force for mental health through specific streams of advocacy and service. Varying in nature and intensity, their direction and accomplishments have constantly been weighed against the original mission: Mental health for "all the world's peoples." This broad charge required a multifaceted approach. Early leaders recognized the diverse ways of making it operational. They saw no conflict between the 1919 heritage of the International Committee for Mental Hygiene, the mental hospital and patient care reform movement, and the post-1948 aims of promoting world peace and "harmonious" international and intercultural relationships. Nonetheless, as indicated in Chapter 12, they felt that the two aims required some conceptual integration. This was accomplished by suggesting that a mentally healthy world requires that people of differing beliefs, ethnicity, nationality, and appearance live together in a peaceful and mutually constructive manner. That legitimated efforts to achieve tolerance, nonviolent conflict resolution, and respect for human rights as well as to prevent and treat mental illness and less than optimal health.

The programmatic issue most obviously connecting the international and intercultural concerns of the WFMH founders with those of the International Committee for Mental Hygiene and the more narrowly defined mental health community was prevention. Focusing on prevention directed attention to (a) early development as it influenced infant and childhood experience and (b) the broad socioeconomic and cultural circumstances of life as they affected such basic determinants of health as reproduction and child caring. There was no doubt in the minds of the founders, as expressed by Rees (1996), that prevention should be the Federation's central advocacy and education thrust.

A second area linking patient care with international harmony was that of human rights. It bore on members of minority groups and victims of abusive governments and minorities, as well as persons diagnosed as mentally ill and detained in mental hospitals. Mental health professionals were seen as agents of society who could abuse or protect human rights. This became a matter of particular interest to ex-patients, including those who styled themselves "users" of psychiatric services or "survivors of psychiatry" (see Chapter 7). In the 1980s UNESCO sponsored Federation attention to the human rights concerns raised by advancing biomedical technology. This was an extension of its earlier attention to individual and cultural adaptations to general technological change (see Chapter 8; Mead, 1953; Brody, 1993b).

A third international and intercultural issue attracting early WFMH attention was the plight of the swelling populations of traumatized refugees from war and collective abuse. Their problems overlapped with those of "voluntary" migrants escaping economic hardship and searching for a better future for their children. Although advocacy for more effective material aid was important, it was clear in the long run that mental health service and research were also essential. WFMH recognized the importance of refugee issues in its founding document and was an advisor to the UN refugee agency in 1957. However, it did not become actively engaged in actual refugee services and research until the 1980s through its affiliation with the Harvard Program in Refugee Trauma (HPRT). It also formed a WFMH committee on the mental health of refugees and other migrants.

By the time that a new international Secretariat was becoming established in Baltimore-Washington in 1981–1983, WFMH advocacy covered a range of loosely interrelated issues. In a release to the newsletter of the American Anthropological Association I included the following among concerns to be addressed at the 1983 World Congress in Washington, DC: "problems of minority groups, migrants and refugees, women with special reference to fertility-related behavior, pregnant mothers and those with very young infants, victims of violence" and "human rights especially in regard to the functioning of social institutions in the mental health field" (AAA, 1981).

Means and Ends

Some Federation activities could be regarded as ends in themselves, whereas others were more obviously means to accomplishing the WFMH mission. A case in point was advocacy to change the attitudes of United Nations leaders (e.g., to make them more sensitive to mental health issues) or to encourage certain actions by United Nations agencies (e.g., to provide psychiatric care for refugees). Some early annual reports listed the development of a network of nongovernmental organizations (NGOs) to work with the United Nations as part of the WFMH mission. In 1948 the International Preparatory Commission encouraged the formation of local and national associations "concerned with mental health problems." These sources of power and initiative can assess needs and effect culturally acceptable change in their areas. Increasing their number and effectiveness could be regarded as an end in itself.

I had thought that a central Federation activity would be bringing the widely dispersed national mental health associations together to exchange information and ideas. It was a surprise, therefore, to learn that WFMH sponsored no regular formal meeting of these member associations. The only possible forum was the annual Assembly that confined itself largely to voting in congress years and was sparsely attended and relatively inactive in intervening years. I resolved to remedy this situation, and at the 1983 Washington World Congress initiated the first Mental Health Association Day. It was intended to bring member organizations together in a formal forum to share experiences and make suggestions for Federation work. Board member Hilda Robbins of the United States agreed to assume the day's organization and direction. Under her inspired and intelligent guidance it was a major success, and with her continued organizational direction it became a regular function of later WFMH World Congresses. She also developed a committee on mental health associations to promote the work. This proved useful in less developed parts of the world, but the leaders of our developing European Council became increasingly reluctant to have non-Europeans help build mental health associations in their territory. As the administrative structure tightened and became bureaucratized, they also preferred that member associations in their region route their communications to the Board and Secretariat through the Regional Council.

Committees and Collaborating Centers

From 1948 through 1967 programmatic initiatives came mainly from the Director's office to the Board. From 1967 through 1983, when there was no Director in the mold of John Rees, they came almost exclusively from the "working president." But as my 1981–1983 term as president reached its midway mark, I realized what others had learned before me: the absence of regular funding and lack of an infrastructure made it impossible to plan an agenda and assign people to carry it out. The WFMH mission, translated into discrete agenda items or operational terms, required volunteers willing to work independently and find their own funds. A model was already present in a task force for the scientific study of victims of violence. In 1983 at the World Congress I began to look for friends and colleagues whose work had already launched them in the direction of research or service in a particular area who felt that they could gain some benefit from affiliation with WFMH and who could initiate and finance their own projects. Later I searched for colleagues in charge of university units that could act as WFMH collaborating centers.

The thrust of both endeavors was toward accomplishing our mission, through decentralization aimed at greater organizational resilience and capacity to work in case of adversity. Working committees, beginning in 1983, were formed by Dr. Henry David (Responsible Parenthood), Dr. Barry Jay (Preventing the Commercial Exploitation of Children), Richard Mollica, M.D. (Refugees and Migrants), and Beverly Long and Hilda Robbins (Prevention). The Committee on Trauma Victims in the Middle East headed by psychologist Dr. Leila Dane and Ahmed El Azayem, M.D., was focused on the region as, initially, was one to combat substance abuse headed by Gamal El Azayem, M.D., of Cairo. By the 1990s some committees, initiated at the enthusiastic request of their would-be organizers, had not gone beyond the point of announcing their presence and perhaps cosponsoring an activity with some other organization. Such a short-lived committee was that on legal affairs and human rights appointed by President Morgan in 1986. Its mission was carried on globally through the work of committed individuals in Europe through a European Regional Council (ERC) committee, at WHO Geneva through Stanislas Flache, M.D., and at United Nations New York (see Chapter 8).

In 1988, during the Cairo conference on Middle East violence (see below), UCLA Professor of Psychology Calvin Frederick, Ph.D., was appointed by 1987–1989 President Gamal El Azayem to head a committee on emergency mental health services. Although the committee did not develop he participated in several meetings on WFMH's behalf including a 1989 Rome conference on kidnapping and hostage-taking. A committee on community care approved by the Board at its post-congress meeting in Auckland in 1989 was headed by John Jenkins, a mental health advisor to the British Department of Health with the collaboration of Edith Morgan. Its initial focus was expected to be the sharing of information from people in different countries regarding the creation of new community mental health services. But it too did not develop, and after two or three years was abandoned. The Committee on Women, co-chaired by Morgan and van Remoortel, was briefly active on a global basis, especially in 1989, but later became an ERC working group.

By the mid-1990s Federation components had multiplied to the point where self-examination became inevitable. Questions were raised about the agenda in terms of its membership recruiting power and attractiveness to foundation and corporate funding sources. The concern thus was not only with the mental health relevance of the Federation's agenda but with its "marketing" potential as an organization depending for its future upon a dues paying membership made up primarily of nonprofessionals as well as occasional grants and gifts. So, at the end of the Federation's first half-century, the matter of program came to be intertwined with that of the organization's ability to attract a membership motivated to support advocacy related to mental health on an international basis. This was one of the issues inconclusively addressed at the Board's 2–4 May 1997 long-range planning retreat (see Chapter 5).

The collaborating centers are discussed in relation to the mental health agenda as described below.

PRIMARY PREVENTION

In its earliest days Federation leaders agreed that one of its unique contributions should be reducing the incidence and frequency of mental disorders. Although there was no scientific agreement about the possibility of primary prevention of mental illness, first principles and available data suggested that this should be possible. General enthusiasm was generated in the 1940s and 1950s about the value of child guidance clinics utilizing psychoanalytically oriented methods of dealing with children and their families. As this enthusiasm paled it was accepted that the origins of disturbed behavior lay not only in the intimate parent-child relationship or in the genes, but in the socioeconomic and cultural circumstances into which people were born, grew, and lived as adults. That required attention to broad issues with no immediate bearing on the care of mentally ill or hospitalized people. It allowed Federation annual meetings and special conferences in the Rees era and afterward to pay attention to such social concerns as urbanization, employment, poverty, education, family planning, and infant development.

Sometimes high levels of abstraction were reached. The August 1975 World Congress for Mental Health in Copenhagen, for example, included papers on "Preventive Health and the Psychology of Economic Growth," "The Relationship between Generations in Contemporary and Future Society," and "No Grandmothers, No Grandfathers—Existential Crises in the Industrial World." That congress issued a long statement entitled "Mental Health and Economic Growth" that called for reforms aimed at protecting the earth and providing optimal cultural, spiritual, and material "living conditions for human well being." One of the two major themes of the 1985 World Congress in Brighton (England) was "Prevention of Mental and Emotional Disability." The other was "Services for the Chronic Mentally Ill." No one doubted that primary prevention (i.e., reducing the actual frequency of disturbance) and to a lesser degree secondary and tertiary prevention (i.e., reducing severity, disability, and chronicity through early intervention) were major elements of the WFMH mission. Its target audiences were influential members of the public, including volunteer members of other organizations, government executives and legislators, WHO officers, and public health officials (see Chapter 8). Past Director Rees observed, in retrospect, that Federation policies had been "shaped increasingly around the concept of prevention and therefore with public health methods, which convinced the health administrators at World Health Assemblies of their value" (Rees, 1966, p. 110).

One aspect of prevention was through the promotion of "positive mental health." In 1995–1996 ERC/WFMH represented the mental health interests of European NGOs in discussions of a proposed European Commission plan to promote mental health as a component of a broad based program on health promotion, education, and training. At the end of the year it was invited to become the European Commission's liaison office for the European Network on Mental Health Promotion.

General Considerations and the Johns Hopkins University Collaborating Center

An important precedent for WFMH prevention advocacy was the 1984 establishment by the U.S. National Mental Health Association (NMHA) of a commission on the prevention of mental and emotional disability. It was chaired by Federation Board member Beverly Long, former president of the NMHA and member of the 1978 Carter administration's Commission on Mental Health. Another member was Hilda Robbins, another former NMHA president and vice president of WFMH's North American region. In the same year a North American regional WFMH Committee on Prevention was founded by Long. In 1986 I took the next step, recruiting the Johns Hopkins Center for Prevention Research directed by psychiatrist Professor Sheppard Kellam, M.D., as our first WFMH collaborating center. This recruitment followed the pattern of finding people in my friendship network who might be willing to join us. Kellam's presence helped stimulate the 1989 formation of a WFMH International Committee on Prevention (supplanting the original regional group) by then North American Vice President Beverly Long and Board member-at-large Hilda Robbins. It was approved by the Board at the 1991 Mexico World Congress.

Another memorandum of agreement, replacing that of 1986, specified the relationship of the Johns Hopkins Prevention Center to the WFMH International Committee on Prevention. Written with major involvement by Long, it was intended to establish a pattern linking collaborative centers to specific committees. As Long put it, "The genuine involvement of the advocate organization, the scientific-academic organization, and government agencies is necessary to move policies toward our goals…[but] the Committee needs to stand as an entity, not as an arm of the Collaborating Center" (1996). Shortly afterward the committee began developing an International Primary Prevention Network. Early in 1993, along with the Vermont Conference on Primary Prevention of Psychopathology, it proposed the establishment of a lectureship in the name of Dr. George W. Albee to be part of the regular program of WFMH world congresses from 1995 onward. On 19 May 1993 the opening discussions of the National Prevention Coalition in Washington, DC, included both Long and Kellam. Both participated in a presentation on 7 December 1993 to mark the release of a new report, "The Prevention of Mental Disorders: A National Research Agenda," prepared by the Coalition and NMHA.

The 1995 Dublin World Congress for Mental Health provided a major opportunity for developing the prevention theme. Kellam, key members of his staff, and colleagues from elsewhere in the world presented a significant program segment on current prevention research that attracted major attention. More than 150 policy makers, mental health administrators, and clinicians attended. Consecutive half-day sessions reviewed preventive intervention trials in the United Kingdom and the United States, research methods, the history of prevention science, policy issues, and the dissemination of knowledge.

The success of this event encouraged Long and Kellam to establish a WFMH International Consortium for Prevention. It included 45 members from seven regions, with representatives from Australia, Canada, the Bahamas, France, Ireland, Israel, Jordan, New Zealand, Slovenia, South Africa, Taiwan, the United Kingdom, and the United States. Discussion produced the following objectives for the new consortium: to develop a worldwide prevention network and political base so policy makers will be empowered to make primary prevention a priority; to identify outstanding prevention scientists around the world; to survey primary prevention activities in WFMH regions with particular attention to the cross-cultural relevance of programs; and to facilitate the initiation by local leaders of culturally appropriate and well-evaluated programs. After the congress a coordinating committee formed to further develop the consortium. Members included Beverly Long, Kellam in his role as director of the Collaborating Center for Prevention Research, and Dr. Patricia Mrazek, formerly of the Institute of Medicine of the U.S. National Academy of Sciences.

Other Prevention-Related Conferences and Initiatives

WFMH representatives attended the 9–11 May 1985 U.S. National Institute of Mental Health (NIMH) conference on prevention research and supported the campaign of WFMH member organization, the NMHA, entitled "Voices of Violence."

A major event, billed as "historic," was a 7–9 February 1986 symposium at the National Autonomous University of Mexico entitled "Prevention and Education in the Field of Mental Health: Implications for Latin America" (see Chapter 9). Cosponsored by WFMH, the university's faculty of psychology and the Mexican Committee for Mental Health (comprising 15 organizations ranging from psychoanalysis to neurology), it was planned and organized by Federico Puente Silva, M.D., WFMH Vice President for Mexico, Central America, and the Caribbean. Collaborating was Dr. Juan José Sanchez Sosa, Director of the Faculty of Psychology and General Secretary of the Committee. At the inaugural ceremonies I welcomed the group along with Jesus Kumate Rodriguez, Undersecretary for Health Services, representative of the president of the republic, Licensiada (Lic). Miguel de la Madrid Hurado, and other Mexican dignitaries. Our WFMH Vice President for South America, Alvaro Gallegos, M.D., of Costa Rica was present as well as Beverly Long and Hilda Robbins in her second term as WFMH Vice President for North America.

On 15–16 November 1993, WFMH president, Puente organized another meeting with prevention significance under the auspices of the short-lived Latin American Council of WFMH (see Chapter 9). This was a conference proposed by the Mexican Ministry of Agriculture and Water Resources and its Department of Wild Fauna and Flora on the human relationship to the natural environment. It was rephrased in terms of preserving the biosphere and enhancing human-environment relationships, all with an easily assumed relationship to mental health. WFMH Treasurer de Vries and I, in addition to Puente, represented the Federation along with a stellar cast of Mexican speakers whose presence reflected Puente's organizational skill. They came both from government and scientific institutions such as the Mexican National Academy of Ecology and the National Museum of Anthropology. The intergovernmental system was also well represented with participants from Unicef, the Food and Agriculture Organization (FAO), Pan-American Health Organization (PAHO), and the United Nations Program for Development. The location of the conference hall in the traffic choked and polluted heart of Mexico City dramatized the importance of educating institutional decision-makers as well as the public in this field.

RESPONSIBLE PARENTHOOD AND POPULATION ISSUES

In its various incarnations the cluster of concerns including women's status and rights, reproductive health, and population growth has been part of the Federation's concern with prevention and human rights. But it has also been regarded as a significant advocacy on its own merit. In January 1962 the Executive Board declared that among the "most important international problems of the twentieth century is the very considerable acceleration of population growth." It noted the tensions associated both with advocacy for and rejection of population planning and concluded that the "ways in which these questions are answered in various societies of the world are of greatest importance to the mental health of the people." "Their significance for human rights" emerged when women began to assert their rights as equal partners. A woman who lacks control over her fertility has considerable difficulty completing her education, maintaining gainful employment, and maintaining independent marital decisions.… The health rationale became the basis for advocating that pregnancy be delayed until the most appropriate time and for preventing high-risk unintended pregnancies" (David, 1995). These issues have been especially significant in the less industrialized world with high levels of female illiteracy. Parents there have seen little value in educating girls, and many girls have dropped out of the educational system before reaching secondary school.

With the 1962 Board statement in mind, as well as the growing focus on population problems by United Nations agencies, WFMH accepted the invitation of the Dutch Federation for Mental Health to hold its 16th annual meeting in Amsterdam in August 1963 on the theme of population and mental health. During this meeting psychologist Dr. Henry David agreed to join the Federation staff as associate director of its Geneva Secretariat (see Chapter 4). One of his initial tasks was to collate and edit major papers from the Amsterdam meeting into a monograph, *Population and Mental Health*, that was subsequently published in Switzerland and the United States (David 1964). In its preface he called for preventive planning so that mental health workers could contribute their special skills to the problems of population growth. He recalled that international consultations during his two years with the Federation had gradually persuaded him that "public health and mental health issues related to population concerns and women's reproductive rights were a central issue of human reproductive behavior and that mental health professionals had something to contribute to this emerging field" (David, 1995).

Henry and I became colleagues in the late 1960s and early 1970s before my association with WFMH. On the basis of my earlier interest in adolescence and in mental health in the less industrialized world (Brody 1964, 1968, 1969b) he invited me to be a consultant to a study by the Prague Psychiatric Research Institute of children born to mothers who were twice denied abortion, once on initial request to an abortion commission and again on appeal. The Prague project that continued to follow the children's lives for many years was ultimately published as a book under WFMH auspices (David et al., 1988). I also assisted him as a consultant in the same year to a project in Budapest trying to discover why Hungarian women seemed to prefer abortion to other means of birth control (David, 1969). Although neither of these projects were connected with WFMH, the interests of its leaders at that time were supportive. President Michael Beaubrun (1972–1974), for example, had encouraged me to study contraceptive use and women's status in Jamaica as a visiting professor in his Department of Psychiatry at the University of the West Indies beginning in 1972. After the 1973 Australia World Congress, he made a special stop to attend a meeting on "Mental Health and Population Education" held by the Mental Health Association of Thailand on 18-19 October 1973. WFMH Vice President Dr. Khunying Ambhorn Meesook (see Chapter 10) was also a leader of the Thai Family Planning Association. In 1985 she had the distinction of being simultaneously president of the Thai Mental Health Association and president of Thai Planned Parenthood. From 1974 to 1978 she served as a member of the UN Economic and Social Council's (ECOSOC) Commission on the Status of Women and was the head of delegations at the United Nations Conferences on Women in Mexico City in 1975, in Copenhagen in 1980, and in Nairobi in 1985.

Douglas Deane, a friend of Henry David, who represented both the Pathfinder Fund and WFMH in Geneva was another WFMH veteran with an interest in the subject. He regarded "the population explosion as the world's number one social problem" with profound mental health implications. Because of my work with Henry, my research on personal fertility control in Jamaica in the 1970s (Brody, 1981b), and an earlier concern with reproductive rights (Brody, 1976), Deane's Pathfinder Fund financed my attendance at the 1979 Salzburg World Congress to present a symposium on wanted and unwanted children. Henry could not be with us, but the participants were all colleagues and friends: Brown University anthropologist and Professor of Community Health, Dr. Lucile Newman, who as a WHO consultant had been a pioneer investigator on the acceptability of contraceptive methods; Yale University psychiatrist Stephen Fleck, M.D.; Yugoslavian psychologist Nila Kapor Stanulovic, Ph.D.; and psychiatrist Zdenek Dytrych, M.D. , the leader of the Prague study. Deane joined me as co- chair. We formulated a resolution that, as a newly elected member-at-large, I presented to the same Salzburg post-congress Board meeting at which the new by-laws were adopted (see Chapter 5). The resolution's major focus was not on the impact of increasing population density on behavior but on women's ability to control their own fertility, which is directly correlated with their education, social status, and autonomy. It was aimed at having all children "wanted." Discussion was milder than I had expected, with the major critique coming from Professor Narendra Wig, M.D., Chairman of Psychiatry at Chandigkhar and later at New Delhi. Naren Wig and I had been colleagues in the first (and last) joint consultation between the Divisions of Mental Health and

Human Reproduction at WHO Geneva in 1970 in which a key player and organizer was Henry David. He wanted to be sure that the resolution did not imply the Federation's encouragement of abortion, and, modified to meet his concerns, it was passed by the full Board.

This topic and the fact that 1979 was the United Nations International Year of the Child offered an opportunity for cooperation with other national and international groups. Among them was the conference of the United Kingdom's National Childbirth Trust where, representing WFMH, I gave the opening address focusing on the interlinked mental health of mother and child in situations of obstetric intervention into normal labor. Another opportunity was presented by the International Society for Psychosomatic Obstetrics and Gynecology, of which I was an executive committee member at the time. We met in Berlin at the March 1980 meeting. The topic of its next congress, "Women in a Changing Society" scheduled for West Berlin 2–6 September 1980, made cosponsorship with WFMH natural. I pressed the Board of Directors to join forces with International Society for Psychosomatic Obstetrics and Gynecology. Although North American Vice President Mary Chase Pell, former president of NMHA, was interested, President Guest and his other advisors were uncertain whether the WFMH-obstetrics/gynecology linkage was good for its public image. The possibility died through inaction.

In June 1981 Henry and I both spoke at a Santo Domingo meeting of the Interamerican Society of Psychology. I had been an early member and was involved in one of its meetings in 1966 in Lima, Peru, while serving on the advisory board for Professor Alberto Seguin's Institute of Social Psychiatry. In Santo Domingo we arranged a symposium entitled "Personal Fertility Control: Collaborative Research in the Americas" with cosponsorship from WFMH and WHO/PAHO.

Inevitably I enlisted Henry David in preparations for the 1983 Washington World Congress. He helped arrange the invitation of United Nations Fund for Population Activities in New York (UNFPA) Executive Director, Nafis Sadik, M.D., to be a plenary speaker at the congress. Newman, who had spoken at the 1979 World Congress, obtained a supporting grant from the New World Foundation of New York on whose board she served; she introduced Dr. Sadik's address. This was the first time that WFMH had devoted significant attention to the issue since the 1963 meeting 20 years earlier it was the first World Congress with a major speaker on the topic of family planning and mental health.

The congress was the site of a chance encounter with fortunate long-term consequences for the WFMH agenda. Henry met Professor S. Wiegersma who 20 years earlier had chaired the organizing committee for the 1963 Amsterdam meeting. Together they formulated the idea of a WFMH committee on responsible parenthood. We discussed it, and as president I endorsed its formation. Board approval came without comment at its postcongress meeting. In 1984 Wiegersma, Director of the Netherlands Foundation for Mental Health, provided seed money for the committee to begin enhancing mental health activities in the interdisciplinary field of population. After some deliberation the objective was restated. It was to pursue the expressed interests of the Federation in this sphere and to bring into closer perspective mental health, public health, psychosocial, and sociocultural aspects of family planning and fertility regulation on an international and cross-cultural basis. Implicit was the idea that respect for her human rights was essential to any woman's mental health.

All subsequent WFMH advocacy in this area was initiated by David or members of his committee. Its international membership, nourished by his indefatigable traveling, included among others the core group that I had recruited for the 1979 symposium. Among them were Newman as co-chair and Fleck from the United States; Dytrych and Zdenek Matejcek, M.D., from Prague; Susan Pick de Weiss, Ph.D., from Mexico City; Kapor-Stanulovic from Yugoslavia; and Meesook from Thailand. Later they were joined by Maria MacDonald, Ph.D., of International Planned Parenthood in London (after a few years she moved to the World Bank); Adriana Baban, Ph.D., from Romania, Lic. Lourdes Garcia from Cuba; and Mogens Osler, M.D., from Denmark. I was a consultant and ex officio member. During the next 13 years the committee joined with colleagues in Cuba, the Czech Republic, Denmark, Mexico, Romania, Thailand, the United States, and Vietnam in cooperative research and/or action projects. It received direct and indirect support from the Cuban Ministry of Public Health, the Czechoslovak State Research Plan, the Danish Family Planning Association, the Ford Foundation, the International Health Foundation, Organon International, the Pan American Health Organization, the Population Council, UNFPA, UNESCO, NIMH, and the European Regional Office of WHO.

During this period of the committee's maximum activity, WFMH benefited from David's international reputation and rich network of connections. In turn he used the Federation's reputation and formal United Nations consulting status as a platform to enhance his work with its major significance for prevention and women's health and rights. He quickly became an important and much needed link to various United Nations, governmental, and NGO activities— utilizing among other groups the meetings of Interamerican Society of Psychology as a connecting mechanism with Latin American colleagues. He also launched a series of meetings under committee auspices that did not diminish in frequency until the mid-1990s.

These meetings are noted in some detail below because they indicate the way in which elements of the WFMH international mental health agenda have typically been pursued by a single committed individual and his/her associates aided informally by members of his or her extended personal and professional network. It reveals the thickness of the relevant interconnections and how they all work in concert for common goals. Typically general Board involvement has been minimal, but most group leaders, in this instance David, have remained in close touch with me by telephone, fax, mail, and in the late 1990's, e-mail. At the same time they have acted with much autonomy and flexibility and their own institutional or personal bases. This committee functioned not only as a component of WFMH but as an extension of the private Transnational Family Institute that David directed from offices in his home in Bethesda, Maryland. While WFMH linked it to other NGOs and elements of the United Nations and provided a framework bringing the far-flung group of international colleagues into a coherent unit with an explicitly mental health mission, the Institute acted as its central office, communications hub, and fund manager.

This was the organism that, shortly after its inception in 1984, obtained a grant from the National Fund for Mental Health of the Netherlands It was to help explore prospects for a WFMH service contract with UNFPA to provide mental health consultation upon request to family planning programs in developing countries. The service contract did not materialize, but Henry began his liaison work as our official representative to the International Population Conference in Mexico City sponsored by UNFPA 6–13 August 1984. Its declaration entitled "Population and Development" adopted on 14 August 1984 made several points germane to the WFMH mission: the principal aim of population policies is to "improve the standards of living and quality of life of the people"; "improving the status of women and enhancing their role is an important goal in itself"; and "all couples and individuals [should be able to] exercise their basic human rights to decide freely, responsibly and without coercion the number and spacing of their children" (UNFPA, 1984).

The WFMH role in advocacy for responsible parenthood in Latin America continued at a 5–7 December 1984 meeting of the Interamerican Society for Psychology in Havana. It was held under the auspices of WHO, PAHO, and the National Health Psychology Group of the Cuban Ministry of Public Health directed by Lic. Lourdes Garcia Aventura. I represented WFMH at the opening ceremonies and along with David and several members of his committee presented several lectures and symposia on various aspects of reproductive behavior. At that time Lic. Garcia was also recruited to membership in our WFMH committee that, mainly through David's work under WHO/PAHO auspices, continued to supply technical assistance for Cuban research on adolescent pregnancy and later, again, with WHO sponsorship, for specialized training in health psychology in general.

At the same time interest in the problem continued to be stimulated by the WFMH top leadership. The 1983–1985 president, Dr. Estafania Aldaba-Lim of Manila, chaired a working group of the International Planned Parenthood Federation on "The Promotion of Family Planning as a Human Right." She also participated in a UNESCO expert's meeting in Dubrovnik, Yugoslavia, on 9–14 December 1984 on "Factors Influencing Women's Access to Decision Making Roles in Political, Economic and Scientific Life and on Measures that May be Taken to Increase Their Responsibilities." She distributed the final version of the Dubrovnik report, issued on 15 April 1985, to Meesok who was the WFMH delegate to the July 1985 United Nations Decade of Women meeting in Nairobi. Meanwhile, in Thailand between 23 February and 2 March 1985, Meesook had helped arrange joint meetings of the Mental Health Association of Thailand, Planned Parenthood Association of Thailand, and the Population and Community Development Association to which David came as a consultant with the aid of a Ford Foundation grant. This was facilitated because another colleague, Khun Mechai Viravaidya, was secretary general of the Population and Community Development Association. During one of David's consulting visits a pilot project was developed with local mental health professionals serving as volunteer moderators of focus groups with adolescents and service providers. One hope was to reduce the incidence of unwanted adolescent pregnancy. By good fortune Lourdes Garcia was in Bangkok for a WHO meeting and could pass along her experience with the then ongoing study in Cuba. The findings from that Ford Foundation funded project were reported at meetings of the United Nations Economic and Social Commission for Asia and the Pacific.

In 1985 on 15–18 April, PAHO held a seminar in Mexico City on "Adolescent Risk Taking Behavior: Health and Psychosocial Implications," to which David, invited in his personal role, also represented WFMH. In May 1985 Committee Co-Chair Newman represented WFMH at a Unicef meeting in Boston on their Child Survival Program, which emphasized family spacing as it affected child survival. On 17–18 June the committee's reach expanded to cosponsor the International Workshop of Longitudinal Studies of Unwanted Children at the University of Oulu (Finland) where the Prague study was presented. Studies at Oulu appeared to confirm that with time and advancing age mental health impairments become increasingly marked in children born to mothers who did not plan their pregnancies compared with children from planned pregnancies.

In 1986 with initial funding from the National Fund for Mental Health in Utrecht, the committee undertook cooperative work in Cuba, Thailand, and Mexico. Along with WHO and the Interamerican Society of Psychology it was invited to cosponsor a seminar in Havana on the psychology of health. Two important impetuses to the process were Lourdes Garcia's appointment to the steering committee of the WHO Task Force on Adolescent Reproductive Health and the interest of the American Psychological Association, which facilitated a meeting of a planning group in their Washington DC offices on 10 March 1986 with the attendance of Rene Gonzalez, M.D., Mental Health Advisor for PAHO. Meanwhile, across the world in Thailand data were being collected in collaboration with the Mental Health Association of Thailand and the Population and Community Development Association. In Mexico UNFPA approved a grant for a two-year study of contraceptive practices and unwanted pregnancies among adolescents to be directed by Dr. de Weiss.

In late 1986 the committee received international publicity when the newsletter of the Population Association of America carried an article about Henry David. It gained further status when Aldaba Lim asked to become a member. She came, at her own request, as a representative of the Adolescent Fertility Education Project of the Girl Scouts of the Philippines. In this role as well as others she addressed a seminar for professionals and volunteers from the ASEAN countries (Indonesia, Malaysia, Philippines, Singapore, Thailand) at a meeting on "Women's Rights and Reproductive Health" in Singapore on 12–15 August 1986. Among its recommendations were the elimination of discrimination against women embodied in legal and health codes, and laws to prevent the physical and sexual abuse of women and children. She contributed a paper entitled "Plight and Rights of Women and Children in the Context of Poverty and Development" for an experts' meeting 14–18 November at UNESCO Paris.

1986 also saw the continuation of several simultaneous streams of WFMH activity concerned with women's health and reproductive behavior, family integrity, and responsible parenthood. As described in Chapter 8 the UNESCO/WFMH/International Social Science Council project on "Women's Rights and Roles and Reproductive Technology" led by Committee Co-Chair Newman with my collaboration was continuing. At United Nations Vienna, WFMH (through its senior representative, Dr. Maria Simon) continued to supply input into various meetings concerned with family health with special reference to women as targets of violence.

Also in 1986 Organon International and the Danish Family Planning Association each granted $2000, matching an earlier grant from the Netherlands Fund for Mental Health to support the committee's projected seminar on family planning for the mentally ill and handicapped. The seminar was organized jointly with the Danish Family Planning Association and the Danish Association for the Mentally Ill and encouraged by WFMH's European region and International Planned Parenthood Federation. Although it was not supported by WHO's Mental Health Section in Geneva, it had participation from the WHO European Regional Office. It took place 8–9 May 1987 in Gentofte, Denmark, and was limited to 50 participants from several Nordic and Western European countries. Its proceedings were published in the same year (Osler and David, 1987). A key seminar organizer, Mogens Osler, M.D., Danish Family Planning Association President and Professor of Obstetrics and Gynecology at the University of Copenhagen, announced that in consequence of the Gentofte seminar the Danish National Board of Social Affairs would produce a pamphlet, "Guidelines on Sexuality—Irrespective of Handicap."

On the occasion of the 21st Congress of Interamerican Society of Psychology in Havana on 28 June–4 July 1987 the committee organized a symposium on service-oriented research in adolescent reproductive behavior chaired by David, who was present as a representative of PAHO/WHO. Other committee members present were Pick de Weiss from Mexico and Lourdes Garcia from Cuba who, with the committee's help, was providing technical assistance to PAHO/WHO.

In 1987 the WFMH World Congress was held in Cairo. That gave Henry the opportunity to further expand the geographic and cultural base of his committee. Shortly thereafter he announced the addition of Dr. Sarah Loza, a sociologist from Cairo.

Major support for the committee's work continued to come from Danish Family Planning Association which cosponsored an informal consultation on "Clinician's Perceptions of Psychological Risks for Abortion" in Copenhagen, 2 June 1989, led by David. At this time Osler became a committee member. In that year WHO's European Regional Office, with the support of UNFPA, also made a grant to Dytrych at the Prague Psychiatric Research Institute to study the psychosocial situation of the young adults who had been "born unwanted" in 1961-1963. In January 1990, with committee support, the Danish Family Planning Association received a grant from the regional office for a study of repeated abortion seeking behavior with Osler as principal investigator. Members of the committee also took advantage of other 1990 meetings to discuss their program. European members conferred during a 10–13 October WHO conference in Tbilisi, Georgia (U.S.S.R.) and the 14–16 November congress of the Mexican Association of Social Psychology. In December 1990 at the invitation of the Vietnamese Women's Union David met with representatives of family planning and women's organizations in Hanoi, Ho Chi Minh City, and neighboring communes over nine days, making arrangements to exchange experiences with WFMH committee member Meesok as well as the Population and Community Development Association in Bangkok.

An important nodal point was the 1991 World Congress for Mental Health in Mexico. The committee participated in planning for its subcongresses on population and one on women's health. Participants in the heavily attended subcongress on population and mental health passed a resolution in support of UNFPA, which had had its U.S. funding cut by the Reagan administration on the grounds that it supported abortion.

A highlight of the year was the award of the University Medal and Citation to Henry from the rector of Charles University, Prague, on 9 April 1991 at a convocation honoring the 30th anniversary of the Psychiatric Research Institute in Prague. This presentation recognized his more than 25 years of international scientific cooperation.

As detailed in Chapter 8 various committee members as well as Dr. Kay Greene, our senior representative to United Nations New York, participated in meetings during 1992 and 1993 of the steering committee of the NGO planning committee for the 1994 United Nations Cairo International Conference on Population and Development. In 1993 members participated in a panel of the Psychosocial Workshop of the Population Association of America in preparation for this conference. That year was marked by the presentation to David by the American Psychological Association's Committee on International Relations of its award for distinguished contributions to the international advancement of psychology. On 5–13 September 1994 he was our representative to the Cairo Conference that reviewed issues of gender equality and the empowerment of women. Thanks to the good offices of former WFMH President El Azayem he also addressed several Egyptian mental health groups during his stay. Thus he was able to carry the Federation's message in this area to parts of the world in which women's status and freedom to manage their own reproductive activities were still narrowly constrained.

In 1995 committee members Dytrych and Matejcek in Prague received the annual award of the Ministry of Health of the Czech Republic for their ongoing research that had been initiated with David. In Mexico sexuality education conducted by committee member Pick de Weiss received strong governmental support, permitting publication of a series of monographs for children, adolescents, teachers, and parents. In Bucharest, new committee member, Dr. Adriana Baban, published a monograph, "Voices of Romanian Women: Perceptions of Sexuality," with the support of the International Health Foundation of the Population Council. In Russia, new member Dr. Valery Chervyakov organized the first baseline comparative study of adolescents' sexual attitudes and behavior with MacArthur Foundation funding.

Although the 1991 Mexico subcongress had been marked by enthusiastic excitement in sessions concerned with family planning, responsible parenthood, and population, this was diminished by the time of the Tokyo Congress in 1993. The Dublin World Congress of 1995 was more disappointing with two sparsely attended sessions on responsible parenthood, one including the director of the local Family Planning Association recruited by David without the assistance of the local planners. In 1996 his involvement in Federation activities was reduced by illness. In 1997 he decided to retire as chairman of the committee that he had founded and had become such an integral element in his life's work and contributed so much to the Federation's advocacy for prevention. He was succeeded by his cochairperson, Lucile Newman.

WOMEN'S RIGHTS, PRIVILEGES, AND STATUS

While the Committee on Responsible Parenthood maintained an active pace, the Federation's concern with the general social status and mental health of women continued to progress through other means. It had been addressed from time to time at world congresses, one of the first being that in Vancouver in 1977 where three sessions addressed the topic, including women's rights and priorities in the Third World. In the late 1980s, with this concern in mind, I arranged the affiliation of the Key Centre for Women's Health in Society of the University of Melbourne, Australia, with WFMH as a collaborating center. It was headed by psychiatrist Professor Lorraine Dennerstein, M.D., whom I had first met when we were both on the board of the International Society for Psychosomatic Obstetrics and Gynecology of which she later became president.

1987 saw the initiation of an ERC project on women and mental health proposed by a group, all of whom already had strong ties to WFMH as well as their national mental health associations. They were Edith Morgan of the United Kingdom, Pirkko Lahti of Finland, Mary J. O'Mahony of Ireland, Josee van Remoortel of Belgium, and psychologist Dr. Inge Schock of West Germany. Its starting premise was the idea that "women are seriously disadvantaged" in ways inimical to their mental health. Another concern was the "strikingly low representation of women amongst senior office holders in WFMH throughout its history" and a commitment to increase women's "active participation in WFMH at all levels." It is true that the only female president early in Federation history was Margaret Mead. Since the establishment of the Baltimore-Washington Secretariat in 1983, however, the trend had changed with Presidents Aldaba-Lim (1983–1985) and Morgan (1985–1987) at the helm in positions to influence the recruitment of other women leaders.

Supplementing this focus, Edith Morgan initiated an international network or "circle" concerned with women's opportunities in the European workplace during the Auckland World Congress in 1989. This effort had an uneven history and, over a few years, evaporated. However, Morgan in London continued to develop projects as part of the ERC/WFMH program on women and mental health. A recurring theme was "good practices in mental health" aimed not only at documenting successful interventions with mentally ill women but at a much broader goal that could be understood in terms of prevention and health promotion. As noted in a 1997 report by her and co-project leader Dr. Heather Scott of the University of Northumbria (United Kingdom), the project "aims to help eradicate the disadvantages and discrimination against women and to help them become more influential in shaping their own lives and those of their fellow human beings." This effort, funded from European granting sources and the European Union's HELIOS II Program, included participants from Albania, Bulgaria, Estonia, and Slovenia in Eastern Europe and Belgium, Finland, Ireland, and Italy in Western Europe. A 28 April–1 May 1995 London conference on women and mental health was attended by representatives of 14 countries.

The culminating Federation point for many of these interests was our delegation to the United Nations Fourth World Conference on Women in Beijing on 30 August–15 September 1995 and its accompanying NGO forum. During the preceding year our United Nations representative Nancy Wallace, C.S.W., and her colleagues had been working hard on preparatory documents for this event. The goal of three international preparatory meetings was to have mental health included in the Beijing agenda. The advocacy focus was two-fold: to have the words "physical and mental health" replace the single word "health" wherever it appeared and to include the provision of counseling services in relevant sections. In the first draft of the platform document in 1992 there was virtually no mention of either, but by the final version health was defined in the original WHO language as complete mental as well as physical and social "well-being and not merely the absence of disease or infirmity." Despite this work there had been no concrete plans for a WFMH delegation, so I telephoned our 1995–1997 president, Beverly Long, and suggested that she lead and organize it. She immediately went to New York to meet with Wallace and her team, and together they made the necessary arrangements. At Beijing they were joined as official observers by Drs. Anie Kalayjian and Ricki Kantrowitz of our WFMH United Nations NY group and Susan Feldman, head of the Melbourne WFMH collaborating center's unit on aging. Although our European representatives chose not to join the WFMH delegation, it was greatly strengthened by the presence of former President Aldaba-Lim attending as part of the government delegation from the Philippines. In Africa our member organization, the Zimbabwe National Association for Mental Health, could not send a delegate but marked the United Nations conference by producing a video on women's mental health.

In Beijing the WFMH group continued its lobbying efforts on the wording of the platform document. A resolution prepared for the conference under Long's leadership and approved by our 1995 Board in Dublin was widely distributed. A workshop entitled "Mental Health and Women in a Global Context" attracted a standing room only audience during the NGO forum held under challenging conditions 30 miles outside of Beijing. During the official United Nations Conference, WFMH representatives led a mental health caucus attended by approximately 100 women from diverse backgrounds.

MENTAL HEALTH AND AGING

Aging has concerned the Federation as a focus for both prevention and treatment. A major preventive effort has been the attempt to keep older people actively engaged with life in the hope that this will reduce the likelihood of cognitive deterioration, depression, and other undesirable concomitants of aging. WFMH regularly addressed the topic at every annual meeting from 1948 on. It first devoted an entire conference to this issue at a plenary session in Brussels in August 1952. Its emphasis, voiced by Professor of Psychiatry van der Horst of Amsterdam, was on the loneliness and social isolation of the aged and practical ways in which to keep older people in contact with others. This became a topic at world congresses after 1977. It was also the topic of occasional special meetings such as one organized in 1979 by Edith Morgan on "Aging in Industrial Society" in Helsinki with the cosponsorship of WHO and the Finnish Mental Health Association.

In the latter phase of the Lin presidency (1974–1979) a scientific advisory committee headed by Board member Gaston Harnois, M.D., included aging issues in its portfolio. It became involved when, in the fall of 1981, WFMH was asked to participate in a United Nations World Assembly on aging in Vienna in the summer of 1982. Although Harnois and colleagues joined in a preparatory meeting and attended the assembly, there were no funds to put together an official delegation with an agenda compatible with the WFMH perspective. I turned therefore to Dr. Gary van den Bos of the American Psychological Association, who agreed to organize a self-financing WFMH delegation to that conference. It was especially pleasing that Bert Kruger-Smith, a friend from the University of Texas' Hogg Foundation for Mental Health, consented to be part of our delegation. With Ralph Cullen and Hogg Foundation support she had conducted a survey of self-help programs for the elderly. She was also a pioneer in creating centers for frail older people, including some with Alzheimer's disease, in Austin, Texas. Using their own resources our delegation participated in the Vienna assembly but had to report that their attempted initiatives concerning emotional support for older people, and the importance of keeping the elderly engaged in meaningful life activities, met with little interest. The main concerns of the intergovernmental, national, and NGO groups in attendance were in economic support, adequate housing and nutrition, and dealing with treatment rather than prevention of the infirmities of old age. However, our review of the matter at the 21 July 1983 Board meeting at NMHA headquarters (where Kruger-Smith and Cullen reported on their survey) led us to appoint Marion Kalousek, M.D., of Vienna as our observer for possible follow-up activities.

Finding a permanent WFMH focal point in this area proved unexpectedly difficult. During the late 1980s and early 1990s I could not find an individual or group whose professional trajectory had already focused on aging and who was willing to work with us on a volunteer basis. However, special opportunities sometimes presented themselves. A "Working Group on Prevention and Reduction of Mental Health Problems in the Elderly" was held under WHO and other auspices in Groningen (The Netherlands) on 29 April–3 May 1985. The major WFMH representative was Dr. Jennifer Newton of MIND, the renamed British national mental health association, along with Dr. G. Anquinet of Belgium and Marten de Vries from nearby Maastricht. They participated in discussions that recognized the trend away from the care of the elderly infirm by their children in favor of independent or institutional arrangements. One scenario encouraged the mutual aid of elderly by other elderly to reduce the increasing need for statutory services. The working group also urged the development of a formal international classification of services and the development of scales to assess minimum standards of care in residential and community services.

At its summer 1986 meeting at Cumberland Lodge (England), the Board adopted a resolution from our United Nations New York representative Yael Danieli. It proposed that the United Nations should adopt a plan of action for the elderly proposed by one of the United Nations' working groups (see Appendix V). In January 1987 as a member of the Hogg Foundation's

National Advisory Council I visited the facility of the Austin (Texas) Groups for the Elderly described in recognition of Bert Kruger Smith's role as the "House that Bert Built." It was a model for groups concerned with maintaining the health and psychosocial integrity of the frail elderly. In Vienna, Dr. Vijaya Rao represented us as well as "HelpAge International" at an 11 February 1988 meeting of the NGO Committee on Aging at the Vienna International Center. Reports focused on issues in developing countries including "the myth of multigenerational families providing answers to the problem." All recommendations included active constructive participation in plans for their welfare by the elderly themselves.

United Nations New York became an especially active center of WFMH advocacy for the mental health of aging people. In the early 1990s after Dr. Kay Greene had developed, for the first time, a team of several WFMH representatives we were represented on the ECOSOC NGO Committee on Aging. When I attended its meeting there was lively discussion from representatives of an eclectic group of organizations about the possible role of the United Nations in influencing national aging programs. On 10–11 January 1995, Dr. Dianne Davis, one of our representatives to the United Nations Department of Public Information as well as our member on the NGO Committee on Aging, organized a conference at United Nations headquarters entitled "Better Living—Adding Life to Years." This was the first in a series of international meetings focused on architectural and city planning initiatives to create integrated neighborhoods that were supportive of older persons. Its goal was not only to encourage community-based care but participation by older people in a full range of community activities. On 16 October 1996 Davis met with the NGO committee in Helsinki during the Second Annual Conference on Gerotechnology. These activities anticipated the 1999 United Nations International Year for Older Persons

Other advocacy and education meetings took place at United Nations Geneva. On 13-14 February 1995 Myrna Merritt Lachenal represented us at a workshop entitled "Population Ageing in Europe and North America." Organized by the United Nations Economic Commission for Europe and the American Association of Retired Persons, it drafted policy recommendations regarding poverty, employment, and integration of older persons in society for the United Nations World Summit on Social Development held in Copenhagen on 6–12 March 1995.

In time the ERC, in the process of developing its own committee structure focused on Europe, named Jenny Steenhaut, a nursing professor at the University of Ghent, to lead its working group on aging. In 1993 she consented to add the general WFMH aging portfolio to her responsibilities. She was our nominal representative, as well as that of ERC, at several conferences. She presented data from the "European Survey of Good Practices in Mental Health Care for the Elderly" at an international meeting on Alzheimer's disease in 1994 and in 1995 a paper entitled "The Social Aspects of Older People with Mental Health Problems" at a Strasbourg meeting of the European Parliament's Intergroup on Health, Ageing and Disability. Although her emphasis was not on prevention, but on the care of already mentally ill and demented people, there was a preventive element in her concern for the relatives who bore the responsibility for the ill. After two years, she withdrew from her general WFMH role, saying that the mental health issues of aging were so determined by regional and local considerations that a Federation committee on the subject was not appropriate.

However, in 1995, a potential WFMH leader in this field with a global outlook appeared at the Dublin World Congress. He was Professor John Copeland, M.D., Director of the Institute for Mental Health and Aging at the University of Liverpool, who was presenting his joint research with former WFMH President Tsung-yi Lin on aging in Taiwan. I attended their session and was favorably impressed. Then he was independently recommended by Marten de Vries. With this encouragement I initiated correspondence and was pleased to learn that he was indeed interested in joining us as a collaborating center. The Board approved his application at its December 1996 meeting in Chile despite the objections of Vice President for Europe John Henderson and the view of ERC/WFMH's Executive Director van Remoortel that the Federation had no need for collaborating centers. Happily, Copeland and I spent time together at the WFMH Western Regional Pacific meeting in Taiwan (see Chapter 10), also in December 1996. At that time he also agreed to form a WFMH working group or committee with its nucleus at his institute.

NONVIOLENT CONFLICT RESOLUTION

This element of our international mental health agenda was directly linked to the original Federation goal of promoting harmonious international relations and could be logically listed under the general rubric of prevention. At the 1983 World Congress I was able to arrange a plenary session devoted to the peaceful resolution of international conflict. The speaker was David Hamburg, M.D., President of the Carnegie Corporation, who discussed leadership in relation to international conflict resolution. He was introduced by Jerome Frank, Ph.D., M.D., Professor of Psychiatry at Johns Hopkins University and a world figure in the antinuclear armaments movement. A keynote by Rector Saedjemoko of the United Nations University in Tokyo drew a standing ovation for its range of approaches to world peace in relation to mental health.

A specific initiative regarding conflict resolution grew from the concern with victims of violence presented at a symposium organized by Dr. Leila Dane at the 1987 World Congress in Cairo. She was executive director of what was then called the Institute for Victims of Terrorism (IVT), changed in June 1989 to Institute for Victims of Trauma. I moderated the symposium as a way of emphasizing the importance we attached to this topic and enlisting the support of the 1987–1989 WFMH president, Gamal El Azayem, M.D., for future activities. His interest and that of his son, Ahmed, clinical director of the family-owned hospital, were aroused, and they developed a relationship with Dane and IVT colleagues strong enough to address the potentially explosive issues surrounding conflict resolution in this part of the world. As indicated in Chapter 10, I had come to know Dr. Gamal and his Sufi background and felt that his efforts deserved Federation support. To facilitate them I recommended the formation of the WFMH Committee on Trauma Victims of the Middle East with Ahmed and Dane as co-chairs. In his combined role as president and father of one of the proposed co-chairs, he quickly approved it. The Board offered no objections or comments.

The new committee's first project was an April 1988 WFMH regional conference sponsored by IVT at the El Azayem hospital. It dealt both with mental health services to victims of community violence and the possibility of preventing such violence. IVT, funded largely by the Dane family, subsidized my travel to provide a strong WFMH presence. The group was small without representation from the larger countries in the region, but the event was a pioneering one and a step toward more direct confrontation with the issue. One outcome was its approval of the "Working Draft Resolution on Mental Health Services to Victims of Community Violence" that Dane had designed ahead of time. Recalling a series of earlier proclamations and recommendations from WHO, the American Psychological Association, and the United Nations' 1985 Declaration of Basic Principles of Justice, which was strongly supported by WFMH (see Chapter 8), it was in essence a call to all WFMH member organizations to become involved in preventing community violence and caring for its victims. This was published in the June 1988 newsletter and adopted without significant discussion at the 1992 Board meeting in Sydney. Although this resolution was clearly relevant to the WFMH mission, it has had no apparent impact on the member associations to which it was directed.

Nonetheless the fact of the resolution's formulation and adoption, and the activities surrounding the 1988 conference, helped create a sympathetic view in the WFMH Eastern Mediterranean region of conflict resolution as a legitimate field of study. The Persian Gulf War with its displaced and traumatized persons caused former WFMH president Gamal to believe that the topic merited further development among mental health practitioners. His immense personal prestige in the area allowed him to begin by talking with the influential religious leaders whose support was essential for this kind of a project. After consulting with Sheik Dr. Mohammed Tantawi, the Grand Mufti of Egypt (the senior Islamic figure in the country who is appointed by the president), and psychiatric colleagues he asked IVT to join forces with him to establish a "Joint Program on Conflict Resolution" under WFMH auspices.

I encouraged this development and participated in a November 1991 conference cautiously entitled, "Examining the Merits of Conflict Resolution as an Academic Discipline: Its Applications to Real Life Situations." The immediate sponsors were WFMH member associations the World Islamic Association for Mental Health and the Egyptian Mental Health Association. Its patron was the grand mufti in the new Dar Al-Iftaa, the Islamic center of Egypt in Cairo. The grand mufti embraced the aim of understanding and promulgating the nonviolent resolution of international and interethnic conflict. In the broadest sense this was to prevent trauma and its consequences for individuals, families, and communities. Among the 200 participants were many ulemas, Islamic scholars from nearby Al Azhar University, some of whom were vocally critical both of the aim and of U.S. participation. One Al Azhar faculty member condemned my role as co-chairman of the opening session with Dr. Gamal because, he said, of the U.S. invasion of Iraq. Gamal defended me with an appropriate quotation from the Koran, and the objector subsided. The conference captured daily media attention and was regarded by most participants to have successfully achieved its goal. That was to acknowledge the applicability of conflict resolution theory and principles to everyday life in the Middle East (Dane, 1992). The "joint program" was also formed, with the official aim of sponsoring education and research on the topic. It was chaired by the two committee leaders with Mideast and North American boards of advisors. A special issue of *Mental Peace*, the journal of the World Islamic Association for Mental Health, was devoted to the conference, which also stimulated the beginning of active planning and negotiation for a subsequent meeting.

A follow-up conference, "Building Tolerance for Diversity," was held in Cairo on 3-5 February 1994 under WFMH and joint program auspices. It was preceded by a year of preparation by the co-chairs of the WFMH Committee on Trauma Victims in the Middle East and cohosted by the grand mufti with the addition of Fathi Arafat, M.D., Director of the Red Crescent Society that had its headquarters in the city. This conference was directed toward reducing the likelihood of traumatizing conflict between cultural (including ethnic and religious) as well as national groups. The program included video presentations of skills training in conflict management in the workplace and of the reconciliation process among children of Holocaust survivors working together with children of Nazi perpetrators. This was marked by mutual, effective communication of Israeli and Palestinian participants. Including an exercise for Arab and Israeli practitioners to identify the steps necessary to facilitate peaceful coexistence, it received wide media attention.

However, after this promising start various reasons made it necessary to defer new joint program projects, including a proposed conference entitled "Conflict Transformation in the Arab World." This may have been, at least in part, a consequence of the bitter refusal of the Egyptian medical syndicate to interact with Israelis and the associated danger to Ahmed El Azayem's professional standing. Although most Egyptian colleagues did not exhibit their hostility toward Israelis and Jews, it appeared just beneath the surface. During a social event, one Board member made a point of telling me that complaints by "the Jews" about the Holocaust were exaggerated because they had not lost more than 20,000 people. Even though Israelis have attended WFMH events in Egypt, both Gamal and Ahmed El Azayem have adamantly refused to visit Israel. Yet their work helped establish peaceful conflict resolution as a WFMH concern, not only in the Middle East but in Europe. In Europe this became a leading issue in September 1994 when it was the theme of the ERC/WFMH annual meeting in Belfast. The meeting came, fortuitously, at the time of an IRA cease-fire. Plenary sessions and workshops dealt with ethnicity and conflict; discrimination and minorities; religion; poverty; unemployment; the family; and marital and sexual violence. Collaborating with the organizing body, the Northern Ireland Association for Mental Health, was the Centre for the Study of Conflict of the University of Ulster. Ahmed and I chaired a special session including Dane and Egyptian, Israeli, Kuwaiti, and Palestinian speakers who explored the use of mental health professionals in conflict resolution in the Middle East.

In the Arab states work in this area continued during 1995 but more directly under the auspices of the new Eastern Mediterranean Regional Council of WFMH, led by the younger El Azayem, as its membership and organizational strength increased. Ahmed and local colleagues, without reference to the committee or the joint program, participated in a conference on 1–4 April 1995 in Kuwait on the rehabilitation of victims of the Iraqi invasion. Through WFMH member associations, the Egyptian Mental Health Association, and the Egyptian Association for Family and Social Conflict Resolution they assisted the Yemen Mental Health Association in developing a support program for Yemeni children traumatized by war. On 4 April 1996 the Eastern Mediterranean Regional Council organized a "Day Without Violence in the Middle East." Other organizers were the Jerusalem-based Association for Social Change and the Containment of Conflict headed by Israeli psychoanalyst, Judith Issroff, M.D., the Child-Family Consultation Center in Jerusalem directed by Palestinian psychologist Dr. Elia Awwad, and the Palestinian Center for Non-Violence headed by Noa Salameh. During a meeting of the Arab Federation of Psychiatrists in Lebanon on 12–15 November 1996, Ahmed organized a symposium on conflict resolution including a paper entitled "The Role of Forgiveness and Reconciliation in Conflict Resolution—Lessons from Lebanon." As Dr. Nancy Dubrow's UNESCO financed project under WFMH auspices on community reintegration of Intifada participants in Gaza was progressing (see Chapter 8), he telephoned me to suggest that Gaza might be the site of a 1998 WFMH anniversary meeting with the theme of conflict resolution.

THE MENTAL HEALTH OF CHILDREN AND ADOLESCENTS

A staple of traditional thought has been the idea that the surest key to avoiding illness in adulthood is the promotion and protection of health in childhood and adolescence. This theme has been alive, with varying intensity, in Federation thinking and activities for its entire existence. During the Rees era, as noted in Chapter 3 and Appendix I, recurrent interest in infant research mirrored that of the professional community at large. The major event was the 1952 Chichester (England) seminar during which the topic was examined by key people from different countries over several days (see Chapter 3) (Soddy, 1955).

World Congresses and annual meetings provided opportunities to address the mental health of children in both the family and school environment. Although every congress included some presentations, a few were outstanding in this respect. At the 1968 congress in London, most presentations dealing with children focused on therapeutic interventions including those with families. Among them, however, were several with prevention as a specific theme. Examples are "Preschool Age, the Time for Psychiatric Prevention" and "Development of Preventive Community Mental Health Programs in the United States and Israel," describing programs with a close liaison between schools, clinics, and family members. Another example concerned the "prevention of damaging stress in children" with special reference to bereavement and deprivation. The 1977 Vancouver World Congress devoted major attention to the influence of mass media (television) on children. Its program on preventive mental health for children and parents included sessions on bonding in early development, socialization in the family, school, and peer groups, and children's services. The high point in congress attention to children and youth was the 1979 gathering in Salzburg that observed the United Nations Year of the Child. Its papers ranged from rights to services; the only session with a directly preventive focus was the one I had arranged with the help of the Pathfinder Fund. Retitled by the program committee to downplay its family planning and contraceptive aspects, it was billed as: "Making Unwanted Children Wanted. Preparation for Parenthood."

As we tried to organize our approach to various topics after 1983 it was apparent that the WFMH mission required a working group or committee concerned with children and adolescents to act as advocates for their rights and concerns. It proved unexpectedly difficult, though, to find someone whose career line would naturally include the organization of such a group with the thought that WFMH affiliation would be beneficial. With this in mind I accepted an invitation to discuss the topic at the June 1984 meeting of the International Association of Child and Adolescent Psychiatry in Athens. However, there were no volunteers to develop a committee. In 1986, while a visiting fellow of the Institute for Advanced Study at Tel Aviv University and a visiting professor in Dr. Phyllis Palgi's Department of Behavioral Science, I met Emanuel Chigier, M.D. He was a pediatrician and adolescent psychiatrist who was a consultant for refugee children in Israel, particularly the adolescents who had come from Ethiopia. My wife and I visited the major center for Ethiopian adolescents and were impressed by his ability to relate to them. He was much interested in WFMH and eventually became a member of our Board and chairman of the WFMH Committee on Children and Adolescents. But his activities remained focused on the organization and cosponsorship of still more conferences. In time he confined his purview to the mental health of adolescents; while he did not develop a group to work with him, he referred to his "committee," and the Board acquiesced in his desire to use the WFMH "committee" name as a cosponsor for some meetings. One of the last as we approached the 50-year mark was the First International Conference on Health and Culture in Adolescence in Jerusalem, 24–27 November 1996. This meeting, attended by 130 professionals representing 33 countries, was "cosponsored by WFMH," but we made no organizational input into its program.

In June 1990 the WFMH International Committee on Prevention organized a five-day meeting at the University of Vermont in Burlington that touched on the issue of children's mental health. In addition to parenting and child development, it addressed a range of prevention-related issues including family planning, prenatal and perinatal nutrition, health care, education, reduction of economic and social distress, racism, delinquency, AIDS, and drug abuse.

Another route to addressing the needs of children and adolescents was through Unicef (see Chapter 8). Nancy Dubrow represented our interests in many Unicef groups and projects concerned with children in extremely difficult circumstances including that of armed conflict. Occasionally, depending on timing and location, other colleagues represented us in such discussions. On 13–15 March 1996 Aldaba Lim was our delegate to a meeting of the Unicef regional office for Asia in Manila on the "Impact of Armed Conflict on Children." This included representatives from the social welfare sectors of Vietnam, Sri Lanka, Cambodia, and the Philippines.

Preventing Commercial Sexual Exploitation

The most visible WFMH advocacy in this area came through the WFMH committee on "Preventing the Commercial Sexual Exploitation of Children." Co-chaired by child psychiatrist Syed Arshad Husain, M.D., a Pakistani located at the University of Missouri at Columbia, and Dr. Mawaheb El-Mouelhy of the Arab Women's Solidarity Association in Cairo, it was approved by the Board in the autumn of 1990. Its goals were (1) To provide information concerning the commercial sexual exploitation of children; (2) to describe the social, cultural and economic factors contributing to the evolution of this phenomenon; (3) to make recommendations to the governments involved about the sequence of legal, cultural and economic measures that could be expected to ameliorate or prevent the commercial sexual exploitation of children within their borders. The committee acquired several members, but its driving force soon became U.S. child psychologist Barry Jay, Ph.D., who maintained a close and continuous relationship with my office. As the committee became more widely known it was invited, in 1992, by the Human Rights Commission of Pakistan and WFMH member; the Pakistan Mental Health Association to conduct a fact-finding mission on trafficking of children in Pakistan and was offered an opportunity to conduct a project in Bangladesh. It also formed linkages with other involved advocacy groups. At Barry Jay's suggestion, committee member Professor Chok Hiew Ph.D. of the University of New Brunswick, Canada, a native of Thailand, was designated WFMH representative to the 30 March–4 April 1992 Bangkok conference of the End Child Prostitution in Asian Tourism organization (ECPAT). Another collaboration was with "Women and Children International, Inc." On 2 October 1993 Jay, along with Dr. Abdul Momem and his wife Nasim Momem, president and director respectively of that organization, met at United Nations New York with Prime Minister Khaleda Zia of Bangladesh. They presented the Prime Minister with a letter signed by the committee (which had been reviewed in my office and circulated to the Board without response), urging her to take action on the sale of Bangladeshi women and children into forced prostitution in Pakistan and other countries of the region. They also urged financial support to repatriate victims to their home countries for rehabilitation there. She agreed in principle to work cooperatively with the Pakistan government to repatriate women and children from Bangladesh held in Pakistani's prisons.

Meanwhile, I approved Jay's suggestion to make Chok Hiew a WFMH consultant to End Child Prostitution in Asian Tourism and our representative to its 1–14 May 1993 conference in Stuttgart, Germany-a country that was alleged to have provided significant numbers of customers for child prostitutes in Asia. He became visible to our members at the Assembly during our 1993 Tokyo World Congress when he presented a resolution in support of the committee's work. It focused on the detrimental health consequences of sexual exploitation of children as well as the need to enforce the United Nations Convention on the Rights of the Child of which WFMH was one of the signatories. The Assembly approved the resolution, and former WFMH President Aldaba-Lim presented it later to the XVI World Law Conference, which endorsed it in September 1993 in Manila. The resolution was also endorsed by WFMH member association, the International Council of Psychologists and the Federation of Bangladeshi Associations of North America.

Many efforts of this committee culminated in 1996 in Jay's active representation of WFMH at the World Congress Against the Commercial Exploitation of Children hosted by the Swedish government in Stockholm on 27–31 August. It brought together government delegations of 118 countries, United Nations agencies, and NGOs concerned about the sale of children for sexual purposes. In addition to Jay, two other members of the WFMH Committee were present. One was Aldaba Lim, attending as an advisor to the delegation of the Philippines government. The other was Hiew representing End Child Prostitution in Asian Tourism. He chaired a workshop, for which Jay was the rapporteur, entitled "The Mental Health of Children in Commercial Sexual Trafficking."

The major WFMH initiative at the Stockholm Congress was a resolution—produced over several drafts by the committee, other NGOs, and the WFMH Secretariat—calling on the World Bank to require impact studies of factors affecting children as a condition for development loans. It also called for protection of children's human rights and denial of development loans that might be used for human trafficking and child prostitution. It also asked the World Bank, when reviewing loan applications, to consider government enforcement practices and prevention programs regarding human trafficking and child prostitution. Aldaba Lim was instrumental in having a reference to the World Bank and other financial institutions included in the conference summary report from the Asian region. She retired from the committee at the end of 1996, and her place was taken by the Honorable Lina B. Laigo, the Philippine government's Secretary for Social Welfare and Development who headed the Philippine delegation to Stockholm. Laigo endorsed the inclusion of the resolution in the agenda of Asian Pacific

Economic Commission leaders. She sent me a letter from Domingo L. Slazon, Jr., Secretary of Foreign Affairs, indicating that the Asian Pacific Economic Commission was primarily a forum for economic cooperation toward free and open trade and investment in the Asia Pacific region and that, social development issues are dealt with indirectly. However, it was clear to us that the economic route could be an effective way of dealing with social issues.

On 22 November 1996 Dr. Elena Berger from my office attended a briefing for NGOs at the Justice Department in Washington, DC, organized by Laurie Robinson, U.S. Assistant Attorney General and head of the U.S. delegation to Stockholm. The WFMH resolution was discussed there as well as in several other settings, including a Geneva meeting of the subgroup on sexual exploitation of children of the NGO Group for the Convention of the Rights of the Child.

THE MENTAL HEALTH OF REFUGEES AND OTHER MIGRANTS

The Rees Era

The traumatic impact of forcible dislocation and uprooting from home, community, and support networks has been, perhaps, the most widely recognized mental health issue of the 20th century. After World War II one of the first agencies of the new United Nations was its Rehabilitation and Relief Agency (UNRRA), with its Displaced Person's Division. In July 1947 it was converted into the International Refugee Organization (IRO).

In August 1948, the Federation's founding document referred to the need to address the mental health problems of displaced persons and others made homeless by forced relocation. Its Second Mental Health Assembly in Geneva on 22–27 August 1949 included a working group on the psychological problems of displaced persons. Its concerns were more those of a reflective social science seminar than an urgent humanitarian group aimed at practical assistance. Its main recommendations were for study of such issues as "the harmful effects of mass living" and the influence of socioeconomic and demographic status on adjustment to refugee camp life. Its first practical recommendation, recognizing the resistance of host populations to accepting strangers in their midst, was to abandon the term "displaced" in favor of "homeless." This designation was regarded as less stigmatizing, i.e., less suggestive of the incoming refugees as "foreign bodies" in the countries of asylum or resettlement. It also recommended exploring the possibility of collaboration in refugee studies with UNESCO and including the problems of homeless or "transplanted" persons (a term for which there was a temporary vogue) as a subject for group discussion in the 1950 and 1951 annual meetings (WFMH, 1948–1949, pp. 63–64).

The Third annual meeting in September 1950 in Paris, with the French League for Mental Hygiene as host, included two papers on the mental health of homeless and transplanted persons, one from Austria, the other from Israel. By that time it was estimated that refugees (including some economic migrants) in Europe alone numbered nearly 10,000,000, with approximately half a million people migrating annually. Special attention was devoted to integrating them into their host communities. Suggested approaches were through vocational guidance, keeping family units together, and encouraging associations of people from the same communities to achieve a measure of self-government and better communications with their home territories. It was also suggested that WFMH should approach the Mental Health Section of WHO or the Social Sciences Division of UNESCO to encourage and coordinate research in this field.

An important part of the 1950 program was a report from psychiatrist H.B.M. Murphy of Canada, assigned by IRO to observer status at the WFMH meeting, about the activities of his organization. He believed that repatriation and, failing that, resettlement were essential prerequisites to any kind of psychosocial rehabilitation. Although IRO was active in efforts to rehabilitate physically disabled refugees in camps before moving them out, the "experience of trying to rehabilitate these people mentally had led to the conclusion that IRO could do little for them until they could be told that this work would get them to a permanent home...after that other types of mental health work might be possible" (WFMH, 1950, p. 96).

Murphy's pessimistic outlook did not fit the long-range optimism of Rees and colleagues. This may have reflected the fact that he was supported by an organization that itself had no future. It was scheduled to disband on 31 March 1951, at which time its functions were to be divided between voluntary organizations in different countries with a United Nations appointed High Commissioner for Refugees (UNHCR) responsible for coordinating the work. This was not good news. The High Commissioner's office, with minimal staff and budget, was to be limited to liaison and coordination.

Murphy also explained that, unlike WHO and UNESCO, IRO had not entered into official relations with the Federation because "its future was so uncertain...it was [also] difficult, or wrong, to think of IRO without realizing the political implications. By assisting politically persecuted refugees IRO inevitably took sides...there had been quite an attempt to use IRO as a political label" (WFMH, 1950, p. 95).

Despite this somewhat discouraging introduction to intergovernmental refugee efforts, WFMH with the freedom of an NGO persisted in focusing major attention on the issue. At the December 1951 Mexico City WFMH Congress the exploration of refugee mental health by several working groups was credited with stimulating wider interest in the issue, including that by governments.

At the 1952 annual meeting a working group of 10 members from five countries continued to define and explore mental health aspects of the refugee situation. Encouraged by the emergence of a stronger than expected UNHCR and enhanced interest from UNESCO and WHO, its first act was to emphasize the importance and continuing nature of the subject. It recommended that it (the working group) be continued throughout the coming year as a nucleus to attract other interested people and that a similar body should be included in future annual meetings. It also recommended the appointment of a qualified refugee expert as part of the WFMH Secretariat to be the focal point for research, practice, and liaison in this area, the formation of a WFMH sponsored refugee issue library, the establishment of a central registry of scientists and other experts, the encouragement of university work , and the establishment of national refugee reception centers staffed with mental health workers.

In 1956 WFMH member association, the Austrian Society for Mental Health, was involved in helping the nearly 200,000 refugees from Hungary who had flooded across Austria's borders. Hans Strotzka and colleagues in the society established a working group for refugees, and this became a topic of that year's annual meeting. Their appeal for money to pay for psychiatrists and social workers was met by a positive response from WFMH affiliated societies and individuals. In his 1958 report to the Federation Strotzka described the difficulties encountered, especially those resulting from hasty selection or faulty training of personnel (Strotzka, 1960). Henry David recalled that Strotzka concluded that most important for preventive purposes were "arrangements for a regular flow of correct information, the encouragement of camp self-government, and programmatic efforts to maintain and/or strengthen the self-respect of refugees" (David, 1969, p. 81). After his experiences with the Hungarian refugees Strotzka was invited to serve as a mental health advisor to UNHCR to help cope with the approximately 18,000 displaced persons remaining in European camps after the massive population movements of World War II. David noted that he was the first mental health specialist with an opportunity to participate in international planning for social action under United Nations auspices.

By 1958, with the WFMH's 11th annual meeting in a Vienna flooded with Hungarian refugees, concern with their mental health had become so intense that it became the meeting's central theme. Its core was the "Conference for Discussion of the Problems of Mental Health of Immigrants." At this meeting Erik Erikson's discussion of identity and uprootedness provided a title for the refugee volume emerging nearly 20 years later from the 1977 World Congress in Vancouver. The importance attached to the theme was indicated by the 1958 list of representatives from United Nations agencies (UNHCR, ILO, UNESCO, WHO, Unicef), governments (Australia, Brazil, Israel, Netherlands, Sudan, Switzerland, United Kingdom, United States), and international NGOs.

Among the areas receiving special attention was the mental health of older refugees. The plenary session papers published in a separate volume (WFMH, 1958) dealt with issues ranging from national responsibility to the sociological aspects of resettlement, common psychological problems, and identity issues. Particular attention was paid to community formation, social integration, and training for combined clinical and social work with refugees.

After 1958 most annual meetings included at least one plenary session on migration and related issues in relation to mental health. By 1960 Strotzka could discuss issues common to refugee populations in different settings (Strotzka, 1961a) as well as the enormous variations in the social atmosphere of various camps (Strotzka, 1961b). Important differences were associated with the personalities of camp officials and counseling personnel as well as the nature of the camp populations, their living circumstances and socioeconomic and cultural conditions outside as well as inside the camps. However, nearly 20 years passed before refugees and migrants again became a high priority concern for the Federation.

The Vancouver Era

President Tsung-yi Lin (1974–1979) had a long history of research in migration, and it was a major professional interest of Morton Beiser, his colleague from the University of British Columbia and North American vice president. Further, the West Coast of Canada was a logical setting for reports involving people from the Pacific Rim and Southeast Asian countries. Significant movements of population had come from those parts of the world to Canada. The 1977 World Congress in Vancouver (see Chapter 10) featured both migration studies and innovative service programs for cultural minorities among its topics. These were eventually published in a volume on the adaptation and resettlement of migrant families and children (Nann, 1982). Beiser organized a regional meeting on migration into Canada before the 1983 Washington World Congress.

The Harvard Program in Refugee Trauma (HRPT)

My own interest in migration research, stemming from experience in occupied Germany beginning in 1946 and later in Brazil during the 1960s (Brody, 1973), led me to organize a conference on the subject in Puerto Rico in 1968 (Brody, 1969a). At that time I was not associated with the Federation. However, one participant was Henry David, who drew on his early experiences with WFMH as well as his current ones as a consultant to the Joint Distribution Committee concerned with continuing problems of Jewish refugees from totalitarian regimes.

After becoming active in the Federation I realized that this was a natural focus for sustained WFMH action beyond holding occasional meetings. With this in mind I telephoned a friend, Richard Mollica, M.D., M.A.R. (Master of Arts in Religion from Yale) of the Harvard Schools of Medicine and Public Health. Rich Mollica, not only a scholar but a social activist, was developing an Indo-Chinese Psychiatric Clinic for Cambodian and Vietnamese refugees into the United States. Some years earlier I had discussed a paper by Fritz Redlich, M.D., Chairman of Psychiatry at Yale, and him on socioeconomic status and treatment for mental illness. Later, while a Fulbright Scholar in England, he had attended a course at Oxford and Cambridge for which I was codirector entitled "Humane Aspects of the British Health System." During our time in England he recalled that I had been Redlich's first chief resident, beginning with my return from military service in Germany in January 1948, and he had been the last chief resident

of Redlich's tenure. With this background, to which he attached considerable emotional significance, he was delighted to reestablish our relationship and agreed to take the initial steps
toward establishing a WFMH committee on refugees. First, though, he felt that I should try to
form a relationship with the office of UNHCR in Geneva.

I followed his advice. During my 12–16 December 1986 visit to Geneva, I engaged Stan
Flache in discussions of possible ways of collaborating in this respect with the United Nations
(see Chapter 8). We visited the UNHCR offices, but their response to the possibility of collaborating with an NGO oriented toward mental health was not encouraging. This visit underscored
the need to develop a WFMH contact group to relate to United Nations and other agencies on
this score. The obvious group was that associated with Mollica's program that, beginning with
the Indochinese Psychiatry Clinic, was transformed by late 1986 into the HPRT. A decade of regular participation in the work of HPRT, both in Boston and outside the United States, began with
my assent to his request to speak on 27 April 1987 to his students at the School of Public Health
on "Behavior in New Environments: Ethnicity and Migration." This marked the initial affiliation of WFMH with HPRT as well as a mutually rewarding collaboration with Mollica and key
members of his team including James Lavelle, M.S.W., Kathleen Allden, M.D., and Svang Tor, a
high status Cambodian refugee who was a key liaison to the Cambodian community in Boston.

HPRT gave WFMH an action arm for promoting refugee mental health, whereas WFMH
through my office gave HPRT regular contact with developing concerns in the United Nations
and in other WFMH regions. New Zealand and Australia, for example, were host to large numbers of refugees from Asia, South and Central America, and Africa, some of whom had suffered
torture as well as uprooting. We facilitated a 1987 consultation by Mollica and Lavelle with
Board member Dr. Max Abbott of Auckland on refugee issues in New Zealand. In the following
year they returned as overseas resource persons for the 12–15 May 1988 first New Zealand
National Conference on Refugee Mental Health under the auspices of WFMH, the Inter-Church
Commission on Immigration and Refugee Resettlement, the Mental Health Foundation of New
Zealand headed by Abbott, and the New Zealand Department of Health. The volume of papers
from that conference, including one by Mollica, notes that it was cosponsored by the WFMH, of
which the New Zealand Foundation was a member (Abbott, 1989).

During that trip Mollica and Lavelle also visited Australia in response to its government's
request to provide technical assistance to its new facility, the Service for Treatment and
Rehabilitation of Torture and Trauma Survivors. It became a WFMH collaborating center with a
presentation by its director, Margaret Cunningham, M.S.W., to the Board in Sydney in 1992. Our
later interchange was mainly with its psychiatrist consultant Professor Derrick Silove, M.D., of
the University of New South Wales who worked closely at times with HPRT.

Meanwhile, through the WFMH network, Mollica was developing contacts with other
refugee advocacy, research, and service groups. They included those with a focus on Africa asso-
ciated with the Institute for Psycho-Ecological Studies of the University of Limburg in
Maastricht directed by Professor of Social Psychiatry Marten de Vries; a subcommittee for
Mexico and Central America chaired by Pablo Farias, M.D.; and one for Hong Kong and the
Pacific Rim chaired by Silove.

WFMH Refugee Work in North and Central America

Opportunities for knowledge sharing and discussion became available with increasing fre-
quency as the importance of the refugee mental health issue became more widely recognized.
Thus, as described in Chapter 10, WFMH cosponsored with our member organization the Hogg
Foundation for Mental Health a 22–25 March 1990 conference in Houston entitled "The Mental
Health of Immigrants and Refugees" (Holtzman and Bornemann, 1990). Defined as a North
American regional meeting it was initiated by regional vice president Beverly Long and orga-

nized by a committee chaired by Hogg Foundation President Dr. Wayne Holtzman and U.S. Refugee Mental Health Office Director Dr. Thomas Bornemann. I was there as a Hogg Foundation National Advisory Council member constituting a link to WFMH. It was my task as keynoter for the conference to tie it to worldwide Federation concerns with the mental health of traumatized refugees. This goal was dramatized by our special guest, Haing Ngor, M.D., an advocate for Cambodian refugees, widely known for his film, *The Killing Fields*.

During the 1991 World Congress for Mental Health in Mexico (see Chapter 9) a major event was a subcongress on refugees. It was repeated in 1993 in Tokyo but given minor billing in Dublin in 1995 and continued only as a few papers in Finland in 1997. In Mexico the first WFMH committee on Southeast Asian migrants was absorbed into a new international committee on the mental health of refugees and other migrants chaired by Mollica and co-chaired by Pablo Farias, M.D., of the Comitan Research Foundation in Chiapas, Mexico. Farias' participation, though, was minimal and brief because of his increasing concern with purely Mexican affairs.

After the intense activity of the 1991 Mexican subcongress, Beverly Long, who had become WFMH honorary secretary, inaugurated a North American regional council committee on refugees, which at a 14–15 January 1992 meeting began work on developing refugee and immigrant mental health resource centers in several parts of the United States. Before the year was over, however, it was clear that the council did not have the resources to carry out a project of this magnitude. Nor did it have a sufficiently strong identity to make it a credible seeker for outside funding. Then the next North American vice president was notable mainly for his failure to become involved. After Long's initial effort, the North American regional council quietly faded away, but Federation concern with refugees did not.

Largely through Long's efforts, the Pew Charitable Trusts granted WFMH $215,000 to support a special project to be led by Farias under our umbrella. Its main goal was to develop the capacity of community agencies in Central America and Southern Mexico to design and implement health and mental health programs. One component focused on psychosocial and mental health community programs for the refugee and displaced populations of the region. The other, focused on the Chiapas-Guatemala border region, involved governmental and nongovernmental agencies from Mexico, Guatemala, El Salvador, Nicaragua, and Costa Rica. By July 1992 the project had attracted the attention of the Mexican government, and Farias was named by the Minister of Education as director of a federal research institute, the Centro de Investigaciones Ecologicas del Sureste, part of a consortium now responsible for administering the project. This accelerated the formalization of a border health association. As he became increasingly absorbed in the organizational complexities of the situation, its already tenuous connection with the WFMH committee was effectively lost. Still, his final report to my office noted that the WFMH sponsored project had provided services for approximately 20,000 people displaced from their communities by revolt in Chiapas. In February and March 1994 group activities for refugee children from Chiapas were developed from materials developed in 1993 in camps for Guatemalans. They were aimed at fostering the expression of emotions "through play and creative activities, development of trust in groups, and narrative skills for children" (Farias, 1994).

Committee on the Mental Health of Southeast Asian Refugees and Sequelae

In the spring of 1988 this committee, headed by Mollica, was formed at my suggestion as a WFMH action arm in the refugee-migrant field. Its initial task was to develop an evaluation protocol to be used in the Cambodian refugee camps in Thailand. Among the members of that initial group were anthropologist Dr. Janice Reid of Australia, an expert on treatment of torture survivors; child and adolescent psychiatrist Massimo Ammaniti, M.D., of Italy (whom my wife and I visited in Australia a year later); Father Koichi Kasuya, a Japanese authority on refugee resettlement; and another old friend, English psychiatrist Douglas Bennett, M.D., a pioneer worker on the rehabilitation of chronically mentally ill persons. The committee voted to conduct as its first major activity an evaluation of the mental health status of the Khmer displaced persons on the Thai-Kampuchean borders. Svang Tor and other Khmer experts living in Boston were recruited to help design the needs assessment aspects of the evaluation.

A grant to HPRT from the Episcopal Church of Boston and a private donor made the first project possible. Between 26 September and 6 October 1988 Mollica and Russell Jalbert, former director of the Federal Assistance Program to U.S. East Coast refugees, conducted a preliminary survey of Cambodians in UNHCR refugee camps at the Thai border with special reference to psychosocial disabilities associated with long stays in the camps. I approved their use of WFMH credentials to enter the camp called Site II with the permission of the United Nations Border Relief Organization (UNBRO) and UNHCR. As a consultant to HPRT (which formed the nucleus of the new WFMH committee) I also helped review and evaluate this first project's findings and plan for the next step. Site II contained 175,000 refugees, and it was clear that a thorough enumeration of their psychiatric problems would require at least another visit. This was accomplished on 1–27 October with a trained assessment team. At this time plans were laid to begin systematic training of indigenous workers to help build a viable mental health system within the camp. Funding was obtained for a third visit to establish a permanent system of training facilities for refugee counselors. With the help of my *Journal of Nervous and Mental Disease* publisher, Williams & Wilkins, the reports of the two visits were reproduced for distribution (Mollica and Jalbert, 1989a; Mollica et al., 1989b). I forwarded them to the United Nations Secretary General in the hope that they would then be passed on to UNHCR, but aside from a routine notice of their receipt there was no acknowledgment.

The first Site II visit (Mollica and Jalbert, 1989a) was the focus of a meeting held 29–30 June 1989 at the Harvard School of Public Health. It was attended by legislators, other government officials, public health experts, representatives from UNBRO, and medical and planning experts from the expatriate Cambodian community of Boston, with some of their professional members receiving further graduate training at Harvard. This meeting was impressive on both scholarly and advocacy grounds; it also displayed Mollica's political skills in bringing the needs of both the Site II Cambodians and those in Boston to the attention of responsible officials. The resulting WFMH-HPRT statement was entitled "Resolving the Mental Health Crisis in the Khmer Displaced Persons Camp in Thailand known as Site Two." A consequence of this conference was UNBRO's designation of WFMH (through Mollica's refugee committee) as its primary consultant in mental health. In April 1989, at UNBRO's formal request, HPRT, identified as a WFMH affiliate, sent a team to Site II to follow its original 1988 recommendations. This visit included the first mental health training of Khmer refugees in the camp. Its report (Mollica et al., 1989b) was accepted by UNBRO as the basis of official guidelines for its response to the mental health crisis of the border Khmer. The committee's report was also presented to the 1989 WFMH Board meeting in Auckland that accepted Mollica's recommendation that to promote the development of a network of region oriented refugee committees his WFMH committee, the first formal Federation-wide service group for refugees, should be redesignated, "Southeast Asian Refugees."

In May 1990 the HPRT/WFMH team implemented the survey recommendations of the second report, "Turning Point in Khmer Mental Health" (Mollica et al., 1989b) by conducting a comprehensive epidemiological survey of 1000 adult households, including children and adolescents, in Site II. This survey was supported by the Ford Foundation and coadministered by HPRT and Lou Harrison & Associates. It focused on the work, disability, and health/mental health status of the Khmer community to help the United Nations prepare it for repatriation to Cambodia. The results of this study were submitted to UNBRO in late spring 1991.

Meanwhile, Mollica's relationships with European colleagues, especially in Italy, demanded more attention. On 11–13 July 1990 (see Chapter 11), Silove, Mollica, and I along with former

WFMH Board member Professor Tolani Asuni, M.D., of Nigeria, addressed a meeting on "Medicine and Migration," cosponsored by Harvard and WFMH and chaired by Luigi Frighi, M.D., Professor of Mental Hygiene at the University of Rome.

At same time the primary HPRT effort at Site II continued. In November 1991, with both the Harvard and the WFMH imprimaturs, a two-volume study of the health, mental health, and social functioning of the Khmer adults and children resident in the camp was issued (Mollica et al., 1991a, 1991b). In consequence the Pew Trust agreed to fund the training of 65 Khmer refugees, including monks, recruited from all border camps to provide family-child interventions and support to the most vulnerable members of the community. The training program begun late in 1991 was conducted primarily by Khmer mental health experts from the United States and Thailand. It was a thrill to acknowledge this work, facilitated by our Federation, with letters of acknowledgment on WFMH letterhead to the Khmer workers who completed the training.

United Nations High Commissioner for Refugees

By 1992, Mollica and colleagues had been moving so rapidly on research and service that they had hardly had time to assimilate what they had been learning. They realized that it was time to stop and take stock. Much of the new knowledge gained in these ventures was discussed at a 29 September–1 October 1992 conference at Harvard entitled "The Science of Refugee Mental Health: Concepts and Methods." Funding from several foundations enabled the participation of key WFMH committee members from Australia, The Netherlands, Italy, and the United States. Among them was psychiatrist Riccardo Colasanti, M.D., a migration specialist attached to the Department of Mental Hygiene at the University of Rome and the Vatican's Committee on Refugees. He obtained funds and edited "Refugee Notes," a committee newsletter that appeared quarterly during 1994 and 1995. We included it without additional mailing cost with the WFMH newsletter.

Soon after the refugee science meeting, Mollica, Lavelle, and I met in Geneva on 14 October 1992 with the UN High Commission for Refugees, Mme. Sadako Ogata, and members of her staff. We agreed on the importance of formalizing a working arrangement between WFMH and UNHCR with HPRT as the instrumental participant. Two months later the Federation Executive Committee meeting at Sheppard Pratt Hospital in Baltimore (13–15 December 1992) officially designated HPRT as a WFMH collaborating center.

Among the people with whom we met in Geneva was Mary Petevi of Cyprus, Senior Resettlement Officer of UNHCR. She was easy to talk with, interested in our perspective, and joined our group at Cape Cod on 4–6 March 1993 for a series of discussions aimed at exploring issues of mental health and sustainable social development in communities devastated by war and oppression. Other guests were Derrick Silove, Louis Kikuchi, Professor Robert Muscat (economic consultant to the government of Thailand), and Hernan Reyes, M.D., of the International Committee of the Red Cross with whom we had met in Geneva. This meeting helped redirect HPRT attention away from an exclusive concern with individual refugees and refugee populations to include the destroyed communities from which they had been displaced and to which most (although not all) aspired to return. It also allowed further clarification of the project agreement with HPRT. A formal tripartite agreement between HPRT, UNHCR, and WFMH was completed and signed in mid-year by Ogata, Mollica, and myself.

Among other features it designated Petevi as the first UNHCR focal point for dealing with mental health issues. This had historical significance. An early consequence of the new agreement was an invitation from UNHCR for WFMH to meet with its representatives and the government of The Netherlands on 17–19 June 1993 at a consultation on the care and rehabilitation of trauma victims from former Yugoslavia—its former components by now separated and embroiled in war with each other. In addition to Mollica, WFMH was represented further by de Vries. In Utrecht guidelines were developed for the evaluation and care of victims of torture, trauma, collective abuse, and war. The project proper began, as described below, in Croatia in 1994. Another consequence was Petevi's leadership of a 19 November 1993 meeting with WFMH President-elect Beverly Long and North American vice president psychologist Dr. Charles Spielberger at the U.S. Office of Refugee Health headed by Thomas Bornemann, who had become a member of our refugee committee. The focus was on how the mental health needs of refugees resettled in the United States might be more completely addressed through coordination with U.S. mental health professionals. Afterward my office made occasional referrals to various U.S. treatment groups. However, this ended as another of the several attempts to develop a North American refugee program that did not succeed, mainly through lack of an adequate infrastructure to carry it out.

Meanwhile, subprojects of HPRT continued. In 1993 my wife and I gained a glimpse of Dr. Allden's study of Burmese student refugees into Thailand as we met with HPRT staff and student refugees at the Institute of East Asian Studies of Chulalongkorn University in Bangkok. I also spoke on human rights and mental health at the University Department of Psychiatry. Here we talked with Professor Supang about her WFMH representation at the March-April meetings of the Asia-Pacific preconference meeting (of the 1993 United Nations World Conference on Human Rights).

Work in Cambodia was continuing. On 10–19 January 1994 HPRT-WFMH conducted a site visit to prepare for the Khmer Mental Health Training and Consultation Initiative funded by two private foundations. The team led by Mollica included Lavelle, Tor, Allden, and Cambodian Savuth Sath, who had lived in Boston for some time. Patrick van der Velde, former director of UNBRO, was a consultant. Meetings were held with a range of international organizations active in the country as well as WHO, UNHCR, the U.S. Agency for International Development, and Khmer working in health-care settings. The group was warmly received by the ministers of health, education, and foreign affairs as well as other representatives of the new government, and it reestablished relations with 32 of the 57 Khmer family-child mental health workers to whom we had given certificates earlier. They were organizing community activities, collaborating with primary care physicians, and in some instances achieving linkages with traditional folk healers. By late spring 1994 the demonstration training program had received the full approval of the Cambodian government. The official opening of the Harvard-WFMH training center took place in Siem Reap province in April 1994 with the recruitment of personnel to initiate a community-based mental health program.

During 1995 the Cambodians founded a mental health association in Siem Reap. By 1996 the Siem Reap Center was so deluged with patients that its meager supply of drugs was not sufficient to meet the demand. Eli Lilly & Company was willing to donate fluoxetine, but Harvard could not ship it to Cambodia for some regulatory reason. The Kingdom of Cambodia's ministry of health, by now familiar with WFMH through its affiliation with HPRT, faxed me a request for the medication. They finally received it after several hours of long-distance telephone calls from Dick Hunter to Cambodia to obtain clearances.

Croatia

On 10–20 March 1994 Jim Lavelle went to Zagreb and Split as a member of a Harvard Medical School group called "Psychologists for Social Change." They taught counseling techniques to mental health professionals and paraprofessionals for use with psychologically traumatized victims of the fighting and forced relocations in former Yugoslavia. This was preliminary to HPRT establishing a project there. In my advisory role I reviewed their grant application that was approved by the U.S. Agency for International Development in early 1995. Its aim was to set up a three-year training program for primary care physicians, teachers, and consultants to the de facto mental health system in Croatia. The work was to be performed with the cosponsorship of UNHCR following the triangular agreement signed by UNCHR with HPRT and WFMH in June 1993. Initial plans were to train and certify up to 120 former Yugoslavian mental health professionals in the psychosocial care of veterans, POWs, displaced persons, and Bosnian refugees into Croatia.

In September 1994 Mollica along with Petevi consulted in Croatia on the development of the program. Major curriculum development was performed in collaboration with local partners, psychiatrists Ljlana Moro, M.D., of the University of Rijeka and Narcisa Sarajalec, M.D., of the University of Zagreb. Kathleen Allden conducted the first phase, training primary care physicians in mental health principles. Later work was coordinated by social worker Mary Mathias from the Indochinese Psychiatry Clinic who in September 1996 established residence in Opatija on the Adriatic a few miles from Rijeka. During that year there were four sessions of four days each for a group of 35 Bosnian (Muslim) and 35 Croatian (Catholic) psychiatrists, psychologists, and social workers. The stated aim was training to deal with victims of organized violence. An unstated goal, accomplished through continuing participation of Bosnians and Croats together in small groups, was collaboration between these individuals from hostile societies and different ethnic backgrounds.

It was my privilege to work with these people, along with Mollica, Lavelle, Matthias, and Croatian and Bosnian colleagues for a week in April 1997. In my combined role as advisor to HPRT and as a WFMH officer I also met with them and U.S. Agency for International Development personnel, their office staffs, and Bosnian and Croatian lecturers in the program. My formal teaching tasks were speaking on the ethical issues involved in refuge work and delivering a brief graduation address when the students received certificates from a Harvard vice president on hand for the occasion; it attested to their having completed 240 hours of instruction. This was an opportunity to emphasize the WFMH concern with intercultural harmony. During the visit we also met with leaders of Mehamet, a volunteer treatment center for Bosnian refugees in Rijeka operated by Bosnian muslims who had come into Croatia before the war. It was an inspiring and emotional experience, and I was grateful for the opportunity.

The Japanese Earthquake Disaster, 1995

A disastrous earthquake struck the Kobe area of Japan on 17 January 1995. More than 5000 people died, and thousands more were left homeless. The emotional sequelae continued for a prolonged period with the dislocation of large numbers of people from their homes into temporary shelters. HPRT was mobilized to help, supported by the Nippon Foundation of Japan working with Dr. Hisao Nakki of Kobe University and anthropology professor Louis Kikuchi of Waseda University in Tokyo. Mollica and Lavelle flew to Kobe in late January to assess the situation, returning again with Allden for two weeks at the end of February to make a more detailed estimate of the need for screening instruments and community intervention. An HPRT working group was organized that included two Japanese physicians, who were graduate students in the Harvard School of Public Health. They visited Kobe every three months during 1995 to perform field work and help local authorities develop a policy for providing humanitarian assistance in case of future disasters. Part of the work involved translating mental health research instruments into Japanese. A central question concerned the role of government in providing for emotional as well as material needs of disaster victims.

Meanwhile, my office was flooded with requests for information on psychological assistance for earthquake survivors. We obtained information from all available sources including the Emergency Services and Disaster Relief Branch of NIMH, WFMH President Puente who had helped provide assistance after the Mexican earthquake of 1985, and our United Nations

New York representative Dr. Anie S. Kalayjian who had participated in relief efforts after the Armenian earthquake of 1988. Materials were sent for distribution to our honorary secretary, Kunihiko Asai, M.D., regional vice president Shimpei Inoue, M.D., and psychologist Nobuko Fuji in Kyoto, one of the first Japanese mental health professionals to offer telephone counseling to survivors. By March 1995 Asai and Inoue reported that more than 20 telephone hotline services were in operation and that emergency psychiatric clinics had been opened in public health centers. Numerous volunteers were active, and the Ministry of Health and Welfare was making long-range plans to continue psychiatric support for people suffering from post-traumatic stress disorders.

The End of an Era

As the end of the Federation's first half-century approached Richard Mollica asked to be relieved of his chairmanship of our refugee committee. He was replaced during the 1997 Finland Congress by psychologist Dr. Solvig Ekblad of the Karolinska Institute in Stockholm with the expectation that she would hold the job for one year and then be succeeded by Derrick Silove. At Richard's request I committed myself to increased involvement with HPRT beginning in autumn 1997, and its collaborative work with WFMH was expected to continue into the indefinite future.

WFMH ADVOCACY FOR HUMAN RIGHTS

The protection of patients' rights is integral to improving the quality of mental health services. Protecting the rights of vulnerable groups such as the very young and the elderly and others at risk for illness or distress also has preventive significance. The basis for subsequent United Nations human rights instruments was article 55 of the United Nations Charter of 1945 that committed it to promote "higher standards of living...solutions of international economic, social, health and related problems, and international cultural and educational cooperation." The United Nations Universal Declaration of Human Rights, proclaimed on 10 December 1948, included many references to health rights. The universality of its proclaimed standards was in perfect accord with WFMH acceptance of an allegiance to humankind as a whole in its founding document issued four months earlier. Among these several deserve particular note (for a detailed review see Brody, 1993b). They include a prohibition against "cruel, inhuman or degrading treatment" (article 5), elaborated in 1966 to include a specific reference to medical research; a reference to the importance of education for the "free and full development of...personality" within one's community; freedom from gender-based discrimination; rights to the benefits of science, adequate medical and social services, safe and healthy working conditions, and, in 1966, "the right of everyone to the enjoyment of the highest obtainable standard of physical and mental health." Children's health rights were included in a 1959 United Nations Declaration of the Rights of the Child, elaborated in later instruments.

Women's health rights including a right to plan a family (Article 16) included in the initial declaration were elaborated in 1967 in the General Assembly's Declaration on the Elimination of Discrimination against Women. The 1979 United Nations International Convention on the Elimination of Discrimination against women also recommended access to family planning services including voluntary sterilization and abortion. These issues were further expounded during 1985–1995 with the same theme. Those relevant to reproductive health and behavior as they bore on infant and child health were further affirmed and elaborated in the 20 November 1989 United Nations Convention on the Rights of the Child. Finally, as noted in Chapter 8, in 1985 the Declaration of Basic Principles of Justice for Victims of Crime and Abuse of Power, with contributions from several NGOs, was passed by the United Nations General Assembly. Following advocacy by WFMH it recognized the importance of mental health impairment in consequence of victimization and the need for mental health services.

As these positive declarations were being formulated, and generally ignored by most of the less industrialized world, the United Nations began to recognize the anxiety engendered in the industrial democracies by the rapid development of biomedical technology. The 1968 United Nations International Conference on Human Rights warned that "while recent scientific discoveries and technological advances have opened vast prospects for economic, social and cultural progress, such developments may nevertheless, endanger the rights and freedoms of individuals and will require continuing attention." That conference recommended that the agencies of the United Nations undertake a study of the problems relating to human rights that arise from developments in science and technology. That recommendation was the basis of WFMH involvement with UNESCO and the International Social Science Council in 1985 (see Chapter 8), culminating in the publication of *Biomedical Technology and Human Rights* under UNESCO/International Social Science Council/WFMH auspices (Brody 1993b).

Although the 1948 United Nations Declaration and its subsequent elaborations, especially in the mid-1960s, were recognized as relevant to Federation interests, "human rights" did not emerge as a specifically identified advocacy issue for WFMH until 23 years after its founding. This may have been in part because, despite the plethora of official declarations, " human rights" often evoked an aversive reaction in influential United Nations and government officials. In fact, some of the covenants asserting children's protection from social and economic exploitation could be described as "expressions of internationally institutionalized hypocrisy insofar as they conceal the existence of several million children...occupying the virtual status of slaves" (Brody, 1993b, p. 27). In more conventional medical contexts, rights issues were concealed behind such topics as "standards" for psychiatric care. I knew this and was cautious when I proposed a Latin American conference on human rights and psychiatry to PAHO. It was to be focused on the rights of people hospitalized in the large, old, understaffed public mental hospitals of the region. After some years a conference touching on the issue did come to pass, but by then it had long been known as "Restructuring Psychiatric Care in Latin America" (see Chapters 8 and 9).

Mental Health, "Freedom of Conscience," and Soviet Abuse of Psychiatry

For the first 20 years of its existence, even as it reiterated its concern for minorities and refugees and its wish to promote harmonious international relations, the Federation paid little attention to the human rights abuses of authoritarian governments. The 24th annual meeting of the WFMH Executive Board in Hong Kong in November 1971 chaired by Morris Carstairs was the first to recognize the totalitarian exploitation of psychiatry. It adopted a statement endorsing that part of the United Nations Universal Declaration of Human Rights affirming every individual's right to enjoy freedom of conscience. The complete statement was prominently displayed in the Autumn 1971 issue of the WFMH bulletin issued from Edinburgh. It declared that all definitions of mental health share "the recognition of each man's freedom of opinion which is based on freedom of conscience-that is, his right to hold and affirm his personal moral values...deprivation of this freedom is both an affront to human dignity and a severe form of mental cruelty." It referred to accusations of misuse of psychiatric diagnosis and treatment, including the enforced mental hospitalization of "persons whose only 'symptoms' have been the avowal of opinions disapproved by their society...these accusations have been directed in particular...against the alleged incarceration of political dissenters in prison mental hospitals in the USSR."

With this beginning WFMH took its first human rights stand: "The World Federation for Mental Health resolutely opposes any such abuse of psychiatric procedures and calls on its

Member Associations throughout the world promptly to investigate all such allegations and to defend the individual's freedom of opinion where it appears to be threatened" (see Appendix V). It made the same demand upon mental health professionals and governments of those countries without voluntary mental health associations (WFMH,1971a).

Evidence quickly appeared that these initial WFMH efforts made a difference. In 1971 a new mental health bill before the Sri Lanka parliament quoted the WFMH statement on "Freedom of Conscience" in its preamble. On 14 March 1972, the *London Times* reported that several prominent Soviet dissenters who had been incarcerated in mental hospitals had been quietly released. The article said that expressions of concern by health bodies in the Western countries, and by the World Federation for Mental Health, could have influenced Soviet authorities. On 8 October 1973 the Soviet health ministry announced that members of the international psychiatric community would be invited to visit the Serbsky Institute in Moscow that had been cited in connection with several cases of alleged wrongful certification of mental illness.

Shortly after this the Executive Board meeting in Sydney, Australia (13 October 1973), passed a resolution endorsing the United Nations Universal Declaration of Human Rights' affirmation of "every individual's right to enjoy freedom of conscience" and "saluted the willingness" of the Soviet Health Ministry "to submit its psychiatric procedures to independent examination. Consequent to these resolutions was an increasing number of "appeals from organizations and individuals for support of causes, petitions and crusades in the name of human rights...in the main concerned with allegations of inhuman treatment of political prisoners, of detention on inadequate grounds or of the misuse of psychiatry for political ends" (WFMH, 1974a). The Federation's response was cautious: "It is often difficult for us to assess to what extent many of these appeals may themselves be politically motivated" (WFMH, 1974a). President Lin's office gave a limited response by reprinting the 1971 Hong Kong declaration in an early 1975 bulletin.

Despite its broad hints to the contrary, major changes did not in fact take place within the Soviet system. In 1974 the Federation again issued a formal condemnation of the Soviet abuse of psychiatry. The U.S.S.R.'s failure to change was addressed at the time of the 1977 Vancouver World Congress by another flurry of resolutions from the Executive Board. One resolution stated that the U.S.S.R.'s "healthy, dissenting citizens...have been forcefully interned in...mental hospitals," condemning the practice and calling for the immediate release of inappropriately hospitalized dissenters. Another resolution called on professionals, governments, and the World Psychiatric Association to take the lead in maintaining worldwide standards for psychiatric practice, agreed to create a task force to study the "misuses of mental health professionals as instruments of political repression," and called specifically for the release of psychiatrist Dr. Semyon Gluzman from a Soviet labor camp where he was imprisoned for objecting to unethical psychiatric practices.

A new phase of vocal Federation human rights advocacy, no longer focused exclusively on the U.S.S.R., began with a 1984 European regional meeting in Copenhagen. Attended by jurists, legislators, other governmental officials, patient advocates, and Federation members from 15 countries (see Chapter 11), its primary concern was the preservation of patient autonomy and the elimination, insofar as possible, of involuntary (compulsory) hospital admission and treatment. These issues were central dilemmas in patient care in the industrial democracies as well as the totalitarian states (Brody, 1988b, 1985).

The Daes Report and Its Sequelae

In 1977 the United Nations Human Rights Commission, prodded by representatives of several governments and NGOs, asked its Sub-Commission on Prevention of Discrimination and Protection of Minorities to produce a set of "principles and guarantees" to protect the rights of people suffering from mental illness. In 1978 the General Assembly added its request. In 1980 a draft declaration was produced by the International Commission of Jurists and the International Association for Penal Reform. In the same year the subcommission established a working group chaired by a Greek lawyer and subcommission representative Erica-Irene Daes to develop the requested principles and guarantees, as well as guidelines, for the protection of persons "detained on grounds of mental ill health or mental disorder." The full title of its first draft, deposited with the commission on 23 August 1984, was "Principles, guidelines and guarantees for the protection of persons detained on grounds of mental ill health or suffering from mental disorder. A contribution to (a) the protection of the fundamental freedoms, human and legal rights of persons who are mentally ill or suffering from mental disorder; (b) the elimination of psychiatric abuses; (c) the promotion of mental health law and medical practice and the improvement of mental health care and mental institutions."

This was in part the United Nations' reaction to the still continuing incarceration in mental hospitals of political dissenters in the U.S.S.R. Its report was intended to lead to an international human rights instrument aimed at protecting these individuals. However, it drew much criticism from psychiatric organizations as potentially damaging to the rights of patients, their access to adequate treatment, their trust in the medical profession, and the ability of the medical profession to help them. Most critics felt that its publication was premature and that it had been prepared without adequate consultation with interested NGOs including WFMH. I felt that the issues had not been made sufficiently clear to the professional community and published a clarifying message in *Psychiatric News*, the official organ of the American Psychiatric Association (Brody, 1987c).

Independent of the Daes report, which had not yet been widely circulated, the WFMH Copenhagen conferees wanted to get a message to the Human Rights Commission. My initial proposal was a resolution requiring that mental hospitals in countries throughout the world be open to inspection by nongovernmental agencies. This was felt to be impractical, especially by the Europeans who preferred that inspections be conducted by governments or the intergovernmental system, i.e., the United Nations. Agreement was reached on a less focused resolution fitting their overall interests in mental hospital practices and depending on the United Nations for enforcement. It declared their widespread concern for the civil rights of people diagnosed as mentally ill and the "coercion and compulsion" to which they were often subjected. And it called upon the United Nations, with the cooperation of all relevant bodies including NGOs, "to establish a body with continuing responsibility" to consider the human rights of people diagnosed with mental disorder "and to work for adequate safeguards which do not of themselves give rise to discrimination." This resolution was presented by WFMH Geneva representative Flache to the 41st Session of the Human Rights Commission in Geneva where it became part of the context of a 6 November 1984 debate between representatives of the U.S.S.R. and other countries on the question of detaining persons who are not mentally ill in mental hospitals for political reasons. Glasnost had not yet arrived, and the resolution made no progress in part because of the argument that it violated the national sovereignty of United Nations member states. It was not until the government of the U.S.S.R. became less restrictive that movement on this issue became possible.

On 12 December 1986, in Geneva, en route home from an International Social Science Council meeting in Paris, I discussed the matter with Flache. At his request acting director Nyamekye of the United Nations Center for Human Rights convened an NGO working group that met on 15 December. In addition to Flache and myself it included John Orley, M.D., of the WHO Division of Mental Health, Tim Harding, M.D., of the University of Geneva's Institute of Legal Medicine, and representatives of the International Commission of Health Professionals for Health and Human Rights, the International Council of Psychologists, and Neil McDermott, a lawyer of the International Commission of Jurists who chaired the WHO working group on human rights.

Their efforts led to a meeting at WHO Geneva (11 May 1987) chaired by MIND national director, and WFMH member Chris Heginbotham, a housing specialist. This was a function of his role as co-chair with Flache of the new WFMH Committee on Human Rights and Legal Affairs appointed by 1985–1987 President Edith Morgan (see below). Additional WFMH representatives included Flache and his Geneva associate, June Spalding. Also present were representatives of Geneva-based NGO groups of psychologists, rehabilitation specialists, jurists, churches, and Quakers as well as Alan Stone, M.D., of Harvard, a visiting professor at the University of Geneva. The group critically reviewed the Daes report, which by then had been submitted to the subcommission and incorporated points made earlier by WFMH representatives. Some were in a paper prepared by Heginbotham, temporarily employed as indicated in Chapter 8 as a consultant for WHO in its effort to provide ideas for the United Nations human rights group (World Health Organization, 1988). Other ideas came from the work of lawyer Larry Gostin and psychiatrist Tim Harding who had attended the 1980 meetings of the International Commission of Jurists and International Association of Penal Reform.

In consequence of this indication of broader NGO interest Flache with the assistance of Deane and Spalding began active efforts to form an NGO committee on human rights/protection of those detained on grounds of mental ill health in Geneva. But by mid-1988, despite many expressions of interest, the number of NGOs required to constitute a formal committee under the aegis of the Conference of NGOs had not been reached, and the effort was abandoned.

Stan Flache's role in pursuing human rights issues at WHO Geneva is detailed in Chapter 8. Following prolonged NGO effort with significant leadership by him and by intergovernmental working groups formed by the commission, a "Declaration of Principles and Guarantees for the Protection of Mentally Ill Persons and for the Improvement of Mental Health Care" was finally formulated and passed by the United Nations General Assembly in December 1991 without a vote. However, since that time specific guidelines have remained to be elaborated and adjusted to the socioeconomic and cultural contexts of various countries to translate the declaration's principles into national legislation. Mechanisms are also needed to monitor the implementation of prescribed measures. One consequence of this work was WHO Director General Hiroshi Nakajima's appointment in 1992 of Flache to the WHO Interdivisional Group on Human Rights of which he eventually became chairman. This is also reviewed in Chapter 8.

Charter 2000: Toward a WFMH Manifesto and Beyond

As the Soviet abuse of psychiatry gradually receded from the public eye and the process of revising the Daes report continued at a slow pace, the general concerns of the 1984 Copenhagen meeting became more prominent. They received special impetus at the 14–19 July 1985 Brighton World Congress with the theme, "Mental Health 2000, Action Programmes for a World in Crisis." The presiding officer was WFMH President Morgan (1985–1987), but the chief organizer and moving spirit was Heginbotham. He had been primed for the task by being part of the United Nations working group attempting to revise the Daes Report. Stimulated by him and Morgan and led by Knud Jensen, the postcongress Board meeting on 19–20 July 1985 passed a resolution based on that from Copenhagen. It called on governments to ensure a "least restrictive environment" for persons "requiring mental health care"; for legal and other rights comparable to the population as a whole; and for a United Nations agency responsible for "abolishing discrimination against and safeguarding the rights of those diagnosed as mentally ill" (see Appendix V).

The major human rights proposal, submitted both to the Brighton Congress and the Board reflected Heginbotham's strong personal views. The document in question was first called "Mental Health 2000" or "Charter 2000", but later was referred to as a "Manifesto." It was intended to provide a comprehensive picture of the rights of psychiatric patients or those at risk of becoming patients. Heginbotham wanted it to be approved by the congress participants or the postcongress Board, as a blueprint to guide WFMH's work into the next century. Much of it was unexceptional, although perhaps unnecessarily detailed. Recommendations for the more usual patient protections included advice about the use of restraint, informed consent, and a series of quasilegal and contractual protections for persons admitted voluntarily to mental health facilities. In addition to a call for increased user (consumer) and NGO participation in the operation of facilities the document warned against the possible conflicts of interest experienced by mental health professionals tempted to "control" the voluntary associations in which they might work. This warning was buttressed by the recommendation that "no single professional group shall exercise undue control over the treatment of patients...the formulation of policy or the allocation of resources."

The special feature of the document was that these recommendations were made in the context of a series of broadly defined socioeconomic "rights" that together constituted the outline of an idealized support system not only for psychologically impaired persons but for the larger population. These were rights to income support, a "free and culturally relevant" education, employment, housing, the elimination of racial discrimination, the provision of general health, leisure, and political opportunity including the provision of "anti-fascist training for all mental health staff." A section on "sexism and mental health" noted that "mental health care for women must challenge the contradictions in society which discriminate against women and ensure that women have the choice to explore how these constraints become part of themselves" as well as asserting that mental health care in the community "is not acceptable if it is at the expense of women's careers." It included specific recommendations for state systems of social security, maintenance of the quality of life, and social stability within nations.

The postcongress Board meeting declined to accept the document as it stood but asked me to collect its comments, "sift" them, and mail them along with my distillate of the siftings to our member associations. I did this, but first, after reading the document and before hearing from others, I wrote Heginbotham on 6 August 1985 stating that this was a MIND, not a Federation, statement, "so broad in places with its social focus that we risk losing some of our leverage in regard to specific goals if it comes to be publicly viewed as the Federation's baby." I also objected to his emphasis on the possible conflicts between professionals and volunteers. Finally I noted that it was much more relevant to the industrial states than to the agrarian and developing world. This last point was later emphasized in the critiques by Board members from these countries.

Most Board members did not respond to the Heginbotham proposal. However, some reactions were lengthy and detailed. Honorary Secretary Jaswant Singh Neki, M.D., an Indian psychiatrist living in Tanzania found it "sectarian" in its developed world perspective, "irresponsible if not actually offensive" in its implication that "freedom and flexibility of organizations" are prerogatives of industrial development, and bordering on "craziness" in its emphasis on "female chauvinism." Aldaba-Lim of Manila felt that it was inappropriate for an international organization and that some of its statements were "contradictory or conflicting." Colleagues from the industrial West were less critical. A consultant from WHO Europe stated, cautiously, that it "might be studied as a strategic paper for policy purposes." European Vice President Jensen, a staunch patient advocate, commented only on the section dealing with commitment and informed consent. He endorsed the usual basic rights as well as the idea that patients should be able to have independent representation before a court to secure their release. More significantly, he supported improved standards of care for all patients as equally important with the recognition of basic rights. Laws and policies regarding mental health, he believed, should be part of a general health care plan for all citizens including prisoners.

Hilda Robbins, the North American vice president reminded me in a letter of 29 August 1985 that she had moved that WFMH "receive" rather than "accept" the document at the end of the Congress. She also recalled that her strong suggestion that the document be marked "draft" had been "just as strongly rejected" by Heginbotham and regretted that "a great many people already have the idea that this is a WFMH publication even though our name is not on it." At the same time she felt that most of the section on increasing the role of voluntary mental health associations was useful.

The various critiques were forwarded to Heginbotham, who by 1986 produced a revision with the help of the MIND policy committee. The document was now entitled "WFMH Manifesto 2000." A major change was the extraction of material about consumer participants to be appended as a separate charter entitled, "Self Determination as a Human Right—Its Implications for Mental Health Services." A timetable suggested the production of a final WFMH policy statement for its 40th anniversary in autumn 1988. This now bulky Manifesto dealt at great length with most issues in the original, including prevention and alternatives to hospitalization and treatment. It was duly forwarded to Board members whose ambivalence was reflected by the fact that no formal action, either to accept it or reject it, was ever taken.

To clarify the situation President Morgan, with the help of Heginbotham and others, organized a conference on mental health and human rights to be held on 9 June 1986 in London immediately preceding the Board meeting at Cumberland Lodge (see Chapter 11). Among the speakers were Tim Harding, M.D., of Geneva, Larry Gostin, J.D., of Boston, and Aldaba-Lim, Flache, Danieli, Mwendapole, and Neki of WFMH. The discussions were interesting but broke no new ground and did not facilitate the contemplation of the Manifesto. At the Board meeting Morgan appointed Heginbotham to co-chair the Committee on Legal Affairs and Human Rights with Gostin, Executive Director of the American Society for Law and Medicine and head of a WHO collaborating center on health legislation at Harvard.

The new committee began its work by preparing terms of reference. These called for it to "(1) plan, draft or assist in the preparation of declarations, guidelines or other national or international documents on the human rights of persons with mental illnesses; (2) investigate and report on abuse of the human rights of persons with mental illnesses; (3) act as an advocate for the human rights of persons with mental illnesses; (4) devise a system for monitoring the implementation of human rights principles and practices." Despite this auspicious beginning the committee did not grow. No new members were appointed, Heginbotham and Gostin—very different in personalities, backgrounds, and styles of work and separated by an ocean—did not collaborate and the committee as an entity lapsed.

Yet, failing a committee effort, the work of individuals under WFMH auspices was notable. Gostin was a brilliant, sometimes acerbic, activist who had been a sometime advisor to Tony Smythe, director of MIND preceding Heginbotham, whose conflict with British psychiatry had nearly lost the organization its government subvention. In 1987 Gostin made an inspection trip to Japan under the joint auspices of WFMH, WHO, and Harvard University. His visit was aimed especially at the nearly absolute powers of private hospital superintendents (Gostin, 1987a and 1987b) (see Chapter 10). In his first volume he reviewed the 1950 Japanese Mental Health Act, proposals for legislative reform, and recommendations by other international visitors. In the second volume he discussed basic principles unanimously adopted by meetings of Japanese and international societies in Kyoto in January 1987. These dealt with a right to humane, dignified, and professional treatment; the importance of encouraging voluntary hospital admission; the right to judicial hearings before involuntary admissions; the right to a free and open environment and free communication; and the right not to be discriminated against on grounds of mental illness. His work with its combined WFMH and WHO auspices contributed to initial changes in Japanese mental health laws, granting greater freedom and autonomy to hospitalized patients and reducing the nearly absolute authority of superintendents.

The follow-up meetings in the autumn of 1988 at which I, along with Max Abbott and others, spoke in Kobe and Tokyo (see Chapter 10) were largely responsible for the Japanese decision to apply for sponsorship of the 1993 World Congress for Mental Health. An important addition to the sponsoring Japanese Association of Psychiatric Hospitals and the Japanese Mental Health Association, was the Japanese Association of Relatives of the Mentally Ill (ZINKAREN). Gostin also wanted to expand the WFMH scrutiny of human rights to the field of general medicine, and at his invitation I prepared an article on the impact of reproductive technologies on women's rights that he edited for the *Journal of Law, Medicine and Health Care* (Brody, 1987b).

Meanwhile, Heginbotham continued to develop his ideas. In May 1987 a British educational charity, "Minority Rights Group, Ltd.," published "The Rights of Mentally Ill People" (Heginbotham, 1987) in pamphlet form. It had much in common with one written by an "advocacy group" at the 1985 Brighton World Congress and circulated but never published. This pamphlet was announced as raising "urgent questions about the nature, diagnosis and attitudes toward those people who are labeled 'mentally ill,' whether their illness is genuine or is induced by torture or inhuman treatment" (Heginbotham, 1987). It was not identified as a publication of WFMH or as one approved by WFMH. However, WFMH approval was implied because Heginbotham was described as a Board member of WFMH representing it on human rights issues at the United Nations Commission on Human Rights and the Sub-Commission.

In early 1988, with recommendations from the 1987 World Congress in Cairo, yet another revision was issued for WFMH Board consideration. This time a more complete title, "Manifesto 2000: Mental Health for All by the Year 2000," clearly indicated in its subtitle that it was issued by WFMH. It still attempted to cover every possible point regarding the identification, hospitalization, and care of mentally and emotionally distressed people and still contained recommendations regarding income, welfare and employment, social security, and "social stability" but in less definitive form. Most Board members did not respond to a request for opinions about this new version, but an ERC/WFMH activist, Dutch psychiatrist Wout Hardeman, M.D., who was deeply involved in the users movement, approved it in a letter of 12 February 1988 as a "well balanced compromise between the consumers' view as adopted by the Brighton Charter and the necessity of mentioning mental illness as a factual entity." He did, however, note elements of Netherlands law incompatible with the draft.

Similarly, former Board member Knud Jensen in a letter of 25 February 1988 noted incompatibilities with Danish law. More importantly he objected strongly to the provision that a psychotic person might be committed because of potential harm to others. Finally, Edith Morgan in a letter of 30 March 1988 raised the crucial question: "Is this a manifesto in which WFMH declares its own beliefs and commitments, or is it a general statement about principles and approaches to mental health in the modern world?" If the former, she believed, WFMH should revise it to become a "statement of intent as well as an exhortation on behalf of people with problems of mental ill health. My own view," she wrote, "is that this Manifesto, like the original one 40 years ago, should commit the Federation to appropriate action in the modern context." She also strongly recommended that any such statement should be "brief, simple and strong," noting as had others that the elaborate detail of the draft meant that it was not universally applicable. By this time, assuming that no more responses from Board members would be forthcoming, I had already voiced similar concerns in an earlier letter to Heginbotham.

The matter came to a head with a meeting at the International Hospital Federation offices in London on 1–2 August 1988 among Dick Hunter, Morgan, Heginbotham, Flache, then President-elect, and myself. Its main purpose was to plan for the 1988 WFMH Board meeting scheduled for London on 3-4 December 1988. However, the Manifesto was prominently on the agenda, which was expected to outline Federation goals for the 12 years until the turn of the century. In its current revision it had become a corollary to WHO's slogan, "Health for All by the Year 2000." The general ambivalence of the group was revealed in its erratic discussion and lack of consensus. When I was asked to summarize our views in writing I reluctantly agreed with no real sense of what had been concluded. However, this seemed to offer an opportunity to impose some order on the process.

Upon returning home I took a copy of the United Nations Universal Declaration of Human Rights and paraphrased it, inserting the relevant ideas from the Manifesto and those gleaned from our discussion. I entitled the product the "Declaration of Human Rights and Mental Health" and, on 8 August 1988, mailed it to the Board, committee chairs and United Nations representatives. It came as no surprise when the London conferees, aside from Dick who was noncommittal, were unanimous in finding it unacceptable. Only three other Board members responded. In October, more than two months later, Chanita Rodney of Israel wrote at length about the difficulties of producing a statement that would be internationally understood and equally applicable; she urged that it specifically mention schizophrenia, the right to "medical" treatment, and the importance of research. On 29 November 1988, three and a half months later, Beverly Long and Hilda Robbins sent a multipage rewritten document that they shared with the rest of the Board. Their accompanying letter endorsed the concept of a comprehensive document for WFMH that respected the practices of people in other countries and cultures. However, their hard work elicited no substantive response from other Board members in anticipation of the December meeting. In the November 1988 Newsletter, distributed before the Long-Robbins material was mailed, I attempted to prepare the ground for that meeting by writing that "two documents may be needed: first, the short version prepared by the Secretary General which could stand, perhaps with additional revisions, as an enduring statement of the Federation's human rights, goals, and ideals; second, a longer document which might be used for planning and policy purposes for the rest of the century."

At the December 1988 Board meeting reactions to my "declaration" were mixed, with the Europeans generally negative and the others passively accepting. However, President Gamal El Azayem of Cairo, always sensitive to opportunities to increase his country's status, saw an opportunity. After the Board had adjourned he suggested privately that the declaration should be presented to the participants in the WFMH 40th anniversary celebration on 17 July 1989 in Luxor, which I had already agreed to attend. The idea was to have it adopted there as the "Declaration of Luxor on Human Rights for the Mentally Ill" (see Chapter 10). This came to pass. At his request I read it to a plenary session peopled largely by professionals from Egypt and surrounding countries, and, in response to his request, they adopted it by acclamation. In this way he appropriated the "declaration" for his country and his presidency. He lost no time in having it translated and printed in both English and Arabic. It was circulated internationally with little delay and was found acceptable in many countries. In response to this fait accompli the Europeans did an about face. Heginbotham, especially, busied himself with revisions reflecting the Federation's concern with the prevention of mental illness and incapacitating emotional distress. The final revision was then, after all, adopted as an official WFMH document by the Board meeting after the World Congress for Mental Health in Auckland 26 August 1989. This version was distributed throughout the world, no longer as the Declaration of Luxor but as the WFMH Declaration of Human Rights and Mental Health. By 1992 it had been translated into Arabic, French, and Spanish. It is included in Appendix V.

El Azayem was succeeded as president in 1989 by Stan Flache. In 1990, after the declaration had been adopted, he decided to reconstitute the defunct Committee on Human Rights and Legal Affairs with himself and Gostin as co-chairs. They proposed the following terms of reference for the new committee that, limiting it to a concern with mentally ill people, overlapped largely with the terms of reference of the previous committee: "The purpose of the Human Rights Committee is to promote and defend the rights, dignity, respect and autonomy of persons with mental illness, to improve their mental health care and appropriate environment. In carrying out its objectives the Committee will (1) plan, draft, or assist in the preparation of declarations, guidelines, or other national or international documents on the human rights of persons with mental illness; (2) investigate, identify, and report on abuse of the human rights of persons with mental illness; (3) advocate for human rights of persons with mental illness; and (4) devise a system of monitoring the implementation of human rights principles and practice." In his joint capacity as committee co-chair and our Geneva representative Flache presented arguments throughout 1991 before the United Nations Commission on Human Rights that ultimately approved the Declaration of Principles for the Protection of Mentally Ill Persons and for the Improvement of Mental Health Care. The declaration was passed by the United Nations General Assembly in November 1991 without a vote. The work of elaborating and adjusting it to the socioeconomic and cultural contexts of regions and countries to translate its general principles into national legislation remained to be done. As noted in Chapter 8, 1992 saw a continuation of work in this field, with Flache playing an active role in the WHO interdivisional group on human rights. In January 1993 WHO Director General Nakajima appointed him as the chair of that group. In that capacity he contributed to preparatory meetings for the 1993 United Nations World Conference on Human Rights.

The 1993 United Nations World Conference on Human Rights

WFMH depended on several colleagues to represent its perspective to this conference. An important precursor was the "Asia-Pacific Pre-Conference Meeting" convened in Bangkok from 22 March to 2 April 1993. Our representative was Dr. Supang Chantavich, Professor of Sociology at Chulalongkorn University in Bangkok, whom I had met at the Harvard School of Public Health through Richard Mollica. It required some discussion to convince her to represent us but having acceded to my request she was a faithful participant and reporter. Despite her efforts the "Bangkok declaration" emerging from this meeting did not accord with WFMH principles. It emphasized the sovereign rights of nations and the importance of state mechanisms of social control, allowing only a negligible role for individuals and NGOs in protecting, promoting, and implementing human rights. WFMH was one of 202 NGOs to complain of the ambiguity of the declaration; its lack of reference to torture, freedom of expression, and the rule of law; and government reservations in ratifying international human rights instruments, especially those concerning the rights of women and children. They endorsed a competing statement, "Human Rights in Asia: The Struggle for Human Dignity," focusing on economic and social rights especially for ethnic minorities and indigenous people violated by authoritarian states. Supang raised mental health issues that were noted neither in the Bangkok declaration nor in the NGO statement. However, she could not evoke a sufficiently positive response to achieve any inclusion of mental health in either document.

Two papers bearing on mental health were submitted to the NGO Human Rights Forum in Vienna on 10–12 June 1993 on behalf of WFMH. One from our new Geneva representative Myrna Merritt Lachenal, R.N., M.N., focused on the relationships among health, well-being, and human rights, including those of disabled persons. The other, a "Joint Statement by International NGOs in Consultative Status with ECOSOC Working in the Field of Mental Health and Rehabilitation," stressed the stigmatized condition of mentally ill and disabled persons and their vulnerability to human rights transgressions, recommending general remedial measures.

The 1993–1995 period marked by WFMH Board preoccupation with administrative and procedural issues saw no formal initiatives in this area. However, the continuing work of many Federation components had human rights significance. At United Nations New York Dr. Kay C. Greene, our senior representative, worked with our representative Dr. Anie Kalayjian, Treasurer for the NGO Committee on Human Rights, on a proposal to create a subcommittee of the conference on NGOs devoted to mental health related human rights issues. Flache in Geneva was working on a counterpart subcommittee with the aim of promoting the implementation of the United Nations Resolution 46/119: "The Protection of Persons with Mental Illness and the Improvement of Mental Health Care." These efforts continued in 1997.

The 1995 Beijing United Nations Forum on Women described above had major significance for human rights. As part of the stream of preparations for this forum, Kalayjian helped organize panels on the prevention of discrimination against minorities and on the rights of women, seen increasingly as a minority group. In a similar vein on 14 February 1995 Douglas Deane represented WFMH at a meeting of the Inter-African Committee, a working group on traditional practices harmful to the health of women and children. Reports from some 20 countries were to be the basis for a workshop at the Beijing forum.

ERC/WFMH participated in the organization of the European Day for Disabled People and collaborated on the report, "Disabled Persons' Status in the European Treaties: Invisible Citizens," dealing with the human rights of persons with disabilities. At UNESCO Paris, largely through our representative Madeleine Riviere, we stayed in touch with the human rights aspects of the bioethics program, and our Committee on Preventing the Commercial Sexual Exploitation of Children was deeply involved in preparations for the 1996 international conference on the topic with its major implications for the human rights of children.

ADVOCACY, PUBLIC EDUCATION, AND RAISING AWARENESS

Annual Meetings, World Congresses, Regional Meetings

Regional and world meetings are well-established ways of transferring knowledge to participants and through them to individuals and institutions. They are also a time-tested means of developing international networks and collaborative relationships. It was therefore surprising to find that this perspective was not universally shared. One of my earliest inquiries into possible Federation funding after my election to the Board in 1979 was in the autumn of that year when I spoke with Dr. Richard Thompson, Projects Officer of the Mental Health Foundation in London. He was candid to the point of bluntness in his negative evaluation of the Federation. A major point was that his foundation could not give money to an organization that did little more than "produce an international congress every two years." I tried to indicate their value.

From 1948 to 1967 when the Geneva office closed Federation annual meetings were hosted by local mental health associations and featured papers and discussions by knowledgeable professionals. They were also stimulating to persons from national mental health associations. Rees frequently attributed the continuing stream of reports from member associations to the circulation of ideas from annual meetings, congresses, and special conferences. He felt that they responded as much to the regular opportunities for personal contact across national boundaries that accompanied these gatherings as from the lectures and published reports. In his Director's report for 1953 he noted that "although we are by no means satisfied with the techniques we employ for running international meetings or congresses, we have the conviction that some real purpose is served by such meetings." He referred to new contacts, new stimulus for work, and particularly the benefit of mental health and professional societies in the country where the meetings are held. Perhaps the most optimistic view was that the interprofessional and international working groups assembled at these meetings generate a kind of experience that is "reflected in the later work of many people in different countries" (WFMH, 1953a, p. 11). By 1960 Rees felt that Federation work , including meetings and congresses, had contributed to changes of public attitudes, especially what he felt was the reduced stigma of mental illness.

The original ethos of the annual meetings was that of international study groups with high value attached to research and science. This reflected the membership on the Board of many university-based scholars for whom scientific investigation and the exploration and integration of ideas had high value. Each annual meeting had a theme. They were also vehicles for a wide array of standard mental health subjects, many of which reappeared regularly at subsequent meetings. Among them were mental health in industry and government, the mental health of children and youth, and child development, as well as topics that were more properly psychiatric such as alcoholism and drug addiction, the role of the nurse, the use of films, and mental health in relation to public health.

The 1973 World Congress in Sydney, celebrating WFMH's 25th anniversary, was arguably the first to include "mass communications" as a significant issue. The nature of leadership in small groups and nations was a particular preoccupation of the Tavistock-influenced Rees and many of his colleagues. Attendance at these meetings was modest, although sometimes as many as several hundred people came. Perhaps because of their small numbers and prior preparation they were quite productive in terms of ideas and publications. Every four or five years they were accompanied by a World Congress. With the 1967 closure of the Geneva Secretariat they could not be maintained in their original form. The new by-laws, however, mandated annual meetings of the Board that were often accompanied by sparsely attended conferences arranged by the local organizers. These are noted elsewhere in accounts of regional activities. Perhaps the most ambitious of these was a two-day symposium entitled "Mental Health in the World" held at the time of the annual WFMH Board meeting on 30 May–1 June 1994 at the Ministry of Health in Madrid under the auspices of WFMH and the Spanish Association of Nurses in Mental Health. This was organized by Board member-at-large Pedro A. Torrejon Garcia of that association and Federico Puente during his 1993–1995 presidency.

The new by-laws proposed at the 1977 Vancouver Board meeting recommended that a World Congress be held every two years, rotating among the regions insofar as possible. This was controversial; members objected to the energy involved and the size that might preclude meaningful exchanges of views. However, the proposal carried the day, and there have been congresses every two years since that in Vancouver in 1977. These have been described elsewhere in this volume. Their sponsorship has, indeed, required a major investment of time, energy, and money. Nonetheless, after 1983 so many national associations have asked to organize one that it has been easy to schedule them at least four years in advance. The first defection was the South African Federation of Mental Health that in 1997 withdrew from its commitment to hold the congress in 2001, but several other groups immediately expressed their desire for the congress. The wish to sponsor a congress has been fueled in part by national and regional desires for the prestige and international visibility attached to having such a meeting. In some instances a congress may have been perceived as a vehicle for furthering personal leadership ambitions. Despite misgivings and difficulties, the world congresses have had major regional impact and attracted a global Federation constituency.

In retrospect several congresses since the founding meeting of 1948 may be said to have had special significance. That in Toronto in 1954 produced the first critical review of Federation activities. The London Congress of 1968 demonstrated that WFMH was alive despite the decline of the years leading to the 1967 Geneva closure. With 2500 participants it was the first to make a substantial profit shared between the U.K. National Association for Mental Health and WFMH. Edith Morgan remembered that it took place during the Russian invasion of Czechoslovakia, and several Czechs stuck in London after the congress had to decide whether to stay or make their way back." Most poignant, "It was just before J.R. Rees' death when he was already old and frail and was a sad figure at the opening ceremony" (Morgan, 1996a).

Perhaps the most important event for Federation revival was the Vancouver Congress in 1977. With more than 2000 registrants it was as heavily attended as that of 1968. It also produced a financial surplus, with the advantage that it did not need to be shared with the Canadian Mental Health Association, which had shocked President Lin by refusing to be a local sponsor (Chapter 10). The Vancouver event permitted the first resurgence of global WFMH activities since the closing of the Geneva Secretariat.

The 1983 Washington Congress represented another rise from a position of financial near destitution to a state permitting renewed programmatic activity on a global basis. As reported elsewhere it was also the scene of several innovations: the first Mental Health Association Day; the first formal involvement of users and self-help groups; the first new topic oriented committee (on responsible parenthood); the decision to make regionalization a priority; and the first Hemingway Memorial Lecture (on psychiatry and spiritual life) by an Islamic scholar.

The 1985 Congress in Brighton was a high point in assertiveness by user and expatient groups, with a declaration noting among other points that there is no such thing as mental illness, that the "'mental health system' endorses…the ideology of an unequal society," and that most psychiatric treatments are harmful (Advocacy Group, 1987).

The 1987 Cairo Congress was the first in the Islamic world. The 1989 Congress in Auckland, the first in New Zealand, brought many foreign visitors their first encounters with the Maori. The largest and in some ways most memorable congresses were arguably those in Mexico City in 1991 and Tokyo in 1993. The 1991 gathering, described in Chapter 9, was dauntingly huge with more than 6000 registrants and an audience of 10,000, mostly Mexican students, at the opening ceremonies. Its basic significance was twofold. First, it established, as an undeniable presence, a progressive mental health force—including patient advocates and community mental health leaders—in opposition to the entrenched traditional psychiatry based in mental hospitals. Second, in accordance with its theme "Science and People: Together for Mental Health," its system of subcongresses invigorated such important elements of the WFMH international agenda as women's mental health, population, refugees, prevention, and human rights. This congress saw the formation of the World Federation of Psychiatric Users.

The Tokyo Congress of 1993 (see Chapter 10) was somewhat smaller with approximately 4000 registrants but continued some of the subcongressional themes, emphasized the relationship between science and the mental health movement underlined in 1991, and was distinguished by its exquisitely organized and presented social programs. It too had a major impact on patient's rights in the country and region.

The 1995 Congress in Dublin, the first in Europe after that in Brighton, was marked, as was Brighton, by significant user participation. In this case, though, with the largest number of user registrants to date, there was no recurrence of their previous insistence on the oppressive nature of psychiatry and the mythological character of mental illness. Instead, as noted in Chapter 11, Board members joined with user leaders in a demonstration in support of community mental health facilities operated with user involvement.

Formal Communications

From the Federation's inception there has been general agreement that one of its functions should be that of an international mental health information clearinghouse, including materials not carried by professional journals. In the Rees era an attempt was made to fill this need for professional and public education by publishing the proceedings of various meetings (see References) as well as by circulating a newsletter. Plans were also made to issue a quarterly magazine or bulletin, but the project was soon abandoned because of lack of financial support. Annual reports ceased after the 1967 closure of the Geneva Secretariat, but newsletters continued through various administrations, sometimes irregularly, but usually on an approximately quarterly basis. I made two unsuccessful attempts to obtain foundation funding for an ambitious project along these lines.

With the shift of Secretariat from Vancouver to Baltimore the newsletters were discontinued for nearly two years, but I revived them in March 1984. With the help of Kathy McKnight we managed to produce five issues yearly until 1990, but by that time other demands had so stretched the capacity of my office that I reluctantly reduced their frequency to four per year. In 1994 we included two WFMH committee bulletins, "Refugee Notes" and "Bulletin of the Joint Program on Conflict Resolution" in the newsletters sent to the entire membership, but the supporting funds ran out after 18 months in both instances.

After a nearly 22-year hiatus I revived an annual report beginning with the year 1989–1990. At first it was typed, photocopied, and distributed to the Board and selected others. It was not until 1992 that, with the help of an anonymous foundation, we were able to print and mail it to the entire membership as well as others. In 1995, with the help of the same anonymous foundation, we initiated a web site and e-mail service for WFMH. In 1996 and 1997 the WFMH presence on the Internet and its availability for instant communication began to tie the Secretariat to outlying individual and organizational members in a new way.

World Mental Health Year, 1960

There have been other special Federation attempts at advocacy and education. The most ambitious, as noted in Chapter 3, was the designation of 1960 as World Mental Health Year. Much of 1958 and 1959 was devoted to its planning, and funds were available to employ a full-time administrator for the project. Kenneth Soddy, M.D., who held the title of Federation "scientific director" for a time, was much involved and hoped that the work of his committee on mental health and value systems would provide at least one major integrating theme for the year. Another hoped-for sequel of the year, never realized, was to establish a clearinghouse for information on relevant projects.

The World Mental Health Year idea was originally suggested by 1954–1955 WFMH President Frank Fremont-Smith as a follow-up to the World Geophysical Year. It was formally conceptualized at the Secretariat in 1957. In 1959 member associations wishing to cooperate began their special activities in April on WHO's World Health Day. The 1959–1960 President Hans Hoff of Vienna described the reasons for its promotion in terms characteristic of the Federation's founding days, seeing it as a balance between the World Geophysical Year focused on the material universe and human efforts to harness its energies. Speaking of the atomic sources of the world's energy future, he declared that "the human way of life will be altered correspondingly with…new potentialities and new responsibilities. Man, having achieved the capacity to destroy his world, will be forced to curb this power or die.… An inevitable shifting of populations is occurring as a concomitant of this process accompanied by vast problems of social adjustment." He listed the problems of "social adjustment, criminality, alcoholism, overpopulation, improvidence…and psychological maladjustment," all as corollaries of the insecurity accompanying technological change (WFMH, 1959a, p. 9).

Brussels Professor of Psychiatry Paul Sivadon, M.D. (WFMH president 1959–1960), declared World Mental Health Year to be a "new starting point in our Federation's work…[it] will find its justification in the future of the Federation and of the mental health movement throughout the world" (WFMH, 1960, p. 9). It was judged by Rees to have been an unqualified success in terms of national responses to suggested improvements in service delivery and the fresh impetus given to the work of national member associations. However, lack of funds made it impossible to conduct the special program of international activities that had been planned.

During 1960 the WFMH Secretariat learned in a piecemeal fashion about World Mental Health Year activities through reports that gradually arrived from many countries. Several entailed increased cooperation between voluntary associations and governments. Approximately 350 new projects, a large proportion of which were scientific, were initiated in 56 countries—approximately 10 more than the actual number of countries in which WFMH had member associations. The culminating event took place in June 1961 after the actual year was over, and a project administrator, Arthur L. Paton, became available. With a grant from the NIMH, 25 WFMH members and Rees and Rumke of the World Mental Health Year Steering Committee met under Dr. Soddy's leadership at Roffey Park for two weeks. The "scientific division," as Soddy's group (himself and one technical assistant) called itself, had records of 225 scientific and technical projects undertaken in connection with World Mental Health Year projects, especially surveys of attitudes to mental disorder and mental health in relation to developing industrialization. The sudden death of Albert Deutsch of the United States, one of the world's premier public communicators on scientific and mental health matters, was a severe blow because he had been expected to write the meeting's final report. The group's ability to do follow-up work was further limited by lack of money and staff, but two reports were eventually completed (WFMH, 1961a; Soddy and Ahrenfeldt, 1967). Soddy, however, was forced to conclude that the effort to have a continuously active scientific division was not feasible: "The Federation cannot aspire to undertake highly organized project activities until adequate finances are forthcoming…there appears at present no likelihood that this condition can be met"

(WFMH, 1961, pp. 27–28). Lack of financial support finally resulted in the dissolution of the WFMH Scientific Committee in 1964 after nine years of effort and an active publishing program.

Problematic Areas of Advocacy Concern

Beginning in the mid-1980s changes in psychiatry and the consumer (user) movement highlighted the Federation's avoidance of two categories of advocacy concern. First was the lack of advocacy for research in the pharmacological treatment of mental illness. This could not have been an issue before the development of psychoactive drugs, which began to be available at the beginning of the 1950s. It reflected in part the possibility of creating conflict with the increasingly influential consumer/user constituency (see Chapter 7). The strongly negative attitude of European leaders, especially Josee van Remoortel, toward "science" or "research" has been noted elsewhere.

An unexpected development was the appearance in early 1997 of what was billed as a "meeting of advocacy associations" in Venice aimed at "building an international network to help those who suffer from mental illness" (conceptualized as brain disease). Addressed by Director Costa e Silva of WHO's mental health division and WHO staff in neuroscience, it was sponsored by Bristol-Myers Squibb, a pharmaceutical firm with which Dick Hunter had already had several contacts in an effort to obtain money. He and Marten de Vries attended for WFMH, along with several U.S. and European consumer representatives, most of whom were veterans of WFMH meetings. In a letter to Marten of 11 February 1997 before the meeting, Dick wrote, "I see our role to help harness the energy in pursuit of a manageable objective, without duplication of effort, to produce something of real value."

The second point of avoidance was the failure to become vigorously involved in the family movement as embodied in such organizations as the Schizophrenia Fellowship and the Alliance for the Mentally Ill—neither of which had existed in an earlier era. The central issue as noted in Chapter 7 was the conflict between the wishes of the patients and their advocates to protect patient autonomy and the fears of their relatives about the possibly untoward consequences of their freedom to be self-determining. Organizers of the 1993 Tokyo Congress were receptive to my efforts to include Diane Frogatt of the Schizophrenia Fellowship in the program. In 1995 at the Dublin World Congress our United Nations Vienna representative, Dr. Maria Simon, gave an energizing paper on the importance of attention to family "carers," in which she noted that there were occasions when involuntary hospitalization was essential to preserving the patient's integrity.

IMPROVING THE DELIVERY OF MENTAL HEALTH SERVICES

Advocacy for Specific Mental Hospital Services and Practices

This stream of Federation activity, directly descended from the International Committee for Mental Hygiene mental hospital reform program, has been most prominent in Europe. It has focused on the use of seclusion, restraints, and alternatives to large mental hospitals—all of which have been in the process of elimination or development in the United States since the end of World War II. Conversely, this aspect of the WFMH agenda has not been as prominent in the less developed regions of Latin America, Africa, and Asia where funds and the political will to effect change have not been available. However, the 1991 World Congress changed the situation in Mexico. Details of several European projects are noted in Chapter 11, and advocacy for improved clinical services through WHO is described in Chapter 8.

An early collaborative project by U.K. investigators was an "International Study of Psychological Problems in General Hospitals" conducted between 1957 and 1959. It was performed as a collaboration among WFMH, the International Council of Nurses, and the International Hospital Federation. The method was the traditional one of discussions by voluntary study groups in 14 countries aimed at a meeting of an international group of experts who could produce a summary report (Barnes, 1961).

Another study, "Good Practices in Mental Health," was initiated in 1977 by Edith Morgan in her capacity as a project officer for the International Hospital Federation. It was designed to collect descriptions of the best mental health services provided in all parts of the world by both statutory and voluntary organizations. Morgan continued to pursue elements of this project during her tenure as Board member, vice president for Europe, and WFMH president.

The 1980 Belgian/Flemish Conference on "Alternatives to Mental Hospitals: A European Workshop" was regarded by many as a nodal point in the formation of the ERC/WFMH. Indeed, as noted in Chapter 5, its emphasis was on a European rather than a global audience. Thus there was no participation by non-European Board members or the Secretariat despite their expressed interest and joint WFMH and International Hospital Federation sponsorship. This project concerned prevention, primary care, and rehabilitation and such alternatives to hospitalization as halfway houses, family care and daycare (see Chapter 10).

Volunteer/Professional/Self-Help/User (Consumer) Relationships

Another issue attracting little attention in many parts of the world has become the relationship of professionals, self-help groups, consumers (service users), and volunteers, both in the advocacy efforts of mental health associations and the actual provision of mental health services. In Europe with volunteers closely associated with salaried mental health association staff members (who tended to regard themselves as volunteers in contrast to psychiatrists), it seemed necessary to have a meeting on the professional/ volunteer relationship as early as 1971. The meeting was convened at MIND in London. In the fall of 1979 another meeting on "Volunteers in Mental Health" brought some 40 delegates, including professionals, to London. With Edith Morgan, then European vice president of WFMH, as coordinator, it was sponsored by the Federation's not yet formally organized European region in cooperation with MIND and the International Hospital Federation. These London meetings, in 1971 and 1979, were part of a move to bring more nonprofessionals into the voluntary mental health movement and to reduce the influence of professionals.

In 1981 after becoming WFMH president I suggested the organization of an "Atlantic basin" meeting to be held the next year in England as a way of bringing consumers and self-help organizations into our framework. In July 1982 in Washington, DC, I suggested to our Board that for the first time we actively recruit self-help and expatient groups to WFMH membership. They agreed with some hesitancy, and afterward I canvassed several self-help and expatient leaders, inviting them to form a panel or to be otherwise involved in our 1983 World Congress in Washington, DC. Several accepted, including Kirsten Nilsson, Director of Fountain House in Stockholm, whose WFMH cosponsored conference was two months earlier (see Chapter 7).

The Atlantic basin conference was held in London 21–23 July 1982, just after the Washington, DC Board meeting. Edith Morgan, with MIND and European colleagues, had assumed the organizing tasks and come up with a title that did not refer to self-help groups and, further, appeared to assume an inherent conflict between people whom I had always regarded as friendly collaborators. However, despite the title, "Professionals and Volunteers: Partners or Rivals?" the meeting focused on opportunities for collaboration. Its success owed much to the support of Stijn Jannes, M.D., WFMH European regional vice president, and Director Miles Hardie of the International Hospital Federation. WHO Europe also gave the meeting its joint sponsorship. As noted elsewhere it was a source of particular pleasure to demonstrate true interprofessional and citizen-professional collaboration in the joint sponsorship and financing by the NMHA, and the

American psychiatric and psychological associations of the travel and participation in the seminar of Judi Chamberlin, a leading representative of the U.S. ex-patient movement (Brody, 1982b). About 50 people, with a large U.S. contingent including American Psychiatric Association Medical Director Melvin Sabshin, M.D., and American Psychological Association Deputy Director Gary van den Bos, Ph.D., participated "vigorously and sometimes passionately" (Brody, 1982c). After the seminar a group convened for several hours at Edith's home where discussions about the planned convocation of national mental health associations at the 1983 Washington World Congress led to a move toward expanding their visibility and participation.

The 1983 World Congress was the first to include spokespeople for consumer/user and self-help groups in our program. WFMH's formal sponsorship of the World Federation of Psychiatrc Users occurred at the Mexico World Congress in 1991.

World Mental Health Day and the Committee of Women Leaders

A major public relations and advocacy/education success aimed at service improvement was the establishment of World Mental Health Day in 1992. It was set after some negotiation as a yearly event on the 10 October, with the cosponsorship of WHO. This was an initiative of Deputy Secretary General Richard Hunter following a suggestion by Robert Leighton of Visionary Productions, a television firm interested in sponsoring global telecasts by WFMH. Its immediate goal was to draw attention to mental health as a cause common to all people across national and cultural boundaries. This aim, essentially raising awareness of mental health as an issue important in all areas of life, has persisted. Its longer-term goal, since muted, was to establish parity for mental health with physical health in health priorities and services. It carries forward the concept of the 1960 World Mental Health Year aimed at sensitizing local and national governments and mental health associations to the mental health needs of their peoples.

The active co-chairs of the first World Mental Health Day, 9 October 1992, were WFMH President Max Abbott and WHO Director General Hiroshi Nakajima, who agreed to WHO cosponsorship at no expense to his agency. This gained the attention of governments looking to WHO for guidance in international health matters. The honorary chair of the first and succeeding World Mental Health Days has been former U.S. First Lady Rosalynn Carter. The first ladies of 16 countries accepted her invitation to join her in an International Committee of First Ladies for Mental Health. For the first three "Days" we had two-hour telecasts broadcast to 127 countries by the U.S. Information Agency Worldnet satellite network. The first telecast required our presence at a studio in Tallahasee, Florida, but after that we broadcast directly from the U.S. Information Agency studios in Washington, DC. These were good opportunities to utilize the presence and knowledge of those of us living near Washington. In 1993 panels of experts in Paris and Washington discussed the global incidence of mental disorders and their consequences. Instances of effective prevention and treatment from several countries were highlighted and examined followed by a challenging live commentary from Virginia Bottomley, the British secretary of state for health.

Unfortunately, even with U.S. Information Agency help the money to support telecasts evaporated after the third World Mental Health Day in 1994. Since then the WFMH role, carried out by the Alexandria office, has been largely in the composition and distribution of planning kits. Although some grants have been obtained, mainly but not exclusively from pharmaceutical companies, funding has continued to be a problem. However, the response has been impressive. On the first World Mental Health Day reports came in from at least 37 countries. Since then it has been adopted as an occasion for government sponsored proclamations and other observances in many parts of the world. These have drawn attention to undersupported public mental hospitals especially in the less developed world. Whether this yearly spotlight has led to any change or whether it has simply substituted for change in the hospitals is not known. But the

Secretariat has taken particular satisfaction in messages about programs in such distant places such as Siberia (in Tomsk, Irkutsk, Khaborovsk, and Vladivostock); the Micronesian island of Pohnpei; Kathmandu, Nepal; Banjul, Gambia; and Mezhuveli in Kerala, India. In 1996 reports were received from 54 countries. It has been, clearly, a consciousness-raising event. Like World Mental Health Year in 1960 there has been no attempt to evaluate its impact in terms of stimu-lating actual improvement of the mental health systems in the participating countries.

In 1995 it was decided, in consultation with Ms. Carter, that her Committee of First Ladies, organized as a symbolic support for World Mental Health Day, be changed to the Committee of Women Leaders, which might include prominent figures in government, first ladies, and royal-ty. In October 1996, as described in Chapter 8, available members of the group from Latin America were brought together for the first time at PAHO headquarters in Washington, DC. In July 1997 in Helsinki women leaders from Europe were brought together. Both occasions were stimulated by the new Nations for Mental Health program of WHO's Division of Mental Health. Their aim was to increase the women leaders' awareness of mental health issues and through them increase the likelihood of positive action by their governments.

Care of Victims of Violence

The first systematic Federation attention to this issue came through its "Scientific Committee on the Study of Victims of Violence," which was formed in 1980 as a task force. It held an initial conference, with joint WFMH, NIMH, and Princeton University Woodrow Wilson School of Foreign Affairs sponsorship, in Bethesda, Maryland, in May 1981. Its mem-bers were Susan Salasin of the NIMH, University of Ottawa Professor of Law Irwin Waller, New York psychologist Dr. Yael Danieli, a student of the Holocaust, and Chairman of the Scientific Advisory Committee Gaston Harnois, M.D, of Montreal. Dr. Robert Rich, Director of the Institute of Government and Public Affairs at Carnegie-Mellon University in Pittsburgh, was added later. Between 1981 and 1983, as reported by Dr. Harnois to the 21 July 1983 Board meeting in NMHA headquarters, members of the task force served as consultants to agencies of the Canadian government including the ministries of justice and of health and welfare. They were also the main panelists at a World Psychiatric Association meeting dealing with victims of violence.

After 1983, with the title changed from task force to committee and, as we initiated an effort that lasted several years for WFMH to become better known at ECOSOC in United Nations New York, the committee acted occasionally in an advisory capacity to the United Nations Crime Prevention and Criminal Justice Branch. As described in Chapter 8 the first major meeting in which members participated was the Seventh United Nations Congress on Prevention of Crime and Treatment of Offenders in Milan, 26 August–6 September 1985, at which the WFMH repre-sentatives were Danieli, Waller, and Dr. Micheline Basil. Chapter 8 also includes a description of the 1985 United Nations Declaration on Justice for Victims of Crime and Abuse of Power and the United Nations New York consultation on the topic organized by Danieli.

After a 31 May 1986 meeting the committee's concerns began to focus on collective victim-ization, and it made plans to convene during annual meetings of the Society for Traumatic Stress Studies. It also contributed to the list of "alternatives to imprisonment" put together by ECOSOC's Alliance of NGOs on Crime Prevention and Criminal Justice. The 11–13 June 1986 Board meeting passed a resolution proposed by Danieli that WFMH should follow the United Nations plans and declarations regarding justice for victims (Appendix V). This passed the United Nations in 1985. By now the committee was chaired by Rich. He convened a meeting in New York City on 24 April 1987 to address implementation of the United Nations declaration, and possible new committee initiatives in the areas of political and social violence and the emo-tional and psychological consequences of "covictim" status.

Another approach to the issue, described under "Nonviolent Conflict Resolution," came with the 1987 World Congress and the 1988 sessions on community violence in Cairo. At the 1988 meeting a resolution calling for attention by all Federation member organizations to victims of trauma was approved by the participants and later presented to the WFMH Board that endorsed it as an element of Federation policy.

As violence against women became more widely recognized as a global health issue it was so recognized by WHO. The May 1996 WHO Health Assembly in Geneva and the meeting of its Executive Board, with the concurrence of WFMH representative Flache, declared that violence is now "a leading worldwide public health problem" especially as it affects women and children. WFMH supported the WHO plan to improve recognition, reporting, and management of the consequences of violence and to "promote research on violence as a priority" for public health work.

Yet another line of advocacy has concerned child victims of war. The WFMH effort in this area was largely carried on through our representative, Nancy Dubrow, especially in her work with Unicef (see Chapter 8). On 26–29 September 1993 WFMH sponsored with Unicef-Germany and other organizations a conference at the Department of Child and Adolescent Psychiatry of the University of Hamburg led by Professor Dr. Peter Riedesser entitled "Children-War and Persecution." It encompassed three major themes. The first theme continued work reported at the WFMH cosponsored conference called "Children of War" in Jerusalem in 1990 (see Chapter 11) and dealt with the therapy of Holocaust survivors and their children and grandchildren. The question was raised as to whether denial of the Holocaust events still persisted in segments of the German population even though its supporting ideology was abandoned. The second theme was the treatment of torture survivors in Latin America, especially Chile and Argentina. Major contributors were David Becker, Ph.D., of the Latin American Institute of Human Rights and Mental Health in Santiago and colleagues who discussed the inappropriateness of the posttraumatic stress disorder concept in dealing with victims of human rights violations. The third theme was the plight of more than 3000 child refugees from Kurdistan, Afghanistan, West Africa, Europe, and other parts of the world residing at the time in Hamburg. This was an impressive gathering marked by considerable emotion, especially from descendants of Holocaust survivors, some of whom had returned to Germany from Israel. On behalf of WFMH I was one of the opening welcomers and moderated the final session. Key speakers included WFMH member Dr. Gillian Straker of the Republic of South Africa who had participated in the Jerusalem meeting and Drs. Bennett Simon and Roberta Apfel of Harvard who had organized that earlier meeting and helped organize this one.

The Treatment and Prevention of Substance Abuse

For many years this problem was approached on religious educational grounds by Dr. Gamal El Azayem, who formed the Committee to Combat Substance Abuse after the 1987 World Congress. He also represented us at many United Nations meetings on the control of narcotics traffic. However, the committee's activities were confined to the Arab states and although well publicized in the Eastern Mediterranean, tended to be unsystematic. This changed with a 24 April 1996 WHO initiative for primary prevention in which several NGOs were involved. It aimed to test models adapted to different cultural and social environments. WFMH was represented by President-elect Marten de Vries whose WFMH collaborating center in Maastricht operated an international program on drug abuse. Eastern Mediterranean region vice president Ahmed El Azayem also attended on behalf both of WFMH and a group of Egyptian NGOs concerned with substance abuse.

Stimulated by this activity Gamal El Azayem's Committee on Substance Abuse met on 27 June 1996 in Cairo and again on 29 August in The Netherlands to establish closer ties with the

Institute for Psycho-Ecological Studies. Marc Morival, M.D., a Belgian psychiatrist affiliated part-time with the Institute for Psycho-Ecological Studies, was appointed co-chair for policy; Regional Vice President El Azayem was appointed co-chair for clinical matters; and Hussein Tuma, M.D., from the United States was appointed co-chair for scientific affairs. Meanwhile, a consortium for the WHO Global Initiative for Primary Prevention of Substance abuse had been formed in Geneva with its founding meeting attended by de Vries and El Azayem. It sent an official representative to the Cairo meeting. WFMH formally became a member of the consortium at a 14 October 1996 session in Geneva.

The globalization of the substance abuse effort pushed by WHO did not diminish Gamal El Azayem's focus on the Arab world. In Cairo, on 28 June 1996, he formed an Arab Federation of NGOs for the Prevention of Drugs and Alcohol from the membership of WFMH's Eastern Mediterranean Regional Council. He was its chairman. After some thought I recommended that the Board give its active support to this endeavor with the proviso that it would not diminish our investment in the global program.

THE DIRECT PROVISION OF SERVICES

As noted on many occasions the WFMH story is that of advocacy and education. Members of its Board and Secretariat, depending upon their own expertise, have provided consultation on request, largely about policy and organizational issues. However, through its components developed after 1981, it has on occasion provided direct clinical, research, and teaching services.

The most outstanding providers of direct research and education services have been our collaborating centers concerned with prevention, refugee work, torture and trauma survivors, and women's health. Outstanding among the committees in this respect have been those concerned with responsible parenthood, substance abuse, refugees, and torture victims (in conjunction with collaborating centers). Others have confined themselves largely to advocacy.

Most regional activities are reported in Chapters 9–11. The major clinical service by a WFMH regional affiliate, continuing as part of the international mental health agenda for many years, has been the National System for Psychological Support by Telephone or Sistema Nacional de Apoyo Psicologico por Telefono in Mexico City, first begun by Federico Puente at the time of the disastrous Mexican earthquakes in 1985. After some years of quiescence it was reopened on 12 October 1992 with cosponsorship from the Mexican Red Cross. In 1993 this project received major financial support from the United Nations Program for Development with the collaboration of the Mexican Ministry of Foreign Affairs. In 1995 there was a sharp increase in calls because of the economic crisis begun late in 1994. The capacity of the system was enlarged with new equipment; an informational pamphlet was published; and the Metro put up free advertisements.

The Mexican group has also extended its service agenda into nearby countries. On 4–6 February 1992, in consequence of contacts made during the 1991 World Congress, President-elect Puente and a team from Mexico conducted a mental health consultation in Belize. This was at the invitation of Dr. Teodoro Aranda, the country's health minister. In May 1992 it responded to a request from the Fondacion Mexicana para la Rehabilitacion del Enfermo Mental-Richmond fellowship for a medical and social audit of the conditions in which patients live in Mexican psychiatric hospitals.

As the Federation's first half century drew to a close the Board's strategic planning retreat in early May 1997 reaffirmed its central thrust as that of advocacy and advocacy-related education. There was, however, some intuitive recognition of the appeal of hands-on work of the type carried on, for example, in regard to refugees. Although this was not made explicit, it appeared possible that if funds to build an adequate infrastructure became available, WFMH as a world body might expand its global advocacy to include more extensive service support, especially in the area of human rights.

RECRUITING NEW MEMBER ASSOCIATIONS: THE HEART OF THE AGENDA

In the continuing concern with Federation components attached to the central office, including the regional councils, the importance of our grassroots base has sometimes been overlooked. In fact, the advent of regional councils has at times inhibited rather than encouraged direct communication among voting member organizations, the Board, and the Secretariat. There has been a tendency to forget that effective change requires the force of an empowered group "on the ground." These issues have been touched upon in Chapters 5 and 9. Recruiting new member organizations has nonetheless remained central, although not usually identified as such, in the international mental health agenda.

The importance of local associations was emphasized by the initiation of Mental Health Association Day at the 1983 World Congress in Washington, DC. This biennial forum has continued largely owing to the efforts of Hilda Robbins. In the later 1980s at her initiative the Mental Health Association Committee was formed with the aim of stimulating and supporting the formation of new mental health associations. On the basis of her long experience Robbins produced a booklet, *How to Organize and Activate an Effective Citizens Advocacy Association* that has been widely used by many groups in and out of the mental health field. Among its sections is one called "The Specifics of Grassroots Lobbying" that highlights the practical aspects of advocacy work. In June 1997, as the Federation's leaders were preoccupied with issues at the top, she was still fighting for the development of a solid base of motivated, empowered mental health associations to give the term "mental health" real meaning in the everyday lives of their members.

References

Abbott, Max (1987, December). Indo-Chinese refugees in New Zealand. *Mental Health News*. Parnell, Auckland: Mental Health Foundation of New Zealand.

Abbott, Max (Ed.) (1989). *Refugee Settlement and Well-being*. Auckland: Mental Health Foundation of New Zealand.

Advocacy Group (1987). *Self Determination as a Human Right—Its Implication for "Mental Health" Services*. A statement prepared by the "Advocacy Group" at the WFMH World Congress, Brighton, England, 1985. Unpublished.

American Anthropological Association (1981, 5 November). *AAA Newsletter*.

Asuni, Tolani (1980, 28 February). Letter to Roberta Beiser.

Barnes, Elizabeth (1961). *People in Hospital*. A book based on the findings of an international study of psychological problems in general hospitals. London: MacMillan & Co. Ltd.; New York: St. Martin's Press Inc.

Beardshaw, V., Morgan, E. (Eds.) (1989). *Mental Health in Torbay*. London: King's Fund (mimeographed).

Beaty, William II (1966, 31 August). Memorandum to officers and governing board members of U.S. committee. Unpublished.

Beaty, William II (1995, 20 November). Interview with author. Ittleson Foundation, New York, NY.

Beaubrun, Michael (1952, 15 April). Carnival, symptom of our frustration. *Trinidad Guardian*.

Beaubrun, Michael (1957). Of alcohol and alcoholics: Script of two addresses on Radio Trinidad (delivered 1956). *Carib Med J*, 19:137–142.

Beaubrun, Michael (1992). Caribbean psychiatry yesterday, today and tomorrow. *History of Psychiatry*, 3:371–382.

Beaubrun, Michael (1994a, 14 July). "Eldra Shulterbrandt, Mental Health Pioneer, a Caribbean Woman Ahead of her Time." Keynote address to Caribbean Federation of Mental Health meeting, St. Thomas. Unpublished.

Beaubrun, Michael (1994b, 26 June). Dr. L. F. E. Lewis 1908–1994. *Sunday Express* (Trinidad).

Beaubrun, Michael (1995, 19 December). Letter to author.

Beers, Clifford (1908). *A Mind that Found Itself*. New York: Longmans, Green.

Beers, Clifford (1924, July). Letter to members of the Organizing Committee, International Congress of Mental Hygiene.

Bell, Luther (1849, 18 August). Letter to G. Peters (Newfoundland). (Cited in Gollaher, 1995, p. 234.)

Bell, Sylvia (Ed.) (1988). *Law and Consumer Issues in Mental Health Law. Volume One of the Proceedings of Conference '87, Mental Health Foundation of New Zealand.* Parnell, Auckland: Mental Health Foundation of New Zealand.

Besterman, Theodore (1951). *UNESCO: Peace in the Minds of Men.* New York: Praeger.

Bethell, John T. (1996, November–December). Frank Roosevelt at Harvard and what became of him later. *Harvard Magazine,* 38–49, 86–87.

Bonnie, R. J. (1982). The psychiatric patient's right to refuse medication: a survey of the legal issues. In A. E. Doudera, J. P. Swazey (Eds.), *Refusing Treatment in Mental Health Institutions—Values in Conflict.* Ann Arbor, MI: AUPHA Press.

British Standing Committee of WFMH (1949–1957). Minutes, 19 March 1949–3 October 1957.

Brockington, Fraser (Ed.) (1954). *Mental Health and the World Community.* London: WFMH. (Twelve papers arising from a symposium in Toronto, August 1954.)

Brody, E. B. (1964). Psychiatry in Portuguese America (Brazil) [Editorial]. *Am J Psychiatry,* 120:959–961.

Brody, E. B. (1966). The psychiatry of Latin America [Editorial]. *Am J Psychiatry,* 123:475–477.

Brody, E. B. (Ed.) (1968). *Minority Group Adolescents in the United States.* Baltimore: Williams & Wilkins.

Brody, E. B. (Ed.) (1969a). *Behavior in New Environments: The Adaptation of Migrant Populations.* Beverly Hills: Sage Press.

Brody, E. B. (Ed.) (1969b). *Mental Health in the Americas. Report of the First Hemispheric Conference* (in Spanish and English). Washington, DC: American Psychiatric Association.

Brody, E. B. (1973). *The Lost Ones: Social Forces and Mental Illness in Rio de Janeiro.* New York: International Universities Press.

Brody, E. B. (1976). Reproductive freedom, coercion and justice: some ethical aspects of population policy and practice. *Soc Sci Med,* 10:553–557.

Brody, E. B. (1978). Lawrence S. Kubie's psychoanalysis. In H. J. Schlesinger (Ed.), *Symbol and Neurosis: Selected Papers of Lawrence S. Kubie* (pp. 1–40). New York: International Universities Press.

Brody, E. B. (1979a, 11 October). Letter to Melvin Sabshin, M.D.

Brody, E. B. (1979b, 1 November). Letter to WFMH Board.

Brody, E. B. (1981a, August). "An Agenda for the 1980s." Inaugural presidential address. World Congress for Mental Health, Manila. Published in Nann et al. op. cit.

Brody, E. B. (1981b). *Sex, Contraception and Motherhood in Jamaica.* Cambridge, MA: Harvard University Press.

Brody, E. B. (1982a). Are we for mental health as well as against mental illness? The significance for psychiatry of a global mental health coalition [Editorial]. *Am J Psychiatry,* 139:12.

Brody, E. B. (1982b). *Professionals and Volunteers: Partners or Rivals?* [Foreword to conference proceedings]. London: King's Fund Publishing Office.

Brody, E. B. (1982c, 27 August). Progress Note to WFMH Board. Unpublished.

Brody, E. B. (1983a, July). *WFMH President's Report to the Board of Directors, 1981–1983*. Unpublished.

Brody, E. B. (1983b). Mental health: more than the absence of illness. *Am J Soc Psychiatry*, 3:20–24.

Brody, E. B. (1983c). World Mental Health: A WHO Social Policy Statement [Editorial book review]. *J Nerv Ment Dis*, 171:67–70.

Brody, E. B. (1985). Patients' rights: a cultural challenge to Western psychiatry. *Am J Psychiatry*, 142:58–62.

Brody, E. B. (1987a). *Mental Health and World Citizenship: The View from an International Nongovernmental Organization*. Austin, TX: Hogg Foundation for Mental Health, The University of Texas.

Brody, E. B. (1987b). Reproduction without sex—but with the doctor. *Law Med Health Care,* 15:152–155.

Brody, E. B. (1987c, 6 February). WFMH and the Daes Report [Letter to Editor]. *Psychiatric News*.

Brody, E. B. (1988a). Culture, reproductive technology and women's rights: an intergovernmental perspective. *J Psychosom Obstet Gynecol*, 9:199–205.

Brody, E. B. (1988b). Patient's rights: science, ethics and the law in international perspective. In S. Bell (Ed.), *Law and Consumer Issues in Mental Health Law. Volume One f the Proceedings of Conference '87, Mental Health Foundation of New Zealand* (pp. 9–12). Auckland: Mental Health Foundation of New Zealand.

Brody, E. B. (1989a). New horizons for liaison psychiatry: biomedical technologies and human rights. *Am J Psychiatry*, 146:293–295.

Brody, E. B. (1989b). Biomedical technology and women's rights. In E. Van Hall, W. Everaerd (Eds.), *The Free Woman: Women's Health in the 1990s* (pp. 34–46). Carnforth, Lancs, UK: Parthenon Publishing Group.

Brody, E. B. (1990a). *Human Rights Aspects of Transactions in Body Parts and Human Fetuses*. Paris: UNESCO (SHS-90/WS/6, Division of Human Rights and Peace).

Brody, E. B. (1990b). Women's rights and the medical use of fetal tissue: an international perspective. *Rhode Island Med J*, 2:53–58.

Brody, E. B. (1990c). Mental health and world citizenship: sociocultural bases for advocacy. In W. Holtzman, T. Bornemann (Eds.), *Mental Health of Immigrants and Refugees* (pp. 299–328). Austin, TX: Hogg Foundation for Mental Health, University of Texas.

Brody, E. B. (1991). *The World Federation for Mental Health, 1948–1991 and Secretary General's Annual Report for 1 January–31 December 1990, Marking a Decade of Progress, 1981–1991*. Baltimore: WFMH (typed for limited distribution).

Brody, E. B. (1993a). *Annual Report of the WFMH Secretary General for 1992*. Baltimore: Office of the Secretary General, World Federation for Mental Health.

Brody, E. B. (1993b). *Biomedical Technology and Human Rights*. Hants, England: Dartmouth Press/UNESCO Publishing. (Published under auspices of WFMH and International Social Science Council; prepared under contract between WFMH and UNESCO.)

Brody, E. B. (1993c). *A Brief History and the Annual Report of the Secretary General for 1993*. Baltimore: Office of the Secretary General, World Federation for Mental Health.

Brody, E. B. (1994). Psychiatric diagnosis in sociocultural context [Editorial]. *J Nerv Ment Dis*, 182:253–255.

Brody, E. B. (1995, March). Message from the Secretary General. *WFMH Newsletter*.

Brody, E. B. (1997). *Annual Report of the Secretary General for 1996*. Baltimore: Office of the Secretary General, World Federation for Mental Health.

Brody, E. B., Redlich, F. C. (Eds.) (1952). *Psychotherapy with Schizophrenics: A Symposium.* New York: International Universities Press.

Cantril, Hadley (Ed.) (1950). *Tensions That Cause Wars*: *Common Statement and Individual Papers by a Group of Social Scientists Brought Together by UNESCO.* Urbana, IL: University of Illinois Press.

Carstairs, G. Morris (1971, May). Letter to the WFMH Executive Board.

Carstairs, G. Morris, Morgan, Edith (1983). Personal communication, Edith Morgan, 1985.

Caudill, W., Redlich, F. C., Gilmore, H., Brody, E. B. (1952). Social structure and interaction processes on a psychiatric ward. *Am J Orthopsychiatry* 22:314. Reprinted in H. Wechsler, et al. (Eds.) (1970). *Social Psychology and Mental Health.* New York: Holt, Rhinehart and Winston.

Chamberlin, Judi (1978a). *On Our Own: Patient-Controlled Alternatives to the Mental Health System.* New York: McGraw-Hill.

Chamberlin, Judi (1978b). The case for separatism. In I. Barker, E. Peck (Eds.), *Power in Strange Places* (pp. 24–26). London: International Hospital Federation.

Chamberlin, Judi (1990). The ex-patients' movement: where we've been and where we're going. *J Mind Behavior,* 11:323–336.

Chisholm, G. Brock (1946). The psychiatry of enduring peace and social progress. *Psychiatry,* 9:1–44.

Chisholm, G. Brock (1948). The future of psychiatry. *Am J Psychiatry,* 104:543–549.

Chisholm, G. Brock (1949a). New vistas of responsibility. *Psychiatry,* 12:191–195.

Chisholm, G. Brock (1949b). Social responsibility. *Science,* 109:27–31.

Chisholm, G. Brock (1957). *Prescription for Survival.* New York: Columbia University Press.

Chisholm, G. Brock (1966). Jack Rees—the man. In J.R. Rees, *Reflections: A Personal History and an Account of the Growth of the World Federation for Mental Health* (p. vii). New York: United States Committee of World Federation for Mental Health.

Cohen, Elizabeth (Mrs. Myer) (1995, 4 September). Letter to the author.

Conferences on Health and Human Relations in Germany. (1950, 1951). Princeton, 1950; Williamsburg, 1950; Hiddesen, Germany, 1951. Unpublished.

Cushman, Philip (1995). *Constructing the Self, Constructing America: A Cultural History of Psychotherapy.* New York: Addison-Wesley.

Dain, Norman (1980). *Clifford W. Beers, Advocate for the Insane.* Pittsburgh: University of Pittsburgh Press.

Dain, Norman (1989). Critics and dissenters: reflections on "anti-psychiatry" in the United States. *J Hist Behav Sci,* 25:3–25.

Dalos, L. P., Keen, C. H., Keen, J. P., Parks, S. D. (1996). *Common Fire: Lives of Commitment in a Complex World.* Boston: Beacon Press.

Dane, L. F. (Ed.) (1992). *The Cairo Proceedings: Report of the First Conference of the Joint Program on Conflict Resolution, Dar Al-Iftaa, Cairo, Egypt, 12–14 November, 1991.* McLean, VA: Institute for Victims of Trauma.

Dane, L. F. (Ed.) (1996). *Building tolerance for diversity.* Proceedings of a February 1994 meeting in Cairo, Egypt. McLean, VA: Institute for Victims of Trauma. Unpublished.

David, Henry P. (Ed.) (1964). *Population and Mental Health. Proceedings of the Sixteenth Annual Meeting, World Federation for Mental Health, Amsterdam, August 1963.* Berne: Hans Huber Publishers.

David, Henry P. (1969a). Involuntary international migration: adaptation of refugees. In E. B. Brody (Ed.), *Behavior in New Environments: The Adaptation of Migrant Populations* (pp. 73–95). Beverly Hills: Sage Press.

David, Henry P. (1992). Born unwanted: long-term developmental effects of denied abortion. *J Soc Issues*, 48:163–181.

David, Henry P. (1994). Reproductive rights and reproductive behavior. *Am Psychol*, 49:343–349.

David, Henry P. (1995). *The WFMH committee on responsible parenthood.* Unpublished.

David, Henry P. (1996b, 20 February). Interview with the author.

David, Henry P., Brody, E. B. (Eds.) (1969). *Proceedings of the Research Planning Conference for Transnational Studies in Family Planning, 18–19 September, Budapest.* Bethesda, MD: Transnational Family Planning Institute.

David, Henry P., Dytrych, Z., Matejcek, Z., Schuller, V. (Eds.) (1988). *Born Unwanted: Developmental Effects of Denied Abortion.* Prague: Avenicum-Czechoslovak Medical Press (under auspices of WFMH).

David, Henry P., Morgall, J. M. (1990). Family planning for the mentally disordered and retarded. *J Nerv Ment Dis*, 178:385–391.

Deutsch, Albert (1949). *The Mentally Ill in America: A History of Their Care and Treatment from Colonial Times, 2nd Ed.* New York: Columbia University Press. (Original work published in 1937.)

Dix, Dorothea (1843, 1847). Memorial to the Legislature of Massachusetts: Boston, 1843, p. 4; Memorial Soliciting Enlarged and Improved Accommodations for the Insane of the State of Tennessee: Nashville, 1847, pp. 1–2. Cited in Grob, G. (1994). *The Mad Among Us: A History of the Care of America's Mentally Ill* (pp. 386). New York: The Free Press.

Dytrich, Z. (1994). Children born to women denied abortion: mental health concerns. In *Proceedings of the 1993 Japan World Congress, WFMH, 23–27 August* (pp. 86–89). Makuhari Messe: Ovta-Reha.

Earle, Pliny (1845). Letter to the editor. *Am J Insanity*, 2:92.

El Azayem, G., Salem, A., Dunbar, S. (Eds.) (1989). *Mental Health Services to Victims of Community Violence. Proceedings of WFMH Working Conference.* Cairo: El Azayem Mental Health Center.

Erickson, Erik (1960). Identity and uprootedness in our time. In *Uprooting and Resettlement Papers Presented at the 11th Annual WFMH Meeting, Vienna 1958.* Geneva: World Federation for Mental Health.

European Newsletter of Users and Ex-Users in Mental Health (1996, Winter). 5:14–15.

European Regional Council of WFMH (1995). *Annual report.* Brussels: ERC/WFMH.

Farias, Pablo (1994). *Report on Chiapas Project to WFMH Secretary General.* Unpublished.

Ferguson, George A. (1993). Psychology in Canada 1939–1945. *Can Psychol*, 3:2–10.

Finnish Association for Mental Health (1995). A Century of Service. *Newsletter of Finnish Association for Mental Health*, 5.

Flugel, J. C. (1948a). *A Hundred Years of Psychology, 1833–1933.* London: Duckworth.

Flugel, J. C., et al. (Eds.) (1948a). *International Congress on Mental Health, London 1948. Volume I: History, Development and Organization.* London: H. K. Lewis & Co. Ltd.; New York: Columbia University Press.

Flugel, J. C., et al. (Eds.) (1948b). *International Congress on Mental Health, London 1948. Volume III: Proceedings of the International Conference on Medical Psychotherapy, 11–14 August.* London: H. K. Lewis & Co. Ltd.; New York: Columbia University Press.

Flugel, J. C., et al. (Eds.) (1948c). *International Congress on Mental Health, London 1948. Volume IV: Proceedings of the International Conference on Mental Hygiene, 16–21 August.* London: H. K. Lewis & Co. Ltd.; New York: Columbia University Press.

Fost, Rosemary (1980, 28 February). Letter to the author.

Frank, J. D., Frank, J. B. (1991). *Persuasion and Healing: A Comparative Study of Psychotherapy, 3rd ed.* Baltimore: Johns Hopkins University Press.

Freeman, Hugh (Ed.) (1969). *Progress in Mental Health. Proceedings of the 1968 International Congress on Mental Hygiene.* London: J. & A. Churchill.

Fremont-Smith, F. (1966). His vision. In J. R. Rees, *Reflections: A Personal History and an Account of the Growth of the World Federation for Mental Health.* New York: United States Committee of World Federation for Mental Health.

Freud, Sigmund (1901). *The Psychopathology of Everyday Life.* London: The Hogarth Press (standard edition, VI, 1960).

Freud, Sigmund (1930). *Civilization and its Discontents.* London: The Hogarth Press (standard edition, XXI, 1961).

Funkenstein, Dan (Ed.) (1959). *The Student and Mental Health: An International View.* Report of a conference held by WFMH in 1956 with the joint sponsorship of the International Association of Universities, Princeton, NJ. Cambridge, MA: Riverside Press.

Glover, Edward (1969). In honor of Lawrence Kubie. *J Nerv Ment Dis*, 149:5–18.

Gollaher, David (1995). *Voice for the Mad: The Life of Dorothea Dix* (pp. 538). New York: The Free Press.

Goldman, Stephen B. (1994). The difficulty of being a gay psychoanalyst during the last fifty years: an interview with Dr. Bertram Schaffner. In T. Domenici, R. C. Lesser, A. Harris (Eds.), *Disorienting Sexuality: Psychoanalytic Appraisals of Sexual Identities.* London: Routledge.

Gostin, Larry (1987a). *Human Rights in Mental Health: Japan.* Boston: American Society for Law and Medicine (sponsored by WHO International Collaborating Center on Health Legislation, Harvard and WFMH).

Gostin, Larry (1987b). Human rights in mental health: a proposal for five international standards based upon the Japanese experience. *Int J Law Psychiatry*, 10:353–368.

Greene, Kay C. (1997). *United Nations, New York, 1990–1995.* Unpublished manuscript written at request of the author.

Griffin, John D. (1989). *In Search of Sanity: A Chronicle of the Canadian Mental Health Association 1918–1988.* London, Canada: Third Eye.

Grob, G. (1994). *The Mad Among Us: A History of the Care of America's Mentally Ill.* New York: Free Press.

Guest, Gowan (1979a, 25 September). Letter to author.

Guest, Gowan (1979b, 26 September). Letter to Dr. Regine Schneider.

Guest, Gowan (1995, 22 November). Letter to author.

Hansard, L. (1904–1993). Cited in Jones, 1993.

Harnois, Gaston (1980, 6 February). Letter to Gowan Guest (from secretary, Executive Board).

Harnois, Gaston (1995, 15 November). Letter to author.

Heginbotham, C. (1987). *The Rights of Mentally Ill People.* Minority Rights Group, report 74 [Pamphlet]. London: Minority Rights Group.

Hollingshead, A., Redlich, F. C. (1958). *Social Class and Mental Illness.* New York: John Wiley & Sons.

Holtzman, Wayne, Bornemann, Thomas (Eds.) (1990). *Mental Health of Immigrants and Refugees* [Proceedings of conference]. Austin, TX: Hogg Foundation for Mental Health, University of Texas.

Inkeles, A. (1969). Making man modern: on the causes and consequences of individual changes in six developing countries. *Am J Sociol*, 75:208–225.

Inkeles, A., Smith, D. (1974). *Becoming Modern.* Cambridge, MA: Harvard University Press.

International Social Science Council Annual Report (1992–1993). Paris: ISSC Publications, UNESCO House.

Jahoda, Marie (1960). *Race Relations and Mental Health.* Paris: UNESCO House (prepared under a contract between WFMH and UNESCO).

James, C. L. R. (1938). *The Black Jacobins.* Great Britain: Redwood, Burns, Trowbridge and Esher. Revised in 1963 as *Black Jacobins: Toussaint L'Ouvertoure and the San Domingo Revolution.* New York: Random House.

Jesperson, Maths (1995a). The user organization in Sweden. In *Deviant*, Netherlands. (Printed in Dutch by an irregularly issued newsletter of the Netherlands user organization.)

Jesperson, Maths (1995b, 4 Autumn). Editorial. *European Newsletter of Users and Ex-Users in Mental Health.*

Jesperson, Maths (1996). *Proposal to the Third European Conference of Users and Ex-Users in Mental Health regarding the Nomination for the Right Livelihood Award.* Unpublished.

Jones, Kathleen (1993). *Asylums and After. A Revised History of the Mental Health Services: From the Early 18th Century to the 1990s.* London: Athlone Press.

Keens-Douglas, Gloria (1994, 30 April). Letter to the author.

Klineberg, Otto (1950). *Tensions Affecting International Understanding.* New York: International Social Science Council.

Klineberg, Otto (1951). Psychological aspects of international relations. In Alfred H. Stanton, Stewart E. Perry (Eds.), *Personality and Political Crisis: New Perspectives from Social Science and Psychiatry for the Study of War and Politics.* Glencoe, IL: Free Press.

Kolding Seminar (1994, 16–18 December). *Our Own Understanding of Ourselves: European Network of Users and Ex-Users in Mental Health* [Report]. Rotterdam: European Desk of the European Network of Users and Ex-Users in Mental Health.

Lacoste, Michel C. (1994). *The Story of a Grand Design. UNESCO: 1946–1993.* Paris: UNESCO.

Lin, Tsung-yi (1978, October–December). President's letter. *WFMH Newsletter.* Vancouver, BC, Canada: WFMH.

Lin, Tsung-yi (1979, April–June). President's letter. *WFMH Newsletter.* Vancouver, BC, Canada: WFMH.

Lin, Tsung-yi (1980, 21 May). Letter to author.

Long, Beverly (1996, 23 May). Letter to author.

Mead, Margaret (1947–1950). Papers of Margaret Mead. U.S. Library of Congress.

Mead, Margaret (1949). The International Preparatory Commission of the London Conference on Mental Hygiene. *Ment Hygiene*, 33:9–16.

Mead, Margaret (Ed.) (1953). *Cultural Patterns and Technical Change*. Paris: UNESCO Publications (produced under contract with WFMH).

Mental Health Observer (1994, Winter). Brussels: ERC/WFMH.

Mental Health Trends in Developing Societies (1971). Proceedings of the WFMH/Singapore Mental Health Association Workshop. Singapore: Koh Choon Hui.

Miller, Louis (Ed.) (1971). *Mental Health in Rapid Social Change*. Proceedings of the WFMH 23rd annual meeting, Jerusalem, 10–12 August, 1970. Jerusalem: Jerusalem Academic Press.

Miller, Milton (1996, 12 January). Letter to author.

Minutes of Governing Board (1947, 1948). International Committee on Mental Hygiene in various months of 1947 and 1948. In papers of Margaret Mead (1947–1950). U. S. Library of Congress.

Mollica, R., Donelan, K., Tor, S., Lavelle, J., Elias, C., Frankel, M., Bennett, D., Blendon, R. (1991a). *Repatriation and Disability: A Community Study of Health, Mental Health and Social Functioning of the Khmer Residents of Site Two. Volume I: Khmer Adults*. Boston: Harvard Program in Refugee Trauma.

Mollica, R., Fish-Murray, C., Donelan, K., Dunn-Strohecker, M., Tor, S., Lavelle, J., Blendon, R. (1991b). *Repatriation and Disability: A Community Study of Health, Mental Health and Social Functioning of the Khmer Residents of Site Two. Volume 2: Khmer Children, 12–13 Years of Age*. Boston: Harvard Program in Refugee Trauma.

Mollica, R., Jalbert, R. (1989). *Community of Confinement: The Mental Health Crisis in Site Two (Displaced Persons Camps on the Thai-Kampuchean Border)*. Baltimore: Williams & Wilkins.

Mollica, R., Lavelle, J., Tor, S., Elias, C. (1989). *Turning Point in Khmer Mental Health: Immediate Steps to Resolve the Mental Health Crisis in the Khmer Border Camps*. Baltimore: Williams & Wilkins (prepared for the United Nations Border Relief Organization by WFMH/Harvard School of Public Health task force on mental health crisis in Site II).

Mora, George (1980). Three American historians of psychiatry: Albert Deutsch, Gregory Zilboorg, George Rosen. In Edwin R. Wallace IV, Lucius C. Pressley (Eds.), *Essays in the History of Psychiatry* (pp. 1–22). Columbia, SC: William S. Hall Psychiatric Institute of the South Carolina Department of Mental Health.

Morgan, Edith (1979, 8 November). Letter to author.

Morgan, Edith (1980). Notes of an exploratory meeting to consider plans for development of European cooperation in mental health, held in Ghent, Belgium, on 30 March. Unpublished.

Morgan, Edith (1981a). Report of WFMH Europe Meeting held on 20–21 March in Central Hotel, Amsterdam. Unpublished.

Morgan, Edith (1981b). *World Federation for Mental Health: European Region*. Report of European Vice President, July 1979–July 1981 (prepared for meeting of WFMH Board in Manila, July–August 1981). Unpublished.

Morgan, Edith (1985, September). *WFMH Newsletter*. Baltimore: Office of the WFMH Secretary General.

Morgan, Edith (1988). *The Formation of the European Regional Council of the World Federation for Mental Health: The Early Years*. Unpublished.

Morgan, Edith (1994, March). *Annual report*. European Section for WFMH. Unpublished.

Morgan, Edith (1996a, 14 March). Letter to author.

Morgan, Edith (1996b, 6, 7, 9 October). Interviews with author. 34 Swain's Lane, London.

Nann, Richard C. (1982). *Uprooting and Surviving: Adaptation and Resettlement of Migrant Families and Children.* Dordrecht: D. Riedel

Nann, Richard C., Butt, D. S., Ladrido-Ignacio, L. (Eds.) (1984). *Mental Health, Cultural Values and Social Development.* Amsterdam: D. Reidel.

Nationale Vereniging voor Geestelijke Gezondheidszorg (1980). *Alternatives to Mental Hospitals.* Gent: Nationale Vereniging voor Geestelijke Gezondheidszorg.

Nemiah, J. (1989). The varieties of human experience. *Br J Psychiatry*, 154:456–459.

Newman, L. F. (1989). Reproduction and technology. In E. Van Hall, W. Everaerd (Eds.), *The Free Woman: Women's Health in the 1990s.* Carnforth Lancs, UK: Parthenon Publishing Group.

Newman, L. F., Brody, E. B. (1987). *The New Reproductive Technologies and Women's Rights and Roles.* Paris: UNESCO House (UNESCO/ISSC/WFMH international working group document commissioned by UNESCO, Division of Human Rights and Peace).

News and Notes (1932). European Reunion on Mental Hygiene and Prevention, and meeting of the European Members of the International Committee for Mental Hygiene held in Paris, 29–31 May. *Bulletin of the National Council for Mental Hygiene of England and Wales*, pp. 22–23.

Norman, Priscilla (1982). *In the Way of Understanding.* Surrey: Foxbury Press.

Nursing Times (1980, 17 April). p. 1.

O'Hagan, Mary (1993). *Stopovers On My Way Home From Mars: A Journey into the Psychiatric Survivor Movement in the USA, Britain and the Netherlands.* London: Survivors Speak Out.

O'Hagan, Mary (1995a, August). Respondent, panel on "healing partnerships." World Congress for Mental Health, Dublin. Unpublished.

O'Hagan, Mary (1995b). *The international user movement and its place in the world wide mental health movement.* Unpublished.

Osler, M., David, Henry (Eds.) (1987). *Sexuality and Family Planning for the Mentally Ill.* Copenhagen: Danish Family Planning Association.

Parsons, Talcott (1952). *Social Structure and Personality.* Glencoe, IL: The Free Press.

Pell, Mary Chase (1979, 13 November). Letter to author.

Perry, Helen Swick (1982). *Psychiatrist of America: The Life of Harry Stack Sullivan.* Cambridge, MA: Harvard University Press.

Pichot, Pierre (1967). Criticism of psychiatry (the Adolph Meyer lecture). *Psychiatria Clin*, 9:133–47.

Pilowsky, Issy (Ed.) (1976). *Cultures in Collision.* Proceedings of the 25th Anniversary World Mental Health Congress. Adelaide: The Australian National Association for Mental Health.

Prince, Raymond (1969). Mental health: the new opiate of the masses? *Soc Sci Med*, 3:276–280.

Rees, John R. (1949, February). Commentary. *WFMH Bulletin*, Number 1, (cited by Edith Morgan in an unpublished letter to WFMH past presidents and Secretariat, 14 September).

Rees, John R. (1966). *Reflections: A Personal History and an Account of the Growth of the World Federation for Mental Health.* New York: United States Committee of World Federation for Mental Health.

Ridenour, Nina (1961). *Mental Health in the United States: A Fifty Year History.* Boston: Harvard University Press.

Rosen, George (1968). *Madness in Society: Chapters in the Historical Sociology of Mental Illness.* Chicago: University of Chicago Press.

Rosenzweig, Saul (1992). *Freud, Jung and Hall the King-Maker: The Expedition to America (1909).* Seattle: Hogrefe and Huber

Rubel, A. J. (1964). The epidemiology of a folk illness: Susto in Hispanic America. *Ethnology,* 3:268–296.

Salonen, Kristina, Lahti, Pirrko, Kosonen, Ylva (1995). *The Finnish Association for Mental Health: A Century of Service* (p. 5). Newsletter of the Finnish Association for Mental Health. Helsinki: Finnish Association for Mental Health.

Sareyan, Alex (1993). *The Turning Point.* Washington, DC: American Psychiatric Press.

Satir, Virginia, Brody, E. B. (1978). Health by the people: right here, right now. In M. Beiser, R. Krell, T. Y. Lin, M. Miller (Eds.), *Today's Priorities in Mental Health: Knowing and Doing.* Miami: Symposium Specialists Medical Books.

Saxton, Calvin I. (1996a). Educating for worldmindedness: the theories of Harry Stack Sullivan, Ruth Benedict, and Brock Chisholm, 1945–1950. (Unpublished doctoral dissertation, University of Connecticut, 1995). *Dissertation Abst Int,* 56, no. 10.

Saxton, Calvin I. (1996b, 18 November). Letter to author.

Schaffner, Bertram (1948). *Fatherland: A Study of Authoritarianism in the German Family.* New York: Columbia University Press.

Schaffner, Bertram (1995, 20 November). Recorded interview by author 8:30–10:00 p.m., 220 Central Park South, New York, NY.

Silva, Pacheco e (1961). The President's foreword. *WFMH Annual Report.* London: WFMH.

Simon, Maria D. (1995). *The perspective of families of the mentally ill on basic issues in psychiatry.* Unpublished paper presented at Dublin World Congress for Mental Health, August.

Simon, Maria D. (1997). *History of WFMH Representation at UN in Vienna.* Unpublished manuscript written at request of author, 30 January.

Soddy, Kenneth (Ed.) (1955). *Mental Health and Infant Development.* New York: Basic Books (report on 1952 WFMH Chichester, England, seminar. Vol. I: Papers and Discussions; Vol. II: Case Histories).

Soddy, K., Ahrenfeldt, R. H. (1967). *Mental Health in a Changing World* (Vol. 1); *Mental Health and Contemporary Thought* (Vol. II); *Mental Health in the Service of the Community* (Vol. III). London: Tavistock (report of international study group convened by WFMH).

Stanton, Alfred, Perry, Stuart (Eds.) (1951). *Personality and Political Crisis.* Glencoe, IL: Free Press.

Steele, Ken (1996, 6 April). In the company of voices. *Fountain House Today.* New York: Fountain House.

Stepan, Margarethe, Lin, Tsung-yi (Eds.) (1960). *Reality and Vision.* Manila: Republic of the Philippines (report of seminar on mental health and family life held in Baguio, The Philippines, 6–20 December 1958).

Stevenson, George (1966). Dr. Rees and WFMH. In J. R. Rees, *Reflections: A Personal History and an Account of the Growth of the World Federation for Mental Health* (pp. xiii–xviii). New York: United States Committee of World Federation for Mental Health.

Strotzka, Hans (1960). Observations on the mental health of refugees. In *Uprooting and Resettlement. Papers Presented at the 11th Annual Meeting, World Federation for Mental Health, Vienna, August 1958.* London: World Federation for Mental Health.

Strotzka, Hans (1961a). Migration and mental health. In E. Thornton (Ed.), *Planning and Action for Mental Health*. London: World Federation for Mental Health.

Strotzka, Hans (1961b). Action for mental health in refugee camps. In E. Thornton (Ed.), *Planning and Action for Mental Health. Papers Presented at the 12th and 13th Annual Meetings, World Federation for Mental Health in Barcelona, 1959, and Edinburgh, 1960*. London: World Federation for Mental Health.

Sullivan, Harry Stack (1946). The cultural revolution to end war. The Second William Alanson White memorial lectures, Major-General G. Brock Chisholm [Editorial]. *Psychiatry*, 9:81.

Sullivan, Harry Stack (1947). The World Health Organization [Editorial]. *Psychiatry*, 10:99–103.

Sullivan, Harry Stack (1948a). Towards a psychiatry of peoples. *Psychiatry*, 11:105–116.

Sullivan, Harry Stack (1948b). Two international conferences of psychiatrists and social scientists. *Psychiatry*, 11:223–229.

Sullivan, Harry Stack (1948c). Mental health and world citizenship. *Psychiatry*, 11:235–261.

Sullivan, Harry Stack (1950). Tensions interpersonal and international: a psychiatrist's view. In H. Cantril (Ed.), *Tensions That Cause Wars: Common Statement and Individual Papers by a Group of Social Scientists Brought Together by UNESCO* (pp. 79–138). Urbana, IL: University of Illinois Press. Reprinted in Sullivan (1964), op. cit., pp. 293–331.

Sullivan, Harry Stack (1964). *The Fusion of Psychiatry and Social Science: Contributions to American Social Science*. New York: Norton.

Sweetser, W. (1843). *Mental Hygiene: or an Examination of the Intellect and Passions Designed to Illustrate their Influence on Health and the Duration of Life*. New York: J. and H. G. Langley. Cited in Rosen, George (1968). *Madness in Society: Chapters in the Historical Sociology of Mental Illness*. Chicago: University of Chicago Press.

Szasz, T. S. (1961). *The Myth of Mental Illness*. New York: Hoeber-Harper.

Thornton, E. (Ed.) (1961) *Planning and Action for Mental Health. Papers presented at the 12th and 13th Annual Meetings, World Federation for Mental Health in Barcelona, 1959, and Edinburgh, 1960*. London: World Federation of Mental Health.

Tormey, J., Brody, E. B. (1978). Values and ethics in medicine. In G. Balis, et al. (Eds.), *The Behavioral and Social Sciences and the Practice of Medicine* (pp. 656–671). New York: Butterworth.

UNESCO (1950). *Toward World Understanding*. Paris: UNESCO.

UNFPA (1984). *Declaration on Population and Development, Mexico City, 14 August*. New York: UN Publications.

van Abshoven, Jan Dirk (1994). Speech at CEDEP Conference, Madrid, 7–9 October.

Veatch, Robert (1981). *A Theory of Medical Ethics*. New York: Basic Books.

Visseur, Pierre (1995). "Marginal memories" (notes mailed to author).

Vitus, Lage (1987). *The role of the national council for mental health and government agencies in developing mental health policy*. Union of South Africa: Unpublished MSocSc Dissertation, UNISA.

Weiner, Dora (1994). "Le geste de Pinel": the history of a psychiatric myth. In Mark S. Micale, Roy Porter (Eds.), *Discovering the History of Psychiatry* (pp. 232–247). New York, Oxford: Oxford University Press.

WFMH (1947). Articles of Incorporation.

WFMH (1948–1952). Executive Board minutes. Unpublished.

WFMH (1951a). *Identity*. Introductory study by scientific committee of Executive Board of WFMH. London: H. K. Lewis.

WFMH (1951b). Minutes of Interprofessional Advisory Committee, Dublin. Unpublished.

WFMH (1953). *Social Provision for Mental Health*. Proceedings of 6th Annual Meeting of WFMH, Vienna (available in German only). Vienna: Wilhelm Maudrich.

WFMH (1955). *Social Implications of Technical Assistance*. Report of a meeting held at United Nations, New York, April 1955. London: H. K. Lewis.

WFMH (1956a). *Mental Health in Public Affairs*. Report on the 5th International Congress on Mental Health, Toronto, 1954. London: H. K. Lewis.

WFMH (1956b). *Family Mental Health and the State*. Papers from the 8th annual meeting of WFMH, Istanbul, 1955. London: H. K. Lewis.

WFMH (1956c). *Mental Health in Home and School*. Papers presented at the 9th annual meeting of WFMH, Berlin, 1956. London: H. K. Lewis.

WFMH (1957a). Director's report. In *WFMH Annual Report for 1956*. London: H. K. Lewis.

WFMH (1957b). *Mental Health Aspects of Urbanization*. Report of meeting at the United Nations, New York, 1957. London: H. K. Lewis.

WFMH (1957c). *Growing up in a Changing World*. Papers presented at the 10th annual meeting of WFMH, Copenhagen, 1957. London: WFMH.

WFMH (1958). *Uprooting and Resettlement*. Papers presented at the 11th annual meeting of WFMH, Vienna. London: WFMH.

WFMH (1959a). *Africa: Social Change and Mental Health*. Report of meeting at United Nations, New York, 1959. London: WFMH.

WFMH (1959b). *Communication or Conflict*. A book on conferences, their nature, dynamics and planning. London: Tavistock.

WFMH (1961a). *Identity, Mental Health and Value Systems*. Scientific Committee of the Executive Board (numbers 1 and 2 in a projected series of cross-cultural studies in mental health). London: H. K. Lewis.

WFMH (1961b). *Mental Health in International Perspective*. A review by an international and interprofessional study group. London: WFMH.

WFMH annual reports. (1948–1949 to 1967).*

WFMH Annual Report. (1949). London: H. K. Lewis.

WFMH Annual Report. (1950). London: WFMH.

WFMH Annual Report. (1951). London: WFMH.

WFMH Annual Report. (1952). London: WFMH.

WFMH Annual Report. (1953). London: WFMH.

WFMH Annual Report. (1954). London: WFMH.

WFMH Annual Report. (1955). London: WFMH.

WFMH Annual Report. (1956). London: WFMH.

* Annual reports are available from The World Federation for Mental Health, 1021 Prince Street, Alexandria, VA 22314.

WFMH Annual Report. (1958). London: WFMH.

WFMH Annual Report. (1959). London: WFMH.

WFMH Annual Report. (1960). London: WFMH.

WFMH Annual Report. (1961). London: WFMH.

WFMH Annual Report. (1962). London: WFMH.

WFMH Annual Report. (1963). London: WFMH.

WFMH Annual Report. (1965). Geneva: WFMH.

WFMH Annual Report. (1966). Geneva: WFMH.

WFMH Annual Report. (1970). Edinburgh: Royal Edinburgh Hospital.

WFMH Annual Report. (1972). Kingston, Jamaica: University of the West Indies.

WFMH Bulletin no. 1. (1948). London: H. K. Lewis.

WFMH Bulletin. (1968a, Spring). Edinburgh: Royal Edinburgh Hospital.

WFMH Bulletin. (1968b, Summer). Edinburgh: Royal Edinburgh Hospital.

WFMH Bulletin. (1970a, Summer). Edinburgh: Royal Edinburgh Hospital.

WFMH Bulletin. (1970b, Autumn). Edinburgh: Royal Edinburgh Hospital.

WFMH Bulletin. (1971a, Summer). Edinburgh: Royal Edinburgh Hospital.

WFMH Bulletin. (1971b, Autumn). Edinburgh: Royal Edinburgh Hospital.

WFMH Bulletin. (1972, Spring/Summer). Kingston, Jamaica: University of the West Indies.

WFMH Bulletin. (1972–1973, Winter). Kingston, Jamaica: University of the West Indies

WFMH Bulletin. (1973, Autumn). Kingston, Jamaica: University of the West Indies.

WFMH Bulletin. (1973–1974, Winter). Kingston, Jamaica: University of the West Indies.

WFMH Bulletin. (1974a, Spring/Summer). Kingston, Jamaica: University of the West Indies.

WFMH Bulletin. (1974b, Autumn). Kingston, Jamaica: University of the West Indies.

WFMH Bulletin. (1974c, Winter). Kingston, Jamaica: University of the West Indies.

WFMH Bulletin. (1975a, 1 May). Kingston, Jamaica: University of the West Indies.

WFMH Bulletin. (1975b, November). Kingston, Jamaica: University of the West Indies.

WFMH Bulletin. (1976, August). Vancouver, BC, Canada: WFMH.

WFMH country reports (1963–1965). Prepared by the Information Department of the World Federation for Mental Health, directed by Dr. Henry P. David, under contract PH 43-64-28 with National Clearinghouse for Mental Health Information, National Institute of Mental Health, Bethesda, MD.

Stutgarden: A Residential Treatment Center for Children. A Special Project Report From Denmark. Based on direct observations and information submitted by Dr. Kurt Palsvig, Director of Stutgarden, Hillerod, Denmark. WFMH/IC/64/478.

Mental Health Services and Resources in The Netherlands. WFMH/IC/8/64/361/REV.

Mental Health Services and Resources in the Czechoslovak Socialist Republic. WFMH/IC/8/64/360/REV.

Integrative Administration at the Sinai Center: A Special Project Report from The Netherlands. Based on direct observations and material submitted by Dr. A. Sunier, Superintendent of the Sinai-Kliniek, Amersfoort, and of the Jewish Federation for Mental Health in the Netherlands. WFMH/IC/8/64/362.

A Rehabilitation Center for Neurotics with Largely Non-Professional Staff: A Special Project Report from Czechoslovakia. Based on material submitted by Dr. Ferdinand Knobloch, Director of the Center for Neurotics in Lobec, and Head of the Psychiatric Department of Charles University Policlinic in Prague, with the assistance of Mrs. Hana Junova. WFMH/IC/8/64/359.

Mental Health Services and Resources in Denmark. WFMH/IC/10/64/476/REV.

The Day Hospital for Children in Paris: A Special Project Report from France. Based on direct observations and information submitted by Dr. S. Lebovici, Director of the Day Hospital for Children in the 13th Arrondissement of Paris, and Dr. P. Chanoit, Deputy General Secretary of the Ligue Francaise d'Hygiene Mentale.

Mental Health Services and Resources in France. WFMH/IC/10/64/476/REV.

Mental Health Services and Resources in the United Kingdom. WFMH/IC/10/64/469/REV.

Statutes in Mental Health and Retardation. Notes on Czechoslovakia, Denmark, France, The Netherlands, Switzerland and United Kingdom. WFMH/IC/10/64/475.

Industrial Rehabilitation of the Physically and Mentally Disabled. A Special Project Report from the United Kingdom. Based on direct observation and information submitted by John Crinnion, M.A., Rehabilitation Officer, Industrial Rehabilitation Unit, Waddon, Surrey, U.K. WFMH/IC/10/64/456.

The Medico-Pedagogic Service of Geneva. A Special Report from Switzerland. Mental Health Services and Resources in Switzerland. WFMH/IC/11/64/481/REV.

Mental Health Services and Resources in West Berlin. WFMH/IC/7/65/648.

Mental Health Services and Resources in Poland. WFMH/IC/7/65/649.

Mental Health Services and Resources in Belgium. WFMH/IC/10/65/778.

Legislation Related to Mental Health and Retardation in Belgium, Poland and West Berlin. WFMH/IC/ll/65/779.

WFMH Newsletter. (1977, March). Vancouver, BC, Canada: WFMH.

WFMH Newsletter. (1978a, January–March). Vancouver, BC, Canada: WFMH.

WFMH Newsletter. (1978b, April–June). Vancouver, BC, Canada: WFMH.

WFMH Newsletter. (1978c, July–September). Vancouver, BC, Canada: WFMH.

WFMH Newsletter. (1979a, April–June). Vancouver, BC, Canada: WFMH.

WFMH Newsletter. (1979b, Autumn). Vancouver, BC, Canada: WFMH.

WFMH Newsletter. (1980, January–March). Vancouver, BC, Canada: WFMH.

WFMH Newsletter. (1981a, October). Vancouver, BC, Canada: WFMH.

WFMH Newsletter. (1981b, December). Vancouver, BC, Canada: WFMH.

WFMH Newsletter. (1982, December). Vancouver, BC, Canada: WFMH.

WFMH Newsletter. (1984–1997). Baltimore: Office of the Secretary General of WFMH. Issued five times yearly from 1984 to 1991, quarterly from 1992 to 1997.

WFMH Newsletter. (1984, March). Baltimore: Office of the Secretary General of WFMH.

WFMH Newsletter. (1985a, March). Baltimore: Office of the Secretary General of WFMH.

WFMH Newsletter. (1985b, September). Baltimore: Office of the Secretary General of WFMH.

WFMH Newsletter. (1988, February). Baltimore: Office of the Secretary General of WFMH.

WFMH Newsletter. (1989, June). Baltimore: Office of the Secretary General of WFMH.

WFMH Newsletter. (1993, August/September). Baltimore: Office of the Secretary General of WFMH.

WFMH Newsletter. (1994, Summer). Baltimore: Office of the Secretary General of WFMH.

WFMH Newsletter. (1995, July). Baltimore: Office of the Secretary General of WFMH.

WFMH Newsletter. (1996, First Quarter). Baltimore: Office of the Secretary General of WFMH.

WFMH: U.S. Committee Inc. (1966). Collection of William Beaty II. Diethelm Library archives, New York Academy of Medicine (arranged and described by Janice Quinter, December 1988).

World Health Organization (1946). *Preamble to the WHO Constitution*. Geneva: World Health Organization.

World Health Organization (1981). *Social Dimensions of Mental Health*. Geneva: World Health Organization.

World Health Organization (1988, 19 July). *Principles for the Improvement of Mental Health Care and the Protection of Persons Liable to be Admitted Involuntarily to a Mental Health Facility Because of a Mental Illness*. Unpublished document prepared by Chris Heginbotham as a WHO paper "for submission to the UN Subcommission on Prevention of Discrimination and Protection of Minorities, for the attention of its Working Group dealing with the rights of those detained by reasons of mental illness."

APPENDIX I

Abbreviated List of WFMH Programmatic Activities for 1948–1962 (condensed from Rees, 1966)

1948

Founding of WFMH at Third International Congress on Mental Health, London. Incorporation in Geneva.

First WFMH Annual Meeting: London (continuation of founding meeting).

1949

Project. Contract by WHO with Secretariat for collection of information on mental health facilities and services throughout the world (1949–1950).

Participation upon invitation in UNESCO specialist meetings: "International Tensions," "Technology and Human Relations," "Adult Education."

Consultation.

WHO/WFMH visit to Philippines by E.E. Krapf, M.D.

WFMH BULLETIN initiated, first bimonthly, changed to quarterly.

Second WFMH Annual Meeting: Geneva.

1950

Project. Contract by UNESCO with Secretariat for a study of the organization, procedure, and functioning of third annual meeting of WFMH by a team of social scientists. With cooperation of UNESCO/University of Michigan Research Center for Group Dynamics/WFMH, participation upon invitation in two UNESCO specialist meetings in Paris: "Demography," "Tensions in International Conferences."

Project. Upon request from United Nations, briefing on mental health problems for medical relief teams for Korea.

Conference. "Health and Human Relations in Germany," Princeton, New Jersey, and Williamsburg Virginia. Supported by the Josiah Macy Jr. Foundation (Director, Frank Fremont-Smith, M.D., WFMH president 1954).

Third WFMH Annual Meeting: Paris.

1951

Project. Secretariat survey to all member associations about their countries' legislation regarding mental retardation.

Conferences. "Health and Human Relations in Germany," Hiddesen-bei-Detmold, West Germany. Continuing conference supported by Josiah Macy Jr. Foundation.

Conferences with United Nations: four dinner conferences among Dr. Rees and possibly other WFMH leaders and United Nations officials in New York and Geneva, supported by Josiah Macy Jr. Foundation.

Fourth WFMH Annual Meeting and Fourth International Congress on Mental Health, Mexico City.

1952

Project. Contract with UNESCO by Secretariat for data collection for conference on education and mental health of children in Europe.

Conference. "Mental Health and Infant Development," Chichester, England, with WHO regional office for Europe; UNESCO; U.S. Public Health Service; International Children's Centre. Support from Grant Foundation, New York.

Publications.

International Catalogue of Mental Health Films

Proceedings, Fourth International Congress on Mental Health, Mexico City, 1951.

Fifth WFMH Annual Meeting: Brussels.

1953

Publications.

Cultural Patterns and Technical Change. Edited by Margaret Mead, WFMH contract with UNESCO (Mead, 1953).

Undergraduate Medical Education in Mental Health and Psychiatry. D. R. MacCalman (publisher not listed, possibly WFMH).

World Mental Health. A quarterly publication succeeding the bulletin. Includes proceedings of fifth annual meeting, Brussels.

Sixth WFMH Annual Meeting: Vienna.

1954

Project. Contract by UNESCO with Secretariat for preparation of a manual on organization of international conferences.

Special Toronto Pre-Congress Symposia. "Mental Health and Public Health," "Mental Health and Child Development," "Industrial Mental Health and Human Relations," "Alcoholism."

Seventh WFMH Annual Meeting and Fifth International Congress on Mental Health: Toronto.

1955

Conference. "Social Implications of Technical Assistance," panel at United Nations New York with cooperation of United Nations Secretariat.

Publications. *Mental Health and Infant Development*. Report on 1952 Chichester seminar, two volumes (publisher not listed).

Eighth WFMH Annual Meeting: Istanbul.

1956

Project. Organized financial aid for work of Austrian Association for Mental Health among Hungarian refugees in Austria.

With UNESCO support an international inquiry on mental health and training of teachers.

Groups organized in London, New York, and Copenhagen to discuss a positive approach to prevention of racial and other forms of prejudice.

Contract with UNESCO for a report on human relations implications in metropolitan planning for United Nations conference on regional planning in relation to urbanization and industrialization scheduled for Japan in 1957.

Meetings of subcommittees of Board on peaceful uses of atomic energy, New York and Copenhagen.

Conferences. "The Effective Functioning of International Discussion Groups and Small Conferences," Eastbourne, England. With Josiah Macy Jr. Foundation.

"Research in Group Processes." New York.

"Student Mental Health," Princeton, New Jersey. With International Association of Universities, supported by Field Foundation and Grant Foundation. Chairman: Dana Farnsworth, M.D., Harvard University. Among approximately 24 seminar members (12 from United States and 12 from other countries) were Margaret Mead, Estafania Aldaba-Lim, Erik Erikson, Frank Fremont Smith, Jack Rees, Dan Funkenstein, and Spurgeon English. See Funkenstein (1959).

Publications (also see References).

Mental Health in Public Affairs. Report on Fifth International Congress on Mental Health, Toronto 1954.

Mental Health and the World Community. Edited by Fraser Brockington. 12 papers from a symposium, Toronto 1954.

Social Provision for Mental Health. Proceedings of Sixth Annual Meeting, Vienna 1953 (in German).

Family Mental Health and the State. Papers from Eighth Annual Meeting, Istanbul, 1955.

Social Implications of Technical Assistance. Report of a meeting held at United Nations New York, 1955.

Student Mental Health. An annotated bibliography. Daniel H. Funkenstein and George H. Wilkie.

Ninth WFMH Annual Meeting: Berlin.

1957

Project. Initiation of World Mental Health Year.

An international study of psychological problems in general hospitals. In cooperation with International Hospital Federation and International Council of Nurses.

Memorandum on peaceful uses of atomic energy (based on subcommittee work of Board) sent to directors-general of UNESCO and WHO, which led to convening of meetings of experts by these agencies.

Conferences. Meetings of subcommittees of Board on peaceful uses of atomic energy, New York and Copenhagen.

"Human Relations in International Administration," held for directors of United Nations agencies, supported by Carnegie Endowment for International Peace. La Tour de Peilz, Switzerland.

"A Positive Approach to Prejudice," organized with Council of Christians and Jews and the Society of Friends, London.

"Mental Health Aspects of Urbanization," panel discussion at United Nations New York.

"The Concept of Mental Health in Different Cultures," New York. Organized by scientific committee of Board.

Publications.

Mental Health in Home and School. Papers from Ninth Annual Meeting, Berlin, 1956.

Mental Health Aspects of Urbanization. Report of meetings at United Nations New York, 1957.

10th WFMH Annual Meeting: Copenhagen.

1958

Projects. Contract with UNESCO for report on teaching of mental health in schools of social work.

Contract with UNESCO for pamphlet, "Race Relations and Mental Health." For publication by UNESCO.

Conferences. "Concepts of Mental Health in Various Religions and Ideologies," scientific committee of Board.

"The Concept of a True International Civil Service." For directors of United Nations Agencies, Vevey, Switzerland. Supported by Carnegie Endowment for International Peace.

"Mental Health in Africa South of the Sahara." Bukavu, Congo. With WHO regional office for Africa and Commission for Technical Cooperation with Africa South of the Sahara.

"Problems of Mental Health of Immigrants." For representatives of governments of immigrant-receiving countries. In conjunction with 11th Annual Meeting, Vienna.

"The Diminution of Prejudice," London. Continuation of 1957 conference.

"Methodology of Attitude Surveys," Princeton, New Jersey. A meeting of a WFMH convened expert group.

"Mental Health and Family Life," Baguio, Philippines, with WHO regional office for the Western Pacific, Asia Foundation, National Family Life Workshop, and Philippines Mental Health Association.

"Psychological Rehabilitation of the Brain-Injured," Helsinki with World Veteran's Federation.

Publications. *Growing Up in a Changing World.* Papers presented at 10th Annual Meeting, Copenhagen, 1957.

11th WFMH Annual Meeting: Vienna.

1959

Conferences. "Social Change and Mental Health in Africa." Panel discussion at United Nations New York.

"Selection of Personnel for International Cross-Cultural Service." Geneva. For personnel officers of United Nations agencies in Europe.

Publications.

Uprooting and Resettlement. Papers from 11th Annual Meeting, Vienna.

Africa: Social Change and Mental Health. Report of meeting held at United Nations New York, 1959.

Communication or Conflict. A book on conferences, their nature, dynamics, and planning arising from 1956 Eastbourne conference.

The Student and Mental Health. An International View.

Mental Health in the Light of Ancient Wisdom. First Mary Hemingway Rees Memorial Lecture by H. V. Dicks, M.D.

WFMH. A Brief Record of Eleven Years.

12th Annual Meeting: Barcelona.

1960

Project. World Mental Health Year involving 400 separate activities reported to WFMH.

Conferences. "International Study of Psychological Problems in General Hospitals," (*a*) conference of representatives of national discussion groups, London; (*b*) conference of specialists, organized with International Hospital Federation and International Council of Nurses, London.

"Malnutrition and Food Habits," Cuernavaca, Mexico. With Josiah Macy Jr. Foundation, WHO, UN Food & Agriculture Organization, UNICEF, and Pan American Health Organization.

"Selection of Personnel for International Cross-Cultural Service," Geneva. Second conference for United Nations agencies in Europe.

Publications. *World Mental Health Films,* International Catalogue, Second Edition. T.L. Pilkington, Ed.

13th Annual Meeting: Edinburgh.

1961

Conferences. International study group to review recent progress and future needs in the field of mental health. Roffey Park, Sussex, England.

"Mental Health and Industrialization." Specialist conference, Paris.

"National Services for Mental Illness and Mental Health." For administrators of mental health services in public health departments, Paris.

Publications.

Identity and Mental Health and Value Systems. Introductory Studies I and II of a series of cross-cultural studies in mental health. Scientific committee of Executive Board of WFMH.

First World Mental Health Year: A Record.

People in Hospital by Elizabeth Barnes. Based on findings of international study of psychological problems of people in general hospitals.

Asylum to Community by E. Cunningham Dax. Development of mental health services in Victoria, Australia.

Hebraic Civilization and the Science of Man. Second Mary Hemingway Rees Memorial Lecture by Henri Baruk.

Mental Health in International Perspective. A review by international, interprofessional study group at Roffey Park, 1961.

14th WFMH Annual Meeting: Paris.

Sixth International Congress on Mental Health: Paris.

1962

Project. WFMH collaborated in preparation of material for technical discussions on mental health programmes in public health planning, World Health Assembly (WHO), Geneva.

Publications.

Prospective Internationale de la Sante Mentale (Mental Health in International Perspective).

Planning and Action for Mental Health. Papers presented at 12th WFMH Annual Meeting, Barcelona (1959) and 13th WFMH Annual Meeting, Edinburgh (1960).

Malnutrition and Food Habits. Report of Conference at Cuernavaca, Mexico, 1960.

Proceedings or Sixth International Congress on Mental Health, Paris, 1961. Amsterdam: Excerpta Medica.

World Mental Health Films. Supplement to 2nd edition (1960) of International Catalogue of mental health films.

APPENDIX II

WFMH Presidents

WFMH PRESIDENTS 1948–1999 (WITH THEIR POSITIONS AT THE TIME OF THEIR PRESIDENCIES)

1948–1949 JOHN R. ("JACK") REES, M.D. (Great Britain) Psychiatrist. Former senior consultant, British Armed Forces

1949–1950 ANDRÉ REPOND, M.D. (Switzerland) Psychiatrist. Director, Mental Hospital in Malevoz

1950–1951 WILLIAM LINE, PH.D. (Canada) Psychologist. Professor and Head of Psychology, University of Toronto

1951–1952 ALFONSO MILLAN, M.D. (Mexico) Psychiatrist. Professor and Chairman of Psychiatry, University of Mexico

1952–1952 M. KAMIL EL KHOLY, M.D. (Egypt) Psychiatrist. Head, Government Mental Health Service

1953–1954 H.C. RUMKE, M.D. (The Netherlands) Psychiatrist. Professor and Chairman of Psychiatry, University of Utrecht

1954–1955 FRANK FREMONT-SMITH, M.D. (United States) Physician. Medical Director, Josiah Macy Jr. Foundation of New York

1955–1956 NILO MAKI, PH.D. (Finland) Psychologist. Professor of Special Education, Helsinki

1956 EDUARDO E. KRAPF, M.D. (Argentina) Psychiatrist. Associate Professor, University of Buenos Aires, Argentina. Left WFMH presidency to direct WHO Mental Health Section.

1956–1957 MARGARET MEAD, PH.D. (United States) Anthropologist. Associate Curator of Ethnology, American Museum of Natural History, New York

1957–1958 GEORGE BROCK CHISHOLM, M.D. (Canada) Psychiatrist. Formerly Director General, WHO, Geneva, Switzerland

1958–1959 HANS HOFF, M.D. (Austria) Psychiatrist. Professor and Chairman of Neurology and Psychiatry. University of Vienna

1959–1960 PAUL SIVADON, M.D. (Belgium) Psychiatrist. Professor of Psychiatry, University of Brussels Brussels, Belgium

1960–1961 A. C. PACHECO E SILVA (Brazil) Psychiatrist. Professor and Chairman of Psychiatry, University of Sao Paulo

1961–1962 GEORGE S. STEVENSON, M.D. (United States) Psychiatrist. Consultant, National Association for Mental Health Inc., New York

1962–1963 PHON SANGSINGKEO, M.D. (Thailand) Psychiatrist. Director-General, Department of Medical Services, Ministry of Public Health

1963–1964 G. P. ALIVASATOS, M.D. (Greece) Psychiatrist. Emeritus Professor of Hygiene, University of Athens

1964–1965 ALAN STOLLER, M.D. (Australia) Chief Clinical Officer, Mental Hygiene Authority, Victoria

1965–1966 CHIEF SIR SAMUEL MANUWA (Nigeria) Lawyer. First Commissioner, Federal Public Service Commission, Lagos

1966–1967 OTTO KLINEBERG, M.D., PH.D. (Canada) Social Psychologist. International Center for Intergroup Relations, Paris, France[a]

1967–1972 GEORGE MORRISON CARSTAIRS, M.D. (Scotland) Professor and Chairman of Psychiatry, Edinburgh University[b]

1972–1975 MICHAEL BEAUBRUN, M.D. (Trinidad) Psychiatrist. Professor and Chairman of Psychiatry, University of the West Indies, Kingston, Jamaica[c]

1975–1979 TSUNG-YI LIN, M.D. (Canada) Psychiatrist. Professor of Psychiatry, University of British Columbia

1979–1981 GOWAN GUEST, ESQ (Canada) Lawyer. Private businessperson[d]

1981–1983 EUGENE B. BRODY, M.D. (United States) Psychiatrist. Professor and Chairman Emeritus of Psychiatry and Director Emeritus, Institute of Psychiatry and Human Behavior, University of Maryland School of Medicine, Baltimore, Maryland; Editor-in-Chief, *Journal of Nervous and Mental Disease*[e]

1983–1985 ESTAFANIA ALDABA-LIM, PH.D. (Philippines) Psychologist and public servant; former Philippines government cabinet member

1985–1987 EDITH MORGAN, M.S.W. (England) Social worker, staff of MIND (Mental Health Association of England and Wales)

1987–1989 GAMAL MADY ABOU EL AZAYEM, M.D. (Egypt) Psychiatrist. Private mental hospital owner and director

1989–1991 STANISLAS FLACHE, M.D. (Switzerland) Public health specialist. Former Assistant Director General, WHO, Geneva

1991–1993 MAX ABBOTT, PH.D. (New Zealand) Psychologist. Director, Mental Health Foundation of New Zealand

1993–1995 FEDERICO PUENTE SILVA, M.D. (Mexico) Psychiatrist. Private practice; part-time faculty of psychology, National Autonomous University of Mexico

1995–1997 BEVERLY LONG, M.P.H. (United States) Mental health association volunteer

1997–1999 MARTEN DE VRIES, M.D. (The Netherlands) Professor of Social Psychiatry, Director, Institute for Psycho-Ecological Research, University of Maastricht

[a]Otto Klineberg was chairman of the WFMH Board (a position no longer extant) for some time before becoming president and in this capacity provided organizational stability during the demise of Francois Cloutier (who had been his nominee) as Federation director general. Klineberg received his M.D. from McGill University in 1925 but never had an internship and never practiced medicine. His Ph.D. is from Columbia University in 1927; Federation reports list him only as having a Ph.D. degree. His career was mainly as a professor of social psychology with a major interest in international relations. The center in Paris with which he was affiliated at the time of his presidency was funded in part by UNESCO.

[b]"Morris" Carstairs, as he was known, would normally have served only one year as president (1967–1968) to be succeeded by Vice President Baltazar Caravedo, M.D., of Lima, Peru, who was the chief medical officer for his country 's psychiatric services. However, a crisis had been building since 1965 with the Federation's progressive move to near-bankruptcy. This was due to several factors. First, Francois Cloutier, M.D., who succeeded Jack Rees as WFMH Director in January 1962 (then changed his title to Director General), embarked on an ambitious program of international travel. Second, although his contract specified that he should engage in fundraising, he delegated this responsibility to a subordinate. Third, the Board remained passive. Fourth, the Federation never recovered from the expense of the 1963 move of its Secretariat from London to Geneva. Once in Geneva expenses were significantly higher than in London. In autumn 1965 Cloutier, confronted with the Federation's impending financial collapse, submitted his resignation. He was succeeded by his deputy, Pierre Visseur, who conducted a markedly reduced operation. By 1967 lack of funds eventuated in the final forced closing of the WFMH Secretariat with the loss of Visseur. Carstairs, formerly Executive Board chairman and then vice president, had succeeded Klineberg as president for a one-year term in 1967. However, the crisis led the Board to request that he remain in the post and undertake an effort at resuscitation. Despite his profound distaste for money raising he was successful in obtaining a sufficient sum from an American business donor to help finance the 1968 20th anniversary congress in London and the 1969 Annual Meeting in Washington, DC. Meanwhile, his Department in Edinburgh supported the everyday work of the Federation, and he served as the first of the so-called "working presidents," who functioned as volunteers in the combined roles of director, Board chairman, and president. This continued until the establishment of the Baltimore-Washington Secretariat in 1983.

[c]Michael Beaubrun, who had been expected to serve as president for four years (in keeping with the agreed-upon arrangements for working presidents) resigned prematurely on grounds of health (glaucoma) after the 1975 Annual Meeting and Congress in

Australia. Available information suggests that another reason for his resignation was the lack of funding to maintain a central Secretariat. His department at the University of the West Indies in Jamaica supplied the major part of the necessary funding during his presidency, but it seems not to have been enough.

[d]Gowan Guest, who had been WFMH treasurer and financial officer for the 1977 World Congress in Vancouver under Tsung-yi Lin, was the first president to serve a two-year term after the new by-laws adopted at the Salzburg Congress in 1979. His office continued to receive support, as had that of Tsung-yi Lin's presidency, from the University of British Columbia. The Vancouver Secretariat was directed on a part-time basis by Roberta Beiser, whose title was changed in 1980 from administrative assistant to executive director. In 1982 Guest resigned from his position as past president, Board member, and member of the incorporated entity in Canada, stating a fear of bankruptcy.

[e]Eugene B. Brody was the first president to have been a president-elect (elected in 1980) after the new by-laws. His office, as president in 1981–1983 and as secretary general in 1983–1987 (when it was moved to Sheppard Pratt), was fully supported by his university. Although the Vancouver Secretariat remained viable and involved in arrangements for the 1983 World Congress in Washington, DC, its functions were progressively assumed by Brody's office staff.

LOCATIONS OF WFMH SECRETARIAT

1948–1961 London. J.R. Rees, M.D., Director (salaried)

1962–1963 London. Francois Cloutier, M.D., Director (salaried)

1963–1965 Geneva. Francois Cloutier, M.D., Director General (salaried)

1965–1967 Geneva. Pierre Visseur, Director (salaried)

1968–1972 Edinburgh, G.M. Carstairs, M.D., Working President (volunteer)

1972–1974 Kingston, Jamaica, Michael Beaubrun, M.D., Working President (volunteer)

1975–1979 Vancouver, Canada, Tsung-yi Lin, M.D., Working President (volunteer)

1979–1983 Vancouver, Canada, Roberta Beiser, Executive Director (salaried)

1983–Present Baltimore-Washington, DC, Eugene B. Brody, M.D., Secretary General (volunteer) and Richard C. Hunter, Deputy Secretary General (volunteer)

APPENDIX III

WHO Regional Designations[a]

Regional Office for Africa. Established November 1950. Executive Board EB 7.R10. Brazzaville approved as site for regional office, January 1952.

Pan American Health Organization/WHO. Agreement between PanAmerican Sanitary Organization and WHO was signed in Washington by director general of WHO and director of PanAmerican Sanitary Organization on 24 May 1949 and took effect 1 July 1949. Second World Health Assembly WHA 2.91.

Regional Office for South-East Asia. Establishment approved on or about 1 January 1949. Provisionally approved New Delhi as site of regional office, November 1948. Executive Board EB 2.R29.

Regional Office for Europe. Copenhagen approved as permanent site subject to conclusion of a satisfactory host agreement with government of Denmark, May 1954. Executive Board EB14.R17.

Regional Office for the Eastern Mediterranean. Integration of WHO with Alexandria Sanitary Bureau was recommended as soon as possible, July 1948. First regional committee held February 1949. First World Health Assembly WHA 1.72.

Regional Office for the Western Pacific. Approved as soon as possible, understanding that expenditure will not be greater than that provided for 1951 budget, May 1950. First regional committee was May 1951. Third World Health Assembly WHA 3.54.

[a]Source: WHO Handbook of Resolutions and Decisions (1948–1972). Compiled by Annette Andkjaer and Franklin Apfel, Communication and Public Affairs, WHO Regional Office for Europe. Courtesy of John Henderson, M.D.

APPENDIX IV

Advocacy, Education, and Network Building Through Regional and Special Meetings 1981–1996

The Federation's mission has been pursued through large international conferences and smaller conferences more focused on issues of regional interest or specific topics deserving examination. After the World Congress for Mental Health in Manila in August 1981 and before the 1997 Congress in Lahti, there were seven additional biennial World Congresses. They were in Washington, DC (1983), Brighton (1985), Cairo (1987), Auckland, New Zealand (1989), Mexico, D.F. (1991), Tokyo (1993), and Dublin (1995). They are described in Chapters 9–11 and further discussed in Chapter 13. In the intervals between World Congresses the Federation programs of advocacy, education, and knowledge transfer included regional and special meetings. The following list contains most of these from autumn 1981 through spring 1997. Omissions, if any, are due to insufficient reporting. Only a few of the meetings to mark World Mental Health Day initiated in 1992 are noted. Meetings sponsored by the United Nations in which WFMH played a major role are discussed in Chapter 8. Some national member organization meetings have been stimulated or enriched by WFMH regional councils. During 1996 the European regional council of WFMH (ERC/WFMH) supported the conferences of WFMH voting member organizations or those interested in becoming members in Spain, the United Kingdom, the Czech Republic, and Bulgaria.

August 1982. "Professionals and Volunteers: Partners or Rivals?" London, United Kingdom. This conference, originally proposed by President Brody as an Atlantic basin meeting aimed to bring together ex-patients, self-help groups, professionals, and other volunteers, was eventually organized and chaired by Edith Morgan and cosponsored by WFMH and MIND (Brody, 1982b).

August 1983. North American regional meeting on migration in Vancouver, British Columbia, Canada, organized by regional vice president Morton Beiser, M.D., in association with the Washington, DC, World Congress for Mental Health.

1–6 July 1984. "Infancy as Prevention," Athens, Greece. Sponsored by the International Study Center for Children and Families. Cosponsored by WFMH with the support of Greek government health and welfare agencies. WFMH was represented by Secretary General Brody who chaired the opening plenary session on prenatal prevention and programmatic care and spoke on family planning in relation to the prevention of illness or less than optimal function.

12–15 August 1984. "Legal Issues in the Commitment and Civil Rights of Mentally Ill Persons," Copenhagen, Denmark. Organized by Knud Jensen, M.D. for the European region of WFMH. Cosponsored by the Danish Association for the Welfare of the Mentally Ill. WFMH Board and Secretariat representatives were Hilda Robbins and Secretary General Brody who spoke on "Patients' Rights: A Cultural Challenge to Western Psychiatry" (Brody, 1985).

30 September–4 October 1984. "Delivering Mental Health Services in a Primary Health Care Context," Beersheva, Israel. A meeting of the WFMH European region cosponsored with Ben Gurion University of the Negev. WFMH Board and Secretariat representation including Stijn Jannes, M.D., WFMH vice president for the European region, and Secretary General Brody.

5–7 December 1984. "Mental Health and Primary Care," Havana, Cuba. Organized by the Interamerican Society of Psychology under the auspices of WHO and PAHO. WFMH as a cosponsor was represented at the opening ceremony by Secretary General Brody who also spoke on the Division of Labor in Health Care with Special Reference to Mental Health. WFMH Committee on Responsible Parenthood sponsored a symposium on reproductive behavior and other lectures by committee chairperson Dr. Henry David and other members.

25–28 March 1985. "Effects of Recent Technological Advances on Human Rights," Barcelona, Spain. Organized by UNESCO and International Social Science Council was cosponsored by WFMH represented by Secretary General Brody, who spoke on human rights issues in psychiatric treatment with special reference to the compulsory administration of neuroleptic drugs.

17–22 March 1985. "International Congress on Stress, Behavior and Coronary Disease," Melbourne, Australia. Organized by the Mental Health Foundation of Australia with cosponsorship from WFMH and several Australian professional associations. WFMH was represented by Board member Professor Graham Burrows, M.D., of Melbourne.

25–29 May 1985. Mexico, D.F. A joint meeting of the Mexican Psychiatric Association, Mexican Society for Psychiatry and Neurology, and American Psychiatric Association. Before the meeting a consortium of Mexican professional societies met under WFMH sponsorship to discuss mental health issues in the region. Groundwork was laid for a new Mexican committee for mental health including 14 societies related to mental health in the region. The first executive was Federico Puente, M.D., followed by Dr. Jose Sanchez Sosa. Dr. Puente chaired the organizing committee for the Mexican Psychiatric Association. Secretary General Brody chaired the American Psychiatric Association committee planning the joint conference.

20–21 July 1985. "Providing a Local Mental Health Service. The Process of Change," Dartington, Devon, England. This meeting followed the 14–20 July 1985 WFMH World Congress for Mental Health in Brighton, England. The topic was addressed by delegates from 16 countries. WFMH President Edith Morgan was the main WFMH representative.

1985. "Meeting the Mental Health Needs of Victims," United Nations New York. Cosponsored by UN Economic and Social Council (ECOSOC). Organized by Yael Danieli, Ph,D., WFMH senior representative to United Nations New York. Additional WFMH representation by Secretary General Brody and Richard Mollica, M.D., who spoke on work with torture survirors in Cambodia.

17–18 June 1985. "International Workshop on Longitudinal Studies of Unwanted Children," Oulu, Finland. Cosponsored by WFMH Committee on Responsible Parenthood, represented by Dr. Henry David.

12–15 August 1985. "Mental Health of Pacific Islanders," Honolulu, Hawaii. Organized by the University of Hawaii with sponsorship from the U.S. National Institute of Mental Health represented by James Ralph, M.D., director of the minority affairs branch. WFMH was a cooperating organization. Secretary General Brody represented WFMH and spoke at opening plenary session.

25 August–5 September 1985. "The Patient with Cancer: Research, Treatment, Supportive Care and Psychosocial Management in Great Britain and the United States," Newbattle Abbey College, Edinburgh, Scotland. Sponsored by WFMH with representation by Board member Professor Knud Jensen, M.D.

7–9 February 1986. "Prevention and Education in the Field of Mental Health: Implications for Latin America. A Tribute to E. B. Brody," Mexico. Organized by Federico Puente, M.D., with cosponsorship of WFMH, National Autonomous University Faculty of Psychology, and Mexican Committee for Mental Health. Participants included major Mexican government leaders, representatives of Mexican associations, PAHO, U.S. National Institute of Mental Health, and, for WFMH, vice president for South America Alvaro Gallegos, M.D., of Costa Rica, vice president for North America Hilda Robbins, and Professor Sheppard Kellam, M.D., director of the prevention research unit at the Johns Hopkins University School of Public Health.

6–9 May 1986. "Family Planning for the Mentally Ill and Handicapped," Copenhagen, Denmark. Cosponsored with Danish Association for Family Planning and WFMH Committee on Responsible Parenthood. Organized by Professor Mogen Osler, M.D., and Dr. Henry David (Osler and David, 1987).

May 1987. "Family Therapy," Prague, Czechoslovakia. Under auspices of ERC/WFMH. Cosponsored with various family therapy associations and Czechoslovak Medical Association.

15–18 May 1987. "The Mental Health of Hispanic Americans," The Simon Bolivar Foundation, University of Illinois, Chicago. Cosponsored by WFMH. WFMH represented by Secretary General Brody and former Board member, Carlos Leon, M.D., of Colombia.

1987. "Mental Health Education," Dublin, Ireland. Mental Health Association of Ireland cosponsored by ERC/WFMH.

23 April 1987. "Meeting the Mental Health Needs of Victims," United Nations New York. Cosponsored by UN Economic and Social Council (ECOSOC). Organized by Yael Danieli, Ph.D., WFMH senior representative to United Nations New York. Additional WFMH representation by Secretary General Brody and Richard Mollica, M.D., of Harvard, who spoke on work with torture survivors in Cambodia, Dr. Richard Rich of Illinois, Chair, and Dr. Susan Salasin of NIMH, founder of the WFMH Scientific Committee on Victims of Violence.

1–4 September 1987. Annual Conference, Mental Health Foundation of New Zealand: Auckland New Zealand, cosponsored by WFMH. WFMH represented by Board member Dr. Max Abbott and Secretary General Brody.

1987. "Migration and Mental Health," Auckland, New Zealand. The Mental Health Foundation of New Zealand with WFMH cosponsorship. WFMH representation by Richard Mollica, M.D., Chair of WFMH Committee on Refugees and Other Migrants and Board member Dr. Max Abbott, Director of the Foundation.

12–15 May 1988. "Refugee Mental Health," Wellington, New Zealand. The Mental Health Foundation of New Zealand in association with WFMH. WFMH represented by Richard Mollica, M.D., and James Lavelle, M.S.W., and Board member Dr. Max Abbott, Director of the Foundation.

25–30 September and October 1988. "The Human Rights of Psychiatric Patients," Kobe and Tokyo, Japan, A regional meeting of WFMH Western Pacific Region to observe the passage of a new Japanese Mental Health Act. Cosponsors with WFMH: Japanese Mental Health Association, ZINKAREN (Association of Relatives of the Mentally Ill), and the Japanese Association of Psychiatric Hospitals. WFMH Board and Secretariat representatives: Board member Dr. Max Abbott (New Zealand), former Board member Hilda Robbins (representing consumers), and Secretary General Brody as well as present and former Japanese Board members including Professor Akira Hoshino and Kunihiko Asai, M.D.

7 April 1988. "Mental Health Services for Victims of Community Violence," Cairo, Egypt. A meeting of the WFMH Committee on Trauma Victims in the Middle East co-chaired by Dr. Leila Dane, and Ahmed El Azayem, M.D., with cosponsorship by the Egyptian Mental Health Association and WFMH. Additional WFMH representation by Dr. Calvin Frederick, chair of WFMH Committee on Emergency Mental Health, and Secretary General Brody, both of whom were program speakers.

10 May 1988. Douglas Hospital Centre, Montreal. Observance of 40th anniversary of WFMH and WHO with UN, Canadian government, and NGO officers during American Psychiatric Association annual meeting. WFMH represented by Secretary General Brody.

1988. "Psychological Trauma in War and Peace," Tel Aviv, Israel. Organized by Tel Aviv University. Cosponsored by WFMH, International Council of Psychologists, and Society for Traumatic Stress. WFMH represented by United Nations Representative Dr. Yael Danieli.

1988. "Youth in Africa," Lusaka, Zambia. Organized by Board member Isaac Mwendapole, M.S.W., for African region of WFMH. Cosponsored by WFMH.

5–6 December 1988. "International Symposium on Quality in Community Mental Health Care." Hosted by King Edward's Hospital Fund for London to mark 40th anniversary of WFMH. Organized by Edith Morgan. Speakers included President El Azayem and several Board members as well as Secretary General Brody.

18–23 January 1989. "The State of the Art in Mental Health and Biological Psychiatry." A "Nile cruise congress" chaired by President Gamal El Azayem. Cosponsored by WFMH with the Egyptian Association for Mental Health to celebrate the 40th anniversary of the founding of both WFMH and the Egyptian association. Speakers included several Board members and Secretary General Brody.

22–25 March 1990. "The Mental Health of Immigrants and Refugees," Houston, Texas. Organized and sponsored by Hogg Foundation for Mental Health and WFMH. WFMH Board and Secretariat participants included North American regional vice president Beverly Long, Committee on Southeast Asian Refugees Chair Richard Mollica, M.D., Central America, Caribbean, and Mexico vice president Jaime Ayala, M.D., and Secretary General Brody.

7–9 June 1990. "European Conference for Relatives of the Mentally Ill," De Haan, Belgium. Organized and cosponsored by Flemish organizations for mental health in collaboration with ERC/WFMH and European Commission.

14–17 June 1990. "Strategies for Meeting the Mental Health Needs of the 21st Century." Mexican Society for Neurology and Psychiatry, Queretaro City, Mexico. Cosponsored by WFMH Central America, Caribbean, and Mexico regional vice president Jaime Ayala, M.D.

25–29 June 1990. "Children in War," Jerusalem, Israel. Organized by Freud Professor Bennett Simon, M.D., and Program Director Roberta Apfel, M.D. (Freud Center, Hebrew University, Jerusalem). Cosponsored by Hebrew University, Israel Psychoanalytic Society, and WFMH. WFMH Secretariat represented by Secretary General Brody who keynoted the section on mental health policy for children.

25 June–1 July 1990. "Improving Children's Lives: Global Perspectives on Prevention," Burlington, Vermont. Organized by the University of Vermont and WFMH Committee on Prevention. WFMH Board representatives and speakers included North American regional vice president Beverly Long and Dr. Max Abbott of New Zealand.

11–13 July 1990. "Medicine and Migration," Rome, Italy. Chaired by Professor Luigi Frighi, professor of mental hygiene, University of Rome. Cosponsored by WFMH with Caritas Diocesana di Roma, Cattedra di Igiene Menale, Universita di Roma "La Sapienza," Associazione Fernando Rielo di Assistenza e Ricerca Sanitaria, Harvard University School of Public Health. WFMH speakers included Richard Mollica, M.D., Derek Silove, M.D., consultant to the new WFMH collaborating center on the rehabilitation of torture victims (University of New South Wales, Sydney, Australia), and Secretary General Brody.

27 September 1990. "International Symposium on Technology, Education, and Health," Mexico, D.F.. Organized by Board member-at-large and 1991 World Congress co-chair Federico Puente, M.D. Sponsored by WFMH. Secretariat representative was Deputy Secretary General R. Hunter.

1 November 1990. "International Symposium on Public Policy Toward Unwanted Pregnancies," Pittsburgh, Pennsylvania. Organized by the University of Pittsburgh Graduate School of Public and International Affairs. Cosponsored by WFMH Committee on Responsible Parenthood, whose co-chair, Dr. Henry David, was WFMH representative.

29 January–2 February 1991. "Development, Technology, Education and Health: Perspectives for the Year 2000," Monterrey, Mexico. Organized by the Mexican Society for Neurology and Psychiatry under the presidency of WFMH Vice President Jaime Ayala, M.D., and cosponsored by WFMH. Secretary General Brody keynoted opening session on "Health Policy Across Cultural and National Boundaries" and spoke with several other groups in Monterrey including the City Council, School of Psychology, and Institute for Children's Care.

23–26 March 1991. "Backgrounds for Violence: The Refugee Experience." A WFMH sponsored symposium during annual meeting of the American Orthopsychiatric Association (WFMH member organization). WFMH speakers were James Lavelle, M.S.W., of the Committee on Refugees, L.F. Newman, co-chair of Committee on Responsible Parenthood, and Secretary General Brody.

25–28 March 1991. "Deaths in Custody," London, United Kingdom. Sponsored by the Institute for the Study and Treatment of Delinquency, King's College, London, with WFMH cosponsorship.

5–8 May 1991. "Mental Health in European Families," Prague, Czechoslovakia. Organized by the Family Therapy Association of the Association of Czechoslovak Medical Societies and the Society for Psychotherapy with the cosponsorship of ERC/WFMH, which also held its annual regional meeting. Several European Board members including former president Edith Morgan were active at this meeting.

6–11 October 1991. "The First International Working Conference on the Mental Health and Wellbeing of the World's Refugees and Displaced Persons," Stockholm, Sweden. Cosponsoring organizations in addition to WFMH included WHO, United Nations High Commissioner for Refugees, International Organization for Migration, Karolinska Institute, and U.S. National Institute of Mental Health, which funded the travel of WFMH participants including WFMH refugee committee chair Richard Mollica, Pablo Farias, M.D., of Mexico, and Secretary General Brody.

1–2 November 1991. "Seclusion and Alternatives: Policies and Experiences," London, United Kingdom. Sponsored by ERC/WFMH. Held in cooperation with Centre for Mental Health Services Development. Chaired by WFMH European regional vice president Josee van Remoortel and addressed by Edith Morgan, founder-president of ERC/WFMH.

12–14 November 1991. "Non-Violent Conflict Resolution," Cairo, Egypt. Sponsored by WFMH in cooperation with Dar Il'Eftaa (Egypt's center for Islamic Religious and Community Affairs), Center for Strategic and International Studies of Washington, DC, and World Islamic Association for Mental Health. It was organized by the WFMH Committee on Victims of Mid-East Violence chaired by Dr. L.F. Dane, director of the Institute for Victims of Violence, and Ahmed El Azayem, M.D., and addressed by former WFMH president Gamal M. Abou El Azayem, M.D., and Secretary General Brody.

12–15 April 1992. "Mental Health in the Pacific Rim." WFMH Pacific regional conference, Sydney, Australia. Sponsored by the Psychiatric Rehabilitation Association of Australia (WFMH member association). Organized by WFMH regional vice president Trevor Elligett, chief executive of the association. Held after an annual WFMH Board meeting, many members of the Board and Secretariat participated.

5–9 October 1992. "Psychology in Health Care Administration and Research," Havana, Cuba. Cosponsored by newly formed Latin American and Caribbean regional council of WFMH led by Federico Puente, M.D., along with the Cuban Society for Health Psychology.

7–10 October 1992. "The Changing Scene in Mental Health Care in Europe: the Reforms of Practice, Policy and Structure." Annual conference of ERC/WFMH, Thessaloniki, Greece. Support by WHO European Region, European Community, Council of Europe, Greek Ministry of Health and Public Welfare, and many local associations and university departments. Among the participants were European region Board members and former Board members including Edith Morgan and John Henderson, M.D.

13–15 November 1992. "The Hidden Power in Psychiatry: Restraints on Mentally Ill People," Blankenberge, Belgium. Joint conference of ERC/WFMH, Flemish Association for Mental Health, and French-speaking confederation of mental health leagues. It examined the disparity between declared policies and the realities of practice in using restraint with mentally ill patients.

28 March–3 April 1993. "Dialogue for Mental Health in the American Continent," San Jose, Costa Rica. This seminar of the Simon Bolivar Program of the University of Illinois was cosponsored by the Latin American and Caribbean Council of WFMH and the Psychiatric Association of Costa Rica. WFMH Board representatives included Federico Puente, M.D.

26–29 September 1993. "Children-War and Persecution," Hamburg, Germany. This conference, a follow-up to that in Jerusalem in 1990, was organized by the Department of Child and Adolescent Psychiatry of the University of Hamburg with cosponsorship of WFMH, Unicef-Germany, and other German organizations. WFMH was represented by Secretary General Brody, who spoke at the opening and moderated the final session.

25–27 November 1993. "Reform of Mental Health Services: New Perspectives of Mental Health Care in Europe," Lisbon, Portugal. ERC/WFMH annual conference.

15–16 November 1993. "Man's Well-Being in Relationship to the Natural Environment," Mexico, D.F. Organized by the Latin American and Caribbean regional council of WFMH in conjunction with the Mexican Ministry of Agriculture and Water Resources and its Department of Fauna and Flora. In addition to Mexican WFMH leaders, the Board and Secretariat were represented by plenary speakers Marten de Vries, M.D. and Secretary General Brody.

10–11 December 1993. "European Conference on Mental Health and Aging," Antwerp, Belgium. Sponsored by ERC/WFMH and Federation for Community Mental Health Centers.

2–5 February 1994. "Building Tolerance for Diversity," Cairo, Egypt. Sponsored by Institute for Victims of Trauma (IVT), El Azayem Medical Centre, and WFMH. Co-sponsored by World Islamic Association for Mental Health, Egyptian Mental Health Association, and Cairo High Institute for Social Work. Follow-up for earlier meeting on nonviolent conflict resolution. WFMH representatives were Dr. L.F. Dane of Institute for Victims of Trauma and Ahmed El Azayem, M.D., who were forming a new WFMH-sponsored entity, the Joint Program for Conflict Resolution.

6–8 April 1994. "Mental Health, Race and Culture in Europe," Bristol, United Kingdom. Organized by the University of Bristol. Cosponsored by ERC/WFMH.

1–4 September 1994. "Conflict and Mental Health." ERC/WFMH annual conference, Belfast, Northern Ireland. In addition to ERC members, the Board and Secretariat were represented by Secretary General Brody and Ahmed El Azayem, M.D., who participated with Institute for Victims of Trauma Director Dr. L. F. Dane in a symposium on nonviolent conflict resolution in the Middle East.

12–14 October 1994. "Fourth Annual European Conference for the Promotion of Mental Health," London, United Kingdom. Cosponsored by ERC/WFMH.

19–20 October 1994. "Mental Health Symposium-Movements on the nongovernmental organization level in the Far East," Kochi, Japan. Cosponsored with University of Kochi by Western Pacific region of WFMH represented by the regional vice president, Professor Shimpei Inoue, M.D.

24–29 October 1994. "Family Mental Health in Africa," Pretoria, South Africa. First conference of African Regional Council of WFMH. Board and Secretariat representation by President Federico Puente, President-elect Beverly Long, regional vice president Isaac Mwendapole, and Deputy Secretary General Richard Hunter.

2–4 December 1994. "International Symposium on Relapse of Schizophrenia," Kaohsiung, Taiwan. Cosponsored by the Western Pacific region of WFMH with the University of Kaohsiung. WFMH representation by Western Pacific leaders and Honorary President Tsung-yi Lin.

11–13 October 1995. "Fifth Annual European Conference on the Promotion of Mental Health," London, United Kingdom. Cosponsored by ERC/WFMH.

10–12 November 1995. "Conference on Mental Health, Restraints and Ethics," Billund, Denmark. Cosponsored by the Danish Society for the Mentally Ill and ERC/WFMH.

9–11 May 1996. "International Conference on Mental Health in the Americas," New York New York. Organized by the American Society of Hispanic Psychiatry with WFMH cosponsorship. Dr. Haydee Montenegro represented WFMH as a discussant.

27–31 August 1996. "World Congress Against the Commercial Exploitation of Children," Stockholm, Sweden. No nongovernmental organization was specified among the sponsors, but WFMH was active through Dr. Barry Jay, secretary of our committee on preventing the commercial sexual exploitation of children, and former WFMH president Dr. Estafania Aldaba-Lim.

18 September 1996. ERC/WFMH general assembly in Brussels with 55 members from 14 countries. It was held in conjunction with a meeting of eight member associations of the forum of European nongovernmental organizations working in the mental health field.

28 September 1996. International meeting of committee of women leaders in mental health, chaired by Rosalynn Carter. Convened by WFMH at PAHO headquarters (Washington, DC). Cosponsored by WHO, PAHO, and Harvard University Department of Social Medicine headed by Professor Arthur Kleinman. It was attended by representatives from 25 countries and several health ministers present at PAHO for their annual meeting as well as officials from the World Bank and other institutions. Its purpose was to advocate for more attention to mental health in national public health policies and to examine initiatives to improve mental health care in Latin America. Speakers included WHO Director General Hiroshi Nakajima and PAHO Director Sir George Alleyne.

3–6 October 1996. "User Satisfaction with Services," Prato, Italy. Held under auspices of European Union's HELIOS II project and ERC/WFMH.

10 October 1996. "Women and Mental Health," New York, New York. This briefing for nongovernmental organizations at United Nations New York, marking World Mental Health Day, was the first event to be coordinated by the newly formed Committee on Mental Health. Cosponsored by WFMH, WHO, and

United Nations Department of Public Information, it was attended by more than 200 people. Moderated by WFMH main representative to United Nations New York, Nancy Wallace, C.S.W., it was addressed by WFMH President Beverly Long and senior representatives from United Nations High Commissioner for Refugees, PAHO, and other organizations.

10–11 October 1996. "Ethics and Psyche," Paris, France. This symposium at UNESCO House marked World Mental Health Day. Organized by the French Federation for Mental Health (WFMH member organization). Cosponsored by WFMH and UNESCO. Organizers as well as speakers were French fed eration president Roland Broca, M.D., WFMH representative to UNESCO Madeleine Riviere, M.D., and UNESCO's bioethics unit director Dr. Georges Kutukdjian. WFMH Past President Federico Puente chaired a session, and Secretary General Brody spoke.

12–15 November 1996. Beirut, Lebanon. Symposium on conflict resolution including "The Role of Forgiveness and Reconciliation in Conflict Resolution-Lessons from Lebanon." Organized by WFMH Eastern Mediterranean vice president and chair of the Eastern Mediterranean Regional Council (EMRC)/WFMH Ahmed El Azayem, M.D., during a meeting of the Arab Federation of Psychiatrists.

15–18 November 1996. Beirut, Lebanon. Sixth International Conference of World Islamic Association for Mental Health (WFMH member organization). Cosponsored by EMRC/WFMH.

24–27 November 1996. "First International Conference on Health and Culture in Adolescence," Jerusalem, Israel. Organized by Emanuel Chigier, M.D., chair of the WFMH committee on adolescents. Cosponsored by WFMH; attended by 130 professionals representing 33 countries.

5–7 December 1996. First regional conference of WFMH's South American region. Concepción, Chile. Cosponsored by WFMH, the Faculty of Medicine of the University of Concepción, and the Chilean Society for Mental Health. It was the fifth annual Chilean congress for mental health and was attended by approximately 350 people including representatives of every South American country except Ecuador. Main organizers were WFMH regional vice president Mabel Vielma, M.D., and Board member-at-large Benjamin Vicente, M.D. WFMH President Beverly Long, President-elect Marten de Vries, M.D., and other Board members participated in the program.

16–19 December 1996. "Mental Health for All: Regional Dialogue," Taipei, Taiwan. Led by regional vice president Professor Shimpei Inoue, M.D., of Kochi Japan, this regional conference of WFMH's Western Pacific Region attracted 750 participants from the region including Hong Kong, Japan, Malaysia, Singapore, and South Korea as well as Southeast Asia, mainland China, and Russia. It was organized by Secretary General Professor Wei-Tsien Soong, M.D., of the Mental Health Association in Taiwan and cochaired by the association's president, Professor Cheuh Chang, Sc.D. Prominent among those present was former WFMH President Professor Tsung-yi Lin. Keynote addresses were given by Professor Norman Sartorius, M.D., president of the world psychiatric association and WFMH Secretary General Brody. Other program participants included former WFMH President Professor Max Abbott and WFMH European regional vice president John Henderson, M.D.

APPENDIX V
Resolutions Passed by WFMH Board

WFMH passed no resolutions as instruments of its policy or advocacy for nearly 23 years. The first was in 1971. Since then, some have been passed at regional meetings or sections of World Congresses and have not come to the Board. An example is a resolution supporting the programs of United Nations Fund for Population Activities passed by the Subcongress on Population at the 1991 Mexico Congress and transmitted to the appropriate authorities through the Secretary General's office.

November 1971 in Hong Kong. The WFMH Board led by President Morris Carstairs adopted its first resolution endorsing the 1948 United Nations Universal Declaration of Human Rights assertion of "freedom of conscience" and condemning the Soviet abuse of psychiatry to stifle the activity of political dissidents.

13 October 1973 in Sydney, Australia: "Alleged Abuse of Psychiatry: A Constructive Proposal." The WFMH Board at the World Congress led by President Michael Beaubrun reaffirmed the "freedom of conscience" aspect of the United Nations Universal Declaration of Human Rights and urged the Soviet Ministry of Health to submit its psychiatric procedures to independent examination.

At the same meeting the following resolutions were also passed.

At the request of Nathan Kline, M.D., chairman of the International Committee against Mental Illness, WFMH notified its member organizations of the importance of psychiatric rehabilitation.

The Executive Board resolved a message of "sympathy and goodwill to all WFMH members and to all those concerned with mental health in Israel and in the Arab countries now tragically locked in conflict." It noted that "the recourse toward violence as a means of settling [this] dispute ... is incompatible with the basic principles of mental health" and called upon all members to work toward "constructive dialogue in order to work out a just and peaceful solution which will respond to the aspirations of all the people of the region."

16 August 1975 in Copenhagen. The Executive Board reaffirmed its declarations of 1971 and 1973 repudiating the abuse of psychiatry as formulated by Louis Miller, M.D., chief government psychiatrist for Israel, "as a means of negativing and suppressing the expression of minority opinions, particularly opinions critical of established ideas and established structures of authority. To deny this right is to do serious harm to the mental health of individuals and of societies." It further expressed the need to review "psychiatric and other practices in relation to the civil rights of all mental patients."

The Board also passed a resolution condemning "all efforts to exclude any nation from participation in the social, cultural and educational agencies of the United Nations as destructive of the principles of the United Nations, the well-being of the human family, and the United Nations itself." This was in response to the 1974 resolutions by the UNESCO general conference that excluded Israel from participation in its work.

27–28 May 1976 in Vancouver, British Columbia, Canada. The WFMH administrative committee recommended to the Executive Board that it endorse the statement: "WFMH protests the Resolution of the United Nations General Assembly which holds that Zionism is a form of racism and racial discrimination." This was later endorsed.

20, 21, 26 August 1977 in Vancouver, British Columbia, Canada. The WFMH Board at the World Congress led by President Tsung-yi Lin passed two resolutions calling upon "the government of the U.S.S.R. for the immediate release of all dissenters who have been inappropriately hospitalized" and "upon all psychiatric and mental health professionals in all countries to ensure that the highest standards of psychiatric practice be maintained throughout the world." It also called for the immediate release from a labor camp of Dr. Semyon Gluzman, a psychiatrist critical of this practice.

Other resolutions supported the mental health association in Taiwan (specifying that it represented only the island of Taiwan), welcomed membership applications from the People's Republic of China, and objected to any attempt by governments or United Nations agencies to determine the membership of WFMH. "Whereas the WFMH receives with the closest attention and highest regard all recommendations and advice from United Nations agencies, including WHO and UNESCO, the fact remains that the WFMH is an independent, non-political, non-governmental organization with its own constitution and rules, from which the WFMH itself cannot deviate. The WFMH, therefore, in principle cannot accept that any outside body should, merely on political grounds, tell the WFMH, as a non-governmental organization, whom it should or should not accept as members."

13 July 1979 in Salzburg, Austria. The WFMH Board, meeting after the Salzburg World Congress, passed a resolution prepared by newly elected Board member-at-large Eugene B. Brody, M.D., with the collaboration of members of the WFMH Committee on Responsible Parenthood, which presented a symposium on the same topic. Beginning with an account of the world's abandoned children and high rates of infant mortality, especially for young mothers, the resolution proposed that "all infants have the right to be wanted; to be born healthy; to continuous loving care; and to acquire the talents and skills necessary to achieve individual and social function." Other rights included those of adults "to achieve optimal family health," which was defined at length. It was resolved that these rights should be a concern of all mental health and psychiatric programs and institutions and groups concerned with the well-being of parents, infants, children, and adolescents. Education should include "intimate communication and the relation of sexuality to reproduction," and related services should include family planning with special counseling for people of reproductive age at risk of impaired mental health. Finally, it was resolved that concerned organizations should monitor the legal-judicial and social structures of the world with the aim of encouraging their publics to modify "policies and procedures which impede reproductive health and diminish the rights of children … making all births intended and all children wanted."

April 12–13, 1980 in Mexico, D.F. The WFMH Board adopted a resolution forwarded by Dr. Grayce Roessler from a workshop during the 1979 Salzburg World Congress on "Food Habits and Mental Health of Children." Its central recommendation was in favor of breast feeding, including education on the topic for caregivers and for WFMH to "go on record as disapproving commercial interest promotions of artificial formula feeding for young infants throughout the world."

May 1981 in Helsinki, Finland. Participants from 10 European countries as well as Canada and the European Office of WHO at a symposium entitled "Old Age and Mental Health" agreed upon a resolution to be presented to WFMH, WHO, and the national governments of the countries represented. It called upon the parties concerned to emphasize the quality of life of the elderly, recognize their contribution to society, develop policies (in relation to financial security, housing, health, and transportation), pursue education and training of the public and therapeutic personnel, pursue research into their needs (in regard to health services, community attitudes, urbanization, migration), and stimulate the self-help potential of elderly people. It was endorsed by the Board at its post-Congress meeting on 1 August 1981 in Manila. In its final form it emphasized the "concept of choice and, when necessary, risk for elderly people …. All participants in approving this strive to secure implementation of these principles in their own country and in the organization with which they are affiliated."

1 August 1981 in Manila. The WFMH Board passed a resolution entitled "A Declaration of the Rights and Responsibilities of Children in a Residential Center." Although regarded as "an ideal which may not be viewed as culturally appropriate in some regions of the world," it was presented as "a set of guidelines which may be used to support the human rights of children who may have been removed from the immediate protection of their families." It was published in the October 1981 issue of the newsletter.

23 July 1983 in Washington, DC. A resolution adopted on children of alcoholic families during the World Congress for Mental Health was aimed at treatment, training, and research in this area. There is no record of it having been submitted to the Board for general approval.

12–13 July 1985 in Brighton, United Kingdom. The WFMH pre-Congress Board passed a resolution on mental health in primary care that had been recommended to it in October 1984 at the WFMH Conference on Mental Health in Primary Care organized by Ben Gurion University of the Negev in Beersheba, Israel. It called for (*a*) mental health associations to assess the implementation of mental health care in primary health care settings with special reference to sociocultural context; (*b*) prevention, evaluation, and treatment of emotional and psychosocial problems to be addressed in the education of all health care personnel; and (*c*) patients and families to have a right of access to information about different models of health care.

19–20 July 1985 in Brighton, United Kingdom. The WFMH post-Congress Board led by President Edith Morgan passed a resolution introduced by Chris Heginbotham calling on all governments to establish flexible mental health services to ensure the care of persons "requiring mental health care" in the least restrictive environment; legal, civil, social, and political rights should be equal to those of the whole population "insofar as possible." It called on the United Nations "as a matter of urgency" to place responsibility within an appropriate agency for "abolishing discrimination against, and safeguarding the rights of those diagnosed as mentally ill." It also recommended that "all bodies relevant to this issue, including non-governmental agencies ... be brought into a cooperative relationship with the United Nations."

11–13 June 1986 at Cumberland Lodge, United Kingdom. The WFMH Board passed two resolutions introduced by United Nations New York representative Dr. Yael Danieli. One, referring to the United Nations General Assembly's Declaration on Victims of Crime, adopted 29 November 1985, stated that "The World Federation for Mental Health adopts the United Nations declaration of basic principles of justice for victims of crime and abuse of power, and is fully committed to its implementation and further development."

The other, to be presented to the United Nations, stated that "WFMH agrees that aging and the implementation of the United Nations Action Plan should be incorporated routinely within the work of all United Nations bodies and agencies, including the five Regional Economic Commissions. The regional Economic Commissions should, in turn, take a more active role in the area of aging, and should establish a focal point for aging in cooperation with other United Nations units and bodies and who would work closely with nongovernmental organizations in the field of aging at the regional and subregional levels."

Another resolution introduced by Board member-at-large and MIND National Director Chris Heginbotham was passed to be released as a WFMH position statement: "Resolved that apartheid is a gross violation of human rights; that apartheid, racism and any discrimination on the grounds of race, color or creed are wholly inconsistent with mental health; and that WFMH affirms its opposition to apartheid and any direct or indirect discrimination against minorities, and states its support of programmes which counter racism and its effects."

20 October 1987 at Cairo. Joe Rogers, representing the National Mental Health Consumers Group (United States) at the Assembly of the Cairo World Congress, offered three resolutions. One called for greater participation of consumers in the activities of the Federation and was accepted by the post-Congress Board. Accepted "in spirit" were resolutions calling all governments and groups to ensure direct consumer-recipient representation in every country's delegation to WFMH congresses and for an advisory panel for Federation policy to include recipients of mental health services.

17 January 1989 at Luxor, Egypt. On the 40th anniversary Nile cruise meeting, the audience adopted by acclamation the "Luxor Declaration of the Human Rights of the Mentally Ill."

26 August 1989. A revised version of the Luxor declaration was adopted by the WFMH Board of Directors during the Auckland World Congress as the "WFMH Declaration of Human Rights and Mental Health" (Fig.1:1). It is a statement of policy regarding not only people defined as mentally ill but those vulnerable to or at risk of mental illness or distress. It recognizes human rights as transcending political, social, cultural, and economic boundaries and applying to the human family as a whole.

9–11 April 1992 at Sydney, Australia. At the Board meeting, a "Resolution on Mental Health Services to Victims of Community Violence" was formally approved. Written by Dr. Leila F. Dane, co-chair of the committee on victims of mid-east violence (co-chair Ahmed El Azayem, M.D.) it had been approved by **a con**ference on the topic in Cairo on 7 April 1988. It gave a background for mental health organizational concern with the subject and in considerable detail recommended that all WFMH member organizations engage in service, teaching, research, and liaison activities concerning preventing community violence and treating its casualties, making community leaders and the public sensitive to the issue. It had been deferred until 1990 so the Board could study it, but it was not approved until after a delay occasioned largely by failure to have it included in the appropriate agendas.

DECLARATION OF HUMAN RIGHTS AND MENTAL HEALTH

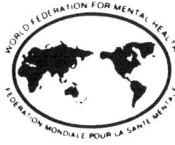

This Declaration, marking the 40th anniversary of the World Federation for Mental Health founded on the 21st of August 1948 and of the United Nations Universal Declaration of Human Rights proclaimed on the 10th of December 1948, was first adopted cn 17 January 1989 as the Declaration of Luxor: Human Rights for the Mentally Ill during the Federation's 40th Anniversary Congress at Luxor, Egypt. The present revision recognizes the Federation's concern not only with people defined as mentally ill, but also with those vulnerable to or at risk of mental and emotional illness or distress. It recognizes that human rights transcend political, social, cultural and economic boundaries and apply to the human family as a whole. It was adopted by the Federation's Board of Directors on the 26th of August 1989 on the occasion of the Federation's biennial World Congress for Mental Health convened in that year at Auckland, New Zealand.

Published by the
World Federation for Mental Health
Office of the Secretary General

DECLARATION OF HUMAN RIGHTS AND MENTAL HEALTH

PREAMBLE

Whereas the 1948 founding document of the World Federation for Mental Health entitled "Mental Health and World Citizenship" regards mental health as involving "an informed, reflective, responsible allegiance to mankind as a whole," built "on free consent" and "respect for individual and cultural differences,"

Whereas persons publicly labelled or professionally diagnosed, treated or confined as mentally ill, or suffering from emotional distress, share, in the words of the 1948 United Nations Universal Declaration of Human Rights, "the inherent dignity" and "the equal and inalienable rights of all members of the human family" and, in the words of the 1948 founding document of WFMH, the "common humanity" of persons everywhere,

Whereas the World Health Organization defines health as "a state of complete physical, mental, social and moral well-being and not merely the absence of disease or infirmity,"

Whereas a diagnosis of mental illness by a mental health practitioner shall be in accordance with accepted medical, psychological, scientific and ethical standards, and difficulty in adapting to moral, social, political or other values in itself shall not be considered a mental illness; and, whereas, persons have, nonetheless, been at times and continue to be inappropriately labelled, diagnosed, treated or confined as mentally ill,

2

Whereas severe mental illness not only impairs an individual's capacity for work, love and play, but impairs, as well, the life of his or her family and community and places a continuing burden of care upon society,

Whereas WFMH has endorsed the principle of user or consumer involvement in the planning, management and operation of mental health services,

Whereas WFMH affirms the fundamental rights and freedoms set out in the 1948 United Nations Universal Declaration of Human Rights and its subsequent human rights instruments,

Whereas WFMH recognizes that while implementing these principles requires note of the cultural, economic, historic, social, spiritual, and other circumstances of particular societies, minimum basic standards of human rights, transcending the limits of political and cultural groupings, shall be observed at all times,

Now, therefore, the Board of Directors of the WORLD 'FEDERATION FOR MENTAL HEALTH proclaims this

DECLARATION OF HUMAN RIGHTS AND MENTAL HEALTH

as a common standard for all peoples and all nations and all members of the human family.

Article 1

Mental health promotion is a responsibility of governmental and nongovernmental authorities, as well as the intergovernmental system, especially in times of crisis. In keeping with the WHO definition of health and recognizing the WFMH concern with optimal function, health and mental health programs shall contribute both to the development of individual and family responsibility for personal and group health and to promoting the highest possible quality of life.

3

Article 2

The prevention of mental or emotional illness or distress is an essential component of any mental health service system. Education in this respect shall extend to all health care providers as well as the public. Preventive efforts also require attention beyond the confines of the mental health care system to include optimal circumstances for development, beginning with family counseling, prenatal and perinatal care, and continuing throughout the life cycle with adequate general health care, opportunities for education, employment and social security. High priority shall be given to research on the prevention of mental disease, illness and ill health.

Article 3

The prevention of mental or emotional illness and distress and the care of those suffering from them requires cooperation between intergovernmental, governmental and nongovernmental health, science, and social welfare systems as well as educational institutions. Such cooperation shall include community involvement and the participation of professional and voluntary mental health associations and consumer and self-help groups. It will extend to research, education, planning and all necessary aspects of the problems which may arise as well as the provision of direct services.

Article 4

The fundamental rights of persons who are labelled, or diagnosed, treated or defined as mentally or emotionally ill or distressed, shall be the same as those of all other citizens. These include the right to coercion-free, dignified, humane and qualified treatment with access to medically, psychologically and socially

4

indicated technology; freedom from discrimination regarding equitable access to therapy or inequitable restraint on grounds of political, socio-economic, cultural, ethnic, racial, religious, gender or age status, or sexual orientation; the right to privacy and confidentiality; the right to protection of personal property; the right to protection from physical or psychological abuse; the right to protection from professional or nonprofessional neglect and abandonment; and the right, for every person, to adequate information about his or her clinical status. The right to treatment shall include hospitalization and outpatient or psychosocial treatment as appropriate, with the safeguards of accepted medical, ethical and legal opinion, and for involuntarily committed patients the rights of impartial representation, review and appeal.

Article 5

All mentally ill persons have the right to be treated under the same professional and ethical standards as other ill persons. This must include efforts to promote the greatest degree of self-determination and personal responsibility on their part. Treatment shall be in settings valued and accepted by the community, in the least intrusive manner, and under the least restrictive circumstances possible. It shall be beneficent in the sense of being carried out in the patient's best interest, not that of the family, community, professionals or the state. Treatment for persons whose capacities for self-management have been impaired by illness shall include psychosocial rehabilitation aimed at reinstating skills for living and shall take account of their needs for housing, employment, transportation, income, information and continuing care after hospital discharge.

5

Article 6

All populations include vulnerable groups at particular risk for mental or emotional illness or distress. Members of such groups require special preventive as well as therapeutic attention and concern for the protection of their health and human rights. They include victims of natural disaster, community and other violence including war, and of collective abuse including state sponsored abuse; and those vulnerable because of residential mobility (migrants, refugees), age (infants, children and elderly people), minority status (ethnic, racial, sexual, socio-economic), loss of civil rights (soldiers, prisoners) and health status. Life crises such as bereavements, family disruption and unemployment also place persons at risk.

Article 7

Inter-sectoral collaboration is essential to protect the human and legal rights of those who are or have been mentally or emotionally ill or at risk of mental ill health. All public authorities must recognize an obligation to respond to major mental health related social problems, as well as to the mental health consequences of catastrophic conditions. Public responsibility shall include the provision of specialized mental health services, whenever possible within the context of primary care facilities, and public education regarding mental health and illness and ways of supporting or coping with them.

Article 8

Nothing in this Declaration may be interpreted as implying for any State, group or person any right to espouse any belief or engage in any activity ' leading to the destruction of any of the rights or freedoms set forth herein.

WFMH October 1989

6

FIGURE 1:1

24 August 1993 at Tokyo. The Board meeting of the World Congress approved a resolution presented by Dr. Chok Hiew representing the committee on preventing the commercial sexual exploitation of children. It focused on the detrimental health consequences of and condemned the sexual exploitation of children as well as emphasizing the need to enforce the United Nations Convention on the Rights of the Child. It urged national mental health associations to influence their own governments to protect children through this convention.

17 August 1995 at Dublin, Ireland. The pre-Congress Board passed a resolution against nuclear testing introduced by Richard Redom, Oceania regional vice president from Australia. It stated that WFMH "has as its mandate the mental and emotional well being of all peoples," and opposed nuclear weapons testing as a threat to mental and physical health. Specifically it deplored "the stated intention of France to resume nuclear testing in the Pacific" and implored President Chirac and his cabinet to immediately rescind this decision.

A resolution proposed from the assembly floor but never acted upon by the Board stated "that given the level of feeling about the issue of WFMH receiving funds from drug companies expressed here tonight the Board should consult widely with the membership on this subject so that a clear policy can be implemented that reflects he views of the grassroots membership." Several months later President Beverly Long invited membership comment on the issue in her message from the president in the newsletter. There were no responses.

Other resolutions included one prepared by President Beverly Long and United Nations New York representatives Nancy Wallace and others for the United Nations Fourth Conference on Women in Beijing in September 1995. Approved by the Dublin Board it listed a range of goals to improve women's health and status, ensuring the inclusion of "mental health needs, services and rights of women in the Platform for Action" (see Chapter 8). Another circulated to the Board for approval was that submitted by Dr. Barry Jay to the 27–31 August 1996 Stockholm World Congress against the commercial exploitation of children.